T0155914

Dr Podcast Scripts for the Final FRCA

Dr Podcast Scripts for the Final FRCA

Edited by

Rebecca A Leslie
Speciality Registrar in Anaesthesia
Severn Deanery, Bristol, UK

Emily K Johnson
Speciality Registrar in Anaesthesia
West Midlands Deanery, Birmingham, UK

Gary Thomas
Consultant in Anaesthesia and Perioperative Medicine
Princess of Wales Hospital, Bridgend, Wales

Alexander PL Goodwin
Consultant in Anaesthesia and Intensive Care
Royal United Hospital, Bath, UK

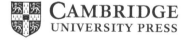
CAMBRIDGE
UNIVERSITY PRESS

CAMBRIDGE
UNIVERSITY PRESS

University Printing House, Cambridge CB2 8BS, United Kingdom

One Liberty Plaza, 20th Floor, New York, NY 10006, USA

477 Williamstown Road, Port Melbourne, VIC 3207, Australia

314-321, 3rd Floor, Plot 3, Splendor Forum, Jasola District Centre, New Delhi - 110025, India

79 Anson Road, #06-04/06, Singapore 079906

Cambridge University Press is part of the University of Cambridge.

It furthers the University's mission by disseminating knowledge in the pursuit of education, learning and research at the highest international levels of excellence.

www.cambridge.org
Information on this title: www.cambridge.org/9781107401006

First published 2011
10th printing 2018

A catalogue record for this publication is available from the British Library

ISBN 978-1-107-40100-6 Paperback

....

Every effort has been made in preparing this book to provide accurate and
up-to-date information which is in accord with accepted standards and practice
at the time of publication. Although case histories are drawn from actual cases,
every effort has been made to disguise the identities of the individuals involved.
Nevertheless, the authors, editors and publishers can make no warranties that the
information contained herein is totally free from error, not least because clinical
standards are constantly changing through research and regulation. The authors,
editors and publishers therefore disclaim all liability for direct or consequential
damages resulting from the use of material contained in this book. Readers
are strongly advised to pay careful attention to information provided by the
manufacturer of any drugs or equipment that they plan to use.

Dedicated to Alan and my parents,
For their help and understanding through my exams
and again through the busy times with Dr Podcast,
and the editing of this book.

EJ

Dedicated to my sister Claire and all of my family,
For their wise words, love and support.

RL

Dedicated to Pat, Dan and Laura.

DGT

Dedicated to my lovely wife Juliette.

AG

Contents

1 – Medicine

2 – Surgery

3 – Emergency medicine and intensive care

4 – Anatomy and regional anaesthesia

Contributors

Sarah F Bell
Speciality Registrar in Anaesthesia
Wales Deanery, Cardiff, Wales, UK

Andrea C Binks
Specialist Registrar in Anaesthesia
Severn Deanery, Bristol, UK

Pascal J Boddy
Specialist Registrar in Anaesthesia
Leicester Deanery, Leicester, UK

Poonam M Bopanna
Specialist Registrar in Anaesthesia
Wales Deanery, Cardiff, Wales, UK

Alison J Brewer
Specialist Registrar in Anaesthesia
Leicester Deanery, Leicester, UK

Michael B Clarke
Specialist Registrar in Anaesthesia
West Midlands Deanery,
Birmingham, UK

William A English
Consultant in Anaesthesia and
Intensive Care Medicine
Royal Cornwall Hospital,
Cornwall, UK

Jonathan J Gatward
Specialist Registrar in Intensive
Care Medicine
Royal North Shore Hospital, Sydney,
Australia

Andrew P Georgiou
Specialist Registrar in Anaesthesia
Severn Deanery, Bristol, UK

Gareth J Gibbon
Locum Consultant in Anaesthesia and
Intensive Care Medicine
Musgrove Park Hospital, Taunton, UK

Santhosh Gopalakrishnan
Specialist Registrar in Anaesthesia
West Midlands Deanery,
Birmingham, UK

James D Griffin
Consultant in Anaesthesia
Torbay Hospital, Devon, UK

Katherine A Holmes
Specialist Registrar in Anaesthesia
South West Peninsula Deanery,
Plymouth, UK

Catherina Hoyer
Specialist Registrar in Anaesthesia
Severn Deanery, Bristol, UK

Corinna J Hughes
Specialist Registrar in Anaesthesia
Oxford Deanery, Oxford, UK

Asim Iqbal
Specialist Registrar in Anaesthesia
West Midlands Deanery, Birmingham, UK

Caroline SG Janes
Specialist Registrar in Anaesthesia
Oxford Deanery, Oxford, UK

Helen L Jewitt
Specialist Registrar in Anaesthesia
Wales Deanery, Cardiff, Wales, UK

Emily K Johnson
Specialty Registrar in Anaesthesia
West Midlands Deanery, Birmingham, UK

Ami Jones
Specialist Registrar in Anaesthesia and
Intensive Care Medicine
Wales Deanery, Cardiff, Wales, UK

Dana L Kelly
Specialty Registrar in Anaesthesia
Oxford Deanery, Oxford, UK

Murli Krishna
Consultant in Anaesthesia and
Pain Medicine
Frenchay Hospital, Bristol, UK

Rebecca A Leslie
Specialty Registrar in Anaesthesia
Severn Deanery, Bristol, UK

Sarah J Love-Jones
Consultant in Anaesthesia and
Pain Medicine
Frenchay Hospital, Bristol, UK

Justin C Mandeville
Specialist Registrar in Anaesthesia and
Intensive Care
Oxford Deanery, Oxford, UK

Imran Mohammad
Specialist Registrar in Anaesthesia
Oxford Deanery, Oxford, UK

Matthew P Morgan
Specialist Registrar in Anaesthesia
Wales Deanery, Cardiff, Wales, UK

Carl J Morris
Specialist Registrar in Anaesthesia
Oxford Deanery, Oxford, UK

Neil J Rasburn
Specialist Registrar in Anaesthesia
Severn Deanery, Bristol, UK

Mari H Roberts
Specialist Registrar in Anaesthesia
Wales Deanery, Cardiff, Wales, UK

Joy M Sanders
Specialty Registrar in Anaesthesia
Wessex Deanery, Winchester, UK

Richard Ll Skone
Specialist Registrar in Anaesthesia
and PICU
West Midlands Deanery,
Bristol, UK

Amy K Swinson
Specialist Registrar in Anaesthesia
London Deanery, London, UK

Matthew JC Thomas
Consultant in Anaesthesia and
Intensive Care
Bristol Royal Infirmary,
Bristol, UK

Matt Thomas
Locum Consultant in Anaesthesia
and Intensive Care Medicine
Frenchay Hospital,
Bristol, UK

Susanna T Walker
Specialist Registrar in Anaesthesia
London Deanery, London, UK

Jessie R Welbourne
Specialist Registrar in Anaesthesia
Leicester Deanery, Leicester, UK

Timothy JB Wood
Specialist Registrar in Anaesthesia
Wales Deanery, Cardiff, Wales, UK

Consultant Reviewing Panel

Rebecca L Aspinall
Consultant in Anaesthesia and
Perioperative Medicine
Bristol Royal Infirmary, Bristol, UK

Ian M Davis
Consultant in Anaesthesia and
Perioperative Medicine
Bristol Royal Infirmary, Bristol, UK

William A English
Consultant in Anaesthesia and
Intensive Care Medicine
Royal Cornwall Hospital,
Cornwall, UK

Sarah J Love-Jones
Consultant in Anaesthesia and
Pain Medicine
Frenchay Hospital, Bristol, UK

Murli Krishna
Consultant in Anaesthesia and
Pain Medicine
Frenchay Hospital, Bristol, UK

Maggie Gregory
Consultant in Anaesthesia and
Perioperative Medicine
Frenchay Hospital, Bristol, UK

Stephen J Mather
Consultant in Anaesthesia and
Perioperative Medicine
Bristol Royal Infirmary, Bristol, UK

James Nickells
Consultant in Anaesthesia and
Perioperative Medicine
Frenchay Hospital, Bristol, UK

S Jane Olday
Consultant in Anaesthesia and
Perioperative Medicine
Frenchay Hospital, Bristol, UK

Caroline D Oliver
Consultant in Anaesthesia and
Perioperative Medicine
Frenchay Hospital, Bristol, UK

Samantha P Shinde
Consultant in Anaesthesia and
Perioperative Medicine
Frenchay Hospital, Bristol, UK

Malcolm C Thornton
Consultant in Anaesthesia and
Perioperative Medicine
Royal United Hospital, Bath, UK

Gary Thomas
Consultant in Anaesthesia and
Perioperative Medicine
Princess of Wales Hospital, Bridgend,
Wales, UK

Matthew JC Thomas
Consultant in Anaesthesia and
Intensive Care Medicine
Bristol Royal Informary, Bristol, UK

Matt Thomas
Locum Consultant in Anaesthesia and
Intensive Care Medicine
Frenchay Hospital, Bristol, UK

Jennifer P Tuckey
Consultant in Anaesthesia and
Perioperative Medicine
Royal United Hospital, Bath, UK

Tom P Simpson
Consultant in Anaesthesia and
Perioperative Medicine
Royal United Hospital, Bath, UK

Ruth E Spencer
Consultant in Anaesthesia and
Perioperative Medicine
Frenchay Hospital, Bristol, UK

Preface

This book has been written entirely by post-fellowship trainees in anaesthesia and it is intended that it should complement the ever-popular Dr Podcasts. The authors have all had recent experience of anaesthetic examinations and were best placed to write about their areas of interest in an exam orientated, concise and relevant manner.

The subject areas mirror those of the podcasts and it is hoped that the contents of the book will prove invaluable for candidates preparing for the Final FRCA examinations. The book can be read either in conjunction with the podcasts, or used as a separate resource to aid revision.

The format is built along the lines of a structured oral examination (SOE) and elements of it reflect the composition of model answers to the short answer questions (SAQs). Key components of the Royal College of Anaesthetists syllabus have been selected for podcasting and publication because they feature regularly in the exam.

In the future, it is hoped that further topics will be introduced to cover more areas of the syllabus and reflect any changes or advances in practice.

Acknowledgements

We would like to thank Sarah Bell and Caroline Janes for helping to get this project off the ground. Thanks to all our consultant reviewers, who are too numerous to name individually, but whose hard work and effort we appreciate greatly. A big thank you to Reston Smith, Chris Seller, Alexandra Marland and Mark Pauling for spending hours in the recording studio.

We thank Cambridge University Press for permission to use diagrams from Fundamentals of Anaesthesia Third Edition and Physics, Pharmacology and Physiology for Anaesthetists First Edition. We also thank the original providers of these diagrams: Tim Smith, Colin Pinnock, Ted Lin, Robert Jones, Matthew Cross and Emma Plunkett.

Chapter

1.1

Bone, joint and connective tissue

1.1.1. Rheumatoid arthritis – Sarah F Bell

You are on the ward reviewing a 55-year-old female patient who is on your list for a total knee replacement tomorrow. She is keen to tell you that she has severe rheumatoid arthritis that is particularly bad in her hands.

What can you tell me about this condition?

The examiners will be looking for some background medical knowledge to start with.

Rheumatoid arthritis is a systemic chronic inflammatory disease that affects 1 to 2% of the UK population. It is more prevalent in women, affecting females three times more than men. The onset is generally between 30 and 55 years. The exact cause of the condition is unknown, but it is thought to involve an autoimmune process. About 70% of cases are positive for HLA-DR4, and 80% of sufferers are seropositive for rheumatoid factor.

How does the arthritis present?

The patient develops a symmetrical polyarthritis. This may be of varying extent and severity. Rheumatoid arthritis tends to affect the hands, feet, knees, elbows, shoulders and neck.

What is the pathological process that occurs?

The pathological process involves synovitis of joints and tendon sheaths. Loss of articular cartilage and erosion of juxta-articular bone leads to joint destruction.

What is Still's disease?

This is the most common childhood form of the disease. It can be particularly debilitating.

Going back to our case, what might be your concerns regarding anaesthetising a woman with rheumatoid arthritis?

I would want to fully assess the extent of the disease since rheumatoid arthritis is a multi-system condition that can have a number of implications for the anaesthetist. I would

Dr. Podcast Scripts for the Final FRCA, ed. Rebecca A. Leslie, Emily K. Johnson, Gary Thomas and Alexander P. L. Goodwin.   Published by Cambridge University Press.

be particularly concerned about any airway, respiratory, cardiac, musculoskeletal or haematological problems. I would need to review her drug therapy since this may also influence the anaesthetic.

If the woman had not told you that she had been diagnosed with rheumatoid arthritis, what might be some of the symptoms of the condition?

Start with the musculoskeletal symptoms and then move on to the extra-articular symptoms if the examiner will let you.

Rheumatoid arthritis generally presents with **symmetrical** joint problems. Patients experience **pain** and **stiffness**. This is worse in the morning and improves with activity. The symptoms may occur as flare ups interspersed with good periods. The patient may have noticed progressive **joint deformities**, particularly affecting the hands. The patient may also describe fatigue, weight loss and low mood. About half of sufferers have extra-articular complications, which can involve the airway, respiratory, cardiovascular, neurological, renal and haematological systems.

So, what signs might you observe in the musculoskeletal system?

The patient may have hand or feet signs such as ulnar deviation, boutonniere or swan neck deformities and Z-shaped thumbs. Subcutaneous nodules might be visible.

What would you ask the woman in your history?

I would take a general and a specific history.

In the specific history I would be looking to ascertain how and when the rheumatoid arthritis was diagnosed. I would ask which joints were involved and to what extent. In particular I would discuss the range of neck and hand movement. I would also want to know about the drug treatments that the patient has tried and is currently taking.

So what can you tell me about rheumatoid neck disease?

The atlanto-axial joint may be affected in rheumatoid arthritis due to erosion of the transverse ligament and breakdown of the odontoid peg. About 25% of patients develop atlanto-axial subluxation. This can lead to acute spinal cord compression or compression of the vertebral arteries. Anterior axial subluxation is the most common type of subluxation and is worsened by neck flexion.

A fixed flexion deformity of the neck may also occur due to fusion of the spine. Osteoporosis is further worsened by steroid medication.

All of these problems may challenge the anaesthetist since manipulation of the airway may be difficult and should be kept to a minimum.

Let's go back to your history. Is there anything else that you might want to discuss regarding the musculoskeletal system?

I would want to ascertain whether either the temporomandibular or crycoarytenoid joints are affected since this might have implications for intubation and airway management. With regards to the temporomandibular joint I would ask about mouth opening. The symptoms of crycoarytenoid involvement might include dyspnoea, hoarseness, stridor and, rarely, upper airway obstruction.

For a total knee replacement I would consider performing a spinal. I would therefore want to find out whether the patient had had any back involvement or operations. I would also ask whether they would be able to get into a suitable position for this technique to be performed.

What other body systems might you ask about and why?

The examiner is looking to test your knowledge of the multiple complications of this disease. If you list at least some of the systems at the start you will indicate that you are planning to talk about them and that you have a thorough grasp of the condition.

I would enquire about the respiratory, cardiovascular, haematological, renal and neurological systems.

With regards to the respiratory system I would be looking for any evidence of pulmonary fibrosis, vasculitis, pulmonary hypertension, pulmonary nodules and pleural effusions. Furthermore the drugs given for the arthritis might have had unwanted pulmonary effects such as fibrotic changes.

Rheumatoid disease can affect the cardiovascular system in a number of ways. The patient is at an increased risk of arteriosclerosis, myocardial infarction and stroke. Mitral valve disease is present in up to 5% of patients. Pericardial disease such as effusions and inflammation may occur. Cardiac conduction defects may also develop.

The haematological system can be affected by the development of anaemia of chronic disease. Sometimes the platelet count is elevated in association with the generalised inflammatory response during a flare up. A leucopenia may also be seen.

And what about the nervous system?

The patient might develop a peripheral neuropathy from the rheumatoid arthritis or the drugs given to modify the condition. It is important to discuss and document any neurological changes, especially if a regional or central neuraxial block is considered, or if the cervical spine needs to be manipulated.

You mentioned the renal system. Can you tell me anything about the changes that might occur?

The patient may develop renal amyloid or a vasculopathy from the rheumatoid arthritis. This might be identified as acute or chronic renal failure.

Can rheumatoid arthritis affect the liver?

Yes. Felty's syndrome occurs when the inflammatory mediators associated with rheumatoid arthritis cause nodular hepatocyte enlargement. This can be associated with splenomegaly and leucopenia.

What about the eyes and skin?

The sclera may be involved. Episcleritis is a feature of rheumatoid arthritis, as is dry eyes. It is therefore important to protect the eyes during general anaesthesia to reduce the risk of corneal ulceration or abrasion. With regards to the skin, rheumatoid nodules are common. Steroids can cause thin, papery skin to develop which needs to be handled extremely carefully to avoid trauma.

Let's consider the drugs that this patient might be taking. Can you suggest any drugs and their unwanted side effects?

Remember not to forget painkillers and the immunosuppressant or disease modifying agents.

The patient might be taking regular non-steroidal anti-inflammatory medications for pain relief. These can cause renal impairment, gastrointestinal ulceration, reduced platelet function and exacerbation of asthma in susceptible individuals.

Azathioprine, methotrexate, gold and penicillamine are all used to suppress the immune system in patients with rheumatoid arthritis. These drugs can cause bone marrow suppression, lung toxicity, liver dysfunction, thrombocytopenia, anaemia and renal side effects.

Steroids are frequently given to patients with rheumatoid arthritis. They have many side effects including hypertension, diabetes, obesity, adrenal suppression, fragile skin, peptic ulcer disease and electrolyte changes.

Anti-cytokine agents can give flu-like symptoms and cause bone marrow suppression.

Having ascertained that this woman has developed hypertension and diabetes since taking regular steroid medication, you find that there are no other extra-articular features of rheumatoid disease. What further information would you want to know in you general history?

I would enquire about previous anaesthetics and whether she has a family history of any problems with an anaesthetic. I would then ask the woman about other medical conditions and go stepwise through the body systems. I would particularly focus on the blood pressure, diabetic control and the cardiovascular history. I would then talk about the medications that the woman was taking and ask whether she had any allergies. Finally I would discuss starvation history and ask about the woman's dentition.

What examination would you perform on this woman?

I would examine the cardiorespiratory, neurological and musculoskeletal systems. I would include a thorough airway assessment in my respiratory examination. I would also look at the condition of the patient's skin and assess their ability to use a patient-controlled anaesthesia (PCA) (i.e., if the disease causes significant pain or deformity of the hands).

How would you investigate this patient prior to surgery?

I would want to review blood tests and an electrocardiogram (ECG) at a minimum. With regard to the blood tests, I would check the full blood count, renal function, electrolytes, liver function and ensure that a valid group and save were available. If I had identified features of respiratory disease in my history or examination I might request a chest X-ray or pulmonary function tests. If I suspected the rheumatoid disease might be affecting the neck I would consider performing a neck X-ray in flexion and extension. If these were abnormal an MRI may be required. With regards to the airway, indirect laryngoscopy might be required if I suspected that the cricoarytenoid movement was impaired.

From your thorough assessment you have found that this 55-year-old woman has rheumatoid arthritis that appears to mainly affect her hands and knees. She has hypertension and diabetes. She takes 20 mg of prednisolone daily along with paracetamol and diclofenac when her arthritis is particularly bad. Her skin appears fragile.

What would be your preferred anaesthetic technique for this patient?

Try and be decisive about what you would want to do for this patient. The examiner wants to see that you have been in this position before and that you are confident of your abilities.

I would consider performing a spinal anaesthetic technique with local anaesthetic and intra-thecal opioid. In addition I would perform femoral and sciatic nerve blocks to provide additional post-operative analgesia. I would offer the patient intra-operative sedation. I would chart regular paracetamol and diclofenac with tramadol for breakthrough analgesia.

What are the potential problems with this technique?

The examiner is not trying to catch you out. They want to know that you can appreciate that there are pros and cons to every anaesthetic.

The spinal might be difficult to perform due to a number of factors. These include problems with patient positioning and altered anatomical landmarks. There is also a potential increased risk of infection, so aseptic technique is vital. The spinal with opioid poses the following risks: nerve damage, post-dural puncture headache, post-operative nausea and vomiting, respiratory depression and urinary retention. It is important that the nurses looking after the patient post-operatively are aware of these potential complications.

With regards to the peripheral nerve blocks these may also be challenging because of altered anatomical landmarks. I would use both a peripheral nerve stimulator and ultrasound to aid location of the nerves. Further risks include nerve damage, failure, intra-vascular injection and local anaesthetic toxicity.

What other anaesthetic techniques might be appropriate for this case?

The patient could have a general anaesthetic with peripheral nerve blockade and or morphine PCA. The general anaesthetic will require consideration of the need for intubation. The risk of aspiration should be weighed up against the potential difficulty of intubation and the risks associated with manipulation of the neck. There are many different ways of achieving an appropriate airway, which include an awake fibre-optic intubation, gas induction, IV induction, rapid sequence induction and insertion of either an endotracheal tube or a laryngeal mask airway (LMA).

A morphine PCA might also be appropriate for severe post-operative pain. Disadvantages of this include nausea and vomiting, respiratory depression and potential under-usage due to the patient being unable to manipulate the device due to their arthritis.

Are you aware of any recent publications regarding post-operative analgesia for total knee replacement?

A review article published in *Anaesthesia* in 2008 by the PROSPECT working group made a number of recommendations. They suggested that a general anaesthetic with a femoral nerve block or a spinal with opioid and a femoral nerve block were the anaesthetic options of choice for a total knee replacement, based on current evidence. They advised paracetamol, non-steroidal anti-inflammatory, residual femoral nerve block and opioid titrated to pain levels for post-operative analgesia. They were unable to advise regarding sciatic nerve blocks due to a lack of evidence.

How would you manage the steroid cover for this patient?

This question is relevant for any patient on steroids. Try and be as clear as possible.

Long-term steroid therapy suppresses the hypothalamic–pituitary–adrenal (HPA) axis. This axis is activated by major stress. It is therefore important to consider steroid replacement therapy for patients presenting for surgery to avoid peri-operative haemodynamic instability due to lack of cortisol.

Patients who take less than 10 mg of prednisolone daily do not require steroid replacement.

Patients who take more than 10 mg of prednisolone daily, or have done so within the past 3 months, should receive replacement therapy. For minor surgery this involves only 25 mg of hydrocortisone at induction. For moderate surgery the patient should receive their normal pre-operative dose of steroids followed by a further 25 mg of hydrocortisone at induction and 100 mg of hydrocortisone the next day. For major surgery the patient should again take their normal pre-operative dose of steroids. The anaesthetist should then give 25 mg of hydrocortisone at induction followed by 100 mg of hydrocortisone daily for 2 to 3 days or until normal gastrointestinal function has returned.

If this patient were taking a different steroid how would you convert the dose?

The 10 mg of prednisolone is equal to 1.5 mg of dexamethasone, 8 mg of methylprednislolone and 40 mg of hydrocortisone.

Further Reading

Fischer HB, Simanski CJ, Sharp C, et al. PROSPECT Working Group. A procedure-specific systematic review and consensus recommendations for postoperative analgesia following total knee arthroplasty. *Anaesthesia*. 2008; **63**(10): 1105–1123.

Fombon F, Thompson J. Anaesthesia for the adult patient with rheumatoid arthritis. *Continuing Education in Anaesthesia, Critical Care & Pain*. 2006; **6**(6): 235–239.

Joint Formulary Committee. *British National Formulary*. 58th edition. London: British Medical Association and Royal Pharmaceutical Society of Great Britain, 2009.

Nicholson G, Burrin JM, Hall GM. Peri-operative steroid supplementation. *Anaesthesia*. 1998; **53**: 1091–1104.

Chapter

1.2

Cardiovascular

1.2.1. Pre-operative assessment and management of patients with cardiac disease – Timothy JB Wood

You are in the pre-assessment clinic seeing a 66-year-old gentleman for a right total hip replacement. The pre-assessment nurse identified a systolic murmur, and the patient suffers from angina and is notably breathless on minimal exertion.

What are the important issues that you would like to explore in the history?

A structured approach is vital, ensuring you mention the routine history so that you don't miss anything out before focussing on the specific cardiac details.

I would introduce myself to the patient and ensure that I am talking to the correct patient and that he is expecting the operation that he is listed for. Then there are a number of general points in the history and some points specific to the cardiac history.

The general history would involve enquiry into:

- Previous general anaesthetics – what were they for and if they presented any problems
- Family history of problems with anaesthetics
- Any regular prescribed or non-prescribed medications
- Any allergies
- Any problems with his gastrointestinal system, particularly heartburn or reflux
- Starvation history
- Any joint problems other than his hips, especially focussing on his cervical spine flexion and extension
- Smoking history
- Alcohol intake.

The cardio-respiratory systems are inextricably linked and would form the focus of my attention in this patient.

Dr. Podcast Scripts for the Final FRCA, ed. Rebecca A. Leslie, Emily K. Johnson,
Gary Thomas and Alexander P. L. Goodwin.   Published by Cambridge University Press.
© R. A. Leslie, E. K. Johnson, G. Thomas and A. P. L. Goodwin 2011.

Specifically I would enquire about the following:

- Whether he suffered from hypertension, was on treatment for it and how well controlled it is.
- Had he ever had a myocardial infarction, and if so, what was done about it, had he had "clot busting" drugs, stents or surgery?
- Does he suffer from angina, and if so, when and how frequently does it tend to occur, and what does he do when it happens?
- How many pillows does he tend to sleep on and does he become breathless if he sleeps lying flat?
- Does he ever get palpitations or become aware of his heart beating in a funny rhythm?
- Has he suffered from sudden blackouts or loss of consciousness that had not been explained?
- Had he ever been told that he had a murmur?
- Does he suffer from asthma or chronic obstructive pulmonary disease (COPD) or any other problems with his breathing?
- How much exercise is he able to do before he is limited, and what is it that limits him? Through specific questioning it should be possible to calculate how many metabolic equivalents (METs) he is capable of.

You mentioned metabolic equivalents, can you tell me more about them and explain their significance?

Metabolic equivalents provide a means of approximating a patient's ability to increase their oxygen delivery to tissues in response to a physical demand. For example, 1 MET is based on the calculation of the basal oxygen requirement of a 40-year-old male of 70 kg at rest and this equates to 3.5 ml of oxygen per kilogram per minute. By enquiring about what the patient is able to do in their daily activities it is possible to estimate how many METs they can achieve.

- 3 METs is equal to light household work or walking 100 yards on the flat
- 4 METs is equal to climbing 2 flights of stairs
- 6 METs is equal to a short run
- Greater than 10 METs is equal to strenuous exercise.

The significance of this is that less than 4 METs is deemed to be a poor exercise tolerance and this group of patients has a higher rate of peri-operative and post-operative cardiovascular and neurological complications. However, often this system is limited due to patient's medical problems such as arthritis or visual impairment reducing their ability rather than cardiorespiratory problems.

What particular aspects in the history and examination would cause you to be particularly concerned about the murmur?

There are three cardinal features of aortic stenosis:

1. Angina
2. Syncope
3. Dyspnoea.

However, the severity of these symptoms do not correlate well with the degree of the aortic disease. Angina occurs due to the oxygen demand of hypertrophied myocardial muscle outstripping supply. Angina occurs in approximately two thirds of patients with critical aortic stenosis, about 50% of these patients will also have significant coronary artery disease. The precise mechanism of syncope is unclear, however, it would appear that, with a relatively fixed cardiac output, it is not possible to meet the increased demand placed on the cardiovascular system by standing or exercise. Thus such activities cause a fall in cerebral perfusion and a "blackout". Shortness of breath on exertion and orthopnoea and paroxysmal nocturnal dyspnoea and pulmonary oedema tend to be late symptoms and reflect pulmonary venous hypertension.

On examination, aortic stenosis classically has a slow rising and low volume pulse. However if aortic regurgitation is occurring simultaneously then the pulse pressure may be increased. A carotid and precordial thrill may be palpated, especially on leaning forward in expiration. The murmur is a harsh late peak systolic murmur heard best at the second right intercostal space. It radiates to the carotids. However these signs change as the severity of the aortic disease increases and the left ventricle fails, therefore reducing the flow through the valve and the murmur becomes less audible. Therefore an echocardiograph is required in order to assess the severity of a valve lesion.

You have mentioned echocardiography. How would you interpret the results of this investigation to form a risk level for different grades of aortic stenosis?

Echocardiography can be used to assess the anatomy of the aortic valve, grade the severity and assess the function of the left ventricle. The best indicator of aortic stenosis severity is the valve area.

- Mild stenosis is equal to an area of 1.2–1.8 cm^2
- Moderate stenosis is equal to an area of 0.8–1.2 cm^2
- Severe stenosis is equal to an area of 0.6–0.8 cm^2
- Critical stenosis is equal to an area of less than 0.6 cm^2.

Occasionally the pressure gradient across the valve is used for grading severity. However this can be misleading as in high output states such as simultaneous aortic stenosis and regurgitation the severity will be overestimated. More dangerously in low output states where there is a failing left ventricle the flow across the valve will be reduced and so will the gradient, thereby underestimating the disease severity.

Also, the left ventricular function will be graded as normal, mildly, moderately or severely impaired based on the subjective assessment of the echo images.

What blood investigations would you request?

The routine investigations would include:

- Full blood count to exclude any significant anaemia and any platelet or leucocyte abnormality
- Coagulation studies, especially if this patient is on warfarin, and determination of blood group

- Measurement of serum electrolytes, urea and creatinine as these are likely to be disturbed by medication that the patient is taking like diuretics
- Specific investigations may be required depending on the history, for example these may include liver function tests and B-type natriuretic peptide.

Can you tell me about B-type natriuretic peptide?

B-type natriuretic peptide is a hormone secreted by cardiac myocytes in response to mechanical stretch. It is increasingly being used as a biomarker for the diagnosis, management and prognostication of cardiac failure. It has been suggested that this marker could be used as a relatively non-invasive risk stratification tool, especially with a patient undergoing major or intermediate risk surgery who does not have the ability to function at greater than 4 METs without symptoms.

B-type natriuretic peptide levels can be elevated due to cardiac causes, pulmonary causes or other causes, for example renal or septic shock. However the cause of the elevation does not appear to alter the prognostic value. Also, if a threshold level of B-type natriuretic peptide that is consistent with a diagnosis of cardiac failure is found in a patient due to be undergoing elective surgery, then this should be postponed until the patient's medical treatment has been fully optimised.

The history is suggestive of severe congestive cardiac failure and angina. How would you investigate this further to decide whether it is safe to proceed to anaesthesia for this patient?

Non-invasive tests:

- ECG – looking for any arrhythmia or evidence of ventricular hypertrophy or myocardial ischaemia and infarcts.
- Exercise tests such as the exercise tolerance test – the patient is exercised on a treadmill to a fixed Bruce protocol while ECG readings are taken looking for ischaemic changes. Alternatively, a simple 6-minute walk test where a patient is asked to walk around a circuit with an oxygen saturation probe attached. The distance achieved over 6 minutes is recorded alongside any desaturation that occurred.
- Cardiopulmonary exercise testing (CPEX) – exercise tests are often limited due to disabilities such as arthritis or visual impairment preventing the patient from sustaining exercise. CPEX testing helps overcome this.
- Echocardiography can be used to establish and define the cardiac anatomy and assess ventricular and valvular function; however, this assessment of left ventricular function represents a static measure and gives no indication of the patients functional reserve.
- More invasive tests to establish the extent, sites and severity of coronary artery stenosis include coronary angiography.
- Dobutamine stress echocardiogram, which has the advantage of as well as looking at the function of the heart, establishes how well it performs under stress due to the dobutamine.
- Also dipyridamole–thallium scan tests can be used to identify areas of the myocardium that are under-perfused whilst the heart is under the relative stress of dipyridamole.

Can you tell me about cardiopulmonary exercise testing (CPEX)?

Cardiopulmonary exercise testing is a means of objective testing to determine a patient's pre-operative fitness. It correlates well with post-operative survival and can be used to identify patients who are at increased risk of adverse post-operative outcome for which surgery may be deemed inappropriate or the patient can be warned of the high risks. It examines the ability of the cardiovascular system to deliver oxygen to tissues during the stress of exercise. This is done by asking the patient to exercise on an ergometer, usually a bike, but the hands can peddle instead if there are difficulties with the lower limbs. At the same time as they are exercising a number of variables are being measured, these are as follows:

- ECG
- Blood pressure
- Expired air flow
- Oxygen uptake from the air
- Carbon dioxide output from the body.

From these variables the volume of oxygen consumed (VO_2) in millilitres per minute and the volume of carbon dioxide produced (VCO_2) in millilitres per minute can be calculated. If the VO_2 and VCO_2 are plotted on the same graph against time there is a point where the rise in VCO_2 becomes disproportionate to the rise in VO_2. This indicates the level of exercise where the body has reached its maximum aerobic capacity. This point is termed the anaerobic threshold. An anaerobic threshold of less than 11 ml/kg/min has been shown to have a higher risk of cardiorespiratory events or death post-operatively. Interestingly, 4 METs equates to about 14 ml/kg/min of oxygen consumption. The advantages of CPEX testing are that it provides an objective number as opposed to a subjective assessment of the patient's ability to exercise and perform daily tasks. It provides a means of assessment for patients that fall in the category of not being able to achieve 4 METs or are unable to exercise due to other limitations. Also, the intensity of the exercise required to reach the anaerobic threshold is much less than that required in other tests to achieve a meaningful result.

Are you aware of any risk scoring systems in anaesthesia?

The simplest and most commonly used scoring system is the American Society of Anesthesiologists' scale to assess physical fitness for anaesthesia or ASA. This system grades patients from I, a normal healthy patient, to V, a moribund patient. The absolute mortality for these grades varies from 0.1% for grade I to 9.4% for grade V.

The Goldman cardiac risk index assesses the likelihood of peri-operative cardiac event in patients having non-cardiac surgery. Goldman identified nine independent factors and gave them weighted scores. The total score for the patient is used as a guide to the incidence of severe cardiovascular complications or death. The highest being a score greater than 25, who have a 56% incidence of death and a 22% incidence of severe cardiovascular complications.

The nine independent factors and scores assigned are:

Third heart sound	11 points
Elevated jugular venous pressure	11 points
Myocardial infarction in the past 6 months	10 points
ECG shows premature contractions or not sinus rhythm	7 points
ECG shows greater than 5 premature ventricular contractions	7 points
Age greater than 70 years	5 points
Emergency procedure	4 points
Intra-thoracic, intra-abdominal, or aortic surgery	3 points
Poor general status or bedridden	3 points

Cardiac surgery is an area with numerous risk scoring systems. Originally the Parsonnet system was used. Then as surgery and anaesthesia developed it was found that most present day cardiac surgeons "out perform" Parsonnet by a factor of 2, reducing its usefulness.

The European System for Cardiac Operative Risk Evaluation (EuroSCORE) was developed in the late 1990s and provides a more robust risk assessment that can be calculated at the bedside.

Intensive care is another area with multiple scoring systems such as APACHE I, II and III; POSSUM; and TISS. These are used to help with risk stratification for individual patients, and also to allow comparisons between different centres of care as it allows for variation in severity of illness for the different patients admitted to each unit and to try and standardise and match different patients in clinical trials.

How could you consider optimising a patient like this for surgery?

Pre-operative optimisation could be either medical, surgical or intensive care.

Medical optimisation involves ensuring that any condition that the patient suffers from is being treated optimally. For the cardiovascular system this requires ensuring angina and ischaemic heart disease are treated and ideally Canadian Class 1 or 2, which means that they can walk at least 150 yards or climb a flight of stairs before their angina occurs. If they have suffered a recent myocardial infarction then at least 6 months should have passed before elective surgery is considered. The patient's coagulation status needs to be considered as they are often on aspirin, clopidogrel or even warfarin because of previous MI, angina, arrhythmia or coronary artery stenting. The indication for these drugs needs to be considered and the risks of stopping them versus the benefits of continuing them during surgery needs to be decided between cardiologist, surgeon, anaesthetist and patient. Arrhythmias should be identified and managed, and heart failure medication should be optimised. The use of peri-operative β-blockade was initially thought to reduce the risk of peri-operative myocardial infarction; however, recent research has indicated an increased risk of peri- or post-operative stroke and other adverse events if the β-blockers are started pre-operatively. Therefore current advice is that β-blockers should be continued if the patient is already on them, but should not be started, with the exception of possibly major vascular surgery where the benefits may outweigh the risks.

Surgical optimisation would be considered when the coronary heart disease enters Canadian Class 3 and above when coronary stenting or coronary artery bypass grafting

(CABG) should be sought prior to elective surgery. Also valvular surgery may be considered particularly if severe or critical aortic stenosis is present. The last surgical optimisation would be the consideration of a pacemaker for patients with arrhythmias.

Intensive care optimisation involves the use of fluid and inotropes under the guidance of invasive monitoring to increase the cardiac output and oxygen delivery to tissues of patients who are undergoing high-risk surgery pre-operatively and continuing through into the post-operative period. Bland and Shoemaker were the first to use this method in high-risk surgical patients and found a significant reduction in mortality in the treatment group. More recently Older and colleagues identified patients at high risk undergoing major abdominal surgery with CPEX testing. The patients with anaerobic thresholds less than 11 ml/kg/min were admitted to intensive care, and invasive monitoring, fluid and inotropes were used to optimise them pre-operatively. Mortality was reduced from 18% to 8.9%.

Further Reading

Bouch C, Thompson JP. Severity scoring systems in the critically ill. *Continuing Education in Anaesthesia, Critical Care & Pain*. 2008; **8**(5): 181–185.

Brown J, Morgan Hughes NJ. Aortic stenosis and non-cardiac surgery. *Supplement Continuing Education in Anaesthesia, Critical Care & Pain*. 2005; **5**: 1–4.

Campeau L. Grading of angina pectoris. *Circulation* 1976; **54**: 522–523.

Cornelissen H, Arrowsmith JE. Preoperative assessment for cardiac surgery. *Supplement Continuing Education in Anaesthesia, Critical Care & Pain*. 2006; **6**(3): 109–113.

Davies SJ, Wilson RJT. Preoperative optimization of the high-risk surgical patient. *British Journal of Anaesthesia*. 2004; **93**(1): 121–128.

Goldman L, Caldera DL, Nussbaum SR. Multifactorial index of cardiac risk in noncardiac surgical procedures. *New England Journal of Medicine*. 1977; **297**: 845–850.

Nashef SA, Roques F, Michel P, et al., European system for cardiac operative risk evaluation (EuroSCORE). *European Journal of Cardiothoracic Surgery*. 1999; **16**: 9–13.

Parsonnet V, Dean D, Bernstein AD. A method of uniform stratification of risk for evaluating the results of surgery in acquired adult heart disease. *Circulation* 1989; **79**: 13–12.

Wong DT, Knaus WA. The APACHE III prognostic system. Risk prediction of hospital mortality for critically ill hospitalized adults. *Canadian Journal of Anaesthesia*. 1991; **38**: 374–383.

1.2.2. Arrhythmias – Rebecca A Leslie

Why do arrhythmias occur?

Arrhythmias occur when the normal conducting system in the heart becomes unstable. The three main mechanisms that lead to this instability in the conducting system are:

- Re-entry circuits
- Enhanced automaticity
- Triggered activity.

Tell me a little more about re-entry circuits

These occur when, in addition to the normal route of conduction via the AV node, there is a second connection between the atria and ventricles. The refractory period in the two connections can be different. This means the action potential will be conducted down one of the connections quicker than the second connection. Subsequently, when the two pathways re-join, the fast connection will have already repolarised, and the refractory period finished, so the action potential from the slower connection is then not only transmitted onwards through the remaining conduction pathway but also transmitted back up the fast connection (retrograde transmission). The impulse can then enter a repeated cycle of activity, cycling through the two pathways so that it repeatedly activates the atria and the ventricles in rapid succession.

Can you give me an example of an AV re-entry tachycardia?

Wolff-Parkinson-White (WPW) syndrome is an example of an AV re-entry tachycardia.

In this condition, there is an accessory pathway called the bundle of Kent, which conducts more quickly than the AV node. This means that the action potential passing through the bundle of Kent reaches the ventricle more quickly than normal AV action potential. This results in a very short P wave. The ventricle activated by the accessory pathway depolarises slowly, giving rise to the characteristic delta wave on the ECG. When the normal action potential conducted through the AV node and bundle of His reaches the ventricle, the rest of the ventricular muscle is depolarised rapidly and the normal QRS complex is produced.

Patients with WPW are susceptible to AV re-entry tachycardias, where there is anterograde conduction through the AV node, and retrograde conduction though the accessory pathway. Occasionally a re-entry tachycardia can occur taking the opposite route, passing antegradely through the accessory pathway and retrogradely through the AV node. When this occurs only the delta waves are seen on the ECG, as the accessory pathway is activating the whole of the ventricular tissue.

What do you mean by enhanced automaticity?

Almost all cardiac cells undergo slow spontaneous depolarisation (automaticity), leading to the initiation of an action potential. However, the sino-atrial node (SA node) fires at the fastest rate, allowing it, in normal circumstances, to act as the pacemaker.

Spontaneous depolarisation results from a slow increase in the permeability of the pacemaker cell membrane to sodium ions, accompanied by a reduction in potassium permeability (phase 4 in the pacemaker action potential). As a result, the intra-cellular concentration of sodium ions gradually increases, bringing the membrane potential towards the threshold potential for depolarisation. The rate of firing of the pacemaker cells can be increased by:

- Increasing the rate of rise of phase 4
- Increasing the resting membrane potential
- Lowering the threshold potential.

This can occur as a result of increased sympathetic stimulation, digoxin toxicity, or ischaemia. In some circumstances, the rate of discharge of a group of cardiac cells can become faster than the normal discharge from the SA node, and it will then act as an ectopic pacemaker, for example in atrial flutter.

The final arrhythmogenic mechanism you mentioned was "triggered activity". What does this mean?

This refers to a spontaneous action potential, or series of action potentials, which occurs following a normal action potential. There are two different types:

1. Early after-depolarisation
2. Delayed after-depolarisation.

Early after-depolarisation normally occurs in slow resting heart rates and is characterised by an additional depolarization, which occurs during the plateau phase (phase 2) of the ventricular action potential, or during repolarisation (phase 3) of the myocardium. Normally, activation of Ca^{2+} channels occurs early in the action potential and causes the plateau phase (phase 2) of the myocardial action potential. The inactivation of these Ca^{2+} channels then causes the repolarisation that occurs during phase 3. However, if the cardiac action potential is sufficiently prolonged, these channels can become reset and re-activated, allowing further inward movement of calcium and a second depolarisation of the cell membrane and a second action potential, called an early after-depolarisation. They result in a prolonged QT interval.

Delayed after-depolarisation involve an after-depolarisation that occurs after repolarisation is complete during phase 4 of the myocardial action potential. These depolarisations may summate to cause a full action potential, and are thought to be the mechanism behind some sustained tachycardias. They are more likely to occur during faster heart rates and with increased intra-cellular Ca^{2+}, their appearance is a feature of cardiac glycoside toxicity.

What factors predispose to arrhythmias?

Remember to classify your answer.

There are several predisposing factors that lead to arrhythmias. These can be classified as those arising from primary cardiac disease and those arising secondary to systemic disease processes.

Predisposing factors arising from primary cardiac disease:

- Myocardial ischaemia especially inferior infarct
- Congenital heart disease
- Excessive vagal tone
- Cardiomyopathies.

Predisposing factors secondary to systemic disease processes:

- Hypoxia
- Hypercarbia
- Hypothermia
- Hypovolaemia
- Electrolyte abnormalities such as hyperkalaemia
- Sepsis
- Pyrexia
- Excessive endogenous catecholamines (pain)
- Excessive exogenous catecholamines
- Thyrotoxicosis
- Tension pneumothorax

- Pulmonary embolism
- Drugs or alcohol withdrawal.

How would you classify arrhythmias?

Arrhythmias can be classified as narrow complex and broad complex arrhythmias. This allows easy recognition and subsequent management.

Narrow complex arrhythmias are those which have a QRS duration of <0.12 seconds, whilst arrhythmias with a QRS duration >0.12 seconds are described as a broad complex arrhythmia. Narrow complex arrhythmias arise above the bifurcation of the bundle of His. Broad complex arrhythmias usually arise from the ventricles. Occasionally they arise from a supra-ventricular site and have broad complexes due to aberrant ventricular conduction.

Which different types of narrow complex arrhythmias do you know about?

Narrow complex arrhythmias can arise at various parts of the conducting system:

- In the SA node: sinus arrhythmias, sinus bradycardia or sinus tachycardia
- In the atria: atrial fibrillation, atrial flutter or atrial ectopics
- In the AV node: AV nodal tachycardia
- In the conducting system between the AV node and ventricles: heart block.

Tell me about the different types of heart block

They can be classified as:

- First-degree heart block
- Second-degree heart block: Mobitz type I and Mobitz type II
- Third-degree (complete) heart block.

First-degree heart block describes a prolonged PR interval >0.2 seconds. Each P wave is followed by a QRS complex. First-degree heart block is normal when it accompanies a vagally induced bradycardia. It is also seen in ischaemic heart disease, hypokalaemia and with the use of digoxin, β-blockers, quinine and some calcium channel blockers. First-degree heart block does not normally progress to other heart blocks, and does not normally require treatment.

In second-degree Mobitz type I heart block the PR interval increases with each successive beat until one P wave fails to be conducted and is unable to produce a QRS complex. The PR interval then resets to normal and the cycle repeats. It is also known as the Wenckebach phenomenon. Mobitz type I AV block is thought to occur due to abnormal conduction through the AV node. It can occur due to periods of high vagal activity (such as sleep) and a permanent pacemaker is not normally required.

In second-degree Mobitz type II heart block most P waves are followed by a QRS complex, and the PR interval is constant but occasionally there is a P wave that is not followed by a QRS complex. It is thought to occur due to an abnormality in conduction below the AV node, in the bundle of His. It can progress to third-degree heart block without warning, so referral to a cardiologist for a pacemaker is required.

In third-degree heart block there is complete interruption of conduction between the atria and the ventricle. As a result the atria and the ventricles are working entirely independently and the P wave bears no relationship to the QRS complex. A pacemaker is required.

What are the indications for temporary cardiac pacing in the peri-operative setting?

Peri-operative pacing is required in patients who do not have a permanent pacemaker if they are about to undergo a general anaesthetic and have the following conditions:

- Complete heart block
- Second-degree heart block
- Trifascicular block (left axis deviation, right bundle branch block and first-degree heart block)
- First-degree heart block with left bundle branch block.

Bifascicular block (left axis deviation and right bundle branch block) is not normally a reason for a temporary pacemaker unless the patient has a history of syncope.

Can you tell me some other indications for temporary pacemakers?

Indications for temporary pacing include the following:

- Symptomatic bradycardia that is unresponsive to atropine.
- Myocardial infarction; acute inferior myocardial infarction may damage the artery that supplies the AV node. This can cause complete heart block and bradycardia. Anterior myocardial infarction can involve the bundle branches in the inter-ventricular septum resulting in bradycardia. Pacing will be required if there is second-degree or third-degree heart block.
- Asystole with P wave activity.
- Post-operative period following cardiac surgery, especially in aortic surgery, ventricular septal defect closure, tricuspid surgery and ostium primum repair.
- Some tachyarrhythmias (AV re-entry tachycardia and ventricular tachycardia) can be terminated by "overdrive" pacing.

Describe ventricular tachycardia (VT)

Ventricular tachycardia is a broad complex tachycardia, defined as a run of at least three consecutive ventricular ectopic beats at a rate of >120 bpm. It arises from either a single focus or multiple foci in the ventricle or from a re-entry circuit. There may be normal capture beats or fusion beats where a normally conducted beat combines with an ectopic beat travelling in the opposite direction.

If adverse signs are present, the patient should undergo DC cardioversion and subsequently an amiodarone infusion should be started to prevent reoccurrence. If the patient is stable a cause should be identified and corrected. If this is unsuccessful then an amiodarone infusion should be started.

What is torsades de pointes?

Torsades de pointes is a specific variant of ventricular tachycardia. It has a classic undulating pattern in the ECG with variation in the size of the QRS complex. It is usually caused by a prolonged QT interval and carries the risk of precipitating ventricular fibrillation and sudden death.

Prolonged QT can be caused by:
- Drugs: quinidine, procainamide, flecainide and tricyclic anti-depressants
- Hypocalcaemia
- Acute myocarditis, especially rheumatoid carditis
- Hereditary syndromes such as Jervell's and Lange-Nielson's syndrome and Romano-Ward's syndrome.

In an emergency, treatment of torsades de pointes involves stopping QT-prolonging drugs, giving β-blockers and magnesium (8 mmol/15 min). Over-ride pacing may be required.

How can a supra-ventricular tachycardia with aberrant conduction be distinguished from ventricular tachycardia?

Narrow complex tachycardias can combine with abnormal ventricular conduction (left or right bundle branch block) to produce a rhythm that is hard to differentiate from VT.
Features that favour a diagnosis of VT include:
- Concordance between all leads
- Capture beats
- Fusion beats
- Extreme left axis deviation
- AV dissociation
- Failure to respond to intra-venous adenosine.

If there is any doubt about the diagnosis, the arrhythmia should be treated as a VT as it has the propensity to progress to ventricular fibrillation.

Describe ventricular fibrillation (VF)

VF is used to describe an ECG that is random and chaotic and has no identifiable QRS complexes. VF can occur after acute myocardial infarction, in electrolyte abnormalities, after electrical shock, or after degeneration of other arrhythmias. It is incompatible with life and requires immediate implementation of the Advanced Life Support protocol. Effective resuscitation relies on prompt delivery of a DC shock, which should be administered as soon as possible and not delayed for intubation or to gain IV access or institute other treatment.

One episode of primary VF (occurring within 48 hours of an infarction) corrected by a DC shock does not require prophylactic treatment. However multiple episodes or secondary VF (occurring after 48 hours of an infarction) should be treated with amiodarone, β-blockers or lidocaine. Implantable cardioverter defibrillators can be placed to deliver low-energy DC shocks in patients who have recurrent episodes of VF.

Further Reading

Houghton AR, Gray D. Making sense of the ECG second edition. London: Hodder Arnold, 2003.

Kirkman E. Myocardial action potential. *Anaesthesia and Intensive Care Medicine.* 2006; 7(8): 259–263.

Nolan J, Deakin C, Soar J, et al. European resuscitation council guidelines for resuscitation 2005. Section 4. Adult advanced life support. *Resuscitation* 2005; **67**: S39–S86.

Richards KJC, Cohen AT. Cardiac arrhythmias in the critically ill. *Anaesthesia and Intensive Care Medicine.* 2006; 7(8): 289–293.

Singh R, Murphy JJ. Electrocardiogram and arrhythmias. *Anaesthesia and Intensive Care Medicine.* 2009; **10**(8): 381–384.

1.2.3. Hypertension – Matthew JC Thomas

You have been asked to see a patient in the pre-operative assessment clinic prior to surgery on a colonic tumour. The nurse reports the patient's blood pressure is elevated at 170/90.

This is likely to be a question on the risks of hypertension and appropriate therapy.

What else would you like to know?

I would like to take a full history from this gentleman, including any previous medical history plus medications. I would focus my history to look for any symptoms of cardiac disease or if the patient had known hypertension. I would then perform a full examination and request appropriate tests. I am looking for potential causes of hypertension and also any evidence of end-organ damage.

What causes of hypertension are you looking for?

One of the commonest causes in a hospital clinic is white coat hypertension, which should be excluded. Another common cause is essential hypertension. Prior to diagnosing essential hypertension it is important to exclude secondary causes of hypertension.

Tell me what you mean by white coat hypertension?

White coat hypertension, which can be induced by both doctors and nurses, is defined as a persistently elevated clinical arterial pressure in combination with a normal ambulatory arterial pressure. It is usually a benign condition. Before a diagnosis of hypertension is made patients should have several blood pressure readings at different times of the day. Obviously this is not always possible in the hospital clinic but some efforts towards this such as repeated readings following some rest are possible.

What are the possible causes of secondary hypertension? Is it common?

Secondary hypertension is rare and is usually identifiable from the history. It can be split into endocrine or renal causes.

Common endocrine causes include the following:

- Cushing's syndrome
- Conn's syndrome
- Hypothyroidism
- Phaeochromocytoma.

Renal causes include:

- Renal artery stenosis
- Glomerulonephritis
- Polycystic kidneys.

If any of these diagnoses are suspected, referral to a specialist clinic would be advised.

Table 1.2.3. Lee's Revised Cardiac Risk Index

Criteria	Points
High-risk surgery	1
Coronary artery disease	1
Congestive cardiac failure	1
Cerebrovascular disease	1
Diabetes on insulin	1
Serum creatinine >177 μmol/L	1
Total	6
Risk of complications (MI, PE, VF, cardiac arrest or complete HB):	Score:
0.4%	0
0.9%	1
6.6%	2
11%	3

MI, myocardial infarction; PE, pulmonary embolism; VF, ventricular fibrillation; HB, heart block.

Assuming this patient has essential hypertension, you stated that you would look for signs of end-organ damage. What do you mean by this?

In many ways the effects of hypertension on organs is more important than the hypertension itself. The principal effects to concern anaesthetists should be developing heart failure, ischaemic heart disease and renal failure. These have been associated with an increased incidence of peri-operative complications and form three of the components of Lee's revised cardiac risk index (Table 1.2.3).

How do you identify this damage?

Ischaemic heart disease can be identified based on a history of angina that has hopefully been investigated using exercise tests and possibly angiography. It may also be evident on a pre-operative ECG.

Heart failure again can be identified from the history, the gold standard test is an echocardiogram.

Renal failure is identified by history but also by elevated urea and creatinine on routine blood tests.

So are you willing to anaesthetise this patient? What is the threshold of blood pressure that you would accept?

This is a controversial area, and each decision should be based on a variety of factors relating to the patient, their condition and the urgency of the operation. There is little doubt that this patient needs blood pressure control, but as this is surgery for cancer I would proceed with the case. The threshold I would accept for urgent surgery is a systolic blood pressure <180 or a diastolic blood pressure of <110.

What have you based those figures on?

The American Heart Association and American College of Cardiology (AHA/ACC) have produced extensive recommendations on the peri-operative management of hypertension. They have suggested that blood pressure <180/110 is not associated with an increased peri-operative risk.

This finding is supported by a meta-analysis and review article published in the *BJA* that suggests that, whilst there may be a small increased risk with hypertension <180/110, it is not clinically significant.

Obviously these numbers should not be used in isolation but should form part of your comprehensive pre-operative assessment.

What problems are associated with hypertension and anaesthesia?

The main risks are that of peri-operative myocardial infarction. These patients often show quite marked cardiovascular lability. Several authors have shown that the vasodilatation of anaesthesia will drop the patient's blood pressure to the same level as a non-hypertensive patient. For example, a normotensive patient's blood pressure falls from 120/70 to 90/40, whereas a hypertensive patient's blood pressure falls from 180/90 to 90/40, demonstrating a much wider range. This leads to what has been described as alpine anaesthesia described by Longnecker et al!

If this patient were undergoing non-urgent surgery, what would you do?

In that situation if the patient has a blood pressure >140/90, which is considered to be hypertension requiring treatment by NICE guidelines, it should be confirmed on a minimum of two occasions and lifestyle advice regarding diet and smoking cessation should be given to the patient. If this is unsuccessful drug therapy should be started.

What drug therapy should be used?

NICE recommend an ACE inhibitor if less than 55 years old. If the patient is older than 55 they recommend a thiazide diuretic or calcium channel blocker.

Further Reading

American College of Cardiology. www.acc.org.

American Heart Association. www.americanheart.org.

Howell SJ, Sear JW, Foex P. Hypertension, hypertensive heart disease and peri-operative risk. *British Journal of Anaesthesia*. 2004; **92**: 570–583.

Lee TH, Marcantonio ER, Mangione CM, et al. Derivation and prospective validation of a simple index for prediction of cardiac risk of major noncardiac surgery. *Circulation*. 1999; **100**:1043–1049.

National Institute for Health and Clinical Excellence. Guidelines on hypertension. http://guidance.nice.org.uk/CG34/NICE Guidance/pdf/English.

Sperry RJ, Longnecker DE. Regional blood flow changes during induced hypotension. *Anaesthesiology*. 1988; **1**: 94–100.

1.2.4. Anaesthesia for patients with ischaemic heart disease and congestive cardiac failure – James D Griffin

Ischaemic heart disease (IHD) is widely prevalent in the adult population in the United Kingdom. Figures from the National Confidential Enquiry into Peri-operative Deaths 2000 show that, in the surgical population, IHD is the leading cause of death within 30 days of a surgical procedure, accounting for 36% of all peri-operative deaths. As a result the anaesthetic management of patients with IHD undergoing non-cardiac surgery is a very important issue and the examiner will be looking for a good understanding of the key principles of management.

Explain the pathophysiology behind myocardial ischaemia in the peri-operative period?

This is quite a dry question. However, key to this question is understanding that myocardial oxygen supply must meet demand. The examiner will want to see relevant physiology linked to clinical practice.

The pathological feature in patients with IHD is atheromatous plaques within the walls of the coronary arteries. Two problems can arise from this. Firstly, myocardial ischaemia, as myocardial oxygen demand exceeds a limited myocardial oxygen supply. Secondly, plaque rupture with thrombus formation, leading to complete or near complete coronary artery occlusion.

Correct, but why is this important during the peri-operative period?

The over-riding principle is to avoid cardiac ischaemia. This is done by ensuring that the supply of oxygen to the myocardium always meets the demand.

In patients who undergo anaesthesia and surgery a number of stresses, including tissue trauma and temperature changes, alteration in organ function as well as the stress and inflammatory responses may combine to produce a range of pathophysiological derangements. In the presence of IHD these derangements may upset the balance of oxygen supply and demand to the myocardium. This may lead to myocardial injury, arrhythmias, ventricular failure or sudden cardiac death. Furthermore the inflammatory response may result in the activation of the vascular endothelium leading to plaque instability, rupture and coronary artery spasm. Changes in platelet function, coagulation and the fibrinolytic system also contribute and predispose to coronary artery thrombosis.

How important are IHD and congestive cardiac failure (CCF) as risk factors for cardiac morbidity and mortality?

This question gives you a good opportunity to show your knowledge on at least one of the clinical risk stratification indices. Many candidates will mention the Goldman cardiac risk index. However this dates back to 1977, and like a number of other scoring systems that followed soon after, its predictive value was poor. Lee's revised Goldman cardiac risk index in 1999 resulted in improved predictive value.

A number of scoring systems have been developed to assess cardiac risk for non-cardiac surgery. In all of them IHD and CCF score highly. The revised Goldman index in 1999 has a better predictive value than many of the other indexes.

Can you give me some more details on the revised Goldman cardiac risk index?

This index is very simple and worth knowing (see Table 1.2.3).

The index identifies six predictors for major cardiac complications, these are as follows:

1. High-risk surgery (which includes any intra-peritoneal, intra-thoracic, or supra-inguinal vascular procedures)

2. IHD

3. CCF

4. Cerebrovascular disease

5. Insulin-dependent diabetes

6. Renal impairment (creatinine >177 μmol/L)

In essence, if a patient fits into three or more of these groups then their risk of perioperative cardiac morbidity or mortality is 11%. It is 7% with two, and under 1% with one or no predictors.

It may be useful to have some knowledge of the American Heart Association guidelines. They also provide a framework for considering cardiac risk in patients undergoing non-cardiac surgery. Furthermore they give guidance on cardiovascular pre-optimisation.

The American Heart Association updated their 1996 guidelines in 2007. They provide a framework for considering cardiac risk in patients undergoing non-cardiac surgery. They assess risk and give guidance on cardiovascular pre-optimisation. Clinical predictors of outcome are assessed. Based on these the patient is placed into a major, intermediate or minor risk group.

The five major clinical predictors are:

1. Myocardial infarction within 30 days

2. Unstable or severe angina

3. Decompensated heart failure

4. Significant arrhythmias

5. Severe valvular disease

The five intermediate predictors included:

1. Myocardial infarction over 30 days

2. Mild angina

3. Compensated heart failure

4. Diabetes

5. Renal insufficiency

Advice is that elective surgery in those with any major clinical predictors is cancelled or delayed for further investigation, medical optimisation or referral for revascularisation. The presence of intermediate predictors necessitates further consideration based on functional capacity, in METs, and the extent of the planned surgery. Patients would then either proceed with surgery or go for further investigations, initially non-invasive. Coronary revascularisation occurring between 6 weeks and 5 years, without the recurrence of symptoms or signs, constitutes a low-risk group.

What is your approach to the anaesthetic management of patients with IHD?

Any management question must be approached logically. Split this into the pre-operative, peri-operative and post-operative management.

This can be split into pre-operative, peri-operative and post-operative management, as well as the detection and treatment of ischaemia if it occurs.

Good, can you tell me about the pre-operative management first?

The aims of pre-operative management are, firstly, optimisation of pre-operative status, which involves appropriate investigations, review of anti-ischaemic medical therapy and occasionally revascularisation, and secondly, consideration of the most appropriate anaesthetic, level of monitoring and post-operative care.

Tell me about pre-operative medical therapy in these patients?

In general all cardiovascular medications are continued throughout the operative period to protect against ischaemic stresses. There is evidence that starting some drugs may carry additional benefit.

Which drugs are these?

Initial evidence for the use of β-blockers in the peri-operative period was compelling. Numerous clinical trials showed that the peri-operative use of β-blockers could lead to a reduction in the incidence of post-operative myocardial ischaemia, myocardial infarction and cardiac mortality. However, controversy still surrounds this issue, the recent publication of some large prospective randomised trials, such as the POISE trial, has presented mixed results for the effectiveness of peri-operative β-blockade. Although a reduction in non-fatal MI was seen in the POISE trial, it came at the cost of an increased stroke and total mortality rate. As a result there may be a move away from the acute initiation of higher dose β-blocker therapy in the peri-operative period. Those already on β-blockers should stay on them of course. Indeed stopping them peri-operatively is associated with a 2.6-fold increase in 1-year mortality.

Statins have been shown to be useful peri-operatively due to their plaque stabilising effects. They have been shown to lower the incidence of peri-operative cardiac events.

There is current interest in α-2 antagonists, such as clonidine. These drugs can moderate the stress response by reducing prostaglandin-mediated noradrenaline output, they also have analgesic properties.

What is your general approach to anaesthetising a patient with IHD?

There is no evidence to demonstrate a consistent advantage with either general or regional anaesthesia. There is also no consistent evidence to support any general anaesthetic agent or technique over another. What is important is not the choice of agent or technique but how the anaesthetic is managed to avoid cardiac ischaemia by ensuring that the supply of oxygen to the myocardium always meets the demand.

It is also important to remember that these patients often have a number of related co-morbidities, such as hypertension, diabetes and smoking-related lung disease.

At all times good communication is required between relevant carers, including cardiologists, critical care and surgical teams.

Can you give me some more details on the anaesthetic and why particular factors are important?

This is an easy question and gives you the opportunity to put physiology into practice.

Supply of oxygen to the myocardium depends on two factors, the coronary artery blood flow and arterial oxygen content.

Coronary artery flow is determined by the coronary perfusion pressure and the duration of diastole. Due to the high myocardial wall tension in systole most myocardial perfusion, especially to the left ventricle, occurs in diastole. Therefore it is the aortic diastolic pressure minus the left ventricular end-diastolic pressure that determines the coronary perfusion pressure. The duration of diastole is dependent on the heart rate. As the heart rate increases, this time is reduced for two reasons: firstly, the length of the cardiac cycle is shorter, and secondly, the proportion of time devoted to diastole in the cycle is reduced.

Arterial oxygen content can be derived for the oxygen content equation:

$$\text{Oxygen content} = (1.34 \times \text{haemoglobin concentration} \times \text{oxygen saturation}) + (0.003 \times \text{partial pressure of oxygen})$$

And so it is dependent on haemoglobin concentration, oxygen saturation and arterial oxygen tension.

What about demand?

Four factors determine myocardial oxygen demand: the pre-load, after-load, the heart rate and the contractility.

What does this mean in practice?

- Avoid hypoxaemia.
- Avoid hypotension, especially diastolic. There should not be a sustained drop of over 20% in the patient's baseline blood pressure.
- Avoid hypertension. This increases after-load and, hence, the myocardial oxygen demand. In fact pressure work increases oxygen consumption much more than volume work. The increased wall tension also causes further compression of the myocardial vessels.
- Avoid tachycardia. This shortens diastole and increases oxygen demand.
- Avoid autonomic stimulation.
- Avoid anaemia.

When are the particular risk times during anaesthesia in patients with IHD, and how can they be managed?

These are occasions which upset the balance between oxygen supply and demand, particularly:

- Pre-operative anxiety. This can cause tachycardia and hypertension. Use anxiolysis or β-blockade.
- Induction of anaesthesia. This may cause hypotension. Reduce induction dose by concurrent use of opiates, such as fentanyl, alfentanil or remifentanil, or the use of midazolam.
- Laryngoscopy and intubation. This may cause hypoxaemia, hypertension and tachycardia. Ensure good pre-oxygenation and adequate anaesthesia or local anaesthetic to the cords for intubation. Consider the use of a short-acting β-blocker such as esmolol. Alternatively avoid intubation and use a laryngeal mask.
- Surgical incision. This causes autonomic stimulation. Use regional anaesthesia. Neuraxial blockade is associated with reduced peri-operative myocardial ischaemia and infarction. However this must be balanced against the risk of hypotension.
- Extubation. Extubate deep or use a short-acting β-blocker to avoid hypertension and tachycardia.
- Post-operative pain must be controlled to avoid stimulation of the stress response.
- Post-operative hypoxaemia. Ensure adequate oxygenation. Patients should receive 3–4 days of supplemental oxygenation after major surgery.
- Avoid anaemia. The optimum level of haemoglobin is a subject of much discussion but is probably around 10 g/dl in this group.
- Pay close attention to fluid balance.

What about specific anaesthetic agents?

Etomidate will cause less myocardial depression than other agents, but others are often used. Ketamine may increase cardiac work and should be avoided.

Rocuronium and vecuronium are considered the most cardiostable neuromuscular blockers.

Isoflurane may be the most appropriate volatile agent. While all volatiles cause vasodilation, cardiac depression and bradycardia in a dose-dependent manner, isoflurane may cause the least of these. In humans isoflurane has never convincingly been shown to cause the coronary steal that is described in animal models.

What about monitoring in patients with IHD?

The level of monitoring should be appropriate to the disease severity and the magnitude of the surgery. It is based around the detection of factors important in the balancing of myocardial oxygen supply and demand, and for the detection of intra-operative ischaemia. For the majority of patients the Association of Anaesthetists guidelines will be enough. These are, ECG, non-invasive blood pressure, pulse oximetry, oxygen, carbon dioxide, vapour analysis and airway pressure. These should be started before induction and continued until recovery from anaesthesia. A CM5 configuration should be used for the ECG electrodes as this is most sensitive to ischaemia in the left ventricle.

More complicated patients may require further monitoring including invasive cardio-vascular monitoring, temperature and urine output. Invasive monitoring includes an arterial line and a central venous pressure line. The use of a pulmonary artery catheter is controversial and less-invasive cardiac output monitors such as oesophageal Doppler and PiCCO may be more appropriate. Consider their uses in patients with very recent myocardial infarction, significant IHD, high-risk procedures and patient with significant left ventricular dysfunction.

Can you tell me a little about the post-operative care of patients with IHD?

Interestingly post-operative ischaemia and myocardial infarction have a peak incidence at 48 hours. The ischaemia is silent in 90% of cases and often occurs in the early hours of the morning. Its aetiology is not simply explained by oxygen supply and demand. However, management in the post-operative period is based around continuing the principles of care outlined previously. Attention to post-operative analgesia is particularly important in reducing sympathetic activity.

Unfortunately post-operative ischaemia in these patients remains common and is associated with the development of significant cardiac morbidity and mortality. As a result the plan for post-operative care should be considered thoroughly pre-operatively, and critical care support sought in advance.

How would you treat an intra-operative acute ischaemic episode?

The management of intra-operative ischaemia should concentrate on, firstly, correcting any deranged haemodynamic variables by manipulation of the depth of anaesthesia and the use of vasoactive drugs. The intra-venous β-blocker esmolol is particularly useful in reducing heart rate and oxygen demand, due to its rapid onset and titratability. Also the use of intra-venous nitrates can be useful as these redistribute myocardial blood flow and may reverse myocardial ischaemia.

As previously mentioned there should be a high index of suspicion for ischaemia in the post-operative period. The diagnosis of myocardial infarction is made on the basis of history, ECG changes and a rise in the cardiac troponins T or I. Standard therapy is then started depending on the diagnosis of the particular acute coronary syndrome. The nature of the surgery may preclude the use of thrombolysis. If so, primary angioplasty is preferred. Cautious heparinisation and the use of anti-platelet agents is usually acceptable.

Can you tell me about the management of patients with CCF undergoing anaesthesia and surgery?

This is a very open question. Run through the management systematically. Start with a good introduction to set the scene.

CCF is an increasingly common condition in the elderly population. Prognosis is poor, with 82% of patients dying within 6 years of diagnosis. As a result it is of no surprise that CCF is a significant risk factor for cardiac morbidity and mortality in all risk stratification scoring systems.

CCF refers to both left and right heart involvement. The commonest causes are ischaemic heart disease, hypertension, valvular disease and alcohol abuse.

The anaesthetic management can be split into pre-operative, peri-operative and post-operative.

Tell me about pre-operative management?

Answer this in exactly the same way as with IHD.

The aims of pre-operative status by appropriate investigations and review of anti-failure medical therapy for the pre-operative management are, firstly, optimisation of and correction of any exacerbating causes, and secondly, deciding on the most appropriate anaesthetic, level of monitoring, and post-operative care.

History and examination are aimed at identifying the presence of, or recent episodes of decompensation (within 6 months is significant). Medical therapy should be optimised to maximise left ventricular function and functional capacity. All anti-failure medication is continued throughout the operative period. Rhythms other than sinus are poorly tolerated, and if they occur efforts should be taken to restore normal sinus rhythms or optimise the rate to around 80 bpm.

Investigations should include the following:

- Blood tests to look for biochemical disturbances, aggravating factors such as anaemia or co-morbidities such as renal impairment.
- 12-lead ECG, to look for arrhythmias.
- Chest X-ray to look for signs of heart failure.
- Trans-thoracic echo may be useful to quantify the severity of the heart failure, and also to look for a possible aetiology, for example valvular disease, wall motion abnormalities or peri-cardial effusion.
- Cardiac catheterisation is sometimes performed if significant coronary artery disease or valvular heart disease is suspected.

Good, can you quantify the severity of heart failure for me?

This is usually based on the ejection fraction:

- Normal ejection fraction 60–80%
- Mild left ventricular impairment: ejection fraction 40–50%
- Moderate left ventricular impairment: ejection fraction 30–40%
- Severe left ventricular impairment: ejection fraction under 30%

What about the peri-operative management?

For major surgery there is little conclusive evidence for choice between general or regional anaesthesia. However for peripheral surgery regional anaesthesia is preferred. Whichever anaesthetic technique is chosen the aim is to minimise negative inotropy, tachycardia, diastolic hypotension and systolic hypertension. Attention should be paid to fluid balance and temperature control and urine output. For all major surgery invasive cardiac monitoring is required including measurement of cardiac output.

Some patients may be considered unfit for surgery. Beware those with an ejection fraction under 30%. They are dependent on their pre-load to maintain ventricular filling, and may also rely on an increased sympathetic tone. These patients live life on a "knife edge" and are extremely sensitive to small changes in their physiology.

In general all anti-failure medication should be given on the morning of surgery. Some anaesthetists may withhold or reduce the dose of ACE inhibitors on the morning of surgery. They can make the patient more prone to hypotension in the operative period. However they should be resumed as soon as possible post-operatively.

All patients should receive supplemental oxygen post-operatively.

Good post-operative analgesia is essential to minimise the detrimental effects of catecholamine release; however, NSAIDs should be avoided due to the susceptibility of these patients to renal failure and their effect on fluid retention.

Have a low threshold for admission to ICU/HDU in the post-operative period. Decompensation may require treatment with inotropes.

Further Reading

American College of Cardiology. www.acc.org.

American Heart Association. www.americanheart.org.

POISE Trial Investigators, Devereaux PJ, Yang H, Guyatt GH, et al. Rationale, design, and organization of the PeriOperative ISchemic Evaluation (POISE) trial: a randomized controlled trial of metoprolol versus placebo in patients undergoing noncardiac surgery. *American Heart Journal*. 2006; **152**: 223–230.

1.2.5. Post-operative management of myocardial infarction – Andrea C Binks

A 46-year-old man who has no past medical history is having a routine knee arthroscopy. He is fit and active and injured his knee while running a half marathon. During the procedure you notice a change in his ECG and he now has T-wave inversion on the monitor. He has not had a 12-lead ECG prior to surgery.

What do you do?

Start with the ABC approach.

My first move would be to assess his airway and breathing. I would increase his FiO_2. If he is breathing spontaneously through an LMA, I would ensure his airway was still patent and I would check his oxygen saturations and expired carbon dioxide levels. If there were any suggestion that his ventilation was inadequate I would elect to ventilate him. I would then check his pulse rate and blood pressure. I would aim to keep his pulse rate less than 100 and keep his blood pressure normotensive for him. I would ensure adequate analgesia and inform the surgeons that there is a problem with the patient and that they should finish the surgery as soon as is practical.

What factors are associated with post-operative myocardial ischaemia?

There are three factors that are associated with myocardial ischaemia in the post-operative period, and these are pain, hypothermia and anaemia. All of these will increase the heart rate, activate sympathetic tone and increase myocardial oxygen consumption in the presence of decreased oxygen delivery.

What would you ask for when the patient is in recovery?

Start with the usual handover and then move on to specifics for this patient.

I would ask for full monitoring of this patient in recovery: comprising ECG, blood pressure and oxygen saturations. I would inform the recovery staff of the events occurring in theatre and ask for a 12-lead ECG. I would continue to ensure good analgesia to avoid tachycardia and I would keep his blood pressure within normal limits for him. When the patient is able to cooperate I would ask the patient specifically about the presence of chest pain or dyspnoea. I would also check a troponin level and a full blood count.

How do you diagnose post-operative myocardial infarction?

Post-operative myocardial infarction (MI) is diagnosed by a rise in troponin levels plus one or more other signs such as new ischaemic symptoms including chest pain or shortness of breath, new pathological Q waves on the ECG, new wall motion abnormality seen on echo or myocardial perfusion imaging, or the need for coronary intervention.

The 12-lead ECG obtained in recovery shows deep T-wave inversion across the anterior chest leads. What would you do next?

Think about where he should be managed, who by, and how.

This is an abnormal ECG consistent with acute myocardial ischaemia, so this patient will need further assessment and treatment. I would contact the cardiologist on call and arrange for this patient to be admitted to a medical area where ECG monitoring could be continued. He will need serial ECGs and serial troponins.

Generally the medical management of a non-ST elevation MI (an NSTEMI) involves medical stabilisation and risk stratification, whereas an ST elevation MI (STEMI) requires reperfusion therapy with anti-fibrinolytics or percutaneous coronary intervention (PCI). Treatment options in the early post-operative period may be limited by the risk of surgical site bleeding.

What factors would suggest this man might need urgent PCI?

This is asking about patient factors that would urge you to call for urgent help from the cardiologists.

If he were haemodynamically unstable or showed signs of cardiogenic shock then urgent PCI would be warranted. In the absence of these signs, ongoing ischaemia on the ECG despite medical management would also prompt more urgent intervention.

Are there any drugs that you could give in recovery that may improve outcome?

Aspirin has been shown to reduce cardiac events in patients with acute coronary syndromes. It also has an anti-inflammatory action which, in addition to its anti-platelet effect, may be beneficial in patients with unstable plaques in the coronary arteries.

β-**blockers** can also be given. The effect of β-blockers is to reduce heart rate, blood pressure and myocardial contractility. This may help to improve myocardial oxygen balance and may reduce the likelihood of plaque disruption. β-blockers also have anti-arrhythmic properties.

A **GTN (glyceryl trinitrate) infusion** can be started and titrated to the patient's blood pressure. Vasodilatation will improve the blood flow to the ischaemic part of the myocardium and may limit the damage that occurs. There has been no proven survival benefit by using nitroglycerin, but it may be helpful for symptomatic relief if the patient has chest pain, and may resolve ongoing ST changes on the ECG.

Anti-coagulation with **unfractionated heparin** is indicated if the risk of plaque rupture is high, and the bleeding risks are acceptable at the surgical site. For example, in patients following neurosurgery, heparin would be absolutely contraindicated, whereas following arthroscopy, the risks and consequences of bleeding are significantly less.

During an acute MI there is plaque instability, which leads to tissue factor expression and subsequent thrombin generation. Unfractionated heparin binds to anti-thrombin III and thus acts as an indirect thrombin inhibitor.

How common is post-operative myocardial infarction?

In low-risk patients without a history of coronary artery disease the incidence of peri-operative MI is about 1%.

In high-risk patients with a history of coronary disease, the risk is reported to be as high as 35%. As the population ages and more complex surgery is performed on increasingly high-risk patients, the incidence is likely to increase.

When is the risk of post-operative MI the greatest?

The incidence of post-operative MI is highest in the first 72 hours post-operatively, when the patient is mobilising fluid given during the operation and when the thrombotic risk is highest. Many post-operative MIs occur at the end of surgery, during emergence from anaesthesia. It is usually seen as ST segment depression on the ECG and is often accompanied by an increase in cardiac troponin levels. The majority of post-operative MIs are not accompanied by chest pain.

Further Reading

Adesanya AO, de Lemos JA, Greilich NB, Whitten CW. Management of perioperative myocardial infarction in noncardiac surgical patients. *Chest*. 2006; **130**: 584–596.

Lee TH, Marcantonio ER, Mangione CM, et al. Derivation and prospective validation of a simple index for prediction of cardiac risk of major noncardiac surgery. *Circulation*. 1999; **100**: 1043–1049.

Priebe H-J. Triggers of perioperative myocardial ischaemia and infarction. *British Journal of Anaesthesia*. 2004; **93**: 9–20.

1.2.6. Cardiomyopathy – Richard LI Skone

This topic, as with many, may start in very broad terms. Be prepared to have a simple classification ready. Although the three classical groups of cardiomyopathies are straightforward and known by most, we have included the two other classifications for completeness.

Tell me what you know about cardiomyopathies

A cardiomyopathy is a disease of the heart muscle. Although the World Health Organisation (WHO) defines them as being cardiac muscle diseases without an apparent precipitating cause, classically they have been described as being idiopathic or secondary to other disease processes.

The five main categories of cardiomyopathies according to the WHO and International Society and Federation of Cardiology Task Force are as follows:

- Dilated cardiomyopathy (DCM)
- Hypertrophic cardiomyopathy (HCM)
- Restrictive cardiomyopathy (RCM)
- Arrhythmogenic right ventricular cardiomyopathy (ARVCM)
- Left ventricular non-compaction (LVNC).

Although they vary in their pathophysiology, any of the cardiomyopathies can present with arrhythmias and/or heart failure.

The examiner may then ask you to focus on one particular type of cardiomyopathy.

Tell me about dilated cardiomyopathy

DCM has a prevalence of 1:2500 people. It is characterized by ventricular chamber enlargement, normal left ventricle (LV) wall thickness and systolic dysfunction. This leads to a progressive decrease in effective contractile function of the myocardium and consequently, heart failure.

The sequelae of DCM include:

- Ventricular and supra-ventricular arrhythmias
- Conduction system abnormalities
- Mitral regurgitation
- Thromboembolism.

The low cardiac output state also leads to activation of the renin–angiotensin system. Eventually DCM leads to heart failure or sudden cardiac death. DCM has a familial cause in 20–30% of cases.

It can also be caused by the following:

- Alcohol
- Infection – Coxsackie virus or HIV
- High output states – pregnancy, thyrotoxicosis, anaemia
- Drugs – heavy metals, cocaine
- Thiamine deficiency
- Phaeochromocytoma.

The prognosis of DCM is quite poor. The Framingham study showed that life expectancy is inversely proportional to the severity of the disease at presentation. The 5-year survival rate is between 40 and 50% once heart failure has been diagnosed.

Tell me about hypertrophic cardiomyopathy

True HCM is an inappropriate and asymmetrical change in the myocardium in the absence of a stimulus, which would usually cause hypertrophy. It is the most common purely genetic cardiovascular disease, and has a prevalence of approximately 1:500 people. 60% of unexplained LV hypertrophy is caused by HCM. It carries a mortality rate of 1% per year and is the most common cause of sudden cardiac death in young people.

It causes ventricular hypertrophy with preserved systolic function, poor ventricular compliance and diastolic dysfunction. Hypertrophy of the septum with outflow obstruction occurs in approximately 20% of cases.

The disease can be asymptomatic or can present in a range of ways including with dysrhythmias, angina, heart failure or sudden death.

Familial hypertrophic cardiomyopathy occurs because of defects in the sarcomeric proteins. This in turn leads to myofibril disarray and fibrosis (even in seemingly unaffected areas). These areas can be pro-arrhythmogenic and lead to ventricular dysrhythmias.

Myocardial ischaemia can occur because of ventricular wall hypertrophy, elevated diastolic pressures and increased oxygen demand.

The left ventricular outflow obstruction occurs because of inter-ventricular septal hypertrophy. The degree of outflow obstruction is often dynamic and can be affected by the patient's volume status.

Predictors of sudden cardiac death (SCD) in HCM include:

- First-degree relative dying of SCD
- Unexplained syncope
- Significant ventricular ectopy
- Massive left ventricular hypertrophy
- Presence of "malignant" genotype.

Tell me about restrictive cardiomyopathy

RCM is the rarest of the three main cardiomyopathies. It is a progressive condition that leads to low cardiac output heart failure, liver cirrhosis, thromboembolism and death. As is implied by its name the pathophysiology involves impaired diastolic filling, which then leads to pulmonary venous congestion and dilated atria. However, normal systolic function is preserved.

Its causes can be idiopathic or secondary to infiltrative diseases such as:

- Sarcoidosis or amyloidosis
- Storage diseases such as haemochromatosis
- Myocarditis
- Metastatic cancer
- Cardiac transplantation.

The commonest cause of RCM worldwide is endomyocardial fibrosis. This disease affects young adults in tropical and sub-tropical Africa.

The prognosis for RCM depends largely on its cause. The outlook for patients with RCM secondary to amyloidosis is significantly worse than for those who have well-managed haemochromatosis. Death is usually due to progressive low cardiac output failure.

It is unlikely that you will be asked about any of the following two diseases. They are here largely for completion.

Tell me about arrhythmogenic right ventricular cardiomyopathy

ARVCM is a rare condition in which the right ventricle tissue becomes replaced by adipose and fibrotic tissue. This leads to ventricular arrhythmias, loss of function or SCD. It has a prevalence of 1 in 5000 people with a largely genetic predisposition. It also has a striking incidence in athletes.

Patients usually present in their 20s to early 40s; 80% will present with either syncope, or sudden cardiac death. Other manifestations include palpitations or rarely chest pains.

Sequelae of the fibrotic changes include ventricular tachycardia, a dilated right ventricle (often aneurysmal) and involvement of the right ventricle outflow tract. It progresses to affect the left ventricle in 50% of patients.

Diagnosis is by echocardiography or cardiac MRI and the fulfilling of a certain number of major and minor criteria. Treatment is with implantable cardiac defibrillators, ACE-inhibitors, β-blockers and anti-coagulation.

Tell me about left ventricular non-compaction

LVNC is a disease that has a greater prevalence than previously believed. It has a genetic basis and consists of left ventricular wall thickening, spongiform trabeculations and a hypokinetic ventricle.

During development the wall of the ventricle goes through a process of "compaction" (at 5–8 weeks of foetal life) where the spongiform wall becomes packed. In this cardiomyopathy the process does not occur. This leaves a bulky, ineffective ventricle with trabeculations, within which blood can pool and form thrombi which lead to systemic complications. The disease itself leads to progressive heart failure and can necessitate a heart transplant.

The examiner may ask about the anaesthetic management of patients with cardiomyopathies. Again, it is important to remember to give an answer that includes giving a SAFE and BALANCED anaesthetic. As well as mentioning the basics of safe anaesthesia it is important to tailor your answer according to the particular cardiomyopathy. The usual structure of taking a detailed history, examining the patient and arranging investigations still stands. Consider any underlying disease that may have caused the cardiomyopathy. Manage any medications that they may be on such as diuretics or anti-coagulants. Remember also that the patients may have implanted cardiac defibrillators.

Further Reading

McKee PA, Castelli WP, McNamara PM, Kannel WB. The natural history of congestive heart failure: the Framingham study. *New England Journal of Medicine.* 1971; **285**(26): 1441–1446.

Report of the WHO/ISFC task force on the definition and classification of cardiomyopathies. *British Heart Journal.* 1980; **44**: 672–673.

Richardson P, McKenna W, Bristow M, et al. Report of the 1995 World Health Organization/International Society and Federation of Cardiology Task Force on the Definition and Classification of cardiomyopathies. *Circulation.* 1996; **93**: 841–842.

1.2.7. Valvular defects – Mari H Roberts

This topic has a high probability of coming up in one of the two SOEs. It is unlikely that there will be time to cover all the valvular defects in detail, and you are more likely to concentrate on one of them. It is important to have a good understanding of the cardiovascular physiological changes that occur with these defects.

You are asked to anaesthetise an 86-year-old male for a dynamic hip screw insertion. He unexpectedly collapsed on getting out of bed and fractured his hip. He has no significant past medical history and has never been in hospital before. On examination the house surgeon identified a systolic murmur over the apex of the heart and had arranged a trans-thoracic echocardiogram. He is unaware of any problem with his heart. The echocardiogram showed a narrowed aortic valve area of 0.8 cm^2 with a mean pressure gradient of 70 mmHg across the valve. His ejection fraction is 45%. How would you assess this patient's fitness for anaesthesia?

In summary, this is an 86-year-old man presenting for an emergency procedure with severe aortic stenosis.

I would start by taking a detailed history from the patient and do a thorough examination. It is important to quantify the patient's exercise tolerance and what symptoms, if any, limit exercise. In particular I would ask about symptoms of angina during exertion, syncope and dyspnoea. I would also ask about symptoms of palpitations, orthopnea and paroxysmal nocturnal dyspnoea.

This gentleman rarely gets out of the house. Has help with cleaning but manages to do his own cooking. What do you think of his functional capacity?

He has very poor functional capacity, less than 4 METs. The fall on getting out of bed could have been syncope caused by his aortic stenosis.

What signs may you find on examination?

The pulse should be checked for its rate, rhythm and character. The patient may be in atrial fibrillation. Classically the pulse is said to be slow rising and of low volume. The classical murmur of aortic stenosis is an ejection systolic murmur, which is either heard best at the apex of the heart or at the second right intercostal space. The murmur may radiate to the carotids.

What other investigations would you like to see?

I would ask for a 12-lead ECG to look for arrhythmias and left ventricular hypertrophy. As the severity of the stenosis increases there may be evidence of left ventricular strain on the ECG with T-wave inversion and ST segment depression.

I would also like to see a chest X-ray looking for left ventricular hypertrophy. However this is often normal until left ventricular failure occurs.

This patient's valve area is 0.8 cm^2. What is a normal aortic valve area?

Normal aortic valve area is 2.5 to 3.5 cm^2.

Can you classify the severity of aortic stenosis on the valve area?

See Section 1.2.1. "Pre-operative assessment and management of patients with cardiac disease" for the classification of aortic stenosis.

What about the pressure gradient across the valve? Is this important?

Using the mean pressure gradient is another way of assessing the severity of the stenosis. A gradient of more than 40 to 50 mmHg is classed as moderate stenosis and more than 50 mmHg as severe. However, once the left ventricle starts to fail the pressure gradient falls and therefore will under-estimate disease severity.

What is the aetiology of aortic stenosis?

Isolated aortic stenosis is more common in males than females and is usually due to either degenerative calcific aortic stenosis or a congenital bicuspid aortic valve. The degenerative calcific aortic stenosis is the commonest form of aortic stenosis in the United Kingdom. It's caused by mechanical stress over time, leading to fibrosis and calcification of the previously normal valve. It tends to occur in the elderly.

A bicuspid aortic valve has two leaflets instead of three. This causes turbulent flow and produces fibrosis and calcification of the valve. It tends to produce symptoms in the fourth to sixth decades.

Worldwide, rheumatic heart disease is the commonest cause of mixed aortic and mitral valve disease.

What are the pathophysiological changes that occur as the valve area decreases?

As the valve area decreases there is increased obstruction to outflow from the left ventricle. The left ventricle initially responds by hypertrophy, maintaining the pressure gradient across the valve. As the valve narrows further and the obstruction increases the hypertrophied ventricle becomes stiff and less compliant. This compromises filling and causes diastolic dysfunction. Filling becomes more dependent on atrial contraction and the cardiac output becomes fixed, with the blood pressure being proportional to the systemic vascular resistance (SVR). Therefore, maintaining sinus rhythm is important as atrial fibrillation can lead to decompensation.

The increased muscle mass of the left ventricle and the increase in the ventricular wall tension causes an increase in left ventricular oxygen requirements. However, myocardial oxygen supply is reduced. This is due to a combination of a low aortic pressure and an increased left ventricular diastolic pressure. This causes a mismatch between oxygen supply and demand and symptoms of angina on exertion.

Eventually, cardiac output and stroke volume fall, and the pressure gradient across the valve falls.

At what valve area would you expect to see significant haemodynamic obstruction?

At about 1 cm^2 or less.

Tell me how you would anaesthetise this patient, and what are your specific concerns with regards to his aortic stenosis?

The examiner wants to know that you understand the specific haemodynamic goals of anaesthetising a patient with aortic stenosis. You may want to start your answer by classifying your management into pre-, peri- and post-operative. However, the examiner may stop you and guide you towards talking specifically about your peri-operative management.

Pre-operatively, I would take a detailed history and examination and arrange investigations as I've already mentioned.

OK. We have already discussed the pre-operative assessment. Tell me how you would anaesthetise this patient?

I would anaesthetise this patient using general anaesthesia. I would prepare my equipment including emergency drugs, and ensure that I have a trained assistant. I would secure two venous cannulae and also an arterial line for invasive blood pressure monitoring, prior to induction. I would induce anaesthesia in theatre so that there is no break in the monitoring. I would pre-oxygenate the patient and then induce anaesthesia using fentanyl 1–2 µg/kg and etomidate. An acceptable alternative would be to do an inhalational induction with sevoflurane. If I used etomidate he is likely to need less than the standard dose of 0.3 mg/kg; therefore, I would titrate to effect. I would use a neuromuscular blocking agent such as atracurium and secure the airway with a cuffed endotracheal tube. To maintain a stable blood pressure during induction I would run a metaraminol or phenylephrine infusion. I would titrate this to maintain blood pressures close to the pre-induction level.

What haemodynamic goals are you aiming for and how would you maintain them?

Anaesthesia has the potential to disrupt the compensatory mechanisms that maintain the cardiac output, and I would aim to maintain haemodynamic stability.

The important considerations are to firstly, maintain the systemic vascular resistance and diastolic blood pressure. This is essential to maintain coronary perfusion. I would use arterial blood pressure monitoring in this patient so I can detect any changes in blood pressure early and treat any hypotension promptly.

Secondly, it is very important to maintain the pre-load at the upper end of normal by giving fluids and avoiding excessive vasodilatation. I would not use spinal anaesthesia in this case since it causes vasodilatation that can lead to a sudden decrease in venous return to the heart and a potentially fatal decrease in cardiac output.

Thirdly, it is important to avoid tachy- or bradycardia. Coronary perfusion occurs mainly during diastole, which is the part of the cardiac cycle that is shortened most during tachycardia. We should aim for a heart rate of 60 to 80 bpm to allow adequate time in diastole for coronary perfusion to occur. However, severe bradycardia should also be avoided since it will decrease cardiac output.

Fourthly, myocardial contractility should be maintained. Anything that depresses this, for example drugs such as β-blockers, or myocardial ischaemia should be avoided.

Fifthly, arrhythmias, in particular atrial fibrillation need aggressive treatment.

I would like to move on to discuss some of the other valvular lesions. Let's start with mitral stenosis

What's the commonest cause of mitral stenosis?

The commonest cause by far is rheumatic fever.

Good, can you tell me what a normal mitral valve area would be?

The mitral valve area is bigger than the aortic. Normally it is 4 to 6 cm^2.

Can you classify the severity of the disease according to the valve area?

Mild	Valve area of 1.6 to 2.5 cm^2
Moderate	Valve area of 1.1 to 1.5 cm^2
Severe	Valve area of less than 1 cm^2

Explain to me what happens over time as the valve area decreases

Narrowing of the valve occurs over a number of years normally but is not clinically significant until the valve area reaches about 2.5 cm^2. Unlike aortic stenosis, symptoms appear relatively early.

As the valve narrows, passive filling of the left ventricle becomes more difficult and atrial contraction becomes more and more important. In fact, its contribution to filling of the left ventricle increases from 15% to 40%. With time this causes atrial dilatation and hypertrophy. As the disease progresses the increase in left atrial pressure causes pulmonary hypertension and right ventricular failure.

Compare this disease to aortic stenosis. What are the haemodynamic goals we are aiming for during anaesthesia with mitral stenosis?

As with aortic stenosis, mitral stenosis results in a fixed cardiac output state that relies on compensatory mechanisms to prevent decompensation. There are a number of similarities between the haemodynamic goals of the two diseases.

As in aortic stenosis, the systemic vascular resistance and contractility should be maintained. We should also avoid tachy- and bradycardias and aim for a heart rate of 60 to 80 bpm. It is also important to maintain sinus rhythm as left ventricular filling may depend upon atrial contraction.

Again, as with aortic stenosis it is essential to maintain normovolaemia and pre-load to allow sufficient flow across the valve. A decrease in pre-load will cause a decrease in left atrial pressure and therefore a decrease in cardiac output.

However, in mitral stenosis we should also avoid any sudden increases in venous return, for example when a tourniquet is applied. This could cause a sudden increase in pulmonary pressures and result in pulmonary oedema.

We should avoid hypoxia, hypercarbia, acidosis and nitrous oxide. All of these increase pulmonary vascular resistance and can lead to right heart failure.

Let's move on to regurgitant lesions

What are the causes of mitral regurgitation?

Causes of mitral regurgitation can be classified as primary and secondary.

Primary causes are most common, in particular rheumatic fever. Other primary causes are mitral valve prolapse and endocarditis.

Secondary causes are less common but include such things as ischaemia of the papillary muscles and dilation of the mitral ring due to left ventricular hypertrophy or dilated cardiomyopathy.

Describe to me in physiological terms what happens in the heart with mitral regurgitation

An incompetent mitral valve will allow backflow into the left atrium during systole. This will result in volume overload of the left atrium and left ventricle.

Mitral regurgitation may be acute or chronic. In acute mitral regurgitation for instance due to papillary muscle rupture, there is no time for compensatory mechanisms to occur. Therefore there is a sudden increase in the volume of the left atrium and also in the left atrial pressure. This causes acute biventricular failure with decreased cardiac output, right ventricular strain and acute pulmonary oedema.

In chronic regurgitation there is time for some compensatory mechanisms which means that symptoms may not appear until late on in the disease. The left atrium dilates in response to the gradual increase in left atrial volume. The left ventricle also dilates increasing the ventricular end-diastolic volume. The function of the ventricle is preserved initially due to blood being off-loaded through the aorta and the mitral valve. However, as the disease progresses, contraction decreases and irreversible left ventricular dysfunction occurs.

Atrial fibrillation is common (75% at time of surgery) but is not as devastating as in mitral stenosis, since ventricular filling is not as dependent on the atrial contraction. In fact there is often a compensatory tachycardia, which decreases the time for regurgitation through the valve.

How can we quantify the severity of the regurgitation?

We can measure the regurgitant fraction. Up to 0.3 is classified as mild and more than 0.6 as severe. Other values to look at are the ejection fraction and the end-systolic diameter. An ejection fraction of less than 60% or an end-systolic diameter of more than 45 mm are indications of significant left ventricular dysfunction, and these patients should be referred for consideration for surgery.

What are the haemodynamic goals we are aiming for during anaesthesia with mitral regurgitation?

The aims are to maintain forward flow and to decrease the regurgitant factor. This is done by firstly, keeping the systemic vascular resistance low. It is important to decrease the resistance to flow out of the left ventricle. This means that vasoconstrictors should be used very cautiously, if at all.

Secondly, as with mitral stenosis, the pre-load should be maintained but sudden large increases in pre-load should be avoided.

Thirdly, we should aim for a relative tachycardia of 80 to 100 bpm. As I mentioned this decreases the systolic duration, which decreases the regurgitant volume per beat. Although time for coronary perfusion is also decreased with tachycardia, mitral regurgitation is a volume over-load and not a pressure over-load, as in the case of mitral and aortic stenosis. Therefore myocardial oxygen demand is not as high and tachycardia does not threaten myocardial perfusion in the same way as it does with mitral and aortic stenosis.

Fourthly, as with all the valve lesions, contractility should be maintained.

What are the causes of aortic incompetence?

These can be classified into acute causes and chronic causes.

Acute causes include:

- Dissection of the thoracic aorta
- Bacterial endocarditis.

Chronic causes include:

- Infection such as rheumatic fever and syphilis
- Connective tissue disorders such as Marfan's syndrome
- Congenital causes such as a bicuspid valve
- Inflammatory causes such as SLE.

Let's concentrate on chronic aortic regurgitation, since this is by far the commonest form. Describe to me the pathophysiology of this condition?

An incompetent valve allows a significant part of the stroke volume to return into the left ventricle during diastole. This causes a decrease in forward flow and volume over-load of the left ventricle.

What happens in the early stages? Are there any compensatory mechanisms?

Initially, the left ventricle dilates. This causes an increase in the length of the myofibril, which as the Frank-Starling relationship describes, causes an increase in myocardial contraction.

The examiner may ask you to draw this curve and explore it further or move on (Figure 1.2.7).

What happens as the ventricle dilates further?

As the ventricle dilates further, the myofibrils stretch further, and contractility is reduced, which may lead to cardiac failure. This is demonstrated on the Frank-Starling curve by the descending part of the curve.

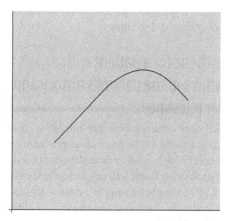

Figure 1.2.7. Frank–Starling curve for isolated muscle fibre. Reproduced with permission from Smith, T., Pinnock, C. and Lin, T. 2009. *Fundamentals of Anaesthesia.* Cambridge: Cambridge University Press. © Cambridge University Press 2009.

What are the different haemodynamic goals when anaesthetising a patient with aortic incompetence?

The aims when anaesthetising a patient with aortic regurgitation are to decrease the regurgitant flow across the valve and, therefore, decrease the left ventricular distension. Also, to maintain subendocardial blood flow.

To do this we must firstly keep the systemic vascular resistance low. This decreases the resistance to left ventricular outflow and therefore decreases the regurgitant factor and maintains cardiac output.

Secondly, the pre-load should be maintained. We should aim for normovolaemia so as to ensure the dilated ventricle is well filled.

Thirdly, unlike aortic stenosis, we should aim for a relative tachycardia. Bradycardia allows more time for regurgitation and, therefore, distension of the ventricle. We should aim for a heart rate of 80 to 100 bpm, which will decrease the regurgitant factor without significantly affecting coronary perfusion.

Fourthly, as with aortic stenosis, the contractility of the heart should be maintained.

If you are doing very well the examiner may ask you about other rarer valvular lesions.

What about tricuspid stenosis. Can you compare this with mitral stenosis?

You can work through the physiology from what you already know.

As with mitral stenosis on the left, tricuspid stenosis causes an increase in right atrial pressure so as to maintain flow across the valve. This leads to right atrial dilatation and hypertrophy. With time this causes right heart failure and symptoms of peripheral oedema and hepatomegaly, compared with the pulmonary oedema that occurs with mitral stenosis.

1.2.8. Pacemakers and implantable cardioverter devices – William A English

This is an important area of anaesthetic practice that is becoming increasingly complex. The examiners will expect a good understanding of the important principles involved in the safe peri-operative management of these patients. Importantly, current guidance from the Medicines and Healthcare products Regulatory Agency (MHRA) highlights that specialist referral to the cardiology team or pacing physiologist is often appropriate if time allows.

You are asked to provide a general anaesthetic for a patient with a permanent pacemaker. Describe the features in the patient's history and clinical examination that are of particular relevance

Safe anaesthetic practice of all patients should start with careful pre-operative review. Patients for all non-emergency surgical procedures should undergo routine pre-admission screening, and patients with permanent pacemakers (PPMs) should be identified at this stage. Many patients with PPMs have multiple medical problems. These will need to be reviewed in detail. In addition, key information regarding the PPM should be sought. Some of this information may be available on a pacemaker card provided to the patient by the pacing clinic.

This includes:

- Device manufacturer
- Model number
- Serial number
- Date of insertion
- Indication for permanent pacing
- Generic pacemaker code including special emphasis on anti-tachycardia, shocking or rate modulation features
- Whether the device is at or approaching replacement phase.

Symptoms suggesting pacemaker malfunction such as dizziness, light-headedness or syncope should be sought.

A general physical examination should be performed with particular emphasis on the presence of cardiac failure.

What routine investigations are required?

A recent 12-lead electrocardiogram is mandatory. The underlying rhythm should be noted together with any signs of pacemaker discharge and electrical capture.

Chest X-ray is not mandatory, although it may be helpful to verify lead continuity and look for signs of cardiac failure.

Serum electrolytes should be measured as electrolyte abnormalities, particularly of potassium, may cause loss of capture. These abnormalities, if present, should be corrected pre-operatively.

Pacemaker interrogation by a pacing physiologist may be required, and this will be discussed in detail later.

Describe the code used to describe pacemakers

It is not necessary to provide all of the detail given in the following answer in order to pass, but some familiarity with this system is required.

A generic five-letter code to describe the functions of pacemakers has been devised.

1. The first letter indicates the chamber being paced (A = atrium, V = ventricle, D = dual).
2. The second letter indicates the chamber being sensed (A = atrium, V = ventricle, D = dual, O = none).

3. The third letter indicates the response to sensing (I = inhibited, T = triggered).
4. The fourth letter indicates programmability (O = none, C = communicating, P = simple programmability, M = multiprogrammability, R = rate modulation).
5. The fifth letter indicates anti-tachycardia functions (O = none, P = pacing, S = shocks, D = dual, P + S).

What are the most common modes of newly inserted pacemakers?

Almost 95% of all newly inserted pacemakers are accounted for by four different modes. These are:

- VVI
- VVIR
- DDD
- DDIR.

What monitoring is required for a patient with a PPM prior to induction of anaesthesia?

AAGBI minimum monitoring standards as suggested for all patients undergoing general anaesthesia should be adhered to. Importantly these include continuous ECG monitoring, pulse oximetry with plethysmography and non-invasive blood pressure monitoring. Although beat to beat evidence of mechanical capture can be gained by monitoring the patient's pulse or observing the plethysmograph trace, consideration should be given to direct arterial pressure monitoring, especially in more complex cases. If a central venous catheter is indicated great care should be taken during insertion, particularly if the PPM has been recently inserted, as the pacing electrode may become dislodged leading to pacemaker failure. Alternatively the femoral venous route may be chosen.

Are there any specific concerns regarding use of suxamethonium?

Muscle fasciculations occur after the administration of suxamethonium. The pacemaker may perceive these as intrinsic cardiac impulses. Depending on the type of pacemaker, this may cause unwanted inhibition of the pacemaker. Suxamethonium should therefore, where possible, be avoided. If it is required, then the pacemaker may be reprogrammed to asynchronous VOO mode or a small "defasciculating" dose of a non-depolarising muscle relaxant may be given a few minutes prior to the suxamethonium.

What is electromagnetic interference?

Electromagnetic interference (EMI) refers to any electromagnetic radiation with the potential to affect implantable devices.

What are the principal sources of EMI within hospitals?

The most important source of potentially damaging EMI in an operating theatre environment is **surgical diathermy**.

Other hospital sources include:

- Magnetic resonance imaging
- Cardioversion/cardiac defibrillation

- Lithotripsy
- Trans-cutaneous nerve stimulation.

What are the potential adverse effects of EMI in patients with PPMs?

Possible responses to external EMI include inappropriate inhibition or triggering of impulses, reprogramming the pacemaker to a back-up mode, which may be asynchronous, or permanent damage to the pacemaker itself.

Is there any safety advantage of using one type of diathermy over the other in this situation?

Wherever possible, surgical diathermy should be avoided altogether. However, where surgical diathermy is deemed essential, the use of bipolar diathermy is preferred as the chance of interference with pacemaker function is less in this mode.

In an elective setting what additional equipment and expertise is required whenever diathermy is to be used in a patient with a PPM?

The Medicines and Healthcare products Regulatory Agency have provided clear guidance on this topic.

If surgical diathermy cannot be avoided, the patient's cardiac follow-up centre should usually be contacted for advice. If the surgical procedure is remote from the PPM site and the device has been checked within the past 3 months then the risk of malfunction is minimal. If the procedure will be close to the implant then the risk of diathermy-induced malfunction is increased. In these instances the patient's follow-up clinic should be asked to advise whether support from a cardiac pacing physiologist will be required before, during and after the surgical procedure.

Steps taken may include:

- Programming a pacemaker to minimise inappropriate inhibition secondary to EMI
- Disabling shock delivery functions and rate response functions that use the minute ventilation or sleep modes of physiological pacing
- Reactivation of these functions after surgery
- Confirmation of device functioning after surgery.

Cardiopulmonary resuscitation equipment must be immediately available during these cases. This must include a defibrillator and access to alternative pacing methods such as temporary external and trans-venous pacing.

How does the advice above differ for emergency procedures?

Wherever possible all the above steps should also be taken for emergency procedures. Where it is not possible for the PPM to be checked before surgery, even greater vigilance is required to detect pacemaker failure and the device should be checked as soon as possible post-operatively.

If diathermy is necessary, what steps must be taken to minimise the chance of pacemaker malfunction?

Bipolar diathermy should be used in preference to monopolar diathermy whenever possible. If monopolar diathermy is unavoidable then its use should be limited to short bursts, keeping the energy level as low as possible. The return plate should be positioned so that the current pathway between the diathermy electrode and the return plate is as far away as possible from the PPM and its leads. In operations involving either mono- or bipolar diathermy the cables attached to the diathermy equipment should be kept away from the PPM.

How is pacemaker failure suspected?

The consequences of pacemaker failure depend upon the underlying cardiac rhythm. This highlights the importance of knowing the original indication for insertion of a PPM. Clearly if the original indication was ventricular standstill then pacemaker failure is potentially lethal. Pacemaker failure results from loss of electrical capture and in the peri-operative period is most commonly caused by EMI. As EMI also interferes with ECG recording recognition of pacemaker failure during EMI relies on monitoring the plethysmograph trace, arterial line trace or patient's pulse. If this is not done then pacemaker failure may initially go unnoticed.

How should pacemaker failure be treated?

If cardiac arrest has occurred then all sources of EMI should be stopped immediately. If PPM failure was due to over-sensing, stopping the EMI storm may help. If cardiac arrest persists, advanced cardiac life support including chest compressions should be commenced immediately. External pacing via pads placed either below the right clavicle and over the cardiac apex or over the left side of the chest in the anterior–posterior position should be attempted. Capture can often be achieved at currents of about 80 mA. Trans-venous pacing will take longer to set up. As will be discussed later, the use of magnets in this setting remains controversial.

If external defibrillation is required in a patient with a PPM what steps are required to minimise device damage and reprogramming?

External defibrillation in patients with a PPM is associated with a high risk of damaging or reprogramming the device. In order to minimise these effects the defibrillation pads should be placed a minimum of 10 cm from the pulse generator. The anterior–posterior position may be used.

What role do magnets have in the management of patients with PPMs undergoing general anaesthesia?

This is an area of controversy. The effect of magnets on the programming of modern pacemakers is unpredictable. Some PPMs will switch to a continuous asynchronous mode when a magnet is applied. This explains why previously they have been thought to be useful in the event of pacemaker failure. However, there is a bewildering array of different responses that PPMs may display after placement of a magnet. Most implantable cardioverter defibrillators will have their shock delivery function inhibited by a magnet, but once again this is not universal behaviour and inhibition of shock therapy will only be effective during magnet placement. Clearly any subsequent VT or VF will need to be treated by external defibrillation.

What follow-up and investigations are required after surgery in a patient with a PPM?

Pacemaker function should be checked by pacing physiologists following any procedure involving surgical diathermy. Rate modulation functions and anti-tachycardia and shock functions will need to be re-activated as soon as possible post-operatively. Until this is done these patients should have continuous ECG monitoring in an appropriate environment.

What are implantable cardioverter defibrillators?

In addition to defibrillating functions, implantable cardioverter defibrillators (ICDs) may also have bipolar anti-bradycardia pacing and anti-tachycardia pacing. The delivery of one shock shortens the normal battery life of 5–9 years by 1 month.

Describe the anaesthetic management of a patient with an ICD undergoing surgery

Detailed pre-anaesthetic assessment is required. The centre that implanted the ICD should be contacted. The indication for insertion and details regarding delivery of counter-shocks should be obtained. The device should be interrogated pre-operatively and the effect of magnet application should be recorded. Many of these patients will have severe cardiovascular disease, including left ventricular impairment.

As for patients with PPMs undergoing anaesthesia and surgery, 12-lead ECG, serum electrolytes and possibly chest X-ray should be performed pre-operatively. Electrolyte abnormalities should be corrected pre-operatively and anti-arrhythmic and anti-failure medicines should be continued.

Defibrillation and anti-tachycardia functions should be disabled if surgical diathermy use is anticipated or the patient is due to undergo lithotripsy or electroconvulsive therapy. Transcutaneous nerve stimulation should not be used.

An external defibrillator should be available. Ideally it should be attached to adhesive pads on the patient prior to surgery. Usual pad placement below the right clavicle and at the cardiac apex will expose the ICD to the minimum induced current. The same advice regarding minimising EMI in patients with PPMs should be applied.

Post-operatively the patient should be managed in either a high dependency or coronary care environment. Continuous ECG monitoring is required until the ICD has been checked and reactivated after surgery.

Further Reading

Medicines and Healthcare products Regulatory Agency. Guidelines for the peri-operative management of patients with implantable pacemakers or implantable cardioverter defibrillators, where the use of surgical diathermy/electrocautery is anticipated. http://www.mhra.gov.uk/ Safetyinformation/ Generalsafetyinformationandadvice/ Product-specificinformationandadvice/ Product-specificinformationandadvice-A-F/Cardiacpacemakersanddefibrillators (implantable)/Guidelinesforimplantable cardioverterdefibrillators-pacemakerperioperativemanagement/ CON2023451.

Endocrine and metabolic

1.3.1. Hormonal and metabolic responses to trauma – Andrea C Binks

A 24-year-old motorcyclist is brought into the emergency department following a road traffic accident. He has sustained a fracture to his right femur and you are asked to take him to theatre for a femoral nailing.

What is the stress response?

The stress response is a cascade of widespread hormonal and metabolic changes that occur in response to trauma. It is a complex neuroendocrine response the net effect of which is to increase catabolism and release endogenous fuel stores.

What can trigger the stress response?

The stress response occurs secondary to an exogenous insult such as trauma. It can also occur following surgery, secondary to burns or severe infection and has been reported to occur following strenuous exercise. The magnitude of the response is related to the degree of initial trauma.

How is the response initiated?

Think about local responses, then systemic responses.

At the site of tissue damage, there is a local release of cytokines, which triggers the acute phase response and local inflammation. Somatic and autonomic afferents are transmitted from the point of tissue damage to the central nervous system via ascending pathways in the spinal cord. These signals trigger the hypothalamic–pituitary–adrenal (HPA) axis releasing cortisol and stimulate the sympathoadrenal response, releasing catecholamines.

What are the characteristics of the resultant state?

The stress response leads to an increase in catabolism, a release of endogenous energy sub-strates and fluid retention, along with an increase in sympathetic tone. In evolutionary terms this mechanism would help to increase an injured animal's chance of survival.

Dr. Podcast Scripts for the Final FRCA, ed. Rebecca A. Leslie, Emily K. Johnson, Gary Thomas and Alexander P. L. Goodwin.   Published by Cambridge University Press.

Can you describe the sympathoadrenal response?

Try and answer these questions from first principles.

This is mediated via the hypothalamus and the autonomic nervous system with the release of adrenal medullary catecholamines. There is also increased pre-synaptic norepinephrine release. This leads to cardiovascular stimulation with resultant tachycardia and hypertension.

Catecholamine effects on other organs include increased brain alertness, increased plasma lactate, increased basal metabolic rate, suppression of insulin release, increased glucagon release and release of renin from the renal juxtaglomerular apparatus. The renin–angiotensin system stimulates aldosterone release, which leads to sodium and water retention.

Can you describe the role of the hypothalamic–pituitary–adrenal axis?

Hypothalamic releasing factors stimulate the anterior pituitary to release adrenocorticotrophic hormone (ACTH), growth hormone and prolactin. Release of ACTH stimulates the adrenal cortex, increasing the production of cortisol. Growth hormone enhances protein synthesis and inhibits protein breakdown, stimulates lipolysis and antagonises insulin. Prolactin is also released, but its role is unclear. Levels of other anterior pituitary hormones including thyroid-stimulating hormone remain essentially unchanged.

The posterior pituitary produces increased levels of arginine vasopressin or ADH, which causes water retention, concentrated urine and potassium loss.

What roles does cortisol play?

Cortisol modulates the overall stress response by its effects on protein catabolism and by its anti-inflammatory effects. Cortisol also antagonises the effects of insulin and growth hormone and has negative feedback effects on the release of CRH from the hypothalamus and ACTH from the anterior pituitary.

Cortisol is released from the adrenal cortex after stimulation by ACTH. This leads to a state of catabolism with protein breakdown, lipolysis, increased glucose production and decreased glucose uptake in peripheral tissues.

Cortisol also exerts anti-inflammatory effects by inhibiting leucocyte migration into damaged areas and inhibits synthesis of various inflammatory mediators including prostaglandins.

Glucocorticoids are required for catecholamines to exert their pressor effects.

What are cytokines, and how do they act?

Cytokines are glycopeptides whose role is in signalling between cells of the immune system and haemopoietic systems. They are produced by activated lymphocytes, macrophages, fibroblasts and endothelial cells in response to tissue injury. Cytokines can be pro-inflammatory (interleukin [IL]-6, and tumour necrosis factor [TNF]-α) or anti-inflammatory (IL-4 and IL-10). Cytokines play an important role in mediating immunity and inflammation by acting on surface receptors of target cells. The effects of the cytokine activation are mostly local but can be systemic. Effects include the production of the acute phase response, fever, granulocytosis, haemostasis, tissue damage limitation and promotion of healing.

What is the acute phase response comprised of?

The acute phase response is the body's response to cytokines produced by the stress response, in particular IL-6, IL-1 and TNF. It comprises increased hepatic synthesis of acute phase proteins such as C-reactive protein, D-dimer, ferritin and complement components. Hepatic synthesis of other proteins such as albumin and transferrin is reduced. Raised prostaglandin E (PGE) levels lead to fever. The response also leads to increased vascular permeability, leucocyte activation and further activation of the hypothalamic-pituitary axis.

What are the potential detrimental effects that the stress response may have?

- Protein catabolism may lead to dramatic muscle loss.
- Hypertension and tachycardia can stress the myocardium and produce ischaemia in susceptible individuals.
- Hyperglycaemia can lead to an impaired immune response and poor tissue healing. It can cause an osmotic diuresis and can lead to organ dysfunction.
- Electrolyte disturbances, particularly hypokalaemia, can cause muscle weakness and promote arrhythmias.
- Fluid over-load as a result of increased ADH activity and exogenous fluid administration can cause congestive cardiac failure. Fluid over-load can also impair wound healing and can lead to anastomotic breakdown and ileus.
- The pro-coagulant state can increase the likelihood of DVT or PE and can make coronary or cerebral ischaemia more likely.
- Altered gastrointestinal motility can cause nausea, vomiting, diarrhoea or constipation and in the medium term can lead to problems with nutrition.
- Immunosuppression increases the likelihood of poor wound healing and increases susceptibility to nosocomial infection.

What is the significance of the stress response for anaesthetists?

The stress response occurs in the majority of patients that anaesthetists deal with in theatre. In elective cases, the onset of the stress response is predictable. In emergency cases, the stress response may well be under way at the time of anaesthetic induction. The goal for the anaesthetist is to try and minimise the undesirable consequences of the stress response.

How can the stress response be modulated?

The stress response can be influenced by choice of anaesthetic technique and anaesthetic agents. It can be modulated by choice of surgical technique. Other methods that may have a role are nutrition, hormone therapy and temperature control.

Tell me how anaesthesia may influence the stress response?

Think of the drugs you use for a general anaesthetic and what effects they may have.

The use of various anaesthetic agents may influence the stress response.

Etomidate inhibits adrenal 11-β-hydroxylase and, therefore, reduces cortisol production. This occurs for up to 8 hours following a single induction dose. Use of etomidate is contentious, as it has been shown to increase mortality when used as an infusion in intensive care patients.

Benzodiazepines may also have an inhibitory effect on steroid production at the hypothalamic–pituitary level, but the significance of this is not known.

Clonidine may decrease sympathoadrenal and cardiovascular responses to surgery.

High-dose opioids can be used to attenuate the stress response.

Injected opioids have been shown to block ACTH release as a result of reduced CRH release at the hypothalamic level. Alfentanil has been shown to reduce cytokine levels after abdominal surgery. However, the relatively large doses required lead to profound respiratory depression post-operatively and may increase the need for post-operative respiratory support.

Using regional anaesthesia may influence the stress response.

Neuraxial blockade is known to block the HPA axis response, by blocking both the afferent activation of the hypothalamus and blocking efferent stimulation of the liver, adrenals and pancreas. Cytokine responses are unaltered, however, as these are stimulated by local tissue damage.

What other methods of altering the stress response are you aware of?

- β-blockers. The use of β-blockers to attenuate the sympathetic response has been proven to be beneficial in high-risk cardiac patients.
- Hormonal. Insulin can be used to modulate the hyperglycaemia which is part of the stress response. Tight glycaemic control remains controversial.
- Steroids. Increased levels of endogenous cortisol present in response to surgery can significantly down-regulate IL-6 production. However, the benefits of using therapeutic steroids to suppress the cytokine response are at a price of increased complications such as wound infection and wound breakdown.
- Surgical techniques. Using less-invasive surgical techniques where possible may reduce the inflammatory response. Cytokine release is lower in laparoscopic surgery compared to open techniques, and potentially leads to quicker recovery and earlier discharge from hospital.
- Nutrition. Enteral feeding has been shown to improve recovery in critically ill patients. Immunonutrition has been of particular use, such as the supplementation of feeds with glutamine, arginine and omega 3 fatty acids.
- Temperature control. The metabolic response to hyperthermia is prevented by maintaining a normal temperature throughout the peri-operative period.

Further Reading

Burton D, Nicholson G, Hall G. Endocrine and metabolic response to surgery. *Continuing* *Education in Anaesthesia, Critical Care & Pain*. 2004; **4**: 144–147.

Desborough JP. The stress response to trauma and surgery. *British Journal of Anaesthesia*. 2000; **85**: 109–117.

1.3.2. Endocrine disease – Helen L Jewitt

What are the presenting features of a pituitary tumour?

Pituitary tumours comprise approximately 10–15% of all intracranial tumours. The vast majority are benign adenomas and arise from the anterior portion of the gland. Tumours can actively secrete hormones; most commonly prolactin produced by 30% of tumours, growth hormone produced by 20% and ACTH by approximately 15%. Conversely there can be decreased or absent hormone secretion resulting in the clinical picture of hypopituitarism.

Pituitary tumours can produce localised or generalised pressure effects. Locally pressure may be exerted on the optic chiasm producing a visual field defect, classically bitemporal hemianopia. Generalised signs and symptoms include vomiting, headache, papilloedema and cranial nerve palsies. Large adenomas can occasionally interfere with the circulation of cerebrospinal fluid producing hydrocephalus and, as a consequence raised intra-cranial pressure. A proportion of asymptomatic pituitary lesions are incidentally detected during imaging for other indications.

What is acromegaly?

Acromegaly is a rare endocrine syndrome caused by excess production of growth hormone by the anterior pituitary gland. Symptoms and signs result mainly from the overgrowth of soft tissue structures. Changes are gradual and include an increase in skull size, coarse and oily skin, prominence of the supra-orbital ridge and large hands and feet.

What potential anaesthetic issues does acromegaly present?

Acromegaly can pose a problem for the anaesthetist both in terms of the effects of the disease on the airway and also the systemic effects.

Pre-operatively any history suggestive of obstructive sleep apnoea should be thoroughly explored. This includes a history of snoring, disturbed sleep and day-time tiredness. The presence of these features suggests the potential for a difficult airway and the risk of post-operative airway obstruction.

Airway problems arise due to hypertrophy of the soft tissues of the upper respiratory tract including the tongue. A quarter of patients have enlargement of the thyroid gland that can exacerbate airway compromise. Despite enlargement of the mandible and other facial structures in acromegalic patients, bag mask ventilation can usually be achieved without difficulty. A large-sized face mask and oropharyngeal airway may be helpful. Obtaining a good view at laryngoscopy may be difficult due to an enlarged tongue and epiglottis. A long-bladed laryngoscope may improve the situation. Passage of an endotracheal tube can be impeded by vocal cord thickening and a reduction in the size of the laryngeal opening. Thorough airway assessment in the pre-operative period is essential and indirect laryngoscopy may add useful information. A fibre-optic technique is appropriate in those cases where difficulty is anticipated.

The systemic effects of acromegaly are predominantly cardiac and endocrine. Acromegaly is an important cause of secondary hypertension and can also result in ischaemic heart disease, cardiomyopathy and congestive cardiac failure. A pre-operative cardiac assessment in the form of a full history, examination and electrocardiogram should be carried out. Patients with evidence of ischaemic heart disease or left ventricular failure should be further investigated with an echocardiogram and angiogram if deemed appropriate. Treatment of these conditions should be optimised prior to an elective surgical procedure.

The endocrine features are glucose intolerance, diabetes mellitus and thyroid dysfunction. Approximately one quarter of patients with acromegaly have diabetes and will require management of their blood sugars in the peri-operative period.

What are the important clinical features of Cushing's disease?

Cushing's disease refers to the condition resulting from excess production of adrenocorticotrophic hormone (ACTH) by a pituitary adenoma. It is clinically difficult to distinguish from other causes of glucocorticosteroid excess such as long-term corticosteroid therapy, ectopic ACTH producing tumours and excess cortisol production by an adrenal tumour. These conditions are collectively referred to as Cushing's syndrome.

Cushing's disease is rare, and 80% of affected individuals are female. Cushing's disease produces multi-system effects, some of which are of major interest to the anaesthetist. Around 80% of individuals are hypertensive, and this can prove resistant to pharmacological treatment. Long-standing hypertension can result in left ventricular hypertrophy and impairment. Obesity, sleep apnoea and gastro-oesophageal reflux are recognised complications of the condition with implications for airway management. There can also be electrolyte disturbances in the form of hypernatraemia and hypokalaemia. Glucose tolerance may be impaired or the patient may develop frank diabetes mellitus.

What are the important considerations for surgery to remove a pituitary lesion?

The principles of anaesthesia for surgery to a pituitary lesion are common to those for any neurosurgical procedure. These are to maintain haemodynamic stability, ensure adequate cerebral perfusion, prevent rapid alterations in intracranial pressure and provide a stable state of anaesthesia that can be rapidly reversed at the end of surgery to allow early neurological assessment. In addition there are some specific issues to consider.

Pre-operative assessment of the patient requires a full history, examination and appropriate investigations to ascertain any pathological effects of the tumour. As explained before these would include syndromes of hormone overproduction, symptoms and signs of raised intra-cranial pressure, visual disturbances or problems relating to hypopituitarism. The patient's past medical and anaesthetic history should be fully explored. The pre-operative assessment should identify and investigate any co-morbidities, either secondary to the tumour or incidental. The patient's cardiovascular, respiratory and endocrine status should be fully optimised including the control of blood glucose and hormone replacement if indicated.

The method of anaesthesia should follow the principles of those for neurosurgical surgery. Some differences in anaesthetic technique will be determined by the surgical approach chosen. Exposure of the pituitary gland and surrounding structures can be achieved via a transsphenoidal approach whereby an incision is made in the nasal septum or by a frontal craniotomy. If a trans-sphenoidal approach is used, a throat pack will need to be inserted to prevent contamination of the airway with blood and debris. A vasoconstrictor agent can be applied to the nasal mucosa to reduce bleeding.

The patient is positioned in a head-up position in theatre. Acromegalic patients are particularly prone to nerve compression syndromes so special care should be taken with positioning and padding.

Balanced anaesthesia can be used with either an inhalational or intravenous technique. The aim is to provide cardiovascular stability throughout the surgery with a rapid wake-up at the end of the procedure. Adequate analgesia must be provided prior to emergence.

Peri-operative complications related to pituitary surgery are uncommon. However the issues to be aware of are haemorrhage, damage to the optic chiasm with consequent visual field defects, CSF leak and post-operative panhypopituitarism. Post-operative airway complications are unusual, but patients with pre-operative airway issues such as obstructive sleep apnoea should be monitored in a high-dependency environment for the first 24 hours.

You are asked to assess a 46-year-old lady for an abdominal hysterectomy. She has a diagnosis of Addison's disease. What do you understand about this condition?

Addison's disease is a clinical syndrome resulting from the destruction of the adrenal cortex. This leads to a deficiency of the adrenal steroid hormones. The majority of cases seen in the UK are due to an autoimmune process. There is an association between Addison's disease and other autoimmune conditions such as pernicious anaemia, vitiligo and thyroid disorders. Alternative causes include infiltration of the adrenal glands by malignancy or infection, infarction due to a compromised blood supply and haemorrhage into the adrenal tissue.

The presenting features of chronic cases are commonly non-specific and include weakness, fatigue, abdominal pain, nausea, vomiting, diarrhoea and weight loss. Signs include postural hypotension and hyperpigmentation of skin creases. Acute presentations are also seen during which the patient is typically profoundly unwell with hypotension, vomiting and weakness. Characteristic biochemical abnormalities are seen; namely hyperkalaemia, hyponatraemia, hypercalcaemia and hypoglycaemia.

How is Addison's disease treated?

Patients require replacement of the adrenal steroid hormones. This is given orally in the form of hydrocortisone and fludrocortisone. Patients should be counselled regarding the importance of taking their medication regularly. Intra-muscular supplementation may be needed in the event of significant gastrointestinal upset.

Addisonian crisis is managed with an airway, breathing and circulation approach. Admission to a critical care area is likely to be necessary for ventilatory support, intra-venous steroid supplementation, fluid resuscitation and correction of serum electrolytes and glucose.

What are the principles of the peri-operative steroid management in adult patients with Addison's disease?

Regular medication should be continued up to the time of surgery. An intra-venous dose of 25 mg of hydrocortisone should be given at the time of induction of anaesthesia. Following minor and intermediate surgery where the patient is expected to resume oral intake promptly in the post-operative period the normal medication regimen can be re-established. After major surgical procedures intra-venous steroid supplementation of 50 mg of hydrocortisone at 6-hour intervals is appropriate until oral intake is restored. Post-operative electrolyte and blood glucose monitoring is important.

Further Reading

Smith M, Hirsch N. Pituitary disease and anaesthesia. *British Journal of Anaesthesia*. 2000; **85**(1): 3–14.

1.3.3. Obesity – Caroline SG Janes

Obesity is a growing problem in the United Kingdom and worldwide with a prevalence of over 20% amongst adults. It presents unique challenges to anaesthetists, which you will be expected to be familiar with for the final exam. It is a topic well suited to both the SAQ and SOE and comes up regularly. The podcast on obstructive sleep apnoea complements this topic. In addition the AAGBI guidelines on the peri-operative management of the morbidly obese patient published in June 2007 should be read prior to the exam.

You are asked to see a 45-year-old female having an umbilical hernia repair pre-operatively. She is 150 cm tall and weighs 120 kg. She has no other co-morbidities, takes no regular medication and has no allergies.

What system is used to classify a person's weight?

The body mass index (BMI) is used as a tool to quantify whether a person is the right weight for their height. The equation used is weight in kilograms divided by height in metres squared. A BMI under 18.5 is considered underweight, 19–25 is optimal. Above 25 is classified as overweight, and above 30 is obese. The term morbid obesity can be used in a patient with a BMI of over 40 with no significant co-morbidities or a BMI over 35 with associated co-morbidities. Super-morbid obesity is a term recently introduced for people with a BMI over 55. The AAGBI guidelines recommend all surgical patients should have their height and weight measured and recorded and the BMI calculated pre-operatively.

Which category of BMI would this patient fall into?

In the long case you will be given all the clinical information beforehand so make sure you work out the BMI if you are given the patient's height and weight.

This lady has a BMI of 53 and is therefore almost in the super-morbidly obese category. Despite having no reported co-morbidities, morbid obesity is a multi-system disorder and she will be a high-risk patient to anaesthetise.

What do you know about fat distribution and the relevance of this to morbidity risk?

Obesity can be of a gynecoid or android fat distribution. Gynecoid fat distribution is more common in women and involves peripheral fat distribution or a "pear-like" appearance. An android distribution tends to predominate in males, involves a more central or "apple-like" fat deposition and is associated with a higher morbidity. For this reason the waist to hip ratio has been developed to further quantify cardiovascular risk. A value of over 0.8 in women and 1.0 in men is typical of an android distribution and signifies a higher risk. The latter results in fat deposition intra-peritoneally and around the neck and airway. Hence, it presents greater challenges both to the surgeon and the anaesthetist.

Tell me more about the effects of obesity on the respiratory system

Obesity causes a tendency to hypoxaemia at rest, which is worsened by the supine position and anaesthesia due to the reduction of the functional residual capacity (FRC). FRC declines progressively with increasing BMI, and a patient with a BMI of over 40 will most likely have an FRC of less than 1 litre. Absolute oxygen consumption is increased and obese patients tend to desaturate more rapidly when apnoeic than non-obese patients. In addition, there is decreased chest wall and lung compliance. The closing volume therefore encroaches on FRC leading to airway closure and ventilation–perfusion mismatch, which in turn causes intra-pulmonary shunting and hypoxaemia. Laparoscopic surgery and Trendelenburg positioning further aggravate these altered mechanics of breathing in the obese patient. Obese patients therefore require a higher fraction of inspired oxygen and higher ventilatory pressures to prevent desaturation. Positive end-expiratory pressure is especially useful to increase FRC and prevent airway collapse.

Added to this, obese patients are at increased risk of obstructive sleep apnoea (OSA), characterised by episodes of apnoea during sleep, snoring and day-time somnolence. They also have increased pharyngeal wall compliance resulting in a tendency of the latter to col-lapse. OSA ultimately leads to desensitization of the respiratory centres to hypercapnia. These patients can therefore be dependent on their hypoxic drive. They can also develop pulmonary hypertension.

Tell me more about the cardiovascular problems encountered in obese patients

To meet the increased metabolic needs of being obese, circulating volume, plasma volume and cardiac output are all increased. This increased circulating volume can in turn cause an increase in pre-load that can eventually lead to dilatation and hypertrophy of one or both ventricles. These changes can progress to systemic and pulmonary hypertension, which con-tribute to the development of coronary heart disease and biventricular failure. They also have a higher risk of post-operative deep vein thrombosis. In addition the risk of sudden death is higher in obesity.

What is the effect of obesity on the metabolic and gastrointestinal systems?

Obesity is a chronic metabolic disorder characterised predominantly by insulin resistance. This is associated with diabetes mellitus and hyperlipidaemia. Obese patients can also develop a fatty liver, sometimes termed steatohepatitis. This is a reversible condition with weight loss but if untreated can progress to cirrhosis and liver failure. Obese patients also have a higher risk of gastric aspiration due to gastro-oesophageal reflux disease and an increased incidence of hiatus hernia.

How would you assess this patient pre-operatively?

I would want to conduct a thorough pre-operative assessment on this patient. In addition to a routine anaesthetic history, I would specifically look for symptoms or signs suggestive of cardiovascular or respiratory dysfunction as these can be masked by a sedentary lifestyle. I would also ask about symptoms of gastro-oesophageal reflux.

I would perform a detailed assessment of her airway. If the patient were male I would ascertain their collar size, as a large collar size increases the risk of OSA and difficult intu-bation. I would also examine her back to see whether regional anaesthesia would be feasible and assess veins for venous access.

I would look for previous anaesthetic charts to check for evidence of any airway problems.

What investigations would you want for this patient?

I would want a full blood count, urea, creatinine and electrolytes, a fasting glucose level, liver function tests and C-reactive protein. I would review her electrocardiogram looking for evidence of ischaemic heart disease or cor pulmonale. If significant cardiovascular disease was suspected, I would request an echocardiogram and a cardiology review. I would also request an arterial blood gas analysis, lung function tests and if appropriate, sleep studies.

What are the practical considerations when listing an obese patient for surgery?

According to the AAGBI, all hospitals should have a named consultant anaesthetist and the-atre nurse responsible for the management of morbidly obese patients. These members of staff are responsible for training all staff to care for these patients and for ensuring availability of specialised equipment. All hospitals should also have local guidelines for the management of the morbidly obese patient.

The patient's BMI should be included on the theatre list so that all staff are forewarned. The operating table and ward bed should be checked to ensure that the patient's weight is below the maximum allowable. Additional personnel should be present in theatre to help with positioning and to help turn the patient in an emergency. Arm boards should be avail-able for optimum positioning, especially if an extra wide table in not available.

Manual handling should be kept to a minimum. Therefore ideally the patient should be anaesthetised in theatre on the operating table, and if appropriate they should position them-selves ready for surgery.

Alternative equipment and monitoring devices should be available. An arterial line may need to be inserted in case the non-invasive blood pressure cuff does not read accurately. Intra-venous access can sometimes be difficult, therefore central venous access equipment and an ultrasound machine should be immediately available.

As both anaesthesia and surgery are more challenging in obese patients the additional time required should be allowed for when booking the case.

How would you anaesthetise this patient for her umbilical hernia repair?

A patient with a BMI of over 50 should always be anaesthetised by an experienced anaes-thetist; I would therefore discuss this case with the duty consultant following my pre-operative assessment and confirm the availability of a high-dependency bed for post-operative care.

I would administer antacid prophylaxis as she will be at increased risk of gastro-oesophageal reflux.

My anaesthetic technique would depend on the size of the umbilical hernia. If the hernia is small I would discuss the possibility of carrying out the surgery under local anaesthesia with the surgical team. If the hernia is large and local anaesthesia is not possible I would opt for a general anaesthetic technique. I would consider using an epidural for post-operative pain relief although this may be technically difficult. This could provide optimal analgesia, reducing the need for systemic opiates.

If the patient had symptoms of gastro-oesophageal reflux I would use a rapid sequence induction and secure the airway with a tracheal tube. I would have equipment available in case it is a difficult intubation. I would thoroughly pre-oxygenate the patient monitoring nitrogen washout and induce the patient in a ramped position with abducted arms. Following intubation I would use pressure controlled ventilation and apply positive end-expiratory pressure. I would fully monitor the patient in accordance with the AAGBI guidelines maintaining balanced anaesthesia with a muscle relaxant, volatile anaesthetic in oxygen and air. If epidural anaesthesia was not possible I would ask the surgeon to infiltrate the wound with local anaesthetic at the end of the procedure. Ultrasound guided rectus sheath blocks and trans-abdominis plane blocks could also be considdered in this event. I would also administer intra-venous paracetamol, diclofenac and fluid ensuring the patient is well hydrated.

I would ensure intermittent calf compression devices are applied intra-operatively to the patient and discuss starting prophylactic fractionated heparin immediately post-operatively with the surgeon.

I would extubate the patient awake and sitting up. The patient may benefit from post-operative continuous positive airway pressure (CPAP) therapy. Further analgesia on the high-dependency area could be provided with patient-controlled analgesia using fentanyl or morphine but should be carefully monitored.

What special considerations should there be for obese patients post-operatively?

Depending on the extent of the hernia, the length of surgery and the patient's conduct during surgery, it may be necessary for them to be nursed on high-dependency or intensive care post-operatively. It will be necessary for a multi-disciplinary approach to their care with the involvement of physiotherapists, dieticians and occupational therapists if they undergo major surgery.

Initially day-case surgery was thought to be unsuitable for obese patients, but, with careful patient selection it is becoming more common and can be very successful. The decision should be made on a case by case basis and depends on other co-morbidities and the type of surgery.

Respiratory problems may persist into the post-operative period. Therefore supplemental oxygen, breathing exercises, physiotherapy and occasionally non-invasive ventilation may be required to alleviate atelectasis and retained secretions and thus prevent the development of a post-operative chest infection. If a patient with sleep apnoea uses a CPAP machine at home they should be asked to bring this in.

Analgesia should be multi-modal including paracetamol and NSAIDs should be used routinely if there are no contra-indications. Regional or peripheral nerve blockade should be used if possible and appropriate. Intra-muscular injections are best avoided in obese patients as they are unpredictable. Opiates can be used with care although they are best avoided in patients known to have OSA.

Many obese patients are diabetic and will require blood glucose monitoring post-operatively. In major surgery a sliding scale with insulin and dextrose to maintain normogly-caemia may be required until the patient resumes a normal diet. This may also be necessary in some non-diabetic patients during the catabolic phase post-surgery.

Obese patients should be nursed post-operatively on a special bariatric bed with a pressure-relieving mattress and a trapeze. Early mobilisation is essential as is post-operative DVT prophylaxis. Well-fitting thromoembolic deterrent (TED) stockings and subcutaneous fractionised heparin should be used routinely even in minor surgery. In major pelvic or orthopaedic surgery continuation of DVT prophylaxis post-discharge should be considered.

Further Reading

Association of Anaesthetists of Great Britain and Ireland (AAGBI) Guidelines.

Peri-operative Management of the Morbidly Obese Patient. June 2007. http://www.aagbi.org/publications/ guidelines.htm#p.

1.3.4. Diabetes – Andrea C Binks

An elderly male with type 1 diabetes is scheduled for an axillo-bifemoral bypass graft.

What would be your anaesthetic management for this patient?

Try and classify this answer. The factors that would influence the anaesthetic management of this patient are the diabetes, the surgical procedure and an elderly patient with possible associ- ated co-morbidities.

I would start with the pre-operative assessment of his diabetes. There are two particular areas I would concentrate on. The first is glycaemic control and the second is assessment of diabetic complications.

Starting with glycaemic control, I would ask about the patient's recent diabetic control, at home and in hospital, and review the patient's notes and any relevant charts at the bedside. There may be evidence of past hospitalisations and clinic reviews by the diabetic physicians. Prior random or fasting glucose measurements and previous HbA1c assays may indicate the adequacy of diabetic control and should be noted. Current medication should be reviewed, including insulin regimens and any oral hypoglycaemic agents.

I would also make an assessment of hydration and general condition by clinical examin- ation and a review of fluid balance charts. I would send a sample of blood for a full blood count (FBC), urea and electrolytes (U&ES), glucose and a blood gas to determine the acid– base status of the patient.

In the acute setting, poorly controlled sugars can cause symptomatic hypoglycaemic episodes or severe dehydration with an acidosis caused by either lactate or ketoacids. Peri- operative hyperglycaemia is associated with an increase in wound infection rate and, in car- diac surgery, with poor neurological outcome.

In patients with poor diabetic control, the surgery should be postponed unless it is imme- diately life-saving.

In the long-term, poor glycaemic control is associated with microvascular complications.

What diabetic complications would you look for?

Try and discuss these in the order of relevance.

First I would assess for coronary artery disease, which is 4–5 times more common in patients with diabetes and may be asymptomatic. Patients are also at risk from peripheral vascular disease, hypertension and cerebrovascular events.

The second complication I would assess is autonomic neuropathy. There are two major manifestations of this, which are of particular concern to the anaesthetist.

The first is disordered cardiovascular responses and the second, orthostatic hypoten- sion. Patients are prone to develop unexpected tachyarrythmias, bradycardia or episodes of hypotension. Hypotension from hypovolaemia or central neuraxial blockade tends to be poorly tolerated in these patients, particularly if there is underlying cardiovascular disease.

Gastroparesis is another concern. Despite fasting, gastric volumes can be quite large, thus increasing the risk of reflux and aspiration on induction.

How would you assess for the presence of autonomic neuropathy?

You can assess for autonomic neuropathy by asking the patient to perform a Valsalva manoeuvre. In the presence of autonomic neuropathy the blood pressure will drop, and because the ability to compensate is lost, the blood pressure will stay low until the intra-thoracic pressure is released. A routine ECG may lose normal heart rate variability.

What other diabetic complications would you ask about?

The third complication I would ask about is diabetic nephropathy. If there is any evidence of this, for example microalbuminuria, then the risk of post-operative renal failure is greatly increased. I would ensure that appropriate haemodynamic monitoring is in place and that fluid balance is maintained.

Next I would assess the respiratory system. Diabetes is associated with a reduced FEV_1 and FVC. There is also a higher incidence of chest infections post-operatively and in the obese patients, COPD is more prevalent.

I would then ask about stiff joints, as 30–40% of patients will have some limited joint mobility. This may lead to difficulties with laryngoscopy and tracheal intubation.

I would ask the patients about eye complications, as patients with retinopathy are at high risk of developing vitreous haemorrhage during hypertensive episodes.

I would then ascertain if there were any associated endocrine disorders such as hypo-adrenalism or thyroid disease.

How would you manage this man's glucose control pre-operatively?

I would ask him to omit his normal morning dose of insulin and then establish an insulin, glucose and potassium sliding scale regimen for the period of his starvation, starting on the ward. He should be the first patient on the morning list. His blood glucose levels should be monitored regularly throughout this period, aiming for a blood glucose of between 7 and 10 mmol/L.

How would you anaesthetise this man?

Think of any diabetic patient you have anaesthetised for a major operation here.

This is a major operation in an elderly diabetic gentleman who is likely to have other co-morbidities as well as complications of his diabetes. The surgical team is likely to have chosen this axillo-bifemoral graft instead of an aortobifemoral graft because it is associated with less haemodynamic instability and does not entail a large abdominal incision. The procedure typically requires three small incisions for the anastomoses (infra-clavicular, left and right groin) and therefore central neuraxial blockade is not an option. He will need a balanced general anaesthetic with close haemodynamic monitoring. The choice of anaesthetic technique must balance the requirement for haemodynamic stability and allow rapid recovery after surgery.

Prior to induction of anaesthesia, I would insert an arterial line for close monitoring of his blood pressure, and would insert a central line and a urinary catheter to facilitate accurate fluid balance management.

If there is any suggestion of autonomic instability and gastroparesis, he will need a rapid sequence induction. His blood glucose should be checked hourly throughout the procedure and the insulin infusion rate adjusted according to the regimen used.

What instructions would you give to the recovery staff regarding his glucose control?

I would ask the recovery staff to continue checking his blood glucose hourly and adjusting his insulin, glucose and potassium infusions according to an appropriately prescribed sliding scale. I would ask that they hand over to the ward staff that the insulin, glucose and potassium infusions should continue until he is eating and drinking adequately and able to take his insulin as normal.

How would you define diabetic ketoacidosis?

Diabetic ketoacidosis is a state of insulin insufficiency that results in high blood sugar levels and the accumulation of organic acids in the blood. It is a serious, often life-threatening complication of diabetes and is characterised by the triad of hyperglycaemia, metabolic acidosis and ketonaemia.

What is the mechanism for ketone production in diabetes?

This is testing knowledge of some of the steps in intermediary metabolism. You need to at least be able to explain the final steps, which lead to metabolic acidosis.

Ketones are produced from Acetyl CoA in the liver mitochondria. Acetyl CoA is the end-product of β-oxidation of fatty acids, and the product of condensation of two pyruvate molecules. Acetyl CoA can be combined with oxaloacetate and then enter into the citric acid cycle of aerobic metabolism. In states of excess fatty acid breakdown such as diabetic ketoacidosis and starvation, there is not enough oxaloacetate to combine with all the Acetyl CoA molecules. The excess Acetyl CoA molecules are diverted into ketone production. The accumulation of the ketoacids β-hydroxybutyrate and acetoacetate are what result in the development of a metabolic acidosis.

How might a patient with diabetic ketoacidosis present?

Think history, then findings on examination.

A patient with diabetic ketoacidosis will present with symptoms and signs of uncontrolled diabetes, namely polyuria, polydipsia, weight loss and dehydration. They may complain of abdominal pain, diarrhoea, nausea and vomiting. On examination they will appear dehydrated with dry skin and a dry mouth. Their conscious level may be impaired. They will be hyperventilating due to the metabolic acidosis. This is known as Kussmaul breathing. There may be the distinct odour of ketones noted on the breath. They may have a tachycardia and be hypotensive.

How would you manage this patient?

Break this down into history, examination, investigations, monitoring and specific treatment.

I would take a history and examine the patient, looking for the signs and symptoms already mentioned.

The investigations I would request initially would be as follows:

- Arterial blood gas for acid–base balance
- Urea and electrolytes, checking for sodium levels, which may be low as an osmolar compensation for the high glucose level
- Potassium level, which may be high on presentation, although total body potassium will be low due to the absence of insulin
- Urinalysis, looking for ketones.

The anion gap is likely to be high due to the unmeasured ketones causing an acidosis.

I would review the plasma urea and creatinine concentrations as indicators of renal impairment or renal failure.

I would also request a full blood count, blood, urine and sputum cultures, a chest X-ray and a 12-lead ECG in order to determine the cause.

I would want to establish ECG, blood pressure, pulse oximetry, and temperature monitoring. I would place a urinary catheter to measure urine output, and check blood glucose regularly.

I would want to transfer this patient to a high-dependency unit where definitive treatment can be given.

Which specific treatments would you institute?

The fluid deficit should initially be replaced with normal saline, starting with 1–2 litres in the first hour and reducing to 300–500 ml/hr thereafter, titrated against response. A central line may be necessary to guide treatment.

An insulin bolus of 0.1 unit per kg should be given followed by an infusion of 0.1 unit per kg per hour. The blood sugar levels should be checked hourly thereafter, and the insulin infusion adjusted accordingly.

Potassium should be added to the replacement fluid when the serum level reaches 4.5 mmol/L.

When the blood sugar level falls below 14 mmol/L, a glucose infusion should be commenced.

If the cause of the diabetic ketoacidosis is established then this should also be treated.

Would you give the patient bicarbonate?

This is a contentious issue.

Bicarbonate has been used in the treatment of diabetic ketoacidosis if the pH is less than 7.0, but it has several inherent problems.

The formulations that are currently available deliver a large sodium load. Also, giving bicarbonate will increase carbon dioxide production. Bicarbonate does not cross the blood–brain barrier so will worsen cerebral intra-cellular acidosis. Bicarbonate will also worsen hypokalaemia, which might provoke cardiac arrhythmias. As the ketoacids disappear, a metabolic alkalosis may develop. Bicarbonate also causes a left-shift of the oxyhaemoglobin dissociation curve. There is no evidence of any outcome benefit to using bicarbonate if the patients pH is greater than 6.8.

Further Reading

Joint British Diabetes Societies. Inpatient Care Group. The management of diabetic ketoacidosis in adults. March 2010. http://www.diabetes.nhs.uk/news.php?o=193.

Lever E, Jaspan JB. Sodium bicarbonate therapy in severe diabetic ketoacidosis. *American Journal of Medicine.* 1983; **75**: 263–268.

McAnulty GR, Robertshaw HJ, Hall GM. Anaesthetic management of patients with diabetes mellitus. *British Journal of Anaesthesia.* 2000; **85**: 80–90.

1.3.5. Calcium and magnesium homeostasis – Sarah F Bell

How is calcium metabolism controlled?

Calcium metabolism is controlled by parathyroid hormone (PTH), vitamin D and calcitonin. Parathyroid hormone is secreted in response to low plasma calcium levels. It causes a rise in plasma calcium and a fall in plasma phosphate. The parathyroid hormone increases bone resorption, enhances vitamin D activity and also reduces phosphate resorption by the kidney.

Vitamin D is produced in the skin in response to sunlight. It is activated in the liver and then kidney to form 1,25-dihydroxy vitamin D. This active form of vitamin D is stimulated by low calcium and phosphate levels and by parathyroid hormone. Active vitamin D increases calcium and phosphate levels by increasing gut absorption and bone resorption. The active vitamin D has a negative feedback effect on parathyroid hormone levels.

Calcitonin reduces plasma calcium and phosphate levels.

What are normal plasma calcium levels?

The normal level is 2.2–2.6 mmol/L. It is important to remember that calcium is 40% bound to albumin and it is the unbound, ionized portion which is active. Calcium measurements should therefore be adjusted for the albumin level. For every 4 g/L of albumin that is below the normal level of 40 g/L, 0.1 mmol/L of calcium should be added to the initial result.

What are the actions of calcium?

Calcium is vital for a number of different body systems. In the haematological system calcium is required for haemostasis. In the musculoskeletal system it is vital for the structural integrity of bone. It plays a key role in the release of acetylcholine at the presynaptic bulb and is also integral to the function of the actin–myosin power-stroke in skeletal muscle contraction. Calcium is also important in cardiac and smooth muscle contraction. Finally in the neurological system, calcium functions as a neurotransmitter and as a second messenger system.

What are the causes of hypocalcaemia?

Calcium levels need to be considered in conjunction with phosphate levels. If calcium and phosphate are low the cause may be removal of the parathyroid tissue, chronic renal failure, hypoparathyroidism or pseudohypoparathyroidism (failure of the target cell response to parathyroid hormone). If the phosphate level is normal or raised the cause might be osteomalacia, overhydration or pancreatitis.

What are the features of hypocalcaemia?

Patients may present with tetany, peri-oral tingling, carpo-pedal spasm and depression. Neuromuscular excitability may also be seen and can be elicited by tapping over the facial nerve causing twitching – this is Chvostek's sign. The ECG findings would be of an increased QT interval.

How can we treat hypocalcaemia?

Mild hypocalcaemia can be treated with oral calcium. Severe symptomatic hypocalcaemia should be treated with intra-venous calcium gluconate 10%, repeated as necessary.

What are the possible causes of hypercalcaemia?

The most common causes of hypercalcaemia are malignancy and primary hyperparathyroidism.

What are the features of hypercalcaemia?

The mnemonic "bones, stones, abdominal groans and psychic moans" helps to remind you of the different systems!

Abdominal symptoms of pain, vomiting, weight loss, constipation are all features. As is polyuria, polydipsia, renal failure and renal stones. Patients may also develop depression and confusion. Furthermore, hypertension and even cardiac arrest may ensue. The ECG may reveal a reduced QT interval.

How would you treat hypercalcaemia?

Calcium levels greater than 3.5 mmol/L or patients with symptomatic hypercalcaemia require treating. Treatment includes rehydration, diuretics and bisphosphonates.

We are now going to discuss magnesium. Can you tell me where most magnesium is located in the body and what the normal plasma concentration is?

It is predominantly an intra-cellular ion with an intra-cellular concentration of 5–20 mmol/L. The normal plasma concentration ranges from 0.5 to 1 mmol/L.

What are the roles of magnesium?

Magnesium is an ion that has a number of therapeutic applications. You need to have detailed, accurate knowledge of its actions.

Magnesium is important in maintaining electrical potentials across cell membranes, it is vital in the function of ATP and the synthesis of DNA, RNA and proteins. It affects calcium metabolism, and hypomagnesaemia is often associated with hypocalcaemia. Intra-cellular magnesium also inhibits calcium influx, and it is therefore described as a physiological calcium antagonist.

Magnesium affects most of the body systems. It is a cardiovascular depressant and can cause a reduction in cardiac output and vascular tone. It has anti-arrhythmic effects and inhibits the release of catecholamines. Magnesium is an anti-convulsant that reduces excitability of nerves and antagonises calcium at the pre-synaptic junction. Magnesium will cause skeletal muscle weakness and in theory precipitate respiratory failure at high enough plasma levels. It is an effective bronchodilator. With regards to the genitourinary system, magnesium is a tocolytic and a mild diuretic. Finally magnesium reduces platelet activity.

How is magnesium stored and how are levels controlled?

Magnesium is the second most common intra-cellular cation, after potassium. It is distributed 65% in bone and 35% in cells. About one third of dietary magnesium is absorbed in the small intestine. The kidneys control the plasma levels by controlling excretion of magnesium. Magnesium is reabsorbed in the ascending limb of the loop of Henle, with only 1% excreted in the urine. Parathyroid hormone enhances both gut and kidney reabsorption, whilst aldosterone increases renal excretion.

What are the causes of abnormal magnesium levels?

Magnesium deficiency is due to magnesium loss from diarrhoea or due to lack of intake, classically in patients receiving total parenteral nutrition (TPN). Raised magnesium levels may be caused by excessive treatment or intake.

What are the effects of hypomagnesaemia?

Paraesthesia, fits, tetany and arrhythmias have all been observed. It is important to remember that hypocalcaemia may also occur. The treatment is replacement of magnesium.

What about hypermagnesaemia?

The effect depends on the plasma level. At plasma concentrations of 4 to 5 mmol/L the patient may lose their tendon reflexes and suffer from muscle weakness. At levels of 7 to 8 mmol/L the patient will have respiratory muscle paralysis and at levels over 10 mmol/L cardiac arrest will occur. Treatment is aimed at reducing levels. Calcium gluconate will antagonise the effects of the magnesium whilst diuresis and dialysis will act to remove the excess.

What are the therapeutic actions of magnesium?

Magnesium has a number of therapeutic roles. It is used in acute asthma to treat bronchospasm. The 2008 British Thoracic Society recommends 2 g of IV magnesium sulphate given over 20 minutes for adults with acute severe asthma who have not had a good response to initial bronchodilator therapy.

Magnesium is used as an anti-arrhythmic in torsades de pointe and ventricular arrhythmias unresponsive to other treatment. Again a 2-g IV bolus should be given but over 10 minutes. Magnesium is also used during surgery for removal of phaeochromocytoma in order to suppress catecholamine release.

Pre-eclampsia and eclampsia is another area in which magnesium now has a role. It is proposed that convulsions are due to cerebral vasospasm and a reduction in cerebral blood flow, which can be counteracted by the magnesium. After the results of the MAGPIE trial in 2002, the World Health Organisation has advised that women with severe pre-eclampsia be given magnesium for prevention of eclampsia. A loading dose of 4 g IV followed by an infusion of 1 g per hour is used in my hospital. Again, levels are monitored closely by checking patella reflexes, respiration rate and plasma concentrations. We aim for a therapeutic range of about 2–3 mmol/L. Magnesium is also indicated for eclamptic seizures, and 4 g is again given as a bolus, although this is reduced if the woman is already on an infusion.

Finally, magnesium is used in cases of tetanus to reduce spasm and autonomic instability. It is again given as a bolus followed by an infusion titrated to symptoms and plasma levels.

Further Reading

Joint Formulary Committee. *British National Formulary*. 58th edition. London: British Medical Association and Royal Pharmaceutical Society of Great Britain, 2009.

Lewis, G. (ed.) The Confidential Enquiry into Maternal and Child Health (CEMACH). Saving mothers' lives: reviewing maternal deaths to make motherhood safer – 2003–2005. The Seventh Report on Confidential Enquiries into Maternal Deaths in the United Kingdom. London: CEMACH, 2007. http://www.cemach.org.uk/ Publications-Press-Releases/Report-Publications/Maternal-Mortality.aspx. British Guideline on the management of Asthma. *Thorax* 2008; **63**: 1–121.

1.3.6. Hypokalaemia and hyperkalaemia – Sarah F Bell

You are most likely to discuss plasma electrolyte disturbances as part of a blood result in a clinical structured oral examination or when looking at an ECG. You might also be asked to discuss your initial management of an abnormal electrolyte result.

Let's start with potassium. How is this ion regulated in the body?

This is a core topic that you should remember from the primary FRCA.

Potassium intake is approximately 50 to 150 mmol per day. Potassium is predominantly an intra-cellular ion, present in concentrations 20 to 30 times higher than in plasma. The plasma potassium concentration is 3.5 to 4.5 mmol/L. Acute regulation of plasma potassium levels is achieved by the actions of insulin which promotes uptake of potassium into cells.

Chronic regulation of plasma potassium levels is achieved by the kidney. Normally all of the filtered potassium is reabsorbed in the proximal tubule. Active secretion occurs in the distal tubule and collecting duct. Aldosterone acts on the sodium–potassium ATPase pump in the distal convoluted tubule to increase potassium excretion. Its release is stimulated by hyperkalaemia and via the renin–angiotensin pathway.

What are the causes of hypokalaemia?

Try and structure your answer whenever possible.

Hypokalaemia may be due to inter-compartmental shifts, increased potassium loss or reduced intake.

Inter-compartmental shifts may be due to alkalosis, insulin, β2 agonists and hypothermia; increased losses may be caused by diuretics, mineralocorticoids, renal tubular acidosis, keto-acidosis, ileal conduit, diarrhoea and vomiting, sweating and dialysis. Reduced intake may be due to lack of potassium in IV fluids or diet.

What are the ECG changes of hypokalaemia?

This question may be posed in the context of an abnormal ECG.

The ECG changes include T-wave flattening and inversion, U waves, ST depression a prolonged PR interval and increased QT interval. There may be progression to arrhythmias and possible asystole.

What are the effects of hypokalaemia?

A reduction in myocardial contractility can lead to heart failure. Generalised skeletal muscle weakness may be a feature, along with ileus and polyuria.

How can we treat hypokalaemia?

Treatment is aimed at replacement of potassium, which can be oral or intra-venous depending on the severity of the condition.

What are the anaesthetic implications of hypokalaemia?

Patients with hypokalaemia are at risk of developing arrhythmias. Elective operations should be cancelled if the potassium level is below 3.0 mmol/L. Emergency procedures may warrant more rapid correction with ECG monitoring in a high-dependency environment. The maximum rate of potassium administration via central venous access is 40 mmol/hr. Plasma levels would need to be closely monitored, and I would aim to achieve a level of 4.0 to 5.0 mmol/L. This is particularly important for patients taking digoxin due to an increased risk of toxicity if the level is below 4 mmol/L.

What are the causes of hyperkalaemia?

Again try and structure your answer!

They can be split into inter-compartmental shifts, reduced excretion and increased intake. Causes of inter-compartmental shifts include acidosis, rhabdomyolysis, trauma, malignant hyperthermia and suxamethonium use in patients with burns and spinal injury. Reduced excretion may be due to renal failure, adreno-cortical insufficiency and drugs such as ACE inhibitors or potassium sparing diuretics. Increased intake might be due to excessive IV potassium or as a consequence of a massive blood transfusion.

What are the ECG changes of hyperkalaemia?

The ECG changes include peaked T-waves, wide QRS and prolonged PR interval, which may progress to loss of P waves, ST depression, ventricular fibrillation and asystole. These changes are potentiated by hypocalcaemia, hyponatraemia and acidosis.

What are the effects of hyperkalaemia?

The patient may present with muscle weakness or gastrointestinal symptoms of nausea, vomiting and diarrhoea. Furthermore they may present with palpitations or cardiovascular collapse.

How can we treat hyperkalaemia?

A potassium level of 6.5 mmol/L or more or ECG changes consistent with hyperkalaemia require urgent treatment to avoid deterioration and cardiac arrest. Calcium chloride 10 ml of 10% iv will provide some cardiac protection by acting as a physiological antagonist to the potassium. A total of 15 U of insulin in 100 ml of 20% dextrose infusion given over 30 minutes, or a similar regimen, will drive the potassium into the cells and, therefore, reduce the plasma potassium level. Additional emergency treatment might include β2 agonists such as salbutamol, which will also move potassium into the intra-cellular space, and dialysis to remove potassium from the plasma. Less acute treatment of hyperkalaemia may include calcium resonium, orally or rectally.

What are the anaesthetic implications of hyperkalaemia?

Hyperkalaemia will predispose the patient to arrhythmias which may be fatal intra-operatively. It is therefore essential to treat symptomatic hyperkalaemia prior to induction of an anaesthetic, as I described earlier. Considerations during anaesthesia would then involve avoidance of suxamethonium (which would transiently increase the potassium level by 0.5 to 1 mmol/L and might be fatal). Acidosis and hypothermia would also worsen the hyperkalaemia by encouraging the shift of potassium from the intracellular space into the plasma. Controlled ventilation would allow potential correction of pH via optimisation of carbon dioxide levels. An arterial line would allow regular monitoring of electrolyte and acid–base status. Neuromuscular blockade may be prolonged and therefore should be monitored.

1.3.7. Hyponatraemia and hypernatraemia – Sarah F Bell

What are the causes of hypernatraemia?

Hypernatraemia is defined as a plasma sodium level of greater than 145 mmol/L. This may be due to sodium excess, water depletion or sodium deficiency with proportionally greater water loss. Causes of sodium excess include hyperaldosteronism, Cushing's disease and excessive administration of hypertonic saline. Water depletion may be due to nephrogenic diabetes insipidus, inadequate water intake and burns. Water depletion greater than sodium loss might be caused by renal diuresis secondary to osmotic diuretics (such as mannitol, glucose or urea).

How does hyperaldosteronism (Conn's disease) or Cushing's syndrome lead to hypernatraemia?

Excessive mineralocorticoid level leads to activation of aldosterone receptors in the distal convoluted tubule within the kidney. This causes increased sodium retention with potassium loss. Cushing's disease is caused by excess glucocorticoid secretion. These hormones can have a weak mineralocorticoid action causing similar effects.

What can you tell me about diabetes insipidus?

This question might form part of a clinical or physiology SOE.

Diabetes insipidus (DI) is due to impaired water resorption from the kidney. It may be cranial or nephrogenic in origin. Cranial DI is caused by reduced anti-diuretic hormone (ADH) secretion from the posterior pituitary and nephrogenic DI is due to impaired response of the kidney to ADH. Cranial DI may develop after a head injury or infection, pituitary tumour or autoimmune disease. Nephrogenic DI may be due to infection of the kidney, hypokalaemia or drugs such as lithium or democlocycline.

Investigations to confirm DI should reveal hypernatraemia with high plasma osmolality and low urine osmolality. A water deprivation test should confirm the diagnosis. A normal response to water deprivation would be an increase in urine osmolality but a patient with DI would have an abnormally dilute urine. In cranial DI, the administration of desmopressin (synthetic ADH) would cause an increase in urine osmolality, whereas with a nephrogenic DI no such response should occur.

The treatment would depend on finding the cause of the DI and attempting to correct this. Intra-venous hypotonic fluids and desmopressin might be required.

What other changes in sodium regulation might you observe after a head injury?

This question has the potential to get very confusing. Try and stick to basic physiology.

Both SIADH and cerebral salt wasting syndrome might occur. In both of these diseases the sodium level may fall. In SIADH the excess ADH would cause increased water reabsorption and a dilutional hyponatraemia with increased total body water. In cerebral salt wasting syndrome excessive sodium and water loss occur together.

Moving back to hypernatraemia, what are its effects?

The symptoms of hypernatraemia depend on the rate of increase and the plasma level reached. The patient may present with the signs and symptoms of dehydration (including thirst, nausea, tachycardia, hypotension, confusion and lethargy). Central nervous system effects may also include seizures, muscle spasms, hyperreflexia and possibly intra-cranial haemorrhage. The patient may be hyperthermic. Pre-renal failure can occur due to a fall in cardiac output.

How should hypernatraemia be treated?

The treatment of hypernatraemia depends on the cause. If water excess is suspected then diuretics would be appropriate. If water depletion is evident then rehydration with fluids containing minimal sodium would be required. If sodium depletion is the cause then treatment with 0.9% N saline is necessary. Patients suffering from diabetes insipidus might need desmopressin.

What are the anaesthetic implications of hypernatraemia?

Elective surgery should be postponed if the sodium level is above 155 mmol/L due to the potential effects of sodium changes in intra-cerebral fluid compartments. If the patient requires emergency surgery then a central line should be placed and cautious correction of the sodium level with regular checks should be commenced.

What are the causes of hyponatraemia?

Hyponatraemia is defined as a plasma sodium level below 135 mmol/L. This may be due to water excess, sodium redistribution, water excess disproportionate to sodium excess or water depletion with greater sodium deficiency.

Water excess may be further split into causes of excess administration of hypotonic IV fluids, drinking too much water or TURP syndrome; or reduced water excretion in the case of SIADH, drugs (such as oxytocin) or the normal physiological response to surgery.

Unbalanced sodium and water excess may be evident in patients with nephrotic syndrome, heart failure or hepatic failure.

Unbalanced sodium and water deficiency is predominantly due to renal compromise due to diuretics, renal tubular acidosis or hypoadrenalism; but it may also be due to diarrhoea and vomiting or pancreatitis. Finally, redistribution of sodium into the intracellular space may be found in patients with hyperglycaemia.

What are the effects of hyponatraemia?

The speed of onset will have some impact on the severity of the condition. Plasma sodium levels of 125–130 mmol/L tend to present with gastrointestinal upset whilst levels below 125 mmol/L lead to neurological symptoms of lethargy, headache, seizures, psychosis and coma. Respiratory depression and muscle weakness may also occur.

How should hyponatraemia be treated?

Management is aimed at treating the underlying cause and cautious correction of the hyponatraemia. This may include fluid restriction and diuretics. In cases of SIADH, democyclidine may offer some relief. The administration of hypertonic saline should be carefully considered due to risk of inadvertent over or rapid correction. Rapid correction of hyponatraemia may lead to central pontine myelinolysis.

What are the anaesthetic implications of hyponatraemia?

Severe hyponatraemia (i.e., less than 125 mmol/L) is a contraindication to elective procedures. In emergency cases severe hyponatraemia should be corrected cautiously with ECG monitoring and regular plasma levels to help guide resuscitation. Invasive arterial and central venous pressure monitoring may also be indicated and the patient nursed in a high-dependency unit or intensive care.

What can you tell me about trans-urethral resection of the prostate or TURP syndrome?

This is a surgical complication that you should be aware of. Try and explain the cause of the problem as this will indicate to the examiner that you really understand the condition.

TURP syndrome occurs in about 5% of operations of trans-urethral resection of the prostate (TURP). The resection of the vascular prostate tissue opens venous sinuses which allow absorption of hypotonic glycine 1.5% irrigation fluid into the systemic circulation. The volume of fluid absorbed depends on the duration of the procedure, hydrostatic pressure of the irrigation fluid (or height of the bag above the patient) and vascularity of the prostate.

What are the features of TURP syndrome?

There are three classical features of TURP syndrome: firstly a dilutional hyponatraemia, secondly fluid over-load and thirdly glycine toxicity.

The symptoms and signs of TURP syndrome are predominantly cardiovascular and neurological. Cardiovascular effects include tachycardia and hypertension followed by hypotension, angina and cardiovascular collapse. Neurological features include confusion, convulsions and coma. A regional anaesthetic technique with an awake patient potentially allows the anaesthetist to monitor the neurological features more closely (they would be masked by general anaesthesia).

How would you treat TURP syndrome?

Treatment involves recognition and resuscitation of the patient. Liason with the surgeon to terminate surgery as soon as possible is essential. Initial management would involve an airway, breathing and circulation approach with assessment and treatments occurring simultaneously. If the patient has airway compromise the airway will need to be secured with an endotracheal tube. Breathing complications such as pulmonary oedema may also necessitate intubation and controlled ventilation. Oxygen should be applied to the awake patient. Treatment of fluid over-load and hyponatraemia involves stopping IV fluids and commencing fluid restriction. Furosemide will promote a diuresis and is indicated if pulmonary oedema is present. Anti-arrhythmics and vasopressors may be needed to combat arrhythmias and hypotension. Hyponatraemia causing encephalopathy will require cautious correction of plasma sodium levels with fluid restriction and possibly hypertonic saline. Invasive patient monitoring should be considered. Due to the potential development of seizures and cerebral oedema, anti-convulsive therapy and measures to reduce raised intra-cranial pressure may be instituted.

Can you tell me more about hypertonic saline?

Hypertonic saline is indicated when several symptoms develop or serum sodium levels fall below 120 mmol/L. Ideally sodium levels should rise by 1 mmol/hr (and not more than 20 mmol over 48 hours). Once sodium levels reach 125 mmol/L or symptoms cease, hypertonic saline should be stopped. The patient will need to be closely monitored during this treatment. A suggested infusion regimen is 1 ml/kg/hr of 3% saline to produce a rise of 1–2 mmol/L per hour in a 70-kg male adult.

Further Reading

Porter M. Anaesthesia for transurethral resection of the prostate. *Update in Anaesthesia.* 2003; **16**(8); 21–26.

1.3.8. Hypothermia – Andrea C Binks

You are asked to assess a patient in recovery who has just had a right shoulder replacement. Their core temperature is 33°C.

What is hypothermia?

It is a fall in bodily core temperature to <35°C, and it can be classified into mild, moderate or severe. Mild <33–35°C and severe <28°C.

What are the physical mechanisms by which heat has been lost from the patient?

This question is testing your knowledge of basic science as well as its clinical application.

Heat loss may occur through radiation, convection, evaporation, and conduction, through respiration and through the influence of anaesthesia.

What is radiation?

Radiation is the transference of heat from a hot object to a cooler object. The extent of heat loss depends on the differential between the room temperature and the body temperature. Radiation accounts for 40 to 50% of heat loss during anaesthesia.

What is convection?

The air layer closest to the body is warmed by conduction. As the air temperature increases, the air rises and is carried away by convection currents. This accounts for about 30% of heat loss, but can be accentuated if the body is exposed to convection currents, for example laminar flow systems.

What is evaporation?

As the moisture on the body's surface evaporates, it loses the latent heat of vaporisation, and the body cools down. This accounts for 20–25% of heat loss. The process is accelerated if there is a large moist area exposed during surgery, for example major abdominal or major orthopaedic procedures.

What is conduction?

Conduction is a process by which heat is passed directly from a warm object to a cooler object by direct contact. During anaesthesia this accounts for only 3–5% of heat loss unless the body is touching an efficient heat conductor such as a metal table.

Can you describe how heat is lost through respiration?

During respiration, heat is lost through evaporation and by warming inspired air. This can account for up to 10% of heat loss. During anaesthesia this process can be minimised by use of heat and moisture exchangers.

Can you describe how general anaesthesia affects heat loss?

The normal responses to heat loss are both autonomically and behaviourally mediated. During general anaesthesia the patient will be unable to move to a warmer environment, exercise, shiver or put more clothes on.

The peripheral vasodilatation produced by anaesthetic agents results in heat redistribution from the warmer core to the cooler peripheries. Anaesthetic agents can also affect the hypothalamic core temperature regulatory centre. The hypothalamic threshold is related to minimal alveolar concentration (MAC), so thermoregulatory responses are not triggered until the temperature has fallen below the normal threshold. During anaesthesia, the patient has reduced metabolic heat production, as muscle activity and brain metabolism are both decreased. There is an additional cooling effect from the use of anaesthetic gases and intravenous fluids.

What are the physiological and clinical consequences of hypothermia?

Try and be systematic here.

The physiological effects of hypothermia principally affect the cardiorespiratory, haematological, neuromuscular, gastrointestinal, renal and metabolic systems.

Initially with mild hypothermia there may be a tachycardia, peripheral vasoconstriction and an increase in cardiac output. Further falls in temperature gives rise to a sinus bradycardia and characteristic ECG changes which include the appearance of a J-wave. Hypothermia also increases the risk of arrhythmias.

Mild hypothermia results in an initial tachypnoea followed by a reduction in minute volume and oxygen consumption.

The oxygen–haemoglobin dissociation curve may shift to the left, resulting in decreased oxygen delivery. Blood viscosity is increased; therefore, the risk of intra-vascular stasis is higher. The enzyme systems of the extrinsic and intrinsic coagulation pathways may be inhibited, resulting in the potential for a coagulopathy.

The metabolic effects are a decrease in metabolic rate of about 6% for every degree fall in core temperature. Enzyme reactions and intermediary metabolism are also affected if core temperature is less than 34°C. This may prolong drug action. This particularly applies to neuromuscular blocking agents.

The patient may have a diuresis due to an increased renal blood flow or the failure of renal tubular reabsorption of sodium and water. The gastrointestinal implications of hypothermia include impaired liver function, the development of an ileus and pancreatitis. The patient may develop hyperglycaemia from reduced insulin secretion and peripheral glucose utilisation.

The clinical complications of peri-operative hypothermia include: shivering in recovery leading to increased oxygen consumption and pain; greater blood loss in theatre and consequent need for blood transfusion; angina, myocardial infarction, ventricular tachycardia and cardiac arrest; increased incidence of wound infection; pressure sores and a prolonged stay in recovery.

How would you manage the patient in recovery?

Hypothermia of gradual onset is best managed with a slow re-warming process at about 1°C per hour. Heat can be applied to the patient using external or internal methods. The easiest method of re-warming is by using forced warm air heating blankets or radiant heaters. Alternatively the patient can be re-warmed by using warm intra-venous, intra-gastric or intra-peritoneal fluids, or by bladder irrigation via a urinary catheter.

The most efficient way of rewarming, but by far the most invasive, is to put the patient on cardiopulmonary bypass or other extracorporeal circuit.

Where have you seen hypothermia being used in a theatre setting?

The examiner is looking to see that you have had exposure to a wide range of anaesthetic specialties.

Hypothermia is used in cardiac surgery when the patient is put onto cardiopulmonary bypass. If hypothermia is used, the patient is typically cooled to a temperature of 28–32°C.

In more complex cardiac surgery, for example surgery on the aortic root, deep hypothermia is induced where the patient is cooled to a temperature of 15 to 22°C, which allows periods of low blood flow or circulatory arrest.

Do you know of any clinical applications of induced hypothermia?

This is asking for any trials you may be aware of in the recent literature.

Induced hypothermia has been proven to be beneficial for out of hospital cardiac arrest survivors. In patients with a return of spontaneous circulation, induced hypothermia has been shown to result in a more favourable neurological outcome than in patients given standard treatment. As a result, the International Liaison Committee on Resuscitation has recommended that all patients with a return of spontaneous circulation following an out of hospital cardiac arrest where the initial rhythm was VF should be treated with induced hypothermia of 32–34°C for 12 to 24 hours.

Are you aware of any other therapeutic uses of hypothermia?

There have been trials looking at therapeutic hypothermia in traumatic head injury, and although hypothermia is effective in reducing intra-cranial pressure and cerebral metabolic rate for oxygen ($CMRO_2$), there has been no outcome benefit shown. This is thought to be due to the increased incidence of infective complications.

Hypothermia has also been used in newborn hypoxic ischaemic encephalopathy, and although there was no benefit seen in those patients with the most abnormal EEGs, there did seem to be some protective effect in patients with intermediate EEG with no increase in complication rate.

Other areas where hypothermia has been trialed are in neurosurgery, in ischaemic stroke and in aortic surgery for spinal protection. Although preliminary studies have suggested some positive effects, no conclusive results have been achieved.

Further Reading

Jacobs S, Hunt R, Tarnow-Mordi W, Inder T, Davis P. Cooling for newborns with hypoxic ischaemic encephalopathy. *Cochrane Database of Systematic Reviews.* 2007; Issue 4. Art. No.: CD003311. DOI: 10.1002/14651858.CD003311.pub2.

Nolan JP, Morley PT, Vanden Hoek TL, et al. Therapeutic hypothermia after cardiac arrest: an advisory statement by the advanced life support task force of the International Liaison Committee on Resuscitation. *Circulation.* 2003; **108**: 118–121.

Sydenham E, Roberts I, Alderson P. Hypothermia for traumatic head injury. *Cochrane Database of Systematic Reviews.* 2009; Issue 2. Art. No.: CD001048. DOI: 10.1002/14651858.CD001048.pub4.

1.3.9. Hyperthermia – Ami Jones

You are called to the emergency department (ED) to assess a 35-year-old patient who has run a half marathon. He is drowsy and his temperature is 42°C. The ED registrar is concerned with the hyperthermia and thinks he needs high-dependency care.

What is hyperthermia?

Hyperthermia is defined as an acute condition that occurs when the body produces or absorbs more heat than it can dissipate.

What can cause hyperthermia?

Be general and brief.

Causes of hyperthermia can be environmental, drug related or related to a medical condition such as sepsis or an acute burn injury.

What form of hyperthermia is this patient suffering from?

This patient is suffering from environmental hyperthermia. This can range from mild heat exhaustion to the more extreme heat stroke. Heat stroke exists in two forms; classical heat stroke and exertional heat stroke. This patient is likely to be suffering from exertional heat stroke, which typically occurs acutely in young fit and healthy patients who have taken part in exercise during high ambient temperatures. Classical heat stroke occurs over several hours or days and tends to occur in the elderly and infirm when ambient temperatures are raised for several days.

How do you differentiate between heat exhaustion and heat stroke?

Heat stroke requires the presence of hyperpyrexia and neurological dysfunction. It typically involves temperatures of greater than $40°C$ and the patient is often confused or unconscious and can be hypotensive, suffer from cardiac dysrhythmias and even cardiorespiratory arrest.

If your diagnosis of heat stroke is correct in this patient, how would you manage him?

I would assess his airway, breathing and circulation; make an assessment of his conscious level and commence cooling of the patient. I would start by externally cooling the patient – place him in a cold environment if possible and begin surface cooling him with cold towels, ice packs and I could consider cold water immersion. As he is severely hyperthermic I could also use internal cooling methods such as cold intra-venous fluids, cold lavage of the stomach, peritoneum or bladder and intra-vascular cooling techniques such as haemofiltration or cardiopulmonary bypass.

Apart from cooling the patient are any other therapies that may be indicated?

Heat stroke patients are often intra-vascularly depleted and require fluid resuscitation guided by cardiovascular parameters and urine output. Cooling reduces heat-induced vasodilatation, and over-resuscitating with fluid can cause circulatory over-load, cardiac failure and pulmonary oedema, especially if the patient has pre-existing heart disease. The patient may therefore also require inotrope or vasopressor support.

What tests might you order on this patient?

If the cause of the hyperthermia is not clear, tests may be indicated to find an underlying cause. A full blood count, U&ES, liver function tests, creatine kinase and a coagulation screen should be taken as a baseline as well as thyroid function tests and a drug screen.

What is this patient at risk of if their temperature is not reduced in a timely manner?

Temperatures of more than 40°C can be destructive to the brain and ultimately progress to multi-organ failure and death. A response similar to that which occurs in the systemic inflammatory response syndrome occurs and can affect all organs within the body resulting in seizures, coma, dysrhythmias, hypotension, disseminated intra-vascular coagulation, rhabdomyolysis, hepatic failure and even cardiorespiratory arrest.

Your CT2 calls you to theatre as they are concerned that the patient on the operating table having an appendicectomy has a very high temperature. The oesophageal probe in situ is recording a temperature of 40°C. What is your differential diagnosis?

As with the other questions, divide these into patient factors, environmental factors etc...

Causes of a high temperature intra-operatively include patient-related, drug-related and environmental-related factors.

The patient is undergoing an appendicectomy so has a potential source of sepsis. Intra-abdominal abscesses can cause significant febrile response which often settles once source control is gained. The patient may also be suffering from sepsis from another source such as a pulmonary or urinary tract infection. Pulmonary embolus can also cause a febrile response. Hyperthyroidism, either pre-existing or acute undiagnosed, should also be considered, as should phaeochromocytoma.

Drug-related factors particular to anaesthetic agents include malignant hyperpyrexia associated with the inhalational anaesthetic drugs and suxamethonium. If the patient usually takes anti-psychotics they are also at risk of neuroleptic malignant syndrome. A febrile response can also occur in response to the administration of blood products or drugs such as N-acetylcysteine.

Environmental factors are those such as a very high ambient temperature, excessive warming by warm intra-venous fluids, air warming blankets or warming mattresses.

What further information would you require?

Think history, investigation and examination.

Further information that I would require would included an assessment of the patient's medical notes; from these I would be able to discover if there were any pre-morbid conditions of note or any current medications, transfusions or recreational drugs which may be implicated in the pyrexia. There may also be a family history of malignant hyperpyrexia recorded in the anaesthetic history or history of problems during previous anaesthetics, although I would hope that this would have been considered when choosing an appropriate mode of anaesthesia and indeed I would make a note of any potential drugs given during the anaesthetic which may have triggered a malignant hyperpyrexia.

I would want to determine the time frame within which the pyrexia has arisen. Examining the observations prior to coming to theatre may show a pre-existing pyrexia which may suggest a septic origin. If the pyrexia has developed de novo, I would want to ascertain how quickly it has risen intra-operatively. A temperature that has gradually increased over the course of 2 to 3 hours is likely to be of a very different origin than one that has increased by a number of degrees over a shorter time period.

I would review any blood tests that had been recorded prior to theatre as a leucocytosis or raised C-reactive protein.

I would also review the patient's vital signs as a tachycardia and high blood pressure would be more in keeping with a malignant hyperpyrexia rather than a sepsis. Further information may be gained from the patient's end-tidal carbon dioxide and inspired/expired oxygen levels as a patient suffering from malignant hyperpyrexia would be hypermetabolic and have an increased oxygen requirement and carbon dioxide production rate out of keeping with that which would be expected from a high temperature alone. Performing a full clinical examination of the patient may also allow me to elicit signs of sepsis or features consistent with a malignant hyperpyrexia such as muscle rigidity.

You have deduced that the most likely cause of the hyperthermia is malignant hyperpyrexia caused either by the suxamethonium or the volatile anaesthetic agent. Describe your initial management

This management is based on an AAGBI document, which should be a well-rehearsed drill.

I would cease all potential precipitant drugs and convert to a malignant hyperthermia "safe" technique. I would ask the surgeon to stop operating and inform him of my suspicions. I would then call for senior help and reassess the patient's airway, breathing and circulation. I would remove the patient from the anaesthetic breathing circuit and hyperventilate them with 100% oxygen and provide anaesthesia with an intra-venous agent such as propofol for the remainder of the operation. I would ask my anaesthetic assistant to prepare 2–3 mg/kg of dantrolene and have further boluses of 1 mg/kg ready. I would commence active cooling of the patient by administering cold intra-venous fluids, switching the warming blanket to a cool temperature and ask the surgeon to perform cold peritoneal lavage. I could also consider extracorporeal heat exchange.

I would insert an arterial line and send blood for gas analysis, potassium, haematocrit, platelet count, clotting and creatine kinase. I would also consider inserting a central venous line and a urinary catheter and perform dipstick urinalysis for myoglobinuria as well as sending a sample to the lab for formal analysis.

How would your management continue for the duration of the operation?

My management from this point would depend on the clinical situation. I would ask the surgeon to complete surgery as quickly as possible, calling in a senior surgeon if necessary. Hyperventilation with 100% oxygen and consideration of giving sodium bicarbonate would help to treat acidosis and hypoxaemia. I would treat hyperkalaemia with glucose and insulin, intra-venous calcium chloride and sodium bicarbonate if levels were dangerously high. If myoglobinaemia were detected I would consider forced alkaline diuresis aiming for a urine output of more than 3 ml/kg/hr, with a pH of greater than 7.0. I could consider giving mannitol to induce a diuresis, although I do not know of any evidence to show that this would improve outcome. I would treat disseminated intravascular coagulation with fresh frozen plasma, platelets and cryoprecipitate as indicated and treat cardiac dysrrhythmias with appropriate drugs such as magnesium, amiodarone and procainamide.

Where would you care for the patient post-operatively?

I would continue invasive monitoring of the patient in the intensive care unit and continue to cool to normothermia and treat evolving symptoms appropriately. Following recovery, the patient will need counselling and referral to the malignant hyperthermia unit at Leeds.

You are called to review a long-term patient on the ICU who is being weaned from a ventilator. He has spiked a temperature of 39.6°C. What are the physiological effects of pyrexia on this critically ill patient?

Be organised and work through systems methodically.

A fever on the ICU is defined as a temperature of greater than 38.3°C. An increase in body temperature has effects upon each system within the body. It increases both oxygen demand and expenditure of energy, approximately 10% for every 1°C increase. This can have a profound effect upon a critically ill patient who may already have insufficient oxygen supplies and will be in a catabolic state and already have high energy demands. The haemoglobin–oxygen dissociation curve shifts to the right which improves off-load of oxygen to the tissues. Cardiovascularly the patient is often tachycardic and can be hypotensive which may require fluid resuscitation and inotropic support.

What aspects of the patient's clinical history may be of importance when trying to determine the cause of the fever?

As the patient is a long-term patient any potential infection is likely be nosocomial in nature. I would want to ascertain how long any invasive lines, catheters or drains have been in situ and determine the duration of ventilation. The route of tracheal intubation is important as a patient who is nasally intubated is at more risk of sinus infections. I would also question the nursing staff regarding the presence of any purulent secretions from tracheal suction or discharge from drain or line sites or indeed any wounds. A history of prior haematological disease, recent foreign travel or prior infection with diseases such as tuberculosis would also be important to ascertain, as would the patient's current acute medical or surgical problems.

What aspects of the patient's clinical examination may give further information?

There may be crepitations or bronchial breathing audible on auscultation of the lungs or dullness to percussion consistent with pleural effusion. There may be a new heart murmur or other evidence of subacute bacterial endocarditis such as splinter haemorrhages or Janeway lesions. Examination of the skin may show evidence of septic emboli, cellulitis or fungal infection of skin folds.

A review of the patient's recent microbiology results may also herald clues as to potential infective pathogens and the trends of inflammatory markers such as C-reactive protein, procalcitonin and platelet count. A raised white cell count may also give an indication of an ongoing infective process.

How might you pharmacologically reduce their temperature?

Anti-pyretic agents such as paracetamol are often administered with good effect. NSAIDs also have an anti-pyretic effect, and although these drugs are also associated with renal dysfunction, they have been proven to lower body temperature, tachycardia and lactate accumulation in septic patients.

1.3.10. Thyroid disease and thyroid surgery – Helen L Jewitt

You are asked to assess a 65-year-old woman for a subtotal thyroidectomy. Describe your pre-operative assessment

To answer this question you should use the same approach as for the pre-operative assessment of any patient, namely by taking a full history, examining the patient and obtaining appropriate investigations.

Your specific priorities in this case are to elicit evidence of the patient's thyroid status and any evidence of airway compromise as a result of their thyroid disease.

I would begin by taking a history from the patient. In the history I would try to elicit symptoms of hypothyroidism such as lethargy and intolerance to cold, or hyperthyroidism such as agitation, intolerance to heat and weight loss. I would find out the reason for surgery and any medications prescribed for the thyroid problem. It is vitally important to establish any symptoms of airway compromise resulting from the thyroid pathology. This includes asking about shortness of breath, swallowing difficulties and noisy breathing. Exacerbation of symptoms of dyspnoea or stridor on lying flat is an important indicator of a potentially difficult airway.

In addition to these specific points I would take a full anaesthetic, medical and surgical history.

My examination would focus on eliciting signs suggestive of hypo- or hyperthyroidism. These may include bradycardia, coarse skin and hair and non-pitting oedema in hypothyroid patients and tachycardia, atrial fibrillation, tremor and eye involvement in patients with hyperthyroidism. I would perform a careful examination of the airway and neck to assess the size of any thyroid swelling, detect obvious deviation of the trachea and establish any retrosternal extension of the mass.

Appropriate investigations in this patient include blood tests: full blood count, urea and electrolytes, thyroid function tests and corrected calcium. A chest X-ray may show deviation of the trachea, and this can be further investigated with a thoracic inlet X-ray or ideally a computed tomography (CT) scan. The latter allows the precise localisation of tracheal narrowing. A pre-operative nasendoscopy is useful for two reasons. It gives some indication of the view of the larynx likely to be obtained during direct laryngoscopy and allows assessment of vocal cord function prior to surgery.

This lady has a large goitre with evidence of retrosternal extension. She is uncomfortably short of breath on lying flat. She is clinically and biochemically euthyroid. A CT scan of her thorax shows a marked deviation and narrowing of the trachea at the level of the upper sternum. Describe your options for the technique of induction of anaesthesia in this patient

There are no absolute right and wrong answers to a question like this but your answer should demonstrate that you are aware of the potential problems with the case and have given thought to how to avoid or address them.

This lady has clinical and radiological evidence of airway compromise due to her thyroid swelling. I anticipate her airway may be difficult both in terms of a potentially difficult view at laryngoscopy and also difficulty passing an endotracheal tube past the narrowing. I would keep the patient in a semi-supine position to minimise airway symptoms and ensure pre-oxygenation for 3 minutes. Potentially suitable techniques include an inhalational induction or awake fibre-optic intubation. Tracheostomy under local anaesthetic is an option but problems might be incurred from excessive bleeding from the vascular thyroid tissue.

In view of the fact that insertion of the fibre-optic scope into the narrowed airway may produce complete obstruction I would use an inhalational technique and intubate under deep inhalational anaesthesia. Topical local anaesthetic applied to the airway will help to reduce airway reflexes. A reinforced endotracheal tube is needed, ensuring that a range of sizes are available to pass beyond the tracheal narrowing. In the event of a failure to secure the airway after inhalational induction, ventilation may be possible via a rigid bronchoscope.

What are the other factors that need to be addressed with patients having thyroid surgery?

Careful eye protection should be used in patients with eye involvement since it may not be possible to close their eyes fully. The eyes should be taped and padded. There is the potential for significant blood loss and limited access to cannulae in the patient's forearms due to the extended position of the arms under the surgical drapes. A large bore cannula with an extension should be available to allow the rapid administration of fluid in the event of haemorrhage. The loss of blood can be reduced by a head-up position or induced hypotension. The surgeon may wish to use a peripheral nerve stimulator; therefore, neuromuscular blockade may affect the ability to test the function of the recurrent laryngeal nerves.

How would you extubate this patient?

I would extubate the patient sitting up, fully awake, having ensured adequate reversal of neuromuscular blockade. Some anaesthetists however prefer to extubate in a deep plane of anaesthesia.

You are called to the ward to see this patient 3 hours after her surgery. She is acutely distressed with oxygen saturations of 78%. How would you proceed?

I would approach this problem with an airway, breathing and circulation approach. Whilst making an initial rapid assessment of the situation I would administer 100% oxygen via a non-rebreathing mask. The potential problems I need to consider are bleeding causing a haematoma around the surgical site, laryngeal oedema and damage to the recurrent laryngeal nerves. The most likely cause is a haematoma and an urgent transfer back to theatre should be organised. The wound can be opened on the ward to relieve the pressure by the haematoma on the airway in severe cases. An unusual cause of post-operative airway compromise in patients with a long-standing goitre is tracheomalacia. These patients should be reintubated promptly and are likely to require further management with a tracheostomy.

What are the consequences of damage to the recurrent laryngeal nerves?

The recurrent laryngeal nerves can be affected by compression, ischaemia or direct injury at the time of surgery. The injury can be unilateral or bilateral, and partial or complete. The recurrent laryngeal nerve supplies all the intrinsic muscles of the larynx except cricothyroid. Complete transection of the nerve results in the vocal cord on the affected side adopting a partially abducted or "cadaveric" position. Partial nerve injury is potentially more worrying as the muscles controlling abduction of the cords are affected to a greater extent than the adductors and the cord lies in the midline. Bilateral partial nerve injury can therefore result in the vocal cords overlapping in the midline producing complete airway obstruction.

Name another major post-operative complication of thyroid surgery aside from airway complications

Inadvertent removal of parathyroid tissue at the time of thyroidectomy can produce hypocalcaemia. This manifests as muscle twitching, tingling around the mouth and tetany in extreme cases. Specific clinical signs can be elicited such as Trousseau's sign whereby carpopedal spasm is provoked by inflation of a cuff around the upper arm or Chvostek's sign where tapping over the course of the facial nerve produces twitching of the facial muscles. Corrected calcium levels should be checked routinely 12–24 hours after surgery and earlier if there is clinical suspicion of hypocalcaemia. Calcium supplementation can be oral in mild cases or intra-venous if the corrected calcium is less than 2 mmol/L. Appropriate intra-venous calcium supplementation is 10 ml of 10% calcium gluconate given over 3 to 5 minutes.

Further Reading

Malhotra S, Sodhi V. Anaesthesia for thyroid and parathyroid surgery.

Continuing Education in Anaesthesia, Critical Care & Pain. 2007; 7(2): 55–58.

1.3.11. Phaeochromocytoma – Caroline SG Janes

You are informed that a 40-year-old female patient is due to have a phaeochromocytoma surgically removed on your list next week. She is coming in to the pre-assessment clinic later this morning.

What is a phaeochromocytoma?

A phaeochromocytoma is a rare catecholamine-secreting tumour. It is usually found in the adrenal medulla and develops from chromaffin tissue, although it can develop in other areas within the sympathetic nervous system. The extra-adrenal tumours are mostly associated with the coeliac, renal, hypogastric, and inferior mesenteric ganglia and the organ of Zuckerkandl.

It is often known as the 10% tumour as approximately 10% are bilateral, 10% are malignant, 10% are familial and 10% occur in childhood. It may present at any age but usually affects people in their 40s and 50s. It is more common in females. Phaeochromocytomas form part of multiple endocrine neoplasia syndrome types IIA and IIB and can therefore be accompanied by medullary thyroid cancer and parathyroid adenoma. Tumours can secrete adrenaline, noradrenaline, dopamine or a combination of these catecholamines.

What are the presenting symptoms?

If you are unsure about the exact signs and symptoms think back to first principles and what happens during maximal sympathetic stimulation.

Persistent hypertension refractory to treatment is the most common presentation. Headache, palpitations, psychosis, panic attacks, nausea, sweating and pallor can also be the presenting complaints. Tachyarrhythmias are more likely if the tumour secretes adrenaline, whereas hypertension, vasoconstriction and ischaemia occur in noradrenaline-secreting tumours. However, some patients do not have an elevated resting blood pressure and up to 70% may also suffer from postural hypotension.

Glucose intolerance is a common feature due to increased glycogenolysis. Acute pulmonary oedema can also occur especially where β-blockade has been started. Prolonged secretion of catecholamines without treatment can result in dilated cardiomyopathy and left ventricular failure. The diagnosis should also be considered in pre-eclampsia, thyrotoxicosis and malignant hypertension.

How is it diagnosed?

A 24-hour urine collection should be tested for free catecholamine metabolites including vanillyl mandelic acid (VMA) and metanephrine. Metanephrine is the most accurate test as VMA can miss up to 20% of tumours. The levels of plasma catecholamines, adrenaline and noradrenaline can also be measured but often yield false negative results due to their short half-lives. A T2-weighted magnetic resonance imaging scan should then be carried out to locate the tumour, starting with the abdomen. MIGB, which is an amine precursor, is taken up by the tumour and can be used to locate tumours in abnormal sites with a 90% pick-up rate.

What are the anaesthetic considerations pre-operatively?

It is imperative that the patient is adequately prepared pre-operatively. This is best done in conjunction with an endocrinologist. Initially the patient should be prescribed an α-blocker. Traditionally phenoxybenzamine, a non-competitive, irreversible α-blocker, has been used. Phenoxybenzamine has a long half-life, allowing plasma volume re-expansion but causes hypertension and is associated with toxic megacolon. Prazocin is now more commonly used for α-blockade.

A β-blocker can then be introduced once α-blockade is complete. This is to avoid exacerbating hypertension and ventricular dysfunction secondary to antagonism of β2-mediated vasodilatation. Atenolol and labetalol are the two most commonly used. β-blockade helps to manage tachycardia, arrhythmias and angina symptoms. Calcium channel blockers are sometimes used and are thought to work by inhibiting noradrenaline-mediated calcium influx in smooth muscle. Magnesium is also used to help in the management of acute episodes.

Pre-operatively the patient's blood pressure should be well controlled and they should be asymptomatic. Twenty-four hour ambulatory blood pressure monitoring can be used to assess this. The aim should be a blood pressure below 140/90 and a heart rate below 100 bpm. Marked postural hypotension should be present with a compensatory tachycardia. The patient may need fluid replacement as the blockade takes place and the vasoconstriction subsides.

The patient is normally fit and well and has a mass on her right adrenal gland which was diagnosed 2 months ago. She is taking prazocin and atenolol which controls her symptoms. She reports occasional dizziness on standing. She has no allergies, and you have no concerns with her airway. Her blood pressure is 135/80, and her heart rate is 90 bpm.

How would you anaesthetise this patient?

The α- and β-blockade should be continued until the evening of surgery and premedication should be given on the morning of surgery – usually temazepam 20 mg. The aim of anaesthesia for phaeochromocytoma excision is to avoid excessive sympathetic stimulation, hypoxia and hypercarbia, by the careful use of drugs to counteract acute changes in the cardiovascular system which may arise.

In addition to the minimum standards of monitoring, invasive monitoring through both arterial and central lines should be obtained prior to induction and large bore intravenous access is mandatory. If available, use of the oesophageal Doppler probe can provide valuable information peri-operatively and help guide fluid therapy and inotropic support. A cardiostable induction and endotracheal intubation can then be carried out. Remifentanil is increasingly used both for induction and maintenance of anaesthesia for its haemodynamic stability. This can be used in combination with a volatile or total intravenous anaesthesia with propofol.

Large swings in blood pressure may occur in response to stimulation and in particular when handling the tumour itself. Anti-hypertensives, anti-arrhythmics, and vasodilators should therefore be readily available. Magnesium sulphate, GTN, phentolamine, sodium nitroprusside and prazosin can all been used for hypertension, and β-blockers can be used to treat tachycardia.

Pain relief depends on the site of surgery. If the tumour is located in the abdomen epidural analgesia should be used with local anaesthetic and opiates. If an epidural is not appropriate a synthetic opioid such as fentanyl, alfentanil or remifentanil should be used until the tumour is excised. Morphine can then be used into the post-operative period.

The patient should be kept warm throughout the operation by use of a fluid warmer and forced air heating. Following removal of the tumour intravenous fluid hydration and vasoconstrictors such as phenylephrine or inotropes may be necessary to maintain blood pressure.

How should the patient be managed post-operatively?

Patients should be nursed in a high-dependency or intensive therapy unit post-operatively with invasive monitoring. Blood glucose should be monitored as they are at risk of hypoglycaemia and often need a glucose infusion initially. Signs and symptoms of an addisonian crisis should be looked for and treated promptly. Elective steroid replacement should be considered especially if both adrenal glands have been resected. An unexpectedly low blood pressure would suggest hypoadrenalism.

How would you manage post-operative hypotension in this patient?

Hypotension post-excision of phaeochromocytoma is very common due to a combination of residual α- and β-blockade, a fall in circulating catecholamine levels, receptor downgrading, and a diminished blood volume. In about a half of cases the hypotension can persist for up to 3 days.

It should be treated with adequate fluid resuscitation and close monitoring, ideally on a high dependency unit. Intra-venous infusions of catecholamines may also be necessary.

How would you manage a patient who is diagnosed with a phaeochromocytoma during pregnancy?

There are two options for managing a pregnant patient with a phaeochromocytoma. The tumour can either be excised during the second trimester or a simultaneous caesarean section and tumour excision can be done in the third trimester. The overall mortality is about 17% and is highest with a normal vaginal delivery. Phenoxybenzamine and propranolol can be safely used during pregnancy for symptom control.

Further Reading

Pace N, Buttigieg M. Phaeochromocytoma.
  British Journal of Anaesthesia CEPD Reviews.
  2003; **3**(1): 20–23.

Gastrointestinal

1.4.1. Enteral and parenteral nutrition – Caroline SG Janes

Tell me about enteral nutrition

The best nutrition is obtained when food is chewed, swallowed and digested. Where possible the oral route for nutrition should always be used. However, when the oral route is considered unsafe then a food source can be delivered directly into the gastrointestinal system, this is termed enteral nutrition.

Enteral nutrition can be administered via a nasogastric or nasojejunal feeding tube or via a percutaneous gastric or jejunal feeding tube. The most commonly used route is the nasogastric route but it relies on adequate gastric emptying.

The nasojejunal route is less commonly used, as it often requires an endoscope for the feeding tube to be positioned correctly. It is thought to be advantageous in patients with severe pancreatitis and some suggest that it may decrease the incidence of nosocomial pneumonia.

Percutaneous enteral feeding tubes are useful when enteral feeding is likely to be required long-term and the ability to protect the airway from regurgitation is impaired, for example in patients with cerebral palsy, head injury or major maxillo-facial surgery. It has the advantage of avoiding the discomfort of a nasogastric tube.

Successful enteral feeding requires the use of feeding protocols. These will vary from centre to centre but in general most protocols insist on a gastric residual volume of less than 200 ml following a 4-hour period of continuous feeding. If the volume is greater than 200 ml prokinetics are often indicated to aid gut motility.

Feeding via the enteral route has benefits beyond the supply of nutrition alone, playing a role in maintenance of gut integrity and protecting against bacterial translocation across the gut wall.

What different types of enteral feeds are available?

The majority of enteral feeds are polymeric and contain 1 kCal/ml. Special feeds are available which are fibre-enriched such as Jevity Plus™. Nepro™ is available for renal patients who are fluid restricted as it contains 2 kCal/ml. Elemental feeds are available for patients with gastrointestinal problems such as short bowel syndrome and pancreatitis. Pulmocare™

Dr. Podcast Scripts for the Final FRCA, ed. Rebecca A. Leslie, Emily K. Johnson,
Gary Thomas and Alexander P. L. Goodwin.   Published by Cambridge University Press.

contains a higher proportion of protein and fat and less carbohydrate and can be beneficial in patients with carbon dioxide retention as its use results in a reduction in the amount of carbon dioxide produced.

What are the complications of enteral feeding?

Enteral feeding can be impeded by a number of problems.

Mechanical problems include:

- The lumen of the feeding tube can become obstructed or displaced
- The tube can cause discomfort
- The tube can cause ulceration.

Metabolic problems include:

- Dehydration or overhydration.
- Hyperglycaemia; blood glucose should be monitored and an insulin sliding scale started where appropriate.
- Hypercapnia; ventilation may need to be increased if the carbon dioxide is seen to rise, especially in feeds with a high carbohydrate load.
- Electrolyte imbalance; particularly in patients who have been without a food source for a prolonged period, in extreme cases re-feeding syndrome may occur and should be treated aggressively.

Gastrointestinal complications include:

- Gastric retention/stasis; prokinetics can be helpful
- Nausea
- Vomiting
- Diarrhoea; high-fibre feeds can be beneficial
- Bloating
- Gastro-oesophageal reflux occurs more commonly with a nasogastric tube and can lead to aspiration and pneumonia.

Alternative causes for the above symptoms should be sought prior to attributing them to the feed. In particular, patients with diarrhoea should be screened for *Clostridium difficile*.

What prokinetics can be used in critical care to improve enteral nutrition?

Metoclopramide and erythromycin are the most commonly used prokinetics in critical care units.

Metoclopramide works by improving gastric emptying but has no effect on prevention of pneumonia or mortality.

Erythromycin improves short-term tolerance of enteral nutrition and reduces gastric residual volumes but its use is limited by concerns over development of antibiotic resistance.

Neostigmine is occasionally used to improve tolerance of enteral feeding but is not licensed for this use.

Tell me about total parenteral nutrition?

The use of total parenteral nutrition (TPN) is generally reserved for those patients in whom enteral feeding is unlikely to be established for at least 7 days or those patients who are intolerant to enteral feeding.

TPN is usually formulated as a lipid emulsion and contains medium-branched amino acids. The nutrient solution consists of water and electrolytes, glucose, amino acids and lipids. Essential vitamins, minerals and trace elements are added or given separately. TPN is hyperosmolar and irritant to veins and is therefore usually given through a central vein via a continuous infusion although some formulations do exist that can be administered via the peripheral route. It is imperative to check electrolytes daily and the levels of trace elements should be adjusted accordingly. This is especially important where the patient is at high risk of re-feeding syndrome (see later).

Patients receiving TPN are at high risk of line infection – meticulous asepsis is therefore required when connecting and disconnecting feeds and the infusion line should only be broken when absolutely necessary. A lumen dedicated to TPN should be allocated on insertion of the central line and used exclusively for TPN throughout. In recent years 24-hourly bags of TPN have been introduced to keep disconnections to a minimum. In some circumstances it may be appropriate to administer TPN and enteral feeds simultaneously – in these special cases it is essential to have the input of a dietician.

What is re-feeding syndrome?

Re-feeding syndrome consists of a number of metabolic disturbances that occur as a result of reinstitution of nutrition to a patient who has been starved or severely malnourished for a prolonged period. It usually occurs within 4 days of starting feeding and is characterised by hypophosphataemia accompanied by a multitude of life-threatening complications such as cardiac and respiratory failure, coma, seizures, rhabdomyolysis and haematological dysfunction.

The underlying cause is a shift from fat to carbohydrate metabolism. This results in a sudden increase in insulin levels which in turn increase cellular uptake of phosphate causing a precipitous fall in extracellular phosphate. Levels of potassium, magnesium, glucose and thiamine also fall. The shifting of electrolytes and abnormal fluid balance increases cardiac workload and heart rate which may cause acute heart failure. Oxygen consumption is also increased. It can be fatal if it is not recognized and treated properly. Electrolyte levels should be checked daily until they are stable. Treatment includes starting feeds slowly and aggressive correction of electrolyte deficiency via the intravenous route. In those thought to be at risk thiamine supplements should be prescribed.

What are immune-enhancing dietary supplements?

The dietary supplementation of glutamine, arginine, fish oils and antioxidants such as vitamin C and E together with selenium has been the focus of much research in the last decade. Unfortunately, the exact role of this immunonutrition is inconclusive and randomised clinical trials of immune-enhanced feeds have failed to show a clear benefit in critically ill patients. Glutamine seems to have the largest body of evidence behind it and benefits have been shown in certain circumstances. Arginine has been shown to be beneficial in cancer patients but may be harmful in the critically ill as increasing arginine levels leads to an increase in nitric oxide production. Its use is therefore not recommended on critical care. Fish oils, such as omega-3 fatty acids, have limited evidence to suggest a survival benefit in acute lung injury but more research is needed. Selenium is the most promising anti-oxidant to have been studied but again more research is needed to confirm benefits in critically ill patients.

Tell me more about glutamine supplementation?

Glutamine is the most abundant non-essential amino acid, it is synthesised and stored in skeletal muscle. It has a central role in nitrogen transport, ureagenesis, ammoniagenesis and regulation of acid–base. It is the sole fuel for lymphocytes, hepatocytes and gut mucosa. In catabolic disease states, as are commonly seen on critical care, glutamine becomes an essential amino acid and patients with severe trauma, sepsis, major surgery and chemo- or radiotherapy often have low levels of glutamine. This can lead to a reduced capacity of immune cells to proliferate and hence impaired immune function.

Evidence so far suggests some theoretical benefits of glutamine administration. Notably, it is thought to improve nitrogen balance and preserve glutamine levels in skeletal muscle, improve immune cell function and cytokine production and protects against bacterial gut translocation. However, so far the effects on nutrition and the immune system have not been translated into fewer infective complications and decreased mortality and strong evidence for any effect on hospital stay or long-term survival is still lacking. The evidence for its use is strongest in burns and trauma patients and those undergoing gastrointestinal surgery. There are conflicting data in its usefulness in septic patients.

Overall the use of glutamine in certain patient groups on critical care seems promising but requires more research. In addition the safety of long-term glutamine administration requires further investigation and an optimal dose has yet to be defined.

What special considerations are there for feeding patients with liver failure, renal failure and pancreatitis?

Patients with liver failure may have marked pre-existing electrolyte abnormalities and may have been on fluid restricted diets to minimise ascites formation. Potassium, magnesium and zinc losses are common in these patients, and they may have profound hyponatraemia despite having high total body sodium concentrations. Plasma sodium levels should be corrected slowly to avoid the risk of central pontine myelinolysis. In patients who have developed encephalopathy feeds with increased branched chain amino acids and reduced sulphur containing amino acids should be administered. These limit further accumulation of ammonia, which is responsible for the encephalopathy.

In patients with renal failure the feeding regimen will need to be tailored to the type of renal replacement therapy being received. In fluid restricted patients low volume/low sodium feeds should be used. In patients with chronic renal failure nitrogen intake will need to be reduced to between 0.5 and 0.8 g N_2/kg/day. In patients on peritoneal dialysis glucose levels should be monitored as the dialysis fluid usually contains glucose.

Feeding regimens in acute pancreatitis have been much debated, it was traditionally thought that TPN should be used and the pancreas should be rested but more recent evidence suggests that this may not be associated with improved outcomes. Post-pyloric feeding has been advocated but it has been shown to stimulate pancreatic enzyme synthesis and secretion as much as gastric feeding. However, some studies suggest that resting the bowel may exacerbate the inflammatory response and worsen the catabolic process of pancreatitis thus increasing protein deficiency. There is therefore increasing support for enteral, polymeric feeding in severe, acute pancreatitis.

Further Reading

Campbell Edmondson W. Nutritional support in critical care: an update. *Continuing Education in Anaesthesia, Critical Care & Pain.* 2007; 7(6): 199–202.

1.4.2. Nutritional requirements and malnutrition – Caroline SG Janes

What is the prevalence of malnutrition?

Malnutrition is the condition that develops when the body does not get the right amount of the vitamins, minerals, and other nutrients it needs to maintain healthy tissues and organ function.

Malnutrition in the developed world is unexpectedly high. Ten per cent of patients at home with cancer or chronic diseases are malnourished. This figure rises to between 30 and 60% for hospital in-patients where in up to a quarter of cases it is severe. In most cases malnutrition progressively worsens during hospitalisation, medical staff must therefore know how to recognize and treat it promptly.

Which patients are most at risk of malnutrition?

The elderly, patients with respiratory disease, inflammatory bowel disease and malignancy are most at risk of chronic malnutrition. In the acute setting, trauma patients and patients with sepsis are at a high risk of malnutrition. Various factors can cause malnutrition; a reduced appetite due to generalised malaise or nausea and impaired gut motility, absorption and digestion of food. Increased protein losses from wounds, for example from fistulae, may also contribute.

How can nutritional status be assessed?

Nutritional status is a multi-dimensional phenomenon that requires several methods of assessment as there are no tests that have both a high specificity and sensitivity.

Anthropometric measures are most commonly used, as they are non-invasive and easy to obtain in mobile patients. (This refers to the study of human body measurement for use in anthropological classification and comparison. The use of such data as skull dimensions and body proportions in the attempt to classify human beings into racial, ethnic and national groups has been largely discredited, but anthropometric techniques are still used in physical anthropology and paleoanthropology, especially to study evolutionary change in fossil hominid remains.)

Height and weight measurements are used to calculate body mass index providing an amount in kg/m^2. A normal BMI is considered to be between 18.5 and 25. Other anthropometric measures such as mid-arm circumference and thickness of subcutaneous skin folds can also be used to estimate fat and muscle mass.

The general appearance of the patient can also help in assessing adequate nutrition.

Muscle function tests such as hand grip dynamometry and respiratory muscle strength can also be used.

Anthropometric measurements are rarely useful in critically ill patients as it is difficult to weigh a patient with poor mobility. In addition low-protein states are common and lead to oedema and water retention causing measurements to be misleading.

Biochemical markers are often used to assess nutritional status but can also be misleading. The most commonly used measure of protein nutritional status in critically ill patients is the serum level of albumin. Other biochemical markers linked to nutritional status include pre-albumin, haemoglobin, transferrin, complement, serum folate, magnesium and phosphorus.

Low levels of albumin in critically ill patients are likely to reflect prolonged physiological stress as well as nutritional status. Therefore, many advocate that albumin should be pre-dominantly considered an indicator of severity of illness rather than an indicator of protein nutritional status. Decreases in the concentration of pre-albumin are mediated by the same mechanism as albumin. However, pre-albumin has a half-life of 5 days and is thus a more immediate indicator of physiological stress and nutrition during hospitalisation than albumin. There may therefore be a role for routine monitoring of pre-albumin.

How can the adequacy of nutritional intake be assessed on critical care?

Nutritional adequacy on intensive care is difficult to assess. One method uses the energy intake, which is usually taken as the kilocalories received on the basis of the feeding regimen prescribed divided by the resting energy expenditure. The latter is best measured by indirect calorimetry in critically ill patients whereby oxygen consumption and carbon dioxide production are measured directly and the values used in a standard equation to yield energy expenditure in kilocalories.

Why is nutrition important in critical care?

Malnutrition in critically ill patients is associated with increased morbidity and mortality. In patients receiving mechanical ventilation it has an adverse effect on all physiological processes. It increases the risk of infection and pulmonary oedema, decreases phosphorus levels needed for cellular energy production, reduces ventilatory drive, and impairs production of surfactant. Patients who are under-nourished are prone to the complications of a prolonged and difficult course of weaning because of muscle fatigue caused by diaphragmatic and skeletal muscle weakness. Randomised control trials show that length of stay is reduced if a source of nutrition is established in critically ill patients. There is also evidence of poorer outcomes in critically ill patients who have limited nutritional reserves prior to admission. Conversely, some studies have shown that both enteral and parenteral feeding have been associated with decreased survival in patients with adult respiratory failure or multi-organ system failure with sepsis but has not been proven.

Overall, however, it is well accepted that nutritional support is a vital part of patient management in critical care units.

What are the nutritional requirements of critically ill patients?

An average adult weighing 70 kg requires about 2000 kCal per day. However, the nutritional requirements of critically ill patients vary widely and are difficult to estimate. This group of patients usually have an increased basal metabolic rate but are often sedated, immobile and ventilated. The requirements are usually worked out using a variety of guidelines and formulae that take into account multiple factors including age, sex and body size as well as disease state and mechanical ventilation. Specialised formulae exist for trauma and burns patients. An early referral to a dietician with critical care experience is vital in managing patients on critical care. Feeding regimens should be reviewed and adapted on a daily basis.

What happens to the basal metabolic rate in major surgery, burns or trauma?

Following major trauma, burns and major surgery a hypermetabolic response to the injury occurs and energy requirements can initially increase by up to 30%. This results in a loss of lean body mass, a compromised immune system, delayed wound healing and loss of muscle strength. Resistance to insulin can develop, causing deranged blood sugar control. There are massive fluid shifts due to loss of fluid and electrolytes caused by diarrhoea, vomiting, naso-gastric drainage and stoma losses, leaky membranes and third space losses. Catecholamine and cortisol levels are also altered further affecting metabolism.

1.4.3. Nausea and vomiting – Alison J Brewer

We are going to talk about nausea and vomiting. Can you tell me which groups of patients are more likely to suffer from this complication?

There are patient factors, surgical factors, anaesthetic and disease factors.
   Patient factors include:

- It is increased in females who carry a two to four times increase in risk over that in males.
- Vomiting is higher during and after menstruation (during the luteal phase), and decreased after the menopause.
- It is generally more common in pregnancy, especially the first trimester.
- It may be greater in obese subjects.
- It is increased in younger patients.
- It is increased in patients who mobilise and eat and drink early.
- Smoking decreases the incidence of nausea and vomiting in patients.
- A past history of post-operative nausea and vomiting (PONV) or motion sickness increases the risk.

Surgical factors include:

- Site of surgery influences risk of PONV. Increased risk includes middle ear, intracranial, squint, intra-abdominal and gynaecological surgery.
- If surgery is prolonged or particularly painful this can also contribute.

What about anaesthetic factors and disease factors?

Anaesthetic factors include:

- Use of emetic drugs such as nitrous oxide, opioids and sympathomimetics and inhalational agents.

- Prolonged anaesthesia.
- Spinal anaesthesia and the associated hypotension also increase the risk.
- Dehydration increases risk.
- Gastric dilation increases the likelihood of nausea and vomiting.

Diseases factors include:
- Problems such as intestinal obstruction increase the probability of vomiting.
- Hypoglycaemia.
- Hypoxia.
- Uraemia.

So what things can we do to prevent post-operative nausea and vomiting?

There is a lot to cover here so classify as pre-, intra- and post-operatively.

Pre-operatively it is important to address dehydration and correct this. Any anxiety should also be allayed at this point.

Intra-operatively patients at high risk should have an anaesthetic that minimises the risk of nausea and vomiting. They should have propofol as an induction agent and nitrous oxide should be avoided. A total intra-venous anaesthetic technique should be considered. The use of neostigmine should be kept to a minimum, as should sympathomimetics. Pain should be avoided by using opiate sparing techniques. I would use paracetamol, diclofenac and local anaesthetic techniques in preference to opiates. The length of surgery should be kept to a minimum and anti-emetics should be used prophylactically.

What are the commonly used drugs that can be used to prevent post-operative nausea and vomiting?

In our hospital the commonly used drugs are cyclizine, ondansetron and dexamethasone.

More widely, the classes of drugs used to treat nausea and vomiting are:
- Anti-histamines
- Anti-muscarinics
- Anti-dopaminergics
- Anti-serotoninergics
- Cannabinoids
- Corticosteroids.

They can be classified by site of action.

Would you like to do that for me then?

Peripherally there are visceral afferents in the bowel wall and myenteric plexus and these are mediated by serotonin (5HT3), where drugs such as ondansetron and granisetron work. These afferents relay to the chemoreceptor trigger zone (CTZ). The CTZ, in the medulla in the area postrema on the floor of the fourth ventricle lies outside the blood–brain barrier and receives afferents from the vestibular apparatus and certain drugs such as opiates, volatiles and sympathomimetic drugs. Dopamine receptor antagonists act here to stimulate the CTZ. NK-1 receptors are also abundant at this site.

There is a vestibular input to the vomiting centre and anti-cholinergic drugs (such as hyoscine) and anti-histamine drugs (such as cyclizine) act here. The vomiting centre is the site of central integration and lies in the reticular formation in the medulla oblongata. It receives afferents from the CTZ, gut and the cerebral cortex. This area contains muscarinic and histamine receptors; therefore, drugs which act at the vestibular apparatus also work here.

Some drugs do not have a defined site of action. These include propofol, whose anti-emetic actions are thought to be due to action on the CTZ. Corticosteroids, such as dexamethasone, have an unknown site of action, but it may be due to a reduced turnover of 5HT3, or a decreased permeability of the blood–brain barrier. Cannabinoids, such as nabilone, are thought to act at the CTZ, but receptors CB-1 and CB-2 have been found and it may exert the anti-emetic effects via these sites.

You mentioned that the chemoreceptor trigger zone is outside the blood–brain barrier, is there any benefit to this location?

Yes. This is so that the area can be directly exposed to blood-borne chemicals and response to these is not delayed.

Can you tell me which anti-emetics you would use and why?

We have a protocol in our department which grades people as low, moderate or high risk for nausea and vomiting. In low-risk patients no anti-emetics are used; for moderate risk, cyclizine 50 mg at induction is given and avoidance of emetic drugs and procedures. In high-risk patients, multi-modal therapy is used with ondansetron 4 mg and cyclizine 50 mg being given, with consideration to using dexamethasone 8 mg. Other techniques, such as using TIVA and regional techniques are also used.

Can you tell me the side effects of these drugs?

Anti-muscarinic drugs have an anti-sialogogue effect so dry mouth and eyes are common. They also cause sedation, amnesia and can precipitate a central anti-cholinergic syndrome. Glycopyrrolate is the only drug that does not cause these central side effects as it is a quaternary structure and does not cross the blood–brain barrier.

Anti-histamines can have an anti-cholinergic effect and cause tachycardia post-injection.

Anti-dopaminergic drugs can cause dystonic and extra-pyramidal effects. They can rarely precipitate the neuroleptic malignant syndrome.

What about the other drugs such as corticosteroids and cannabinoids?

Corticosteroids have little side effects in one-off use but can cause steroid psychosis and metabolic disturbances such as fluid retention, hypokalaemia and hyperglycaemia. Cannabinoids cause sedation and psychosis, and the use is limited to chemotherapy patients in view of the side effects.

Why is a combination of drugs used?

This improves the efficacy of the drugs over monotherapy as the cause of nausea and vomiting is likely to be multifactorial and using drugs that act at different sites is likely to have the best outcome. The number needed to treat is about five in the best multi-modal therapy. However this does vary according to the underlying rate of post-operative nausea and vomiting in the patient and surgical risk group. For example the number needed to treat to prevent PONV in gynaecological surgery is much lower than in general surgery.

What is number needed to treat?

This is the number of patients that need to be treated to have a reduction in symptoms. It gives an indication as to the size of the treatment effect and is calculated by 1/absolute risk reduction.

Do you know of any other non-pharmacological ways of reducing nausea and vomiting?

Ginger is thought to help with nausea and vomiting, as is hypnotherapy. Acupuncture at the P6 point distal to the wrist crease between the flexor carpi radialis and palmaris longus tendons reduces the incidence of vomiting.

What are the sequence of events that occurs to allow vomiting?

Vomiting is the retrograde passage of gastric contents through the mouth. In order for this to happen the body must undergo a sequence of events to prevent aspiration from happening. The afferent limb of the reflex of vomiting is coordinated in the vomiting centre. The efferent limb has motor output via the cranial nerves to the upper GI tract and through the spinal nerves to the diaphragm and abdominal muscles. A sensation of nausea is experienced followed by sympathetic activity, such as hyperventilation, sweating, peripheral vasoconstriction and tachycardia. Salivation is as a result of parasympathetic activity. The glottis closes and the breath is held in mid-inspiration. Vagal impulses cause a relaxation of the proximal stomach and then a retrograde giant contraction causing small bowel contents to be forced into the stomach. Expulsion is preceded by retching in many cases, and the oesophageal sphincters and diaphragm relax allowing the gastric contents to be expelled.

Why do we want to reduce the incidence of nausea and vomiting in patients?

Nausea and vomiting is the most common side effect of anaesthesia and surgery and causes considerable patient morbidity. The patient is at risk of aspiration, especially if drowsy post-surgery. They are also at risk of dehydration and electrolyte imbalance. The act of vomiting increases the intra-cranial and intra-ocular pressure as well as worsening pain and increasing the risk of wound dehiscence and herniation.

Tell me about the electrolyte imbalances?

In vomiting the gastric content is lost and this contains hydrogen, potassium, and sodium ions and water.

So what happens to compensate for this loss?

There is renal compensation to restore the pH. To compensate for the volume loss there is aldosterone release, in response to the sodium and extracellular fluid depletion, to cause sodium and water retention in exchange for potassium and hydrogen ions. A metabolic alkalosis develops in vomiting.

1.4.4. Oesophageal reflux – Michael B Clarke

Describe the anatomy of the oesophagus

The oesophagus is a muscular tube connecting the pharynx to the stomach. The upper third of the oesophagus consists of an outer longitudinal and an inner circular layer of striated muscle. The lower two thirds consist of smooth muscle. The inner lumen consists of stratified squamous epithelium.

There are two oesophageal sphincters: the cricopharyngeus muscle acts as the functional upper oesophageal sphincter. It has a high resting intra-luminal pressure (6.7–13.3.kPa). The lower oesophageal sphincter is a functional entity rather than an anatomical one. It results from thickened, tonically contracted smooth muscle at the lowest 2–4 cm of the oesophagus. It has a resting pressure 2–3.3 kPa above the gastric pressure, which prevents gastro-oesophageal reflux.

What is the "barrier pressure" and what is its significance?

Barrier pressure is the lower oesophageal sphincter pressure minus the intra-gastric pressure. The significance is that the lower oesophageal sphincter pressure is reduced by pregnancy and drugs such as atropine and suxamethonium and that the intra-gastric pressure is increased in the fed state. When one encroaches on the other, barrier pressure fails and reflux is possible.

Describe the anatomy of the stomach

Functionally, the stomach is made up of the fundus, the body and the antrum. The wall of the stomach consists of four layers: serous, muscular, submucous and mucous. There are three layers of visceral muscle fibres: longitudinal, circular and oblique. Each muscle layer forms a syncytium acting as a unit. Between the stomach and the duodenum is the pyloric sphincter, a junction formed by thickened circular smooth muscle.

The stomach has an intrinsic and extrinsic nerve supply. The extrinsic nerve supply is from the sympathetic and parasympathetic nervous systems. The sympathetic supply (via the coeliac plexus) inhibits motility. The parasympathetic supply (via the vagus nerve) stimulates motility.

The intrinsic nerve supply is responsible for peristalsis and is formed by the Meissner's plexus which is submucosal, and the Auerbach's plexus which lies between the circular and longitudinal muscle layers of the stomach.

How is gastric emptying normally controlled and what are the causes of delayed gastric emptying?

As always with this sort of question a classification will aid your answer and impress the examiner.

The physical state and chemical composition of a substance affects the speed at which it is emptied from the stomach. Liquids empty more rapidly than solids. The rate of emptying of solids depends on the rate at which chyme is broken down into small particles. Increased gastric volume produces distension which provokes vagal reflexes leading to increased gastric emptying. Both gastric distension and high protein content of food stimulate gastrin secretion which enhances gastric emptying. Nutrients in the duodenum activate chemoreceptors which inhibit gastric emptying, allowing time for further digestion and absorption in the small intestine. Hypertonicity, fatty acids and hydrogen ions activate the secretion of cholecystokinin, secretin and gastric inhibitory peptide, which inhibit gastric emptying

Many factors cause delayed gastric emptying and can be classified as physiological, pathological and pharmacological.

Physiological:

- Pain
- Anxiety
- Pregnancy
- Obesity
- Advanced age.

Pathological:

- Gastrointestinal obstruction
- Electrolyte abnormality, e.g. hypercalcaemia, renal failure
- Diabetes
- Gastritis
- Raised intra-cranial pressure
- Migraine.

Pharmacological:

- Opioids
- Anti-cholinergics
- Sympathomimetics
- Dopaminergics
- Alcohol.

What is gastric acid, and what stimulates its production?

To help you answer the second part of this question a simple diagram of a parietal cell including the three main receptors and the hydrogen ion pump will impress the examiner and will aid you if a further question about drug actions is asked (Figure 1.4.4a,b).

Gastric secretions include hydrochloric acid, pepsin, gastrin, mucus and intrinsic factor. The parietal cells secrete hydrochloric acid and intrinsic factor. These cells are located in the body and fundus of the stomach. A pH of 1–1.5 is needed for optimal pepsin activity as well as providing a degree of anti-microbial activity. Pepsin initiates protein digestion. Intrinsic factor is necessary for vitamin B12 absorption in the terminal ileum and mucus is essential for protection of the mucosal cells.

The three most important factors that act on the parietal cell to stimulate hydrochloric acid production are histamine (via H2 receptors), acetylcholine (via M1 muscarinic receptors) and gastrin (via gastrin receptors). These receptors are located on the basolateral

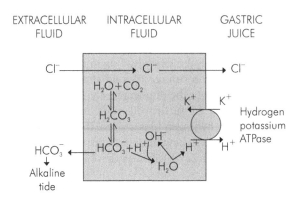

Figure 1.4.4a. Acid production in parietal cells. Reproduced with permission from Smith, T., Pinnock, C. and Lin, T. 2009. *Fundamentals of Anaesthesia.* Cambridge: Cambridge University Press. © Cambridge University Press 2009.

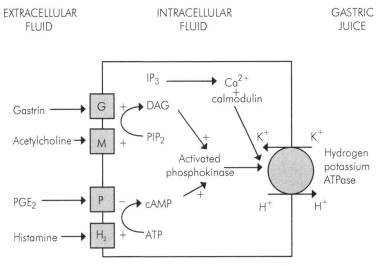

Figure 1.4.4b. Modulators of gastric acid production. Reproduced with permission from Smith, T., Pinnock, C. and Lin, T. 2009. *Fundamentals of Anaesthesia.* Cambridge: Cambridge University Press. © Cambridge University Press 2009.

membrane of the parietal cell. The apical membrane contains an ATP-dependent hydrogen ion pump (Figure 1.4.4.a).

The three receptors on the basolateral membrane utilise second messenger systems. Acetylcholine and gastrin increase intra-cellular concentrations of calcium via inositol triphosphate activation. The histamine receptors activate adenyl cyclase via G-stimulatory proteins. This results in an increase in cyclic AMP levels. Increased calcium and cyclic AMP causes activation of specific protein kinases which increase the activity of the hydrogen ion pump.

Hydrogen ions are produced by the reaction of carbon dioxide with water under the influence of carbonic anhydrase. The hydrogen ions are then actively transported into the lumen by the hydrogen–potassium ATP-dependent pump. Bicarbonate ions pass across the basolateral membrane in exchange for chloride ions via an anti-port mechanism.

PGE_2 inhibits the production of gastric acid. It has a protective function, stimulating the production of mucous and bicarbonate.

Physiological control of gastric acid production may be considered in terms of cephalic, gastric and intestinal factors.

Cephalic factors, such as anticipation, sight, smell and taste, are mediated via the vagus. This occurs before food ingestion and can be responsible for up to 50% of gastric acid production.

The gastric phase is initiated by the entry of food into the stomach. Acid secretion is stimulated in several ways. Distension of the stomach activates mechanoreceptors stimulating vagal reflexes, gastrin release from G cells and acid secretion from parietal cells. The acidic pH enhances pepsinogen secretion mediated by local reflexes.

The intestinal phase is initiated as chyme enters the duodenum, stimulating further gastrin release, but this is of minor importance compared with cephalic and gastric factors.

What factors predispose to vomiting or regurgitation and aspiration of gastric contents?

Vomiting is an active process. As it is more likely to occur during the lighter planes of anaesthesia it is more common during induction of, or emergence from, anaesthesia. It should not occur during maintenance of anaesthesia.

Regurgitation is a passive process. Therefore it may occur at any time and is not always immediately apparent. Because regurgitation usually occurs during deep anaesthesia, laryngeal reflexes are absent and the risk of aspiration is high.

Factors associated with vomiting and regurgitation include:

- Non-elective surgical procedures
- Difficult airway or intubation
- Light anaesthesia
- Gastrointestinal reflux
- Hiatus hernia
- Upper or lower gastrointestinal pathology
- Obesity
- Opioid medication
- Alcohol
- Lithotomy position
- Pregnancy.

A patient with a known hiatus hernia presents for an emergency laparotomy. What drugs would you use pre-operatively to reduce the risk of regurgitation and aspiration?

My aims in this case would be to promote gastric emptying, reduce gastric acid production and neutralise gastric acidity.

To promote gastric emptying I would give metoclopramide. Its prokinetic actions are mediated by antagonism of peripheral dopaminergic receptors and selective stimulation of gastric muscarinic receptors. This results in an increased lower oesophageal sphincter tone and relaxation of the pylorus.

To reduce gastric acid production I could use either a H_2 receptor antagonist such as ranitidine or a proton pump inhibitor such as omeprazole or lansoprazole. Ranitidine is a competitive antagonist of H2 receptors at parietal cells. The gastric pH is raised and the volume of secretions is reduced. It does not affect the lower oesophageal sphincter. Omeprazole reversibly blocks the hydrogen ion pump in the apical membrane of the parietal cell, the final common pathway of gastric acid secretion. Again, it does not affect lower oesophageal sphincter tone. Proton pump inhibitors have a greater potential to achieve absolute inhibition of acid secretion compared with H2 receptor antagonists.

I would use an antacid such as sodium citrate to raise the pH of gastric contents immediately before induction. Also, 30 mmol of sodium citrate just prior to induction is another alternative.

1.4.5. Pancreatitis – Matt Thomas

This is presented as a short case scenario, but could also be used as a long case with the history and examination findings provided along with blood results and radiology.

The surgical registrar asks you to see a previously well 61-year-old man with a 2-day history of epigastric pain and vomiting. He has oxygen saturations of 92% on 5 L/min of oxygen, a heart rate of 115 bpm and a blood pressure of 85/50 after 2 litres of saline. He is tender in the epigastrium and right upper quadrant. What is the differential diagnosis?

The differential diagnosis of an acute abdomen with shock is wide. In this case I would consider particularly gastric, duodenal, biliary, and pancreatic pathology, with the possibility of more remote causes of peritonitis, aortic disease or even an MI in the back of my mind.

The amylase is 2200. What do you think the diagnosis is and how could you confirm this?

An amylase of more than three times the upper limit of the hospital's reference range is usually said to be diagnostic of pancreatitis, but as amylase levels fall rapidly over 3 to 4 days this needs to be considered in the light of the duration of symptoms. A value of 2200 is high nevertheless, and pancreatitis is likely, even given that other pathology, such as a perforated duodenal ulcer, may also increase amylase. It can be confirmed by measurement of lipase, if available, as the pancreas is the only source of lipase, and this test has greater overall accuracy. Ultrasound or CT of the pancreas may show pancreatic swelling, and contrast enhanced CT is particularly good for confirmation. These tests are also useful to determine the cause of pancreatitis (if gallstones) or to exclude other pathology in uncertain cases. An ECG, cardiac enzymes and chest X-ray should be done in all cases for the same reason.

You've mentioned gallstones. What are the other common causes of pancreatitis?

Overall, gallstones account for about 50% of cases and alcohol for another 20–25%. Pancreatitis in women is more likely than this to be gallstone related and in men it is more frequently due to alcohol. In up to 20% of cases no cause is found. Other less common causes include drugs, trauma, endoscopic retrograde cholangiopancreatography (ERCP), infections particularly viral and including HIV, hypertriglyceridaemia, hyperparathyroidism, malignancy and autoimmune diseases.

What is the underlying pathophysiology?

This remains controversial but is believed to be unregulated activation of trypsin within pancreatic acinar cells. Local cell damage and inflammation results, with activation of complement and kinin pathways and stimulation of neutrophils and macrophages. This results in leucocyte migration and release of further pro-inflammatory cytokines and reactive oxygen species leading to further acinar cell injury and necrosis. About 20% of cases are severe in which the local inflammation leads to systemic inflammatory response syndrome (SIRS) and extra-pancreatic organ dysfunction, or there is a local complication such as pancreatic pseudocyst, pseudoaneurysm, necrosis or abscess.

Can you predict which attacks will be severe? Have you heard of any scoring systems, for example?

There are a number of scoring systems using a variety of clinical, laboratory and in some cases radiological factors, perhaps indicating that predicting the course of pancreatitis on admission is difficult. In the United Kingdom the Glasgow score is often used, where a score of 3 or more predicts a severe attack, although strictly speaking this requires 48 hours to complete. Other predictors after 48 hours include an APACHE II score of 8 or more, a CRP of more than 150, and unresolving or progressive organ failure. The mortality rate in patients with organ failure persisting for more than 48 hours exceeds 50%. Before 48 hours prediction is harder, but a pleural effusion on chest X-ray, BMI greater than 30 and a clinical impression of severity all predict severe acute pancreatitis. Finally, the CT severity index, which may be calculated on the day of admission if a CT is done, shows good correlation with complications, sepsis, need for ICU care and mortality.

What are the components of the Glasgow score?

If you really want to remember these try using the mnemonic PANCREAS for pO$_2$, age, neutrophils (i.e., WCC), calcium, renal (urea), enzymes (LDH or ALT), albumin and sugar (glucose).

The Glasgow score uses eight parameters: pO$_2$, age, white cell count, calcium, urea, either ALT or LDH, albumin and glucose. Each may be scored as 0 or 1. I can't remember the cut-off values to score points, but if 3 or more points are scored within the first 48 hours the attack is a severe one. Practically speaking the number of failing organs, and the severity of failure, is a good indicator of the severity of the attack.

This man's score predicts severe acute pancreatitis, and ultrasound shows a stone in the common bile duct. Will you admit him to the HDU?

Yes, I would admit for three reasons. Firstly, whatever the score predicts, he currently is seriously unwell with evidence of organ failure in that he is hypotensive despite fluid resuscitation and is hypoxic. Secondly, he is likely to get worse over the next 24 to 48 hours, especially as there is a difficult balance between fluid required for haemodynamic and renal support and his precarious respiratory function. Finally, as I have said, mortality from severe acute pancreatitis with organ failure is high and a ward environment is inappropriate because early resuscitation is likely to reduce the risk of complications.

How will you manage him once in your HDU?

Management of severe pancreatitis is aimed at the support of organ function and prevention of complications, as there is no therapy for pancreatic inflammation once established. Adequate early resuscitation with oxygen and fluid is probably the most effective way of reducing the risk of later organ failure. I would insert arterial, central venous and urinary catheters and a nasogastric tube. I would use oxygen, and NIV or IPPV as appropriate, aiming for pO_2 above 8 kPa. I would check central venous saturation and arterial lactate and resuscitate with fluid and noradrenaline with an initial target CVP of greater than 8 and MAP of 65 mmHg, as in the Surviving Sepsis Guidelines.

Yes, early intervention is important. Is there anything else?

Analgesia is important, and this could be provided with either morphine or even an epidural if the benefits were thought to outweigh the risks. Nutrition is vital as this will reduce the incidence of infectious complications, and I would begin enteral feeding as soon as haemodynamic stability was achieved, ideally with the first 12 to 24 hours. DVT and stress ulcer prophylaxis should be used in the absence of contraindications. Once stable, the cause of the pancreatitis should be addressed. If the cause of pancreatitis is gallstones, or another form of biliary obstruction, which might also be indicated by raised liver enzymes, then ERCP may be indicated.

There's a lot there to talk about. I'll take your last point first: how soon should ERCP be done? Is it an easy procedure?

Ideally within 72 hours of the onset of pain in severe acute pancreatitis with suspected or proven gallstone aetiology. This will allow sphincterotomy with or without stenting to relieve obstruction. It should also be done if there are dilated bile ducts, jaundice or cholangitis. It requires screening facilities and can be difficult to tolerate and to perform, so in most critically ill patients elective intubation and ventilation will be required.

Why go for a general anaesthetic when most ERCPs are done with sedation?

Patients in the HDU with severe acute pancreatitis have compromised respiratory function, large distended painful abdomens with a significant risk of a full stomach and are often confused. Sedation would carry risks of loss of the airway, aspiration, further hypoxia and worsening confusion.

What about cholecystectomy?

This should wait until organ failure has resolved, but ideally will be done during the same admission to prevent recurrent pancreatitis.

Nutrition is a contentious issue. Is enteral nutrition really safe?

It is true that older strategies emphasised "resting the gut" and avoiding enteral nutrition which was thought to increase pancreatic inflammation. However, recently the advantages of enteral nutrition have become clearer, in particular maintenance of gut barrier function, a reduction in septic episodes, fewer surgical interventions and fewer non-infectious complications, and a difference in mortality in meta-analysis. It is also cheaper than TPN, especially when a shorter hospital stay is taken into account.

Most evidence is from trials of nasojejunal feeding, although direct comparisons of NG and NJ feeding suggest they are equivalent and NG feeding is possible in up to 80% of cases. However, gastric outflow obstruction and ileus are common in severe acute pancreatitis so enteral feeding may be difficult to establish and underfeeding is a serious risk, as is regurgitation, vomiting and aspiration. If adequate NG or NJ feeding cannot be established within 3 to 5 days then parenteral supplementation or TPN should be used as calories are ultimately more important than the route.

Practically speaking, how would you attempt to establish feeding?

I would start using the NG route, and use prokinetics early and in combination if aspirates are high in the first 24 hours. If there is no improvement in the next 24 hours I would move from NG to NJ feeding. If this is poorly tolerated, for example if there is abdominal pain, distension, reflux, nausea or vomiting, then I would supplement with parenteral nutrition ideally including glutamine. It's important to agree this between all those likely to be involved in the patient's care, especially surgical colleagues.

What about probiotics?

Well, although the principle of preventing potentially pathological bacterial overgrowth in the gut is intuitively sound, and there is some experimental support, a recent Dutch trial published in the *Lancet* in 2008 found an increase in mortality in the probiotic group. I would not use them.

Well, we could discuss your choice of resuscitation fluid, or your use of surviving sepsis targets, or even whether an epidural would ever be indicated in this situation. However, time is pressing. So tell me, what are the complications of pancreatitis?

These may be divided into local and systemic complications. Systemic complications arise earlier and are essentially extra-pancreatic organ failures; these are responsible for most early deaths. ARDS, acute kidney injury and gut failure and the abdominal compartment syndrome are most common and, as with other causes of the systemic inflammatory response, patients are more susceptible to infections. Of local complications, pancreatic necrosis may also develop early. Other local complications may take a week or 2 to develop and include pseudocysts, pseudoaneurysm, and pancreatic abscess. There may be a late failure to improve or deterioration if necrosis becomes infected. There may also be therapy-related complications particularly from ERCP.

Tell me more about pancreatic necrosis

The extent of pancreatic necrosis seen on CT is a guide to the severity of the condition. However, what is really significant is the fact that the leading cause of morbidity and mortality is infected pancreatic necrosis, and somewhere over 50% of patients with severe pancreatitis will develop infected necrosis by the second or third week of their illness, so there has been a lot of interest in preventing infection. Most infecting organisms are gut-derived Gram-negative and anaerobic bacteria, hence the interest in probiotics. This might also be why enteral feeding has the beneficial effects it does as it preserves mucosal barrier function. There is also the thorny question of anti-biotic prophylaxis.

Ah, yes, I wondered when you would mention that. Anti-biotics are often used. Should they be?

Yes, broad-spectrum anti-biotics are often started in severe acute pancreatitis with the intention of reducing the incidence of infected necrosis and mortality. There is evidence from RCTs both for and against prophylaxis. Many factors might explain this, including the anti-biotics used and whether they penetrate pancreatic tissue adequately, patient selection, outcome measures and the quality of the trials. Findings from meta-analyses are similarly confusing, probably relating to trial selection, where there is a suggestion that higher quality trials are associated with reduced or no treatment effect. A recent Cochrane review concluded more and better quality research is needed. Current UK guidelines do not make a definitive recommendation, but there is growing recognition of the problems of anti-biotic resistance and bacterial and fungal overgrowth associated with prolonged prophylactic courses. Use of anti-biotics should be targeted at high-risk individuals according to the clinical context, pending definitive trials. Patients with multi-organ failure would generally be considered high risk.

What about selective decontamination of the digestive tract?

As far as SDD is concerned, there is insufficient evidence to recommend routine use, but some units use it in prolonged episodes complicated by recurrent infection.

So what will you do for this man? Will you start anti-biotics? Let us say it is day 5 and he is now ventilated and on noradrenaline, with a creatinine of 350 and rising, despite successful ERCP on day 3. CT shows about one third of his pancreas is necrotic.

Infection is unlikely if less than 30% of the pancreas is necrotic. This man has evidence of progressive multi-organ failure. In this situation I would start anti-biotics after taking blood cultures and also a CT-guided fine needle aspiration (FNA) of the necrosis. I'd be guided by microbiological advice, but meropenem would be an appropriate choice, and plan a course no longer than 14 days. If FNA cultures were negative I would stop the anti-biotics. Fungal cover is usually not necessary unless there have been previous anti-biotics used or other risk factors such as TPN use or surgical intervention.

What is the role of CT scanning?

As said before, the CT severity index is a good prognostic guide early in the course of the disease, but unless there are other diagnostic indications for a CT it should not be done purely for staging purposes. Necrosis may develop throughout the first week, so early CT may under-estimate the final extent and severity. A CT should be done if there are new or persisting symptoms, signs, sepsis or organ failures as local complications may have occurred and require intervention. CT is also indicated where infected pancreatic necrosis is suspected to get samples for culture before starting antibiotics.

So when is surgery indicated?

This is a question best decided by consultation with surgical colleagues. Cases of infected necrosis will not resolve without necrosectomy, but it is best to wait as long as possible to be sure that necrosis has delineated. Rarely, extensive apparently sterile necrosis may need debridement. The surgical technique will depend on local expertise, and there appears to be no difference in outcome between open and laparoscopic approaches. Some patients need an open abdomen, repeat laparotomies or continuous drainage of the pancreatic bed. Other local complications, such as pseudocyst or pseudoaneurysm, may be dealt with surgically or radiologically, depending on the precise anatomy and available expertise.

Thank you, we'll finish there

Further Reading

Al-Omran M, Albalawi Z, Tashkandi M, Al-Ansary L. Enteral versus parenteral nutrition for acute pancreatitis. *Cochrane Database of Systematic* Reviews. 2010; Issue 1: Art. No.: CD002837. DOI: 10.1002/14651858.CD002837.pub2.

Frossard J-L, Steer M, Pastor C. Acute pancreatitis. *Lancet.* 2008; **371**: 143–152.

UK Working Party on Acute Pancreatitis. UK guidelines for the management of acute pancreatitis. *Gut.* 2005; **54**: 1–9.

Villatoro E, Mulla M, Larvin M. Antibiotic therapy for prophylaxis against infection of pancreatic necrosis in acute pancreatitis. *Cochrane Database of Systematic* Reviews. 2010; Issue 5. Art. No.: CD002941. DOI: 10.1002/14651858.CD002941.pub3.

Whitcomb D. Acute pancreatitis. *New England Journal of Medicine.* 2006; **354**: 2142–2150.

Chapter

Haematological

1.5.1. Blood groups – Rebecca A Leslie

What is a blood group system?

Blood groups result from different antigens expressed on the surface of red blood cells (RBCs). There are a number of different blood group antigens, and those produced by the same gene are called a blood group system. Two of the most important blood group systems are the ABO system and the Rhesus (Rh) system as these are the main systems responsible for transfusion compatibility. However, these are only 2 of 29 blood group systems which have currently been identified. Examples of other systems are the Kell, Kidd, Lutheran and Duffy systems. The importance of these other blood groups systems should not be underestimated.

Tell me more about the antigens and anti-bodies in the ABO blood group system

The ABO system describes four different blood groups:

- Blood group A which has A antigens (agglutinogens) on their RBCs
- Blood group B which has B antigens on their RBCs
- Blood group AB which has both A and B antigens on their RBCs
- Blood group O which has no antigens on their RBCs.

Figure 1.5.1 shows the relative frequencies of the ABO groups in the United Kingdom.

Early in life individuals develop anti-bodies (called agglutinins) in the plasma against non-self antigens. These anti-bodies do not require exposure to different types of blood, but instead develop because antigens similar to A and B antigens are found in the gut and in some foods which individuals are exposed to. This is thought to occur early in neonatal life. As a result, anti-A anti-body is present when the A antigen is absent and anti-B anti-body is present when the B antigen is absent. Therefore in summary, individuals who have blood group A with A antigens expressed on their RBC will have anti-B anti-bodies within their blood. Similarly, individuals with blood group O will have anti-A and anti-B anti-bodies, and those with blood group AB will have no anti-bodies.

Dr. Podcast Scripts for the Final FRCA, ed. Rebecca A. Leslie, Emily K. Johnson, Gary Thomas and Alexander P. L. Goodwin. Published by Cambridge University Press.

Blood group	Naturally occurring antibodies (IgM)	UK (%)
O	Anti-A, anti-B	47
A	Anti-B	42
B	Anti-A	8
AB	None	3

Figure 1.5.1. Relative frequencies of ABO groups. Reproduced with permission from Smith, T., Pinnock, C. and Lin, T. 2009. *Fundamentals of Anaesthesia.* Cambridge: Cambridge University Press. © Cambridge University Press 2009.

This explains why patients with blood group AB are the ideal recipients, as they have no antibodies that will agglutinate ("clump") the donor blood. Equally blood group O is the ideal donor blood because once the antibodies are removed from the plasma, there are no antigens expressed on the RBC surface to agglutinate with antibodies in the recipients blood.

Can you tell me about the inheritance of A and B antigens?

A blood group is encoded on a single pair of genes, with each gene being one of three alleles: A, B or O. These alleles are inherited by Mendelian dominance. Therefore a patient with blood group A could have the genotype AA or AO, whilst a patient with blood group B, could have the genotype BB or BO. However an individual with blood group O must have the genotype OO, and blood group AB the genotype AB.

Tell me more about the Rhesus blood group

The Rhesus blood group system is the second most important after the ABO blood group system. It is very complex and comprises of many different antigens, including C, D and E antigens. D antigen is the most important antigen as it is felt to be the most antigenic. When a patient is described as being "Rhesus positive", this term normally is being used to describe the presence of D antigen on the individual' RBC.

In contrast to the ABO blood group system, anti-D anti-bodies are not normally found in the blood of Rhesus D-negative individuals. Instead anti-D anti-bodies only develop if the individuals blood comes into contact with Rhesus D-positive blood. This can occur by either an inappropriate blood transfusion or by the entry of fetal Rhesus D- positive blood into the circulation of a Rhesus D-negative mother. These anti-D anti-bodies will cause potential problems if the individual subsequently receives transfusion of further Rhesus D-positive RBCs.

What causes haemolytic disease of the newborn?

If a Rhesus D-negative mother gives birth to a Rhesus D-positive baby, as explained above, it is likely she will develop anti-D anti-bodies due to exposure to a small amount of the foetal RBCs (normally occurring at birth). The anti-D antibody is an immunoglobulin G (IgG) of small molecular mass (150 kDa) and is able to cross the placenta and enter the foetal circulation. This means that in future pregnancies the anti-D anti-bodies could cross the placenta and cause haemolytic disease of the newborn in Rhesus D-positive babies.

How do we prevent haemolytic disease of the newborn?

In the post-partum period we administer a single dose of Rhesus immune globulin to prevent sensitisation of the mother. This practice has reduced the incidence of haemolytic disease of the newborn by 90%.

How is a "group and save" performed?

Initially the patients ABO and Rhesus blood group is determined by combining the patient's blood with monoclonal typing reagents; anti-A, anti-B, anti-A+B and anti-D. Next, to ensure the correct ABO blood group has been identified, a reverse group is performed. This is where the patient's serum is mixed with both the group A and group B red blood cells. For example if the patient's blood is type A, when it is first combined with anti-A anti-bodies agglutination ("clumping") will occur; however, there will be no agglutination when it is combined with anti-B anti-bodies. Next to ensure that it definitely is blood group A, a sample is combined with blood known to be group A to ensure there is no agglutination, and a sample is combined with blood known to be group B, to demonstrate agglutination.

Next the blood is screened for the presence of anti-bodies. The sample is combined with a sample of red blood cells which are known to carry all common red blood cell antigens. If the test is positive, then the anti-body is identified by testing the patient's serum against a panel of individual RBCs.

How is a crossmatch performed?

After a "group and save" has been performed, samples from donor blood is combined with samples of the patient's blood to ensure no reaction occurs. This is particularly important to detect anti-body/antigen interactions which may occur due to other, less common blood group systems.

When would you consider giving your patient a blood transfusion?

The purpose of giving a blood transfusion is to improve the oxygen-carrying capacity of the blood. A blood transfusion is not without risk, and each patient should be assessed, on an individual basis, prior to considering a blood transfusion.

In accordance with the recent AAGBI guidelines I would tend not to transfuse anyone who has a haemoglobin >10 g/dl; however, it is important to recognise that there are situations where a blood transfusion in these patients might be appropriate.

It has been suggested that even in the elderly and those with cardiorespiratory disease a haemoglobin >8 g/dl is sufficient. However, if their haemoglobin were below this level or if they were symptomatic they should be transfused.

A haemoglobin <7 g/dl has been identified as a trigger for transfusion.

How would you give a blood transfusion?

The British Committee for Standards in Haematology (BCSH) has issued guidelines on the administration of blood transfusions. The AAGBI have also published a guideline for blood transfusion and the anaesthetist. I follow both these guidelines in my clinical practice:

- Confirm identity of patient (all patients receiving blood must be wearing an identification name band). Minimum patient identifiers are first name, last name, date of birth (DOB) and unique hospital number.
- Check the blood compatibility label to ensure the blood is the correct for the patient.
- Inspect the bag to ensure integrity of plastic casing.
- Administer the blood using a blood administration set with an integral mesh filter (170–200 microns).
- Transfusion should be completed within 4 hours of leaving the blood fridge.
- Details of the blood transfused must be recorded on the anaesthetic chart or in the medical notes.
- The patient should be monitored regularly during the blood transfusion.

How can the need for an allogenic blood transfusion be minimised in surgical patients?

Remember to classify your answer.

The need for a blood transfusion can be reduced by pre-operative and intra-operative measures.

Pre-operatively, appropriate assessment is key to minimising the need for a blood transfusion:

- Elective surgery in anaemic patients should be postponed until they have been appropriately investigated and treated.
- Patients on anti-coagulants should have their medications stopped for the pre-requisite prior before surgery.
- Early haematological advice should be sought in patients with bleeding and coagulation disorders.

Intra-operative blood loss can be minimised by:

- Use of tourniquets
- Local infiltration of vasoconstrictors
- Regional anaesthesia
- Using a hypotensive anaesthetic technique
- Pharmacological therapy; tranexamic acid and desmopressin (in patients with von Willebrand disease or mild haemophilia A).

What are the risks of blood transfusion?

The risks associated with a blood transfusion can be classified as immunological, infectious and physiological risks.

Immunological:

- Immediate haemolytic transfusion reaction. This occurs due to ABO incompatibility and is normally due to a human error. Anti-bodies in the recipient's blood interact with antigens on the donor blood causing agglutination of donor cells. This leads to microvascular blockage and haemolysis.
- Delayed haemolytic transfusion reaction. These reactions occur when a patient has developed a red cell anti-body due to a previous pregnancy or transfusion and the low

titre of this anti-body escaped detection in the "group and save". These reactions can present up to several days after the transfusion and symptoms and signs include fever, jaundice, fatigue, a drop in haemoglobin and haemaglobinuria.

- Febrile non-haemolytic transfusion reaction. This is the most common type of transfusion reaction. It occurs as a result of recipient anti-leucocyte anti-bodies. These reactions present with an increased temperature, and – when severe – nausea, vomiting, rigors and collapse.
- Anaphylaxis.
- Urticarial reactions. These occur due to plasma proteins in the donor blood.
- Transfusion-related acute lung injury (TRALI). This is defined as an acute lung injury with occurs within 6 hours of transfusion in the presence of no other risk factors for ARDS. It is most common after FFP transfusion. It is caused by anti-leucocyte anti-bodies in the donor blood. Unlike ARDS, it tends to resolve within 48 hours of the transfusion.

Infectious:

- Hepatitis B, hepatitis C, HIV, HTLV, malaria, cytomegalovirus, brucellosis, bacterial contamination and prion diseases can all be transmitted through contaminated blood; however in the UK the risk is small.

Physiological:

- Electrolyte disturbance: hyperkalaemia, hypocalcaemia and acidosis.
- Congestive cardiac failure can occur in susceptible patients.
- Dilutional coagulopathy.
- Dilutional thrombocytopenia.
- Hypothermia.

How can we reduce the need for allogeneic blood transfusion?

There are several techniques available. These include:

- Intra-operative cell salvage
- Pre-operative autologous donation
- Acute normovolaemic haemodilutional donation.

When would you consider using intra-operative cell salvage?

I would consider use of intra-operative cell salvage:

- Anticipated blood loss of >1000 ml
- Patients with a rare blood group or multiple anti-bodies
- Patients with low haemoglobin or increased risk of bleeding
- Patient objections to the use of allogenic blood (Jehovah's witness).

Further Reading

Association of Anaesthetists of Great Britain and Ireland (AAGBI) Guidelines. Blood Transfusion and the Anaesthetist – Red Cell Transfusion 2. June 2008.

http://www.aagbi.org/publications/guidelines.htm#b.

British Committee for Standards in Haematology (BCSH). Guideline on the Administration of Blood Components. First published 2009. http://www.

bcshguidelines.com/4_HAEMATOLOGY_
GUIDELINES.html?dtype=
Transfusion&dpage=0&sspage=
0&ipage=0.

Kirkman E. Blood groups. *Anaesthesia and
Intensive Care.* 2010; **11**(6): 232–235.

1.5.2. Anaemia and abnormal haemoglobins – Sarah F Bell

*Haematology is a topic that comes up again and again in the final exam since it is vital that we
have a good understanding of key topics such as anaemia. Questions could come up anywhere
in the exam so be prepared!*

**You are reviewing a 77-year-old woman with rheumatoid arthritis for a revision of
her total hip replacement. She has no other medical conditions. Her blood results reveal
a haemoglobin concentration of 9 g/dl with a mean corpuscular volume (MCV) of 80 fem-
tolitres/cell and a mean corpuscular haemoglobin (MCH) of 30 picograms/cell. The white
cell count is 6 × 10⁹/L and her platelet count is 450 × 10⁹/L.**

What can you tell me about the haematology results?

This woman is anaemic. The normal haemoglobin concentration for a woman is 11–15 g/dl
and 13–16 g/dl for men. The MCV and MCH are within normal limits, indicating that the
anaemia is normochromic and normocytic.

What is the difference between the MCV and MCH?

The mean cell volume, or MCV, is a measure of the average red blood cell volume.

The normal reference range is typically 80–100 femtolitres/cell. In contrast, the MCH is
the average mass of haemoglobin per red blood cell in a sample of blood. A normal value is
27 to 31 picograms/cell.

What are the clinical features of anaemia?

The features will, to a certain extent, depend on the speed at which the anaemia has developed. If the red blood cell concentration has fallen slowly, the patient may compensate and
be asymptomatic. Non-specific symptoms such as fatigue, headache and syncope may occur;
as may dyspnoea, angina, intermittent claudication and palpitations. These features will be
more pronounced in an acute situation, and the patient may become confused.

On examination the patient may again have non-specific signs such as pallor, tachycardia, flow murmurs and ankle oedema due to cardiac failure. More specific signs may further
define the cause of the anaemia. For example koilonychia (a disease of the nails, sometimes
referred to as "spoon nails") may be found in iron-deficiency anaemia, jaundice might indicate haemolysis, bone deformities may be found in thalassaemia and leg ulcers in sickle cell
disease.

What are the causes of anaemia?

*This question can be answered in a number of different ways depending on how you want to
classify the causes. This is one way. Describing the type of anaemia is another (i.e., normocytic
or macrocytic).*

I would split the causes into reduced production of red blood cells, increased breakdown
(haemolysis) and blood loss, which might be acute or chronic.

There are many potential causes of reduced production of red blood cells. Deficiencies of key components of red blood cells such as iron, vitamin B_{12} or folate will cause reduced production; as may chronic diseases (such as malignancy or infection) or endocrine conditions such as hypothyroidism or adrenocortical insufficiency. Bone marrow infiltration due to leukaemia or myelofibrosis may also cause reduced production, as may aplastic anaemia. Furthermore, reduced erythropoietin secretion, alcoholism, liver and renal disease may all decrease production of red blood cells.

Increased red blood cell breakdown can be subdivided into conditions that are inherited or acquired.

Inherited diseases may affect the red cell membrane leading to increased sequestration in the spleen. This may occur in hereditary spherocytosis. The abnormal haemoglobin containing cells observed in patients with thalassaemia or sickle cell disease are less deformable but will also become sequestrated in the spleen. Finally, metabolic defects such as glucose-6-phosphate dehydrogenase deficiency will also cause inherited haemolytic anaemia (due to altered cell membrane characteristics triggered by oxidative stress).

Acquired red blood cell breakdown can be classified into autoimmune, isoimmune, and non-immune conditions.

In autoimmune conditions the body's immune system attacks its own red blood cells. Warm and cold haemolytic anaemias may occur. In the cold condition the anti-bodies only bind to red blood cells at low body temperatures of about 28–31°C. The test for the presence of anti-bodies against red blood cells is the direct Coombs test. Certain drugs can also stimulate the productions of anti-bodies against red blood cells. Isoimmune conditions include Rhesus or ABO incompatibility. Non-immune causes of haemolytic anaemia include red cell membrane defects such as paroxysmal nocturnal haemoglobin and diseases affecting the liver and kidneys. Mechanical trauma or destruction of red blood cells may occur in patients with microangiopathic haemolytic anaemia, valve prostheses, march haemoglobinuria or sepsis.

What blood tests would you consider for investigating anaemia?

The blood tests would depend on the type of anaemia present.

If the patient presented with a hypochromic, microcytic anaemia then causes such as iron deficiency, anaemia of chronic disease or thalassaemia should be considered. Appropriate initial investigations would include assessment of iron status. In iron-deficiency anaemia a low serum ferritin, low serum iron and high total iron binding capacity would be expected. Haemoglobin electrophoresis would identify thalassaemia.

A macrocytic anaemia should be investigated by assessment of vitamin B_{12} and folate levels. If abnormal, testing for parietal cell and intrinsic factor anti-bodies will aid diagnosis of pernicious anaemia. Furthermore, tests such as thyroid function, liver function and a pregnancy test should also be considered.

A normochromic, normocytic anaemia might be due to acute blood loss, anaemia of chronic disease, aplastic anaemia, combined deficiency, haemolytic anaemias or endocrine disorders. Investigations would therefore include B_{12} and folate levels, iron studies, evidence of haemolysis such as elevated serum bilirubin and lactate dehydrogenase. The blood film should be assessed for sickle cells, parasites and reticulocytes. The platelet count and white blood cell count and morphology might also be investigated. Endocrine tests such as thyroid, pituitary and adrenal function might be appropriate in some cases.

What are the potential physiological effects of anaemia?

There are a number of effects of anaemia. Firstly there will be a reduced oxygen carrying capacity leading to fatigue, dyspnoea and in susceptible patients, angina. Secondly, the cardiac output increases to maintain oxygen flux which can cause palpitations and tachycardia. Thirdly, anaemia leads to an increase in 2,3-DPG and a shift of the oxyhaemoglobin dissociation curve to the right.

There will also be the effects of the disease or condition causing the anaemia.

What can you tell me about vitamin B_{12} deficiency?

Vitamin B_{12} deficiency causes a macrocytic anaemia due to abnormal DNA synthesis (specifically thymine). The deficiency may be caused by inadequate dietary intake, impaired absorption, chronic fish tapeworm infestation and drugs such as metformin that interfere with absorption. The impaired absorption may also be due to intrinsic factor deficiency or surgical resection of the terminal ileum.

Treatment requires identification of the cause of the deficiency and then replacement.

And what about folic acid deficiency?

A deficiency of folate will occur if the body's requirements increase, dietary intake is inadequate, or when the body excretes more folate than usual. Circumstances in which folate requirements increase include pregnancy, lactation, malabsorption syndromes, renal and liver disease. Many drugs interfere with folate utilisation including anticonvulsants, metformin, sulfasalazine and methotrexate.

What are the causes of iron-deficiency anaemia?

Iron deficiency may be due to chronic bleeding, inadequate intake, malabsorption and drugs which interfere with iron absorption. Gastric acidity enhances the solubility of iron and therefore the availability of iron-derived from food. Achlorhydria or alkaline drugs such as antacids can therefore interfere with iron absorption, as can medications such as H_2 receptor antagonists.

You are the registrar on-call for emergency theatres and are called to see a patient with acute appendicitis. She is a 24-year-old Afro-Caribbean who tells you that her only medical condition is sickle cell disease.

What can you tell me about this condition?

Sickle cell disease is caused by an alteration in the amino acid sequence for haemoglobin. Specifically it is due to the substitution of glutamic acid by valine in the sixth amino acid of the β-chains. The condition has an autosomal inheritance. Heterozygotes are described as having sickle cell trait and possess both normal and abnormal chains, whilst homozygotes contain only abnormal genes and are said to have sickle cell disease.

Sickle cell trait confers relative resistance to malaria and is therefore thought to have evolved in certain at-risk populations.

The condition is most prevalent in African and Asian populations. In the American black population the incidence of sickle disease is less than 1%, whilst the incidence of sickle cell trait is up to 10%.

How do you diagnose sickle cell disease or trait?

The diagnosis is made by taking a full history (including family history) and examining the patient. The sickledex test is a quick laboratory test, but this will not differentiate between disease and trait. The gold standard test is haemoglobin electrophoresis which will provide the clinician with a definite diagnosis.

What are the differences between sickle cells and normal red blood cells?

The haemoglobin in a sickle cell has the potential to polymerise and precipitates when deoxygenated. This leads to formation of the sickle shape, which is more rigid than the normal flexible red blood cell. The sickle cell thus increases blood viscosity and the possibility of thrombosis in the face of a reduction in flow. The sickle cell also has a reduced lifespan. The partial pressure at which the haemoglobin in sickle cells polymerises depends on whether the patient has disease or trait. In patients with the disease this may occur at partial pressures below 6 kPa (and so can happen continuously), whilst in trait the haemoglobin will sickle at lower partial pressures of 2.5 to 4 kPa. Oxygen affinity is normal when the cell is not polymerised.

What features of sickle cell disease would you look for in your pre-operative assessment of this patient?

The features can be divided into those associated with haemolysis, impaired blood flow and end-organ damage.

The haemolysis associated with sickle cell typically causes a normochromic normocytic anaemia. The symptoms and signs of anaemia may be present, depending on its severity. There may be an associated hyperbilirubinaemia and jaundice. Patients may also develop gallstones. Furthermore bone marrow hyperplasia can lead to skull and long bone enlargement.

The altered blood flow has a number of effects on the different organ systems. There can be chronic changes and acute crises precipitated by conditions such as hypothermia, dehydration, infection, exertion and hypoxaemia.

With regard to the neurological system the patient may have a history of stroke or present with acute neurological lesions. The respiratory system may be affected by pulmonary infarcts, pulmonary hypertension and right ventricular failure. Acute chest syndrome may occur with symptoms of pleuritic chest pain, fever, tachypnoea and pulmonary infarcts. The kidneys may be affected by infarction and the development of papillary necrosis and renal impairment. The musculoskeletal system may also be prone to infarction and avascular necrosis. The gastrointestinal system may be affected by bowel ischaemia and splenic infarction or hyposplenism. These patients often require vaccination against pneumococcus, haemophilus and meningococcus and may require prophylactic anti-biotics. The cardiovascular system may be affected by high output cardiac failure due to anaemia and increased risk of thrombotic events. Finally the patient may have ulcers due to impaired blood flow, retinopathy due to arterial occlusion and priapism.

Additional features of sickle cell anaemia include an increased susceptibility to infections such as salmonella, osteomyelitis and delayed growth and development in children.

What would you look for if the patient only had sickle cell trait?

The patient may be asymptomatic, but I would still look for features of sickle cell disease, because trait in combination with other haemoglobinopathies can produce more rigid cells that may sickle at a higher partial pressure of oxygen (for example HbCS).

The surgeons are keen to proceed with the case. Are there any pre-operative measures that you would instigate before taking the patient to theatre?

I would want to take a full history and examine the patient. I would then review the full blood count, U&Es, liver function tests and ECG before going to theatre. I would check that blood was available for the patient if required. (In severe cases an exchange transfusion might be performed pre-operatively to reduce the haemoglobin S concentration to below 40%, but this would depend on the urgency of the case and the patient's condition.) I would want to avoid precipitation of a sickle cell crisis and so would aim to prevent hypoxaemia, dehydration, hypothermia, acidosis and pain.

What would be your concerns intra-operatively?

Again, I would aim to prevent hypoxemia, dehydration, hypothermia, acidosis and pain. In general I would also avoid using a tourniquet, although this would not be required in an appendicectomy!

What can you tell me about thalassaemia?

This disease is due to a lack of expression of a globin chain in the haemoglobin due to deletion or mutation. This leads to reduced production of α- or β-chains. The severity of the condition is related to the pattern of inheritance of haemoglobin since one β- and two α-genes are inherited from each parent.

The condition is more common in Mediterranean, African and Asian populations.

In β-thalassaemia the condition may not be immediately identified as foetal haemoglobin does not contain β-chains. Heterozygotes will have a mild anaemia whilst homozygotes develop a severe anaemia with craniofacial bone hyperplasia, hepato-splenomegaly and cardiac failure. Haemosiderosis will develop if the condition is treated with repeated blood transfusions.

The α-thalassaemia patients are usually anaemic, the severity of which depends on the number of gene deletions.

Let's talk about anaemia during critical illness. Have you heard of the TRICC trial, and what were the important findings?

The TRICC trial stands for Transfusion Requirements in Critical Care. It compared a transfusion trigger of 7 g/dl (with a target haemoglobin of 7–9 g/dl), with a trigger of <10 g/dl (and target of 10–12 g/dl) in patients whose haemoglobin concentration was 9 g/dl during the first 3 days of an ICU stay. Interestingly, the 30- and 60-day mortality was similar for both groups. Furthermore there was a significantly lower mortality with the restrictive strategy among younger patients (below 55) and less ill patients (APACHE score < 20). This has led to the use of lower transfusion triggers in intensive care units.

Why do critically ill patients become anaemic?

Critically ill patients are often anaemic. There are many possible reasons for this. Haemodilution due to crystalloid- or colloid-based fluid resuscitation and or blood loss due to occult haemorrhage or frequent blood sampling often contributes. Additional causes include reduced red cell survival due to the systemic inflammatory response syndrome causing cell destruction or altered membrane characteristics, or reduced red blood cell production due to bone marrow suppression. Alterations in B_{12} and folate metabolism, inappropriately low circulating erythropoietin concentrations and abnormal red blood cell maturation may all be caused by inflammatory cytokines interrupting normal pathways and thus leading to anaemia.

How can we manage anaemic patients on the intensive care unit?

There are a number of measures that can be incorporated into managing anaemia. These include attempting to reduce red cell loss by restricting blood sampling and controlling haemorrhage, using appropriate transfusion triggers and recognising and treating any deficiencies promptly.

What would you consider to be exceptions to the restrictive strategy now employed?

Patients with chronic or acute ischaemic heart disease may require a transfusion trigger of less than 8 g/dl (rather than 7 g/dl).

Further Reading

Association of Anaesthetists of Great Britain and Ireland (AAGBI) Guidelines. Blood Transfusion and the Anaesthetist – Red Cell Transfusion 2. June 2008. http://www.aagbi.org/publications/guidelines.htm#b.

Association of Anaesthetists of Great Britain and Ireland (AAGBI) Guidelines. Blood Transfusion and the Anaesthetist – Intra-operative Cell Salvage. Sept 2009. http://www.aagbi.org/publications/guidelines.htm#b.

Herbert P, Wells G, Blajchman M, et al. A multicenter, randomized, controlled clinical trial of transfusion requirements in critical care. *New England Journal of Medicine.* 1999; **340**: 409–417.

1.5.3. Abnormalities in coagulation and haemostasis – Justin C Mandeville and Emily K Johnson

Disorders of coagulation include those at risk of excessive bleeding and those at risk of excessive thrombosis.

A 23-year-old man needs an urgent laparotomy for a ruptured spleen. The team is happy that there are no other injuries, but he has mild haemophilia.

The patient is tachycardic but otherwise stable, and has large bore intravenous access and a bag of colloid is being infused.

You have time to take a brief history. What questions might you ask him?

I would take a brief general history and specifically ask about his haemophilia. I would ask particularly about previous episodes of bleeding, previous surgical procedures, any regular treatment he receives and any recent blood tests he might have had.

I would also like to be sure which factor was deficient. In haemophilia A this would be factor VIII, and in haemophilia B it is factor IX. If, for example he has haemophilia A, it would be useful to know a recent factor VIII level – a level of 50% or more would be reassuring, but may still require replacement in active haemorrhage. I would also ask about previous blood transfusions as this may impact upon the time taken to perform blood crossmatch.

What might a full blood count and coagulation studies show in this patient at this point?

As the blood loss is acute and there may not have been much fluid given yet it is possible that there will be little fall in the haemoglobin or haematocrit, though the platelets may fall through consumption. In haemophilia A the activated partial thromboplastin time is likely to be raised but the bleeding time and prothrombin would be normal.

The surgeons are keen to start straight away. Would you be happy to do that?

This is a balance between how quickly you can optimise the patient and make arrangements to safely proceed and the risks to the patient of delaying his surgery.

The patient is exhibiting signs of hypovolaemia, and although the blood pressure is stable, a fall in blood pressure is often a late sign of hypovolaemia in a young person. The tachycardia alone suggests he has lost at least 15% of his circulating volume as a result of acute blood loss. Therefore I would like to assess the patient myself regarding his volume status, and ensure adequate fluid resuscitation prior to induction of anaesthesia.

I would ask for senior support with this case, and I would also contact the haematologist for advice regarding specific blood products. I would request that 6 units of blood be crossmatched immediately, ready to give in theatre. As well as intravenous access, I would establish invasive arterial blood pressure monitoring prior to induction and ideally, central venous access.

Can you tell me about the blood products you mentioned that might be of use in the peri-operative period?

Consider those specific to the haematological problem and those you might use in any major haemorrhage.

I would have packed red cells available if there were signs or evidence that blood loss was in excess of around 2 litres.

In an elective case factor VIII levels should be normalised for at least a week before major surgery. In emergencies such as this, factor VIII concentrate should be given as soon as possible. Haematologists should be closely involved, as a proportion of haemophiliacs have been found to have antibodies to factor VIII. Both fresh frozen plasma and cryoprecipitate contain some factor VIII so could be used if there is a delay in obtaining factor VIII concentrate.

I would aim to use other blood products as indicated by the severity of haemorrhage, in accordance with local and national transfusion guidelines, aiming to give FFP and platelets early in order to reduce potential coagulopathy. I would send intra-operative samples for full blood count, coagulation studies and fibrinogen, and if blood loss continues I would request fresh frozen plasma and platelets. If the fibrinogen was low I would correct it using cryoprecipitate.

In the case of inadequate haemostasis post-operatively I would be careful to avoid dilutional anaemia, as this is known to impair coagulation and some centres advocate the maintenance of a haemoglobin level of 10 g/dl.

If thromboelastometry was available, I would use it to guide my blood product administration.

Do you know of any drugs that may be useful in the management of this patient?

Drugs that may be useful include:

- Desmopressin can be useful in patients with haemophilia. It works by stimulation of (VIa) receptors, which both improves platelet function and induces endogenous von Willebrand factor and factor VIII production.
- Antifibrinolytics may be of use, some haemophiliacs will already be taking oral tranexamic acid.
- Recombinant factor VIIa can be used in massive haemorrhage to regenerate the thrombin burst.

I would also avoid non-steroidal anti-inflammatory drugs due to their antiplatelet effect.

It would be important to avoid the intra-muscular route of administration for any drugs, to avoid intra-muscular haematomas.

How else may you limit the need for excessive transfusion in this patient?

Consider pre-op, intra-op and post-op measures.
Pre-operatively:

- Avoid excessive use of blood for volume replacement as a young and otherwise fit man is likely to be able to tolerate considerable haemodilution. As far as possible I'd try to reserve transfusion until the surgeon has achieved haemostasis.
- Attempt to correct coagulation abnormalities as much as possible before theatre to reduce bleeding, consider replacement of electrolytes (particularly calcium), correction of acidosis and avoidance of hypothermia.
- Prepare a cell-saver or equivalent autologous transfusion device for use.

At induction and intra-operatively:

- Take special care with intubation so as not to traumatise the airway and cause further bleeding.
- Consider the use of a topical vasoconstrictor to reduce nasal bleeding if a nasogastric tube was necessary.
- Perform central line insertion under direct ultrasound guidance, avoiding the subclavian route.
- Maintain a normal temperature.
- Consider intra-operative cell salvage.

Post-operatively:

- Continue care on a HDU with continuous monitoring and regular blood sampling.
- Promptly address any abnormalities in coagulation and liaise regularly with haematologists.
- Consider accepting a haemoglobin of greater than or equal to 7 g/dl in accordance with AAGBI transfusion guidelines.

What is your definition of massive transfusion?

There are many definitions so pick one you know and stick with it.
Massive transfusion is when the equivalent of one blood volume is transfused within 24 hours.

What are the complications of massive transfusion?

The complications of massive transfusion include those common to any blood transfusion so it is worthwhile learning a list!
Complications of massive transfusion:

- Errors in blood administration: human error, patient identification problems, inadequate cross checking procedure
- Incompatibility of blood: such as ABO, Rh or other antigens in un-crossmatched blood or patients who have received multiple previous transfusions
- Acute haemolytic reactions
- Anaphylaxis
- Delayed reactions
- Fluid over-load
- Transmission of infective agents – bacterial, viral or prions
- Citrate-related hypocalcaemia
- Hyperkalaemia
- Acidosis
- Dilutional coagulopathy
- Impaired oxygen delivery
- Transfusion-related acute lung injury: recipient neutrophil activation in alveolar membranes
- Disseminated intra-vascular coagulation
- Hypothermia.

Can you tell me more about thromboelastometry?

Thromboelastometry is becoming increasingly popular, and you should be able to describe the technique and give a basic interpretation of the results. To demonstrate a good understanding and help explain your answer it would help to draw a normal trace (Figure 1.5.3; Table 1.5.3).
Thromboelastometry is a bedside test used to assess a patient's coagulation. It involves a pin being rotated in whole blood to analyse the process of coagulation. Clot forms on the pin and a graph is created that shows the change in torque over time. It looks at the time taken for the thrombus to form, the tensile strength and the elastic properties of the clot.

Table 1.5.3. Thromboelastography measurements and interpretation

Measurement	Explanation	Interpretation
Clotting time or R time	Time from start to curve reaching 1 mm wide Coagulation factor activation	Prolonged in factor deficiencies, with anti-coagulants and thrombocytopenia
Clot formation time or K time	Time for the graph to widen from 1 mm to 20 mm Coagulation factor amplification	Prolonged in fibrinogen and platelet deficiencies
Maximal clot firmness or maximal amplitude (MA)	Curve width at its widest point	Reduced in fibrinogen and platelet deficiencies
α-Angle	Line from midline to 1 mm point tangential to the curve – indicates speed of clot formation Coagulation factor amplification	Abnormal in clotting factor deficiencies, platelet dysfunction, thrombocytopenia and low fibrinogen
Lysis time	Measured by decrease from maximal amplitude – a decrease in >15% indicates fibrinolysis Lysis is measured at 30 minutes and 60 minutes after MA is recorded	Reduced in poor platelet function and fibrinolysis
Lambda angle	Angle showing lysis rate	

A NORMAL THROMBOELASTOGRAPH

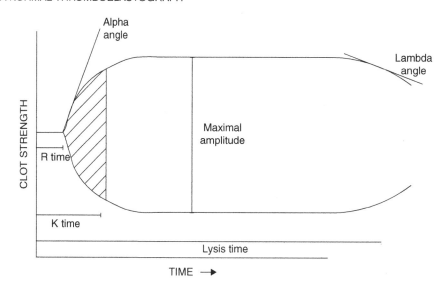

Figure 1.5.3. A normal thromboelastograph.

The measurements and their significance are as follows:
- Time taken to start the clot formation
- Rate of formation
- Maximum strength of the clot
- Time taken for fibrinolysis to start (and its rate and extent) can all be used to assess requirement of clotting factors, platelet or fibrinogen replacement.

Can you tell me about another important inherited disorder of coagulation?

There are a number you could mention, but by far the most common is von Willebrand disease.

Von Willebrand disease is a relatively common disorder of coagulation that is due to either insufficient or ineffective von Willebrand factor. Von Willebrand factor is a glycoprotein which binds to other proteins in the coagulation cascade (Factor VIII). Those with type 1 disorder have only around 75% of normal von Willebrand factor levels; type 2 patients are divided into three subtypes and all have qualitative defects in the factor, but may have normal levels; type 3 patients have an autosomal recessive absence of the factor and therefore very severe disease.

Patients are at risk of bleeding from mucosal surfaces, which is different from haemophilia when bleeding is usually into joints or the peritoneal cavity.

If this patient had von Willebrand disease instead, how might your management have differed?

Pre-operatively I would have attempted to ascertain which type of von Willebrand disease the patient had, and whether he had recent VWF levels checked. Again, I would be in close liaison with a haematologist and seek their advice about timing of administration of drugs and blood products. If they were in agreement I would give 0.3 micrograms per kilogram of DDAVP (desmopressin – which promotes the release of VWF) as soon as possible, as this can help restore clotting function within an hour and has an action lasting about 6 hours.

A normal bleeding time and APTT do not necessarily mean normal VWF levels. If DDAVP is used, the coagulation should be checked after an hour but it may be of little help in some subtypes of the disease.

Intra-operatively, I would use either 1 unit/5 kg of cryoprecipitate, or 20 ml/kg of fresh frozen plasma, as both of these measures have been shown to raise factor levels by 15% or more.

I would not use factor VIII concentrate, as this contains no von Willebrand factor. Post-operatively DDAVP and blood products should be used to maintain von Willebrand factor levels until the risk of haemorrhage has resolved.

Can you give any examples of disease states that result in bleeding tendencies?

Classify your answer, for example mention diseases causing impairment in coagulation factors, platelets and vascular endothelium.

Disorders that result in clotting factor deficiencies include:

- Advanced liver disease
- Disseminated intra-vascular coagulation.

Those resulting in platelet dysfunction or reduced numbers of platelets include:

- Disseminated intra-vascular coagulation
- Haematological malignancy
- Autoimmune platelet diseases

- Splenomegaly
- Uraemia
- Liver disease.

Also there are diseases involving the vascular endothelium, for example:

- Amyloidosis
- Sepsis.

Can you clarify what, in terms of a coagulation disorder, would prevent you from performing regional anaesthesia?

Mention any guidelines you might know about such as the ASRA guidelines for patients receiving regional anaesthesia.

I would avoid regional anaesthesia in the following cases:

- Abnormal APTT, INR or bleeding time, unless the benefits of using it clearly outweighed the risk
- Platelet levels of 80×10^9/L or below.
- On antiplatelet drugs, or had stopped taking them less than a week previously, though non-steroidal anti-inflammatory agents are generally considered safe.
- Known coagulation disorder, whether or not their laboratory results were normal, as it is possible to have a normal coagulation screen but abnormal coagulation.
- Patient received a prophylactic dose of low molecular weight heparin within the past 12 hours.
- Patient received a treatment dose of low molecular weight heparin within the past 24 hours.

Following regional anaesthesia, the first post-operative dose of low molecular weight heparin should not be given until 4 hours after the block. Any catheters used should not be removed until 12 hours after the dose and any subsequent dose should not be given until 2 hours after catheter removal.

Oral anticoagulants, mainly warfarin in this country, should not be given peri-operatively where regional anaesthesia is used. Anyone on warfarin pre-operatively should stop it long enough in advance for the INR to normalise. It is important to remember that INR mainly assesses factor VII activity and not factors II and X so that a normal INR does not necessarily mean normal coagulation.

Are there any patients in whom you would be particularly concerned about peri-operative venous thrombosis?

Categorise into patients with specific risk factors, and patients with specific thrombophilias.

All patients admitted to hospital must undergo a venous thromboembolism risk assessment, and this should be documented.

Those at risk include any patient with the following:

1. A previous history of thrombosis whether or not they had a proven thrombophilia
2. Diabetes

3. Obesity
4. Malignancy
5. Hyperviscocity syndromes.

Particular thrombophilias that raise alarm because of high thrombotic risk would include:

1. Activated protein C resistance (for example factor V Leiden deficiency)
2. Protein C deficiency
3. Protein S deficiency
4. Antithrombin III deficiency
5. Antiphospholipid syndrome.

I would consult a haematologist about the management of these patient groups.

Those with a high risk of thrombosis should be managed with measures to reduce venous stasis, such as graduated or pneumatic compression stockings, leg elevation, early mobility and leg exercises. Also, intravascular coagulation can be prevented by using drugs such as unfractionated or low molecular weight heparins, or antiplatelet agents.

Further Reading

Association of Anaesthetists of Great Britain and Ireland (AAGBI) Guidelines. Blood Transfusion and the Anaesthetist – Red Cell Transfusion 2. June 2008. http://www.aagbi.org/publications/guidelines.htm#b.

Carless PA, Henry DA, Carson JL, et al. Transfusion thresholds and other strategies for guiding allogeneic red blood cell transfusion. *Cochrane Database of Systematic Reviews.* 2000; Issue 10. Art. No.: CD002042. DOI: 10.1002/14651858.CD002042.pub2.

Hebert PC, Wells G, Blajchman MA, et al. A multicenter, randomized, controlled clinical trial of transfusion requirements in critical care. Transfusion Requirements in Critical Care Investigators, Canadian Critical Care Trials Group. *New England Journal of Medicine* 1999; **340**: 409–417.

Horlocker T, Wedel TT, Rowlingson DJ, Enneking JC, Kayser F; American College of Chest Physicians. Regional anesthesia in the patient receiving anti-thrombotic or thrombolytic therapy: American Society of Regional Anesthesia and Pain Medicine Evidence-Based Guidelines (Third Edition). *Regional Anesthesia and Pain Medicine.* 2010; **35**(1): 64–101.

Stainsby D, MacLennan S, Thomas D, Isaac J, Hamilton PJ. Guidelines on the management of massive blood loss. *British Journal of Haematology.* 2006; **135**: 634–641.

UK Blood Transfusion & Tissue Transplantation Services. Guidelines for the Blood Transfusion Services in the UK, 7th edition. http://www.transfusionguidelines.org.uk/index.aspx?Publication=RB.

1.5.4. Anti-coagulant, anti-platelet and anti-fibrinolytic agents – Susanna T Walker

Can you classify anti-coagulants?

Remember, as with everything, you should classify the drugs if possible as you will be less likely to forget any.

Anti-coagulant drugs can be classified into those that inhibit platelet function, those that affect the clotting cascade, and those that lead to the breakdown of a clot once it has formed.

Let's start by talking about anti-platelet agents. Can you tell me about all the drugs you know of that inhibit platelet function

There are several drugs that affect platelet function, all of which work in slightly different ways. It is helpful to have an understanding of platelet function to understand how these drugs work.

Platelets are activated when they are exposed to the subendothelial matrix of a damaged vessel wall. Activation leads to degranulation of the platelets and then a process of aggregation where platelets stick to each other, and clot formation follows. Von Willebrand factor and Factor VIII are essential for the initial phase of platelets sticking to the vessel wall. The degranulation process leads to release of thromboxane A_2, which increases platelet aggregation and also causes localised vasoconstriction of the vessel. Distal to the clot, vessel walls release prostacyclin, which has the opposite effect to thromboxane A_2, preventing platelet aggregation and leading to vasodilatation. This aims to localise and minimise the clotting process.

Thrombin, produced as part of the clotting cascade, increases the activity of platelets by increasing the production of glycoprotein IIb/IIIa receptors. These receptors are required for binding of fibrinogen to platelets, leading to cross-linking of platelets, and strengthening the clot formed.

Adenosine diphosphate (ADP) is also released from the platelets in the degranulation process. This has a positive feedback effect on the platelets by binding to an ADP receptor on the platelet surface. This increases platelet activity by enabling the glycoprotein IIb/IIIa receptor to transform into its active form and therefore facilitate binding of fibrinogen to the platelets.

Drugs that affect platelet function include (Figure 1.5.4a):

1. **Non-steroidal anti-inflammatory drugs (NSAIDs).** e.g., aspirin. These work by inhibiting cyclo-oxygenase enzymes therefore reducing production of thromboxane A_2 from arachidonic acid, thus inhibiting platelet aggregation and preventing localised vasoconstriction of the vessel.

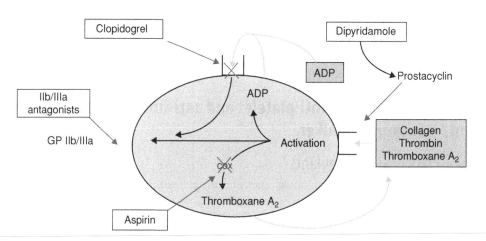

Figure 1.5.4a. Sites of action of anti-platelet agents.

2. **Clopidogrel.** This works by irreversibly blocking the ADP receptor and therefore indirectly reduces platelet activity and inhibits activation of the glycoprotein IIb/IIIa receptor.
3. **Dipyridamole.** This inhibits platelet phosphodiesterase, which normally breaks down cyclic AMP within the platelets. High levels of cyclic AMP prevent activation of platelets, thereby reducing platelet adhesion to vessel walls. It also increases the effects of prostacyclin, thus further preventing platelet aggregation, and leading to vasodilatation.
4. **Abciximab.** This is a synthetic anti-body, which binds strongly to the glycoprotein IIb/IIIa receptor, therefore preventing binding by fibrinogen.
5. **Prostacyclin.** As previously mentioned, this is produced endovascularly leading to localised vasodilatation and inhibition of platelet aggregation. It can be given as a continuous infusion to anti-coagulate a haemofiltration circuit in a patient unable to receive heparin. It may also be used for its vasodilating properties, such as in patients with Raynaud's disease.
6. **Dextrans.** These are large chain carbohydrate molecules, which may be given for fluid resuscitation. They have an inhibitory effect on von Willebrand factor and therefore have an anti-coagulatory effect.

Can you describe, with the help of a diagram if you wish, exactly how anti-inflammatory drugs work to inhibit platelet function

It's always worth drawing a quick diagram if you can, but make sure you make it a big, clear diagram (Figure 1.5.4b).

Membrane phospholipids are broken down to arachidonic acid by phospholipase A. This is then converted to prostaglandin H_2 by cyclo-oxygenase enzyme, and then converted on by a variety of enzymes to thromboxane A_2 in platelets, prostacyclin (PGI_2) in the vascular endothelium and various prostaglandins (PGE_2, $PGF_{2\alpha}$, PGD_2) at other sites. There is an alternative pathway enabling arachidonic acid to be converted to leukotrienes by lipoxygenase enzyme, which is not affected by NSAIDs. It is thought that a relative excess of leukotrienes due to an inhibition of cyclo-oxygenase may be the cause for the wheeze precipitated by NSAIDs.

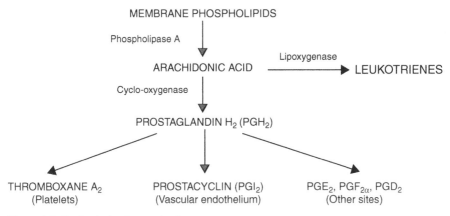

Figure 1.5.4b. Synthesis of prostaglandins.

What is the difference between aspirin and other NSAIDs with regards to duration of action?

Aspirin leads to an irreversible inhibition of the cyclo-oxygenase enzyme, whilst other NSAIDs lead to reversible inhibition. This therefore means that the effect of aspirin lasts for the lifetime of the platelet, whilst the other NSAIDs only have an effect whilst the drug is in the system in its active form. When given in a low dose, aspirin specifically has an effect on platelet cyclo-oxygenases but not on vessel wall cyclo-oxygenase, therefore having an anti-coagulant effect on platelets, whilst retaining the production of vessel wall prostacyclin.

Which groups of patients are routinely started on aspirin and clopidogrel or other antiplatelet agents?

Aspirin and clopidogrel are most commonly used for their anti-platelet effect in patients who are at risk of myocardial infarction or cerebrovascular accident. Both these drugs are routinely started in patients who have had percutaneous coronary intervention with insertion of a coronary stent.

There are two types of stent that are commonly used – drug-eluting stents and bare-metal stents. Both types lead, in the initial stage, to bare metal being exposed in the coronary vessel, which is highly thrombogenic and prone to in-stent thrombosis. Prevention of this is therefore extremely important. Drug-eluting stents have the effect of reducing intimal proliferation, and are therefore used to reduce the rates of in-stent re-stenosis. However, the drug that is released has the effect of prolonging the time that bare metal is exposed, therefore increasing the risk of in-stent thrombosis for a longer period. It has been suggested that dual anti-platelet therapy should be continued for at least a year in patients with drug-eluting stents. A study has shown that premature cessation of anti-platelet therapy is the strongest predictor of subsequent stent thrombosis. The overall recommendations are that if non-cardiac surgery is known to be necessary within a year of stent insertion then a bare-metal stent should be used in preference to a drug-eluting stent. In a patient who has recently had a stent inserted, elective non-cardiac surgery should be avoided until clopidogrel can be safely stopped.

Can you now tell me about the drugs that exert an effect on the clotting cascade that you mentioned in your initial classification?

Once again, it is easier to understand how these drugs work by having an understanding of the clotting cascade (Figure 1.5.4c). Try and describe the clotting cascade and then relate the drugs to this when discussing how they work.

The classical description of the clotting cascade consists of a series of clotting factors that are present within the plasma in an inactive state. Activation of one leads to activation of the next in a cascade fashion. Various co-factors are required at certain stages of the pathway. The purpose of the cascade is to produce thrombin, which converts fibrinogen into fibrin, leading to clot formation. The clotting cascade is classically quoted as having two limbs – the intrinsic pathway and the extrinsic pathway. These then converge to form the final common pathway. The intrinsic pathway consists of factors XII, XI and IX, and is activated by blood coming into contact with subendothelial connective tissues. The extrinsic pathway consists

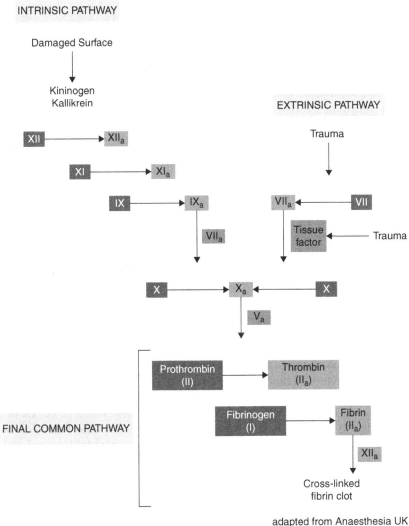

INTRINSIC PATHWAY

Damaged Surface

Kininogen
Kallikrein

XII $\longrightarrow$ XII$_a$

XI $\longrightarrow$ XI$_a$

IX $\longrightarrow$ IX$_a$

VII$_a$

X $\longrightarrow$ X$_a$

V$_a$

EXTRINSIC PATHWAY

Trauma

VII$_a$ $\longleftarrow$ VII

Tissue
factor $\longleftarrow$ Trauma

X$_a$ $\longleftarrow$ X

Prothrombin
(II) $\longrightarrow$ Thrombin
(II$_a$)

Fibrinogen
(I) $\longrightarrow$ Fibrin
(II$_a$)

FINAL COMMON PATHWAY

XII$_a$

Cross-linked
fibrin clot

adapted from Anaesthesia UK

Figure 1.5.4c. The classical clotting cascade.

of factors III and VII and is activated by tissue damage much more rapidly than the intrinsic pathway. Its purpose is to help promote activation of the intrinsic pathway.

The final common pathway starts by activation of factor X, which occurs as the end result of both pathways. Activated factor X converts pro-thrombin to thrombin, which in turn converts fibrinogen to fibrin, as already mentioned.

Drugs that affect the clotting cascade can be classified into:

1. Vitamin K antagonists, which would include warfarin and phenindione
2. Factor Xa inhibitors, which can be subdivided into:

2.1. Unfractionated heparin

2.2. Low molecular weight heparins, such as enoxaparin

2.3. Oligosaccharides, such as fondaparinux

2.4. Heparinoids, such as danaparoid sodium

3. Direct thrombin inhibitors, which can be subdivided into:

3.1. Bivalent compounds, such as lepirudin

3.2. Univalent compounds, such as argatroban

4. Others. For completeness we should also include activated protein C as a drug that may affect the clotting cascade. This is a naturally occurring inhibitor of the clotting cascade. More recently, it has been used in the intensive care setting for its potential role in treating patients with severe sepsis.

Tell me how warfarin works

Warfarin and phenindione are both coumarin derivatives. Coumarin is a naturally occurring compound found in some plants that is toxic and was noted to have anti-coagulant properties.

Warfarin works by inhibiting the reduction of vitamin K. Vitamin K is required in its active, reduced, form as a co-factor in the γ-carboxylation of glutamic acid residues in the production of Factors II, VII, IX and X in the liver. Inhibition of vitamin K production therefore leads to inhibition of clotting factor production. As this process requires inhibition of the synthesis of new clotting factors, warfarin may take up to 72 hours to have a full effect on the clotting cascade.

The effects of warfarin need to be carefully monitored on a regular basis by checking a patient's prothrombin time, or INR (international normalised ratio).

It is important to note that, since warfarin is metabolised by the liver, factors leading to liver enzyme induction or inhibition will have an effect on the levels of warfarin. For example, alcohol, and some anti-biotics such as erythromycin lead to an inhibition of metabolism and therefore an increase in warfarin levels. Conversely, drugs such as barbiturates and carbamazepine induce liver enzymes and therefore reduce the levels of warfarin.

How does heparin work? What is the difference between unfractionated heparin and low molecular weight heparin?

Heparin is a naturally occurring sulphated glycosaminoglycan, which has been found in various sizes within mast cells and liver cells. Heparin has its effect by increasing the activity of anti-thrombin III (a naturally occurring inhibitor of the clotting cascade) by up to 1000 times. When anti-thrombin III binds to thrombin, an inactive complex forms. Antithrombin III also inactivates other factors including II, IX, X, XI and XII. Unfractionated heparin inhibits factor Xa at low concentrations, but will also inhibit these other factors as blood concentrations rise. It is usually administered as a continuous infusion (although occasionally as subcutaneous injections) to achieve therapeutic blood levels, and its effect wears off within about 4 hours of stopping the infusion. Monitoring of the activated partial thromboplastin time (APTT) is required to adjust the infusion rate. This is a measure of the intrinsic clotting cascade.

Low molecular weight heparins, such as enoxaparin and tinzaparin, are the smaller weight fractions (ranging from 2000 to 8000 daltons) of the heparin. They are more effective at inhibiting Factor Xa than unfractionated heparin, and have minimal effect on other factors. For this reason, their effectiveness cannot be measured using the APTT. Levels of Factor Xa can be measured, although this is not routinely done. They have the benefit over unfractionated heparin of having a longer half-life, and so can be given as a once daily injection.

What can you tell me about heparin-induced thrombocytopenia?

If you're asked about this you're doing well!

There are two causes of thrombocytopenia related to the use of heparin. These can be divided into Type I and Type II.

Type I is a non-immune mediated thrombocytopenia, which is reasonably common following the use of heparin. It does not usually cause any problems, and the platelet count usually recovers quickly even when the heparin isn't stopped.

Type II, however, is an immune-mediated process with much more serious consequences. It usually occurs after exposure to unfractionated heparin, although it may also be associated with use of low molecular weight heparin. It occurs when heparin complexes with platelet factor 4, forming antigenic material to which anti-bodies form. Binding of the anti-bodies leads to platelet activation, generation of thrombus, and a resultant thrombocytopenia. This therefore causes a pro-thrombotic state, and so these patients are at risk of severe thrombotic events such as stroke, PE, MI and limb ischaemia. The platelet count rarely drops very low, and therefore patients are less at risk of bleeding. This condition may occur 5–15 days after heparin has been given, even if it is no longer being administered. It is important to consider the condition in patients with an unexplained thrombocytopenia, in patients with thrombosis associated with thrombocytopenia, and in those with necrotic lesions at the site of previous heparin injections.

If a patient is suspected of having heparin-induced thrombocytopenia (HIT), a "HIT Screen" can be sent to look for immune complexes. The result from this can take some days, so in the meantime the patient should have any heparin or low molecular weight heparin stopped. An alternative anti-coagulant should be started, such as a direct thrombin inhibitor (lepirudin or argatroban), or an alternative Factor Xa inhibitor (danaparoid sodium or fondaparinux). Once the platelet count has recovered to acceptable levels, warfarin therapy can be considered for long-term anti-coagulation if required.

What is danaparoid sodium?

Danaparoid sodium is a low molecular weight heparinoid and is effective first line treatment for heparin-induced thrombocytopenia.

Unlike low molecular weight heparin (LMWH), danaparoid is very unlikely to react with heparin-associated anti-platelet anti-bodies, and so does not cause the HIT syndrome itself. Like LMWH, its activity can be monitored by measuring plasma Factor Xa levels.

What recommendations do you know of regarding patients taking anti-coagulant medications and performing a central neuraxial blockade?

It is relatively common for patients receiving some form of anti-coagulation to require a central neuraxial blockade for surgery. Clearly a patient that is fully anti-coagulated with any form of anti-coagulant should not receive a neuraxial block, as the risk of epidural haematoma formation would be too great.

For patients receiving warfarin, it is generally accepted that an epidural can be sited if the INR is less than 1.5.

For patients receiving unfractionated heparin as an infusion, at least 4 hours should have elapsed between stopping the infusion and placing an epidural catheter.

For patients receiving low molecular weight heparin, at least 12 hours should have passed since the last dose before inserting, or removing, an epidural catheter. Another 2 hours should pass after inserting or removing an epidural catheter before giving the next dose of low molecular weight heparin.

For surgery where large doses of heparin may be given intra-operatively, such as vascular surgery, some anaesthetists are cautious about siting an epidural catheter. However, large observational studies have shown no increased incidence of epidural haematoma formation.

Finally, many patients come into hospital taking anti-platelet agents. It is generally accepted that a patient taking low dose aspirin can have an epidural sited without the need to stop taking aspirin. However, there is more concern about the use of clopidogrel. Most anaesthetists would agree that ongoing clopidogrel use would contraindicate the placing of an epidural. It should have been stopped for at least 7 days before attempting to site a central neuraxial block to minimise the risk of epidural haematoma.

In any patient with a degree of anti-coagulation, it is much safer to perform a single shot spinal technique than a technique involving the much larger epidural needle. This should be considered if it is considered appropriate.

Are you aware of any methods available for checking a patient's coagulation status?

There are a multitude of tests that can be performed to assess a patient's coagulation status. These can be divided into lab-based tests, and near-patient tests.

The lab-based tests would include:

1. **INR (international normalised ratio).** As already mentioned, this is a measure of the extrinsic pathway, and is used predominantly as a measure of warfarin activity.
2. **APTT (activated partial thromboplastin time).** This has also been mentioned earlier and is a measure of the intrinsic pathway. It is used as a measure of heparin activity.
3. **Thrombin time.** This is a measure of the final common pathway. It will be affected in patients with abnormal or deficient thrombin.
4. **Platelet count.** Coagulation may be deficient if a patient has a low platelet count. Pre-operatively we would generally aim for a platelet count of greater than 100 million/ml of blood.
5. **Platelet function assay.** This assesses platelet function. Patients with a normal platelet count can have abnormal clotting if their platelets are not functioning normally. Platelet function may be affected by anti-platelet agents, hereditary diseases, or other factors, such as a very high serum urea.

The near-patient tests would include:

1. **Bleeding time.** This is performed by making a standardised incision and timing how long it takes for clot formation. This is predominantly an assessment of platelet function.

2. **Activated clotting time (ACT).** This is most commonly measured in vascular and cardiac theatres. It is a quick assay of clotting that measures time for clot formation. A normal result would be 100–150 seconds. Prolonged values may represent abnormal clotting as a result of heparin given intra-operatively, or a coagulopathy.

3. **Thromboelastogram (TEG).** This is another quick test that can be performed in theatre or on the ITU if the correct equipment is available. It gives an indication of time to clot activation which acts as a surrogate measure of clotting factors; strength of clot which acts as a measure of platelet function; and breakdown of clot, which may be more rapid than normal in conditions such as DIC. This can therefore be used to tailor the coagulation factor replacement to the defect detected. There are some newer reagents that are used with the TEG that can enable near-patient assessment of platelet dysfunction as a result of anti-platelet agent use.

Finally, can you tell me about the fibrinolytic agents?

The fibrinolytic agents are plasminogen activators. During the process of clot breakdown, inactive plasminogen has to be converted to the active plasmin, which can then break fibrin down to fibrin degradation products, thus dissolving the clot. Fibrinolytic agents initially form a fibrino–plasminogen activator complex. This then goes on to convert further plasminogen molecules to active plasmin. There are many examples of fibrinolytics including streptokinase and alteplase. They are generally given to dissolve clot in a life-threatening situation such as a myocardial infarct or pulmonary embolus. They carry with them the risk of serious bleeding, and so there are situations where the risk of administration outweighs any potential benefit of treatment.

Further Reading

Howard-Alpe GM, de Bono J, Hudsmith L, et al. Coronary artery stents and non-cardiac surgery. *British Journal of Anaesthesia*. 2007; **98**(5): 560–574.

1.5.5. Prevention, diagnosis and management of fat embolism, DVT and PE – Ami Jones

An orthopaedic senior house officer asks you what factors increase the risk of a patient suffering from a venous thromboembolism as he is unsure whether or not he should prescribe prophylaxis for one of his patients.

Classify into patient factors and operation factors – there is NICE guidance on this subject that you should be aware of.

Patient-related factors include:

- Age of greater than 60 years
- Immobility
- History of continuous travel of more than 3 hours – 4 weeks before or after surgery
- A central venous catheter in situ
- Obesity
- Personal or family history of VTE
- Pregnancy
- Use of oral contraceptives.

Disease-related factors include:

- Active cancer or cancer treatment
- Acute heart or respiratory failure
- An acute medical illness
- Severe infection
- Inflammatory disease
- Myeloproliferative disease
- Recent myocardial infarction or stroke
- Inherited thrombophilias such as Factor V Leiden.

What can be done to reduce a patient's risk of suffering from a venous thromboembolism?

You might want to divide your answer into physical and mechanical methods or pre-, intra- and post-op.

Pre-operatively all patients should be risk-stratified for VTE and then fitted with well-fitting thigh or knee length graduated compression stockings and those at increased risk should receive low molecular weight heparin. The risks and benefits of stopping pre-existing established anti-coagulation should be considered.

Intra-operatively it is important to keep the patient well hydrated and pay careful attention to positioning. Whilst on the operating table intermittent pneumatic compression devices can be applied to the calves for the duration of the operation.

Regional anaesthetic techniques have been shown to reduce the risk of VTE.

Post-operatively keeping the patient well hydrated and encouraging early mobility reduces risk of VTE.

How would you classify the risk of venous thromboembolism in a 58-year-old obese female, with a history of breast cancer 5 years previously who is undergoing total knee replacement?

This patient has risk factors given that she is obese and is undergoing lower limb arthoplasty. As she is undergoing knee arthroplasty tourniquet-induced venous stagnation may also be an issue.

What prophylaxis might you provide her with?

She should receive both mechanical prophylaxis with compression stockings and receive LMWH at a time suitable to allow for safe regional anaesthesia.

What prophylaxis might you prescribe for a 23-year-old female who is fit and well, of a normal BMI undergoing an elective excision of an ovarian cyst?

The patient is low risk and is undergoing a low-risk procedure, therefore good hydration, early mobilisation and thrombo-embolic deterrent (TED) stockings.

You are asked to assess a 35-year-old man in the emergency department who had a DVT confirmed 2 days ago. He is complaining of chest pain and shortness of breath and has oxygen

saturations of 92% on room air. The emergency medicine registrar is concerned that he is suffering from a pulmonary embolism (PE).

What clinical features may support this diagnosis?

Clinical symptoms of pulmonary embolism include:

- Dyspnoea
- Cyanosis
- Pleuritic chest pain
- Cough
- Haemoptysis.

Clinical signs include:

- Raised jugular venous pulse
- Tachycardia
- Tachypnoea
- Hypoxaemia
- Fever
- Accentuated pulmonary second heart sound
- Third heart sound
- Right ventricular heave.

Baseline blood tests have been sent, what results would support a diagnosis of PE?

- Raised white cell count
- Increased erythrocyte sedimentation rate
- Increased transaminases with normal bilirubin
- Raised troponin
- Positive D-dimer has good sensitivity but poor specificity.

What might his ECG and chest X-ray show?

ECG changes:

- Right axis deviation
- Right bundle branch block
- Atrial fibrillation
- T-wave inversion anteriorly
- ST abnormalities
- Right ventricular strain pattern of S1 Q3 T3.

Chest X-ray changes:

- Cardiomegaly
- Pleural effusions
- Hilar dilatation
- Pulmonary oligaemia if the PE is massive.

What tests could be arranged to confirm the diagnosis?

There are a number of tests that aid diagnosis of PE:

- Spiral computerised tomographic pulmonary angiography (CTPA) is the most accessible and effective form of imaging.
- Ventilation–perfusion scans are another form of diagnostic imaging which can be employed with reasonable accuracy, but this tends to be used in patients in whom a CT scan is not ideal, for example pregnant women.
- The gold standard test is pulmonary angiography but this is more invasive and difficult to organise and is usually reserved for patients in whom CTPA is inconclusive.
- Echocardiography can also be used to rapidly evaluate a patient who is shocked to evaluate the likelihood of PE.

What might an echo show in a patient with a massive PE?

An echo classically shows:

- Dilated hypokinetic right ventricle
- Dilated pulmonary artery
- Paradoxical septal shift or so called "kissing" ventricles
- Tricuspid regurgitation
- Right sided pressure
- Volume overload.

What would be appropriate treatment for this patient?

Any patient with suspected VTE should receive immediate therapeutic anti-coagulation therapy, which will prevent the propagation of clot and reduce the risk of recurrent PE. Massive PE requires immediate treatment with intra-venous thrombolysis. Patients with intermediate or high probability of PE should receive intra-venous heparin prior to imaging. Unfractionated heparin should also be given where rapid reversal of effect may be needed. Otherwise LMWH should be used and it is equally efficacious, easier to use and requires less monitoring.

As you are on the phone to your consultant the nursing staff calls you over urgently as the patient has become unresponsive and looks deeply cyanosed. Describe your initial actions.

I would assess his airway, breathing and circulation and call for further assistance. I would open his airway and give 100% oxygen via a non-rebreather mask and if he was making no respiratory effort I would commence manual ventilation. If no pulse was palpable I would commence external cardiac compressions as per the current ALS guidelines, gain intra-venous access and obtain a three-lead ECG reading. I would administer boluses of intra-venous vasoactive agents and deliver direct current external shocks as indicated by the patient's heart rhythm.

Would his arrest alter how you would treat his PE?

He now fulfils the criteria of massive PE and requires immediate intra-venous thrombolysis with a 50-mg bolus of alteplase, providing he has no contraindications to thrombolysis. He will also require endotracheal intubation, ventilation, fluid resuscitation and insertion of invasive monitoring and may require administration of vasoactive drugs, providing he regains his output.

The patient does well and makes a full recovery. What tests might he need to undergo following his discharge from hospital?

He needs investigation of potential inherited thrombophilic disorders such as Factor V Leiden, protein C&S deficiency and anti-thrombin deficiency.

You are asked to review a 24-year-old man in recovery who has just undergone intramedullary nailing of a fractured femur. Nursing staff are concerned because he is desaturating to 88% when he takes his oxygen off and he is quite confused, even though it has been almost an hour since he woke from his general anaesthetic.

Outline your initial assessment of this patient

Follow a structure for the assessment of any patient in the recovery room.

I would ensure that the patient's airway, breathing and circulatory status were adequate, that he was receiving supplementary oxygen and had IV access. I would then make an assessment of his conscious level using the Glasgow Coma Scale (GCS) and ask to check the patient's blood sugar.

Once I was sure that his vital signs were sufficient I would move on to review the anaesthetic chart making particular note of any pre-morbid conditions or physiological abnormalities that were present pre-operatively. I would ascertain what type of anaesthetic the patient underwent, whether any regional techniques were employed, what drugs and fluids were administered to him and assess how stable the patient had been intra-operatively as well as making a note of any untoward incidents. With the anaesthetic being fully reviewed possible causes of the patient's clinical condition may become more apparent, for example a high spinal block or incomplete reversal of neuromuscular blockade. As this patient has sustained a long bone fracture I would examine the admission notes to see if there were any other significant injuries sustained which may be of relevance to his current condition.

The patient has sats of 97% on 8 litres of oxygen, and his airway is patent. His respiratory rate is 30 breaths per minute, his pulse rate 120 beats per minute and his blood pressure 130/80. His GCS is 13 as he is confused and is opening his eyes to voice and moving all four limbs appropriately. He is previously fit and well and broke his femur playing football with no other injuries sustained. He received a general anaesthetic alone along with 2 litres of crystalloid and 15 mg of morphine, paracetamol and a non-steroidal anti-inflammatory drug. The anaesthetic proceeded uneventfully, the procedure taking 70 minutes in total. You note that his saturations were 95% pre-operatively on room air.

What is your differential diagnosis?

Be systematic.

The patient is tachycardic, tachypnoiec, has a moderate oxygen requirement and is confused.

He may have been slightly hypoxic prior to surgery. Working through systems, his respiratory compromise could be due to basal atelectasis or retained secretions, pneumonia, fat embolus, aspiration pneumonitis, pulmonary embolus (although this would not be high on my differential diagnosis list as he had only recently been admitted to hospital), drug or transfusion reaction.

His altered conscious level could be due to the effects of general anaesthesia, hypoxia, hypercapnoea, a coexisting undiagnosed head injury, fat embolism, excessive opiates, sepsis, meningitis, an undiagnosed ketoacidosis or a hypoglycaemia.

Other conditions such as stroke, intra-cerebral haemorrhage or space occupying lesion would be much less likely given his age and premorbid state.

A pre-existing chest infection exacerbated by a general anaesthetic or a fat embolism could account for these symptoms and signs.

What do you think is the likely cause and what other tests or examinations would you want to perform to confirm this?

Given the history of a long bone fracture and subsequent fixation and the combination of respiratory difficulties and neurological impairment I think that the most likely diagnosis would be fat embolism syndrome.

The triad of pulmonary, neurological and cutaneous signs is a common presentation and I would examine the patient for a petechial rash on the trunk or upper limbs. I would also perform a full respiratory and neurological examination on the patient to rule out other focal abnormalities. I would take blood for arterial blood gas analysis as well as a full blood count, U&Es, a CRP, liver function tests and a coagulation profile. I would ask the hospital laboratory whether they were able to perform analysis of blood, sputum and urine for fat globules as these are classically said to be present although there is no evidence that they are truly diagnostic. I would also order a chest X-ray and an ECG as fat embolism can result in bilateral hazy consolidation. I would consider imaging the patient's brain to rule out other causes of acute confusion. Fundoscopy in this patient may show retinal haemorrhages.

If all tests point to the diagnosis of fat embolism being correct, how would you manage this patient?

Treatment of established fat embolism is mainly supportive and takes the form of respiratory and haemodynamic support. Early fixation of the fracture is thought to avoid recurrent embolisation, but surgery is usually postponed until the patient is stable. There is evidence to suggest that steroids may reduce the incidence and severity of hypoxia. The main approach to managing a patient with fat embolism depends on a high index of suspicion, making the correct diagnosis and ruling out other important causes such as a traumatic brain injury.

What is the physiological mode by which fat embolism syndrome occurs?

There are two main theories. The first is the mechanical theory that suggests that fat droplets from the bone marrow enter intermedullary vessels and move through the pulmonary circulation into the systemic circulation via arterio-venous or intra-cardiac shunts. Once in the arterial system they become emboli that result in petechial haemorrhages and cerebral symptoms. The second theory is the biochemical theory, which suggests that free fatty acids from the endothelial layer cause endothelial disruption resulting in peri-vascular haemorrhage and oedema.

Further Reading

Baker PL, Pazell JA, Peltier LF. Free fatty acids, catecholamines, and arterial hypoxia in patients with fat embolism. *Journal of Trauma* 1971; **11**: 1026–1030.

British Thoracic Society Standards of Care Committee Pulmonary Embolism Guideline Development Group. British Thoracic Society guidelines for the management of suspected acute pulmonary embolism. *Thorax*. 2003; **58**(6): 470–483.

Johnson KD, Cadambi A, Seibert GB. Incidence of adult respiratory distress syndrome in patients with multiple musculoskeletal injuries: effect of early operative stabilization of fractures. *Journal of Trauma*. 1985; **23**: 375–384.

Morton KS, Kendall MJ. Fat embolism: its production and source of fat. *Canadian Journal of Surgery*. 1965; **8**: 214–218.

National Institute for Health and Clinical Excellence (NICE). CG92 Venous thromboembolism - reducing the risk. www.nice.org.uk/guidance/CG92.

Rokkanen P, Alho A, Avikainen V, et al. The efficacy of corticosteroids in severe trauma. *Surgery Gynecology & Obstetrics* 1974; **138**: 69–73.

Hepatic medicine

1.6.1. Hepatic failure – Matt Thomas

This topic is presented as it might be encountered in the clinical science SOE, but could be met in the clinical section as a case-based discussion.

What are the major functions of the liver?

The liver is the largest gland in the body and many of its most important functions are metabolic, but there is also a significant immune function and an essential role in coagulation.

Tell me more about the metabolic role of the liver

The liver has a role in almost all areas of metabolism, including carbohydrates, fats, proteins and urea, bilirubin and vitamins, not to mention drug and hormone metabolism. Regarding carbohydrates, the liver has a key part in glucose homeostasis; it stores glucose as glycogen and is the major site of gluconeogenesis from amino acids, lactate, pyruvate, and glycerol. The liver is the site of much protein synthesis, including albumin, clotting factors II, VII, IX and X, acute phase proteins, complement and cytokines, for example thrombopoietin. It is also the major site of urea synthesis from amino acids and ammonia. The liver synthesises and excretes bilirubin from haem breakdown products. The formation of bile is essential for elimination of lipid-soluble toxins and cholesterol and for the digestion and absorption of lipids and lipid-soluble vitamins. Some vitamins are stored in the liver, for example A, D, E and B12, while others, for example vitamin D, require the liver for their effect. Finally the liver is the site of phase 1 and 2 metabolism of drugs and other toxins.

Please tell me about the immune functions of the liver

Not only does the liver protect the systemic circulation from the onslaught of material from the gut but it also has effects on systemic innate and adaptive immunity. Kupffer cells are modified macrophages within hepatic sinusoids that remove endotoxin and other antigens and pathogens derived from the portal circulation. Hepatic dendritic cells are potent phagocytes and cytokine releasers when stimulated. The liver synthesises complement and IgA is

Dr. Podcast Scripts for the Final FRCA, ed. Rebecca A. Leslie, Emily K. Johnson,
Gary Thomas and Alexander P. L. Goodwin.   Published by Cambridge University Press.

taken up and released into the biliary tree. Balancing the activation of the immune system, the liver has an important role in the development of immune tolerance to self.

And what about coagulation?

Well, the liver synthesises both pro- and anti-coagulant proteins, and is a source of thrombopoietin, a stimulator of platelet synthesis. The pro-coagulants produced are factors II (prothrombin), VII, IX and X. Factors VII, IX and X are crucial in the generation of thrombin from prothrombin when bound by tissue factor in the initiation of clotting. The liver also makes proteins C and S, which are part of the natural anti-coagulation pathways. Synthesis of all these proteins is vitamin K dependent.

How do you define liver failure? What are the consequences?

Be succinct with your definitions. Refer to your previous answer about the functions of the liver to give the open-ended question about consequences a structure.

Liver failure may be chronic, acute-on-chronic or acute.

Acute liver failure is a syndrome of jaundice, encephalopathy and coagulopathy that occurs in individuals with no pre-existing liver disease. It is usually further divided into fulminant (or hyper-acute), acute and sub-acute liver failure according to the time between the onset of jaundice and the onset of encephalopathy, with intervals of 1 week, 2 to 4 weeks and 5 to 26 weeks respectively. This classification does have aetiological and prognostic importance.

Chronic liver failure does not have a widely accepted definition, but is most often used to refer to signs of impaired hepatic function on a background of cirrhosis. A number of scoring systems using clinical and/or laboratory data may be used to classify chronic liver disease of which the Child-Pugh score and the Model for End-stage Liver Disease (MELD) are most common.

Acute-on-chronic failure occurs when there is progressive jaundice, coagulopathy and encephalopathy on a background of chronic liver disease.

What kinds of data are used for the scoring systems you mention?

The Child-Pugh score uses bilirubin, albumin, INR, the extent of ascites and the presence of encephalopathy. The MELD score uses bilirubin, creatinine and INR.

Thank you. Now return to the consequences of liver failure

Liver failure is the loss of its major metabolic and immune functions. Hypoglycaemia is common as glucose stores are depleted and gluconeogenesis impaired. Protein synthesis is markedly reduced with falls in serum albumin, acute phase proteins and clotting factors, the latter contributing to the coagulopathy of liver failure (as does a reduced absorption of vitamin K). Urea synthesis is impaired and systemic ammonia levels rise; this is thought to contribute to the development of encephalopathy. Jaundice develops as unconjugated bilirubin accumulates because of impaired glucuronidation. Immunity is impaired, particularly innate immunity, leading to increased bacterial and fungal infections.

So what are the clinical consequences?

Clinical features that accompany acute liver failure are: hypoxaemia, hypotension with a high cardiac output, low SVR state and abnormal cerebral, splanchnic and renal blood flows and consequently organ function, anaemia and thrombocytopenia, acute renal failure, acidosis and hyperlactataemia. There may also be worsening of the complications of chronic liver disease in acute-on-chronic failure. Infection, cerebral oedema and multi-organ failure are the leading causes of death in acute liver failure, which with the exception of paracetamol induced failure, carries a very high mortality in the absence of transplantation.

Can you expand on the complications of chronic liver disease?

These are essentially the complications of cirrhosis. Those of particular interest are portal hypertension and its sequelae such as varices and splenomegaly, ascites, hepatorenal syndrome and hepatopulmonary syndrome. There may also be additional complications associated with particular causes of cirrhosis, for example, cardiomyopathy associated with alcoholic liver disease.

Let's move back to acute liver failure. What are the common causes in the UK?

The aetiology of acute liver failure does vary according to type, but considering all together the most common cause in the UK is paracetamol overdose followed by viral infections and idiosyncratic drug reactions. In up to one in six cases no cause is found. Acute-on-chronic liver failure is commonly precipitated by sepsis, variceal bleeding, or hypotension and hypovolaemia from any cause, and by drugs including alcohol, diuretics and sedatives.

Which viruses and drugs are involved?

The viruses are hepatitis viruses A to E, and others such as cytomegalovirus (CMV), Epstein-Barr virus (EBV) and varicella zoster virus (VZV), though patients maybe seronegative. One common drug precipitant, especially in younger patients, is ecstasy (MDMA).

And what causes chronic liver disease?

Chronic liver disease is an increasing cause of mortality in the UK and is now the fifth most common cause of death. The commonest cause in the UK is alcohol. Other causes are non-alcoholic steatohepatitis (often associated with diabetes and obesity), chronic viral infections, metabolic and autoimmune diseases and drug reactions.

Now I would like to consider a couple of clinical scenarios. First, take me through your assessment and management of a 25-year-old man presenting with 3 days of jaundice and 1 day of marked confusion and epistaxis. He has a history of severe depression and IV drug use and recently lost his job.

A clear and sensible structure to your answer is a good way of impressing the examiner while ensuring you do not forget important details. In this case there are two parts to the answer: assessment and management. Answer each in turn.

The history is suggestive of acute liver failure, although a similar picture could arise from severe sepsis or endocarditis and these may be difficult to distinguish.

This patient may be seriously unwell, so I would begin my assessment with a rapid review of vital systems using an ABCDE approach to identify immediately life-threatening problems. Then I would take a history from the patient if possible and friends or relatives if not, paying particular attention to potential causes of liver failure, in this case paracetamol overdose or other drug and alcohol use, and exposure to hepatitis B and C. I would examine the patient further, looking in particular for signs of chronic liver disease.

He does not have any signs of chronic liver disease, and looks as you suggest, seriously unwell

Next I would order investigations to confirm my provisional diagnosis of acute liver failure, ascertain the aetiology and assess the severity, and to try to exclude alternatives. In this case I'd like a full blood count, clotting screen and fibrinogen, urea and electrolytes, liver function tests, calcium, magnesium and phosphate, paracetamol levels, arterial blood gases with lactate, an ECG and chest X-ray, and an ultrasound of the liver to assess size and patency of the portal vein and common bile duct. Blood should also be taken for culture and tested for hepatitis viruses A, B and C and HIV, and urine tested for blood, protein and a drug screen. While waiting for results I would give oxygen, resuscitate with IV fluid, and start N-acetylcysteine (NAC) and broad spectrum anti-biotics.

I am interested in your use of N-acetylcysteine and anti-biotics. Can you explain yourself?

Paracetamol overdose is the most common cause of hyperacute liver failure and is readily treated with NAC, which has a wide therapeutic range and may be of benefit in late presentation and some would say even other forms of liver failure. I would give anti-biotics because sepsis is difficult to exclude clinically as a cause or consequence of this patient's condition and mortality increases with each hour delay in administration, and also because prophylactic anti-biotics are indicated in severe liver failure.

Which anti-biotics do you suggest?

I would use tazocin, for its Gram-positive and especially Gram-negative cover and fluconazole as up to 30% of infections in acute hepatic failure are fungal.

I see. Now, it turns out that his paracetamol level is high and there is no history of recent IV or other drug use. He has a GCS of 9, and a bilirubin of 250, INR of 10, creatinine 450, and pH 7.2. Please continue.

The most likely diagnosis is that of paracetamol-induced fulminant hepatic failure, and this man has evidence of multi-organ failure. I would manage this patient in an intensive care unit. Management includes both treatment and supportive care. Regarding the latter, I would intubate and ventilate to protect his airway and control carbon dioxide as he has a very high risk of developing cerebral oedema and raised intra-cranial pressure. Fluid resuscitation is required and I would use 0.9% saline and colloid, with vasopressors as necessary to keep mean arterial pressure above 65 mmHg in the absence of ICP and jugular saturation monitoring.

Sedation is necessary and agents like propofol and alfentanil are appropriate. Other support-ive care, such as early nutrition and stress ulcer prophylaxis should be started and anti-biotics continued. Treatment with NAC should also be continued and the patient referred to a liver transplant unit.

Do you know the criteria for transplant in this case?

The King's College criteria for paracetamol overdose is either a pH of less than 7.25, or all of the following three signs, a prothrombin time greater than 100 seconds, creatinine greater than 300 μmol/L and grade 3 or 4 encephalopathy. These are usually applied after resuscita-tion, and the local transplant unit will advise on whether or not transfer is appropriate.

Would you put in a central and arterial line and would you correct the INR to do so?

Yes I would insert a central and arterial line. However, the INR is a key prognostic tool and should not be artificially corrected even to gain central venous access. Platelets may be given if low.

Right. Now let's turn to a different patient presenting for elective hemicolectomy for carcinoma. They have alcoholic liver disease with ascites and are still drinking. What are the potential problems?

The presence of ascites signals significant disease as the liver normally has a large functional reserve. As a result peri-operative problems are more likely, in particular the risk of acute-on-chronic liver failure or hepato-renal syndrome. Other problems may be considered system by system. The liver metabolises most drugs used in anaesthesia, and drug effects are likely to be pronounced and elimination delayed. Ascites will reform post-operatively and must be accounted for in fluid balance calculations as significant hypovolaemia and electrolyte disturbance may result. It can also compromise respiratory function. Patients are frequently malnourished and need intensive nutritional support both before and after surgery. From a cardiovascular viewpoint this patient may have a cardiomyopathy, or show the low blood pressure typical of cirrhotics. Hypotension and low cardiac output may compromise liver or renal function. They may be anaemic, thrombocytopenic or coagulopathic, which may lead to problems with bleeding and with regional anaesthesia. In chronic liver disease pulmonary shunts develop and ascites compromises respiratory function, and many of these patients are also smokers. This makes pulmonary complications like hypoxia and pneumonia more likely.

Yes, and can you think of anything else?

As mentioned, patients with liver disease are sensitive to the effects of opiates and anaes-thetics and there is a risk of encephalopathy. There is an increased risk of infections such as peritonitis, pneumonia or wound infections, so antibiotic prophylaxis must be given. There may be electrolyte problems associated with drugs like diuretics used for ascites. And the effects of alcohol withdrawal must never be forgotten and benzodiazepines and an alcohol withdrawal score should be used.

So how can you optimise this patient for surgery?

In the first instance I would want to make a full assessment taking a history and examining the patient and getting a FBC, clotting screen, U&Es and LFTs, blood gases and ECG done at a minimum, with a group and save or crossmatch according to the starting haemoglobin. An echo would be useful. From these the Child-Pugh score can be calculated which will give a rough indication of the risks associated with surgery so that the patient may be fully informed. Pre-operative assessment would be best done well before surgery to allow any problems to be sorted out beforehand. The opinion of a hepatologist and any other relevant specialist should be sought to see if there was anything that could be done to improve the patient's medical condition.

Briefly tell me how would you approach the anaesthetic?

Very carefully! This patient is at high risk of morbidity and mortality and should have consultant anaesthetic and surgical involvement and HDU care peri–operatively. I would use arterial and central venous pressure monitoring in addition to basic AAGBI and temperature monitoring and avoid hypotension and hypovolaemia. A urinary catheter and hourly urine output monitoring is also essential as fluid management is challenging especially in the presence of ascites. Propofol is suitable for induction and agents with minimal hepatic metabolism and rapid offset are ideal for maintenance, for example desflurane and remifentanil. Atracurium would be a reasonable choice for neuromuscular blockade. The relative merits of epidural versus fentanyl PCA with local infiltration or transversus abdominis plane blocks will depend on several factors, including clotting problems, presence of respiratory disease and the size and position of the surgical incision. Paracetamol may be used as long as liver function is carefully monitored. Other post-operative care will focus on avoiding precipitants of acute-on-chronic liver failure.

Further Reading

Hanje A, Patel T. Preoperative evaluation of patients with liver disease. *National Clinical Practice. Gastroenterology & Hepatology.* 2007; **4**: 266–276.

Lai W, Murphy N. Management of acute liver failure. *Continuing Education in Anaesthesia, Critical Care & Pain.* 2004; **4**: 40–43.

Marrero J, Martinez F, Hyzy TR. Advances in critical care hepatology. *American Journal of Respiratory and Critical Care Medicine.* 2003; **168**: 1421–1426.

Vaja R, McNicol L, Sisley I. Anaesthesia for patients with liver disease. *Continuing Education in Anaesthesia, Critical Care & Pain.* 2010; **10**: 15–19.

Wiklund R. Preoperative preparation of patients with advanced liver disease. *Critical Care Medicine.* 2004; **32** (Suppl 4): S106–S115.

1.6.2. Jaundice – Dana L Kelly

This topic is likely to be encountered in the basic science structured oral exam but could also form part of a case-based discussion in the clinical structured oral exam. The basic science should be quick to cover, leading plenty of time for the structured oral exam to discuss causes and implications of jaundice. It is important to be structured as this topic can potentially cover a vast amount of medicine and clinical anaesthesia.

Could you please define the term *jaundice*?

Jaundice (or icterus) is the yellow discolouration of the skin, the conjunctival membranes overlying the sclera, and other mucous membranes caused by hyperbilirubinaemia.

Jaundice is not noticeable clinically until the bilirubin concentration is over at least 35 μmol/L.

It is derived from the French for yellow – *jaune*.

Please describe the normal formation and metabolism of bilirubin?

Bilirubin is formed when haemoglobin is broken down in the reticulo-endothelial system. The polypeptides of the haemoglobin molecule are cleaved from haem, an iron-containing prophyrin derivative. The haem is then in turn catabolised to biliverdin, a green tetrapyrrolic bile pigment.

Bilirubin is created by the activity of biliverdin reductase on biliverdin. Bilirubin, when oxidised, reverts to become biliverdin once again. This cycle, in addition to the demonstration of the potent anti-oxidant activity of bilirubin, has led to the hypothesis that bilirubin's main physiologic role is as a cellular anti-oxidant.

Regarding the metabolism of bilirubin, lipid-soluble unconjugated bilirubin is bound to albumin and transported to the liver. Hepatic conjugation occurs, converting unconjugated bilirubin into water-soluble conjugated bilirubin.

The conjugated bilirubin is then excreted into bile and stored in the gallbladder. Some of the conjugated bilirubin remains in the large intestine and is metabolised by colonic bacteria to urobilinogen, which is further metabolised to stercobilinogen, and finally oxidised to stercobilin.

Some of the urobilinogen is reabsorbed and excreted in the urine along with an oxidised form, urobilin. Stercobilin and urobilin are the products responsible for the colouration of faeces and urine, respectively. The remaining urobilinogen is reabsorbed from the gut and undergoes entero-hepatic re-circulation.

Could you classify the causes of jaundice?

There are four potential causes of hyperbilirubinaemia; increased bilirubin production, impaired conjugation, congenital abnormalities of bilirubin transport, obstruction of bile drainage.

To look at these in turn:

Increased production occurs with haemolysis. Free bilirubin concentrations rise, but rarely to very high levels (e.g., <50 μmol/L). This is because the liver has substantial reserve to handle the increased production.

Impaired conjugation occurs for many reasons, e.g., hepatitis, cirrhosis, drug-related hepatic failure. Unconjugated bilirubin is raised and urinary urobilinogen may be raised, as the liver is unable to excrete it.

Congenital abnormalities of bilirubin transport are rare, except for Gilbert's syndrome. This affects 5–10% of the population, and results in an isolated unconjugated hyperbilirubinaemia.

Obstruction of bile drainage can occur due to both extra-hepatic and intra-hepatic causes, and will result in a rise in conjugated bilirubin levels. Extra-hepatic causes for biliary outflow obstruction include gallstones or pancreatic malignancy. Intra-hepatic causes include infective and alcoholic hepatitis, liver cirrhosis, primary biliary cirrhosis and primary sclerosing cholangitis. Cholestasis can occur in pregnancy or can be caused by certain drugs, e.g., contraceptives, neuroleptic agents or steroids. Itching is common, and classically the patient reports dark urine and pale stools, due to the urinary excretion of conjugated bilirubin.

Importantly, a single condition could be responsible for more than one mechanism occurring, e.g., hepatocellular damage. For this reason I believe it is more useful to classify jaundice using the above physiologically based system rather than the classic system of pre-hepatic, intra-hepatic and post-hepatic jaundice.

What are the implications of a high bilirubin for an anaesthetist?

Hyperbilirubinaemia can lead to issues with monitoring, particularly with the use of pulse oximeters. Bilirubin has a similar absorption coefficient to deoxygenated haemoglobin. This may result in artificially low saturation readings when using pulse oximetry.

Clearly the specific implications of jaundice in the peri-operative period are linked to the underlying aetiology. Establishing the cause of jaundice is extremely important because of specific accompanying morbidity depending on the underlying diagnosis, e.g., extreme anaemia in haemolysis, or cardiomyopathy in alcoholic cirrhosis.

It is also important to establish if the patient has an isolated hyperbilirubinaemia, or if the raised bilirubin represents a global impairment of hepatic function. In particular, the coagulation function should be considered, as the liver is responsible for the synthesis of the majority of the protein clotting factors. Coagulation can be significantly impaired, particularly with an intra-hepatic cause for jaundice. This clearly has implications for surgery, but also regarding the application of regional or neuraxial techniques.

It is important to establish if patients with jaundice have an active infective hepatitis. Not only has anaesthesia in the acute phase of hepatitis been shown to worsen long-term hepatic function, there are clearly issues related to infection control and protection of theatre staff from the transmission of blood-borne infections.

The action of anaesthetic drugs can be significantly affected in patients with jaundice. This can be due to hepato-cellular damage leading to impaired ability to eliminate drugs using normal mechanisms (e.g., cytochrome P450 enzymes being converted to inactive cytochrome P420), or due to reduced liver protein synthesis leading to alterations in drug pharmacokinetics.

Anaesthesia in the presence of severe liver dysfunction can predispose to the development of hepato-renal syndrome. This is a life-threatening condition that consists of a rapid deterioration in renal function in individuals with cirrhosis of any cause. Deteriorating liver function due to acute stress (such as surgery and anaesthesia) can result in acute renal failure occurring in the immediate post-operative period. The underlying cause remains unclear, although the risk seems particularly high if serum bilirubin concentrations exceed 180 μmol/L.

Two types of hepato-renal syndrome have been identified. Type 1 hepato-renal syndrome results in a rapidly progressive decline in kidney function, with a very high associated mortality (>50%). Type 2 hepato-renal syndrome is associated with development of ascites that is resistant to management with diuretics. Management recommendations include maintaining intra-vascular volume with large quantities of fluid and administration of mannitol to increase urine output.

High levels of bilirubin can directly depress myocardial conduction leading to significant conduction delay and resultant bradycardia.

Neurological function can be significantly impaired, a situation which can be worsened by general anaesthesia. Hepatic encephalopathy is caused by accumulation in the bloodstream of toxic substances that are normally removed by the liver. It is managed by suppressing the production of the toxic substances in the intestine. This is most commonly achieved with high doses of laxatives. Hyperbilirubinaemia is not normally responsible for a reduced conscious level except in cases where there is a defective blood–brain barrier such as in neonates or in central nervous system infection.

What do you know about neonatal jaundice?

Neonatal jaundice is usually harmless: this condition is often seen in infants around the second day after birth, lasting until day 8 in normal births, or to around day 14 in premature births. Serum bilirubin normally drops to a low level without any intervention required. However, rarely unconjugated hyperbilirubinaemia in a neonate can lead to accumulation of bilirubin within brain tissue. This phenomenon is known as kernicterus, with consequent irreversible brain damage.

The neurotoxicity of neonatal hyperbilirubinaemia manifests because the blood–brain barrier has yet to develop fully, and bilirubin can freely pass into the brain interstitium. Neonates are at increased risk of hyperbilirubinaemia since they lack the intestinal bacteria that are involved in the breakdown and excretion of conjugated bilirubin in the faeces. Instead the conjugated bilirubin is converted back into the unconjugated form by the enzyme β-glucuronidase and a large proportion is reabsorbed through the entero-hepatic circulation, leading to a relative unconjugated hyperbilirubinaemia.

Please consider the following case

A 34-year-old man has presented for a day-case knee arthroscopy. He plays rugby regularly and has no significant medical history. He takes no regular medications. The extremely keen orthopaedic F1 has taken some pre-operative blood tests that show the following: Hb 13.4 (13–16 g/dl), WCC 5.5 (4–11 $\times$ 10^9), platelets 350 (150–400 $\times$ 10^9), MCV 92 (76–96 fl); Na^+ 140 (135–145 mmol/L), K^+ 4.2 (3.5–5 mmol/L), urea 5 (2.5–6.7 mmol/L), Cr 75 (70–150 μmol/L); bilirubin 38 (3–17 μmol/L), ALT 14 (3–35 IU/L), AST 20 (3–35 IU/L), alkaline phosphatase 42 (30–300 IU/L).

What is the likely diagnosis?

These tests show an isolated hyperbilirubinaemia. I would ideally like to see a conjugated/unconjugated differential, but in view of the clinical history, the results suggest the patient has Gilbert's syndrome.

Tell me more about Gilbert's syndrome

Gilbert's syndrome is most common hereditary cause of increased bilirubin. It is found in up to 5–10% of the population. It has an autosomal recessive pattern of inheritance. The main symptom is otherwise harmless jaundice, caused by elevated levels of unconjugated bilirubin in the bloodstream. This is related to the reduced activity of the enzyme glucuronyltransferase, which conjugates bilirubin and some other lipophilic molecules. Conjugation renders the bilirubin water-soluble, after which it is excreted in bile into the duodenum. Gilbert's syndrome is caused by a 70–80% reduction in the glucuronidation activity of the enzyme uridine–diphosphate–glucuronosyltransferase isoform 1A1.

In patients with Gilbert's syndrome, mild jaundice may appear under conditions of exertion, stress, fasting and infections, but the condition is otherwise usually asymptomatic. The unconjugated bilirubin in Gilbert's syndrome rarely exceeds 50 μmol/L.

Are there any implications of Gilbert's syndrome for the anaesthetist?

It is important to be certain that other more serious causes of hyperbilirubinaemia have been considered and excluded.

It is also important to be aware that patients with Gilbert's syndrome may have altered capacity to metabolise certain drugs. Of particular note is the association of Gilbert's syndrome and increased sensitivity to paracetamol toxicity.

What would be your concerns if a patient developed jaundice post-operatively?

I would take a detailed history and perform a thorough examination. A new-onset jaundice immediately post-operatively would raise concerns of haemolysis related to an adverse drug reaction or blood-product transfusion reaction. It would be important to conduct an analysis of the anaesthetic technique applied, particularly related to the use of volatile anaesthetics. Classically halothane is known to cause hepatotoxicity, although this agent is now used rarely in the United Kingdom.

Hepatitis of unknown aetiology has been reported following the use of isoflurane and sevoflurane. I would also want to ensure there was not hepatic damage as a result of severe intra-operative hypoxia or hypotension, which should be evident on the anaesthetic record. I would consider infection, as sepsis can present as a derangement of hepatic function. Depending on the operation, I would want to exclude surgically induced iatrogenic biliary obstruction. I would also consider a pre-exisiting medical or surgical condition that may have not been apparent pre-operatively.

Can you tell me more about halothane hepatotoxicity?

Two types of hepatotoxicity are associated with halothane administration. These are termed type I (mild) and type II (fulminant).

Type 1 hepatotoxicity is common affecting up to 25–30% of individuals who receive halothane. It is benign and self-limiting. The diagnosis is made by mild transient increases in serum transaminase and occasionally by altered post-operative drug metabolism. Type 1 hepatotoxicity is not characterized by jaundice or clinically evident hepatocellular disease. Type 1 probably results from reductive biotransformation of halothane rather than the normal oxidative pathway. It does not occur following administration of other volatile anaesthetics.

Type II hepatotoxicity, or halothane hepatitis, is associated with massive centrilobular liver necrosis that leads to fulminant liver failure. It is a very serious condition characterised by marked jaundice and grossly elevated serum transaminase levels. There is an associated mortality of >50%. It appears to be immune mediated. Halothane metabolites bind liver proteins and, in genetically predisposed individuals, anti-bodies are formed to this metabolite–protein complex. Volatile anaesthetics other than halothane also have the potential to cause type 2 hepatotoxicity. This risk is directly related to the relative degree of their oxidative metabolism. Approximately 20% of halothane is oxidatively metabolised, compared to 0.2% of isoflurane. Hence halothane carries a higher risk of hepatotoxicity.

Further Reading

Mastoraki A, Karatzis E, Mastoraki S, et al. Postoperative jaundice after cardiac surgery. *Hepatobiliary Pancreatic Disease International.* 2007; **6**: 383–387.

Reisman Y, Gips CH, Lavelle SM, Wilson JH. Clinical presentation of (subclinical) jaundice – the Euricterus project in the Netherlands. United Dutch Hospitals and Euricterus Project Management Group. *Hepatogastroenterology.* 1996; **43**: 1190–1195.

Walton B, Simpson BR, Strunin L, et al. Unexplained hepatitis following halothane. *British Medical Journal.* 1976; **1**: 1171–1176

Weitz J, Kienle P, Bohrer H, et al. Fatal hepatic necrosis after isoflurane anaesthesia. *Anaesthesia.* 1997; **52**: 892–895.

Neurological and muscular

1.7.1. Myasthenia and muscle diseases – Helen L Jewitt

You are scheduled to anaesthetise a 37-year-old lady with myasthenia gravis for a thymectomy. What are the anaesthetic implications of this condition?

Although relatively uncommon in routine practice, myasthenia gravis is one of a group of muscle diseases with a number of anaesthetic implications, making the subject a popular exam topic. Your knowledge is explored through discussion of these issues. A useful way to introduce your answer is with an opening statement explaining the basis of the disorder and the main clinical features.

Myasthenia gravis is an autoimmune disease affecting the neuromuscular junction. The patient produces IgG anti-bodies against their own acetylcholine receptors. There is a reduction in the number of active receptors at the neuromuscular junction. The clinical picture is of weakness of the ocular, bulbar and proximal limb muscles, which is exacerbated by exercise. Women are affected more commonly than men, and there is an association with other autoimmune conditions and abnormalities of the thymus.

Describe your pre-operative assessment of this patient

My pre-operative assessment would consist of a routine anaesthetic assessment in addition to specific assessment of the patient's myasthenia. With respect to the myasthenia, my aims are to establish the duration and severity of the patient's symptoms and the regimen of medication required to produce symptomatic improvement. It is vital to establish the degree of bulbar involvement as this has implications on the risk of reflux during general anaesthesia.

The presence of significant respiratory involvement is important as these patients are more likely to require ventilatory support post-operatively. Respiratory function tests may be appropriate to quantify the degree of respiratory muscle impairment.

How would you optimise the patient?

Those with poorly controlled symptoms should have their pharmacological treatment optimised before surgery. This includes anti-cholinesterases, steroids and other

Dr. Podcast Scripts for the Final FRCA, ed. Rebecca A. Leslie, Emily K. Johnson, Gary Thomas and Alexander P. L. Goodwin.   Published by Cambridge University Press.
© R. A. Leslie, E. K. Johnson, G. Thomas and A. P. L. Goodwin 2011.

immunosuppressant agents. Very rarely a severely affected patient will require pre-operative plasmapheresis. The patient's normal anti-cholinesterase dose should be continued up until the time of surgery. Sedative premedication should be avoided as it can worsen respiratory failure. However, the judicious use of benzodiazepines is appropriate in anxious patients. Patients with significant respiratory involvement are likely to have a poor cough and will benefit from pre-operative physiotherapy. A critical care bed should be available post-operatively for patients with severe or unstable disease.

Describe the conduct of your anaesthetic

Thymectomy is carried out either via a median sternotomy or a minimally invasive thorascopic technique. In either case general anaesthesia with endotracheal intubation is required.

Induction:

- Standard induction with propofol and opiate.
- Ideally avoid the use of non-depolarising neuromuscular blocking drugs.
- This is because patients are very sensitive to the effects of these drugs, due to the destruction of acetylcholine receptors.
- If essential, non-depolarising neuromuscular blockers should be used at a reduced dose, for example one tenth of the normal intubating dose.
- In such cases drugs such as atracurium, which are rapidly metabolised, are preferable.
- Other techniques to avoid the need for neuromuscular blocking drugs, such as high-dose opiates, or the use of topical local anaesthesia applied to the airway, can be employed.
- A rapid sequence induction can be performed if indicated by patient factors such as a full stomach or predicted difficult airway.
- Patients are relatively resistant to the effects of suxamethonium.
- This is because reduced numbers of active receptors lead to a resistance to depolarisation.
- Evidence suggests that a dose of 1.5–2 mg/kg produces reliable intubating conditions.
- The return of full neuromuscular function in the form of a train of four without fade should be confirmed after suxamethonium if a non-depolarising agent is to be administered subsequently.

Maintenance:

- Maintenance of anaesthesia with volatile or a total intra-venous technique is appropriate.

Emergence and post-operatively:

- Neuromuscular monitoring is essential if neuromuscular blocking drugs are used.
- Full recovery of neuromuscular function must be confirmed prior to emergence.
- If possible the use of reversal should be avoided.
- Giving reversal effectively gives the patient an additional dose of anti-cholinesterase, which can theoretically provoke a cholinergic crises.
- Post-operative analgesic drugs which can produce respiratory depression should be used cautiously.

What factors can be used to predict the likelihood of this patient requiring post-operative respiratory support?

There are several factors associated with an increased incidence of respiratory failure post-operatively.

These include:

- Disease duration of more than 6 years
- A daily pyridostigmine dose of more than 750 mg
- Coexisting chronic lung disease
- Pre-operative vital capacity of less than 2.9 litres
- Major body cavity surgery.

What are the other post-operative concerns?

These patients need effective analgesia, chest physiotherapy and the early re-establishment of their normal medication.

What do you understand by the terms myasthenic and cholinergic crises, and how would you differentiate between the two?

These two similarly named but unrelated conditions are commonly asked about together, often the question will ask you to compare and contrast them.

A myasthenic crisis results from a relative lack of anti-cholinesterase.

It may be precipitated by missed doses of medication, surgery or intercurrent illness. It is characterised by sudden, rapidly worsening weakness.

A cholinergic crisis is provoked by administration of an anti-cholinesterase. Acetylcholine levels in the plasma are increased leading to weakness with prominent muscarinic effects. These include bradycardia, increased salivation and sweating, pupillary constriction, abdominal pain and diarrhoea.

A dose of short-acting anti-cholinesterase such as edrophonium will improve the features of a myasthenic crisis but exacerbate a cholinergic crisis.

What is myasthenic syndrome?

Myasthenic syndrome is also known as Lambert–Eaton's syndrome and is a para-neoplastic condition. It is most often associated with small cell carcinoma of the lung. It is characterised by proximal muscle weakness more commonly affecting the lower limbs. This weakness is seen to improve with activity in contrast to that seen in myasthenia gravis. There can also be autonomic effects in the form of hypotension, urinary hesitancy and constipation.

The syndrome is thought to result from anti-bodies that are directed against the calcium channels in the pre-synaptic membrane of the neuromuscular junction. The inactivation of these channels leads to a decreased pre-synaptic release of acetylcholine in response to an action potential. Anti-cholinesterases do not improve the clinical features of the syndrome.

Individuals with myasthenic syndrome are sensitive to both depolarising and non-depolarising neuromuscular blocking agents.

A 40-year-old male presents for arthroscopy of the knee. He has a diagnosis of dystrophia myotonica.

What is myotonia and what do you understand about this disorder?

Myotonia is a term to describe the failure of muscle to relax following contraction. In dystrophia myotonica there is an abnormality of sodium conductance within the muscle fibre leading to prolonged contraction.

What are the clinical features?

Most books have a long list of clinical features. Aim to organise your answer by systems, concentrating on those that have potential anaesthetic implications.

There are a characteristic group of clinical features. These include:

- General features: frontal balding, cataracts and muscle wasting affecting the sternocleidomastoid and proximal limb muscles
- Bulbar: poor swallow, slurred speech and recurrent aspiration
- Respiratory: muscle weakness, poor clearance of secretions, a restrictive lung deficit, long-standing hypoventilation, obstructive sleep apnoea and cor pulmonale
- Cardiovascular: cardiomyopathy, conduction defects
- Gastrointestinal: oesophageal dysmotility, delayed gastric emptying
- Endocrine: association with diabetes and hypothyroidism.

What are the potential issues relating to anaesthesia in this patient?

The concerns relate to the patient's underlying cardiac and respiratory disease, their sensitivity to anaesthetic drugs and the risk of precipitating myotonia in the peri-operative period. Appropriate investigations such as ECG, echocardiogram, arterial blood gases and lung function tests should be used pre-operatively if there is a suspicion of cardiorespiratory problems.

Patients are acutely sensitive to sedative and hypnotic agents such that premedication should be avoided and induction agents used cautiously. Local or regional techniques should be used wherever possible. If general anaesthesia is used, antacid premedication is recommended and intubation is likely to be required due to the risk of aspiration. Depolarising muscle relaxants are avoided due to a risk of precipitating myotonia. Invasive monitoring is used in cases with significant cardiomyopathy. Intra-operatively, maintenance of normothermia is important as cold and shivering are recognised triggers for myotonia.

Post-operatively a period of observation in a critical care setting is appropriate

What is muscular dystrophy?

The muscular dystrophies are a group of inherited muscle diseases. They are characterised by gradual destruction of skeletal muscle. Importantly there is also commonly involvement of cardiac muscle. There is a spectrum of severity depending on the genetic mutation and the degree of muscle involvement.

The classification of these disorders is based on the pattern of inheritance, which can be sex-linked, autosomal dominant or autosomal recessive. The most common form of muscular dystrophy is Duchenne's, which has a sex-linked recessive inheritance and therefore mainly affects boys. It is the most severe form of the disease and presents with the onset of muscle weakness between the ages of 3 and 5 years. This weakness is progressive and most patients are confined to a wheelchair by their early teens. Life expectancy is approximately 25 years, with death resulting from cardiac or respiratory failure.

Becker's muscular dystrophy has a similar inheritance pattern but a milder clinical picture.

Autosomally inherited forms of the disease include facioscapulohumeral dystrophy which shows a dominant pattern and limb-girdle dystrophy which is recessive.

Although these syndromes are infrequently encountered in routine practice, there are certain types of surgery where you would expect to more frequently encounter them. These include scoliosis correction and treatment of contractures.

What are the clinical features?

There can be severe respiratory muscle weakness, which may be exacerbated by a restrictive deficit due to kyphoscoliosis. Impaired clearance of secretions and recurrent chest infections are common.

Cardiomyopathy is a common finding, and there is a significant risk of peri-operative arrhythmias.

Exposure to suxamethonium can provoke rhabdomyolysis and significant hyperkalaemia due to potassium efflux from cells. Suxamethonium must therefore be avoided. There are concerns regarding a possible association between muscular dystrophy and a reaction similar to malignant hyperpyrexia on exposure to suxamethonium or volatile agents. This is based on case reports and has so far not been substantiated by prospective studies. Volatile agents are advocated by some for short cases but are generally avoided for lengthy procedures.

Further Reading

Driessen, JJ. Neuromuscular and mitochondrial disorders: what is relevant to the anaesthesiologist? *Current Opinion in Anaesthesiology*. 2008; **21**(3): 350–355.

Thavasothy M, Hirsch N. Myasthenia gravis. *Continuing Education in Anaesthesia, Critical Care & Pain*. 2002; **2**(3): 88–90.

Chapter

1.8

Respiratory

1.8.1. Pneumothorax – Matthew P Morgan

This topic would be suited to the clinical sciences SOE. As it is a potential intra-operative anaes-thetic emergency, you should be able to answer these questions confidently, to a high standard and give the impression that you could deal with such a situation in a logical, calm fashion.

What is normally found in the inter-pleural space?

Don't let such questions put you off track. By now you will understand the mechanics of breath-ing very well and should be able to talk generally about this important potential space.

The pleura is a double-layered sac which surrounds both lungs and mediastinum, being composed of an outer parietal and an inner visceral layer. Between these layers is a potential space normally containing a small amount of serous fluid although pathologically an accu-mulation of air or fluid can occur leading to a pneumothorax or pleural effusion respectively. Whilst the visceral pleura has only an autonomic nerve supply, the parietal pleura has an innervation derived from the intercostal nerves.

Why is this space so important even in health?

Again, try and think through the basics of respiratory physiology to show that you are not only a safe clinician, but one who has a sound knowledge of the basic sciences.

This space is normally maintained at a subatmospheric pressure of between minus 0.5 and minus 1.5 kPa, depending upon the level on the chest that is measured. This negative pressure is due to the elastic recoil of the chest wall springing outwards and the elasticity of the lungs pulling inwards, factors which are also important in determining functional resid-ual capacity. The regional differences in inter-pleural pressures from the top to the bottom of the lung are due to the effect of gravity on lung mass with lower regions being under less neg-ative pressure than those at the apex. This in turn has important consequences when examin-ing a pressure volume compliance curve and explains why, under normal circumstances, the upright lung is ventilated greater at the bottom compared with the apex. It can be seen there-fore that the pleura and the pleural space are essential for forming the changes in pressure which ultimately cause lung expansion.

A 20-year-old man with a history of asthma is admitted to hospital with pleuritic chest pain and dyspnoea. A plain chest radiograph shows evidence of a 3-cm pneumothorax.

Dr. Podcast Scripts for the Final FRCA, ed. Rebecca A. Leslie, Emily K. Johnson, Gary Thomas and Alexander P. L. Goodwin.   Published by Cambridge University Press.

How would you classify and treat this pneumothorax?

The British Thoracic Society has published guidelines on the treatment of pneumothoraces and these should be included in your reading list before the exam. SOE questions often result from topical or controversial guidelines from professional societies, and you should review such publications in the lead-up to your finals.

Pneumothoraces can be divided into those occurring spontaneously and those occurring traumatically either as a result of direct or indirect trauma.

Spontaneous pneumothoraces can be further classified into:

1. Primary, where no underlying lung disease is present
2. Secondary, where lung disease is present.

Therefore, in this case the patient has a spontaneous secondary pneumothorax probably as a result of a plural bleb rupture. According to the British Thoracic Society's guidelines, a trial of aspiration should be performed followed by insertion of an intercostal drain should aspiration be unsuccessful. If the pneumothorax was less than 2 cm deep and without breathlessness, the guidelines suggest that intervention would not be required. A high inspired oxygen concentration would be helpful not only to reduce the chance of hypoxia, but to increase the speed of air reabsorption by forming a large partial pressure gradient for nitrogen between the alveoli and the pleural space.

Would your management be different if this patient required a general anaesthetic with positive pressure ventilation?

When reading guidelines such as in the previous question, always think how this may apply to you as an anaesthetist.

Not only is positive pressure ventilation a risk factor for developing indirect traumatic pneumothoraces as a result of barotrauma, but it can also dramatically worsen an existing small pneumothorax. Although humans normally inspire by creating a negative inter-pleural pressure and therefore suck air into their lungs, positive pressure ventilation uses the exact opposite mechanism, forcing air under pressure into the lungs. This can result in both the enlargement of small pneumothoraces and the life-threatening complication of a tension pneumothorax where a flap of pleura effectively forms a one-way valve allowing expansion of the pleural space but not deflation. This firstly rapidly enlarges a pneumothorax resulting in lung collapse, hypoxia and increased inspiratory pressures. Secondly, as the pneumothorax increases in size, high positive pressure will be transmitted to the contralateral hemi-thorax causing displacement and great vessel compression. This will result in a dramatic decrease in pre-load and eventually cardiovascular collapse. Therefore, before instituting positive pressure ventilation, an intercostal drain should be inserted and attached to an underwater drainage system and nitrous oxide avoided.

What is an underwater drainage system, what are its components and how does it function?

An underwater drainage system is attached to an intercostal drain to ensure drainage of pleural contents whilst minimising the risk of air entrainment. There are two main types in use, a one-bottle system and a three-bottle system, each of which consists of two main elements. Firstly, a tube is attached to the intercostal drain and positioned around 3–5 cm below the surface of a water filled bottle. This tube should be wide enough to minimise resistance to flow and have a volume of at least half of the patient's vital capacity to ensure water is not drawn into the plural cavity during large volume breaths.

Secondly, the bottle should be watertight, clear and have a volume of water above the entry tube equal to half a vital capacity breath to prevent air in-drawing during deep breathing. The whole arrangement should be placed 50–100 cm below the level of the chest to prevent fluid entrainment. Finally, low level suction can be applied to aid resolution of resistant pneumothoraces.

What are the advantages of the three-bottle system that you mentioned?

As always, if you mention something, be prepared to have follow-up questions on the subject. By realising this tendency of examiners, it is even possible to direct your own SOE to an extent.

This allows fluid and air to be drained separately and accurately measured. Using the one-bottle system for this purpose would gradually alter the mechanics of the system as fluid is drained into the same bottle, which is providing an underwater seal. The water level would gradually increase over time leading to increased resistance to air drainage.

You are asked to see a patient on the intensive care unit with adult respiratory distress syndrome on a background of chronic obstructive pulmonary disease. She has just had an internal jugular central line inserted using a high approach under real-time ultrasound guidance. The nursing staff report that her oxygen saturations have reduced and her peak inspiratory pressures increased since the insertion of the central line.

What are the likely causes of this deterioration?

This patient is clearly at high risk of traumatic pneumothorax both from direct causes, including the insertion of a central venous catheter, and from indirect causes such as barotrauma. A pneumothorax following central venous cannulation can occur if the parietal pleura is breached during needle insertion and is particularly common when cannulating the subclavian vein. Although a high approach does reduce the risk of a pneumothorax occurring, the pleura can extend 3–5 cm above the clavicle cranially, thus a direct traumatic pneumothorax is not impossible.

Whilst ultrasound guidance is now recommended by the National Institute for Health and Clinical Excellence for central venous cannulation, using an out-of-plane approach can still result in a double puncture of the internal jugular vein or a lateral placement and hence cause pleural injury. An indirect traumatic pneumothorax is normally associated with barotrauma leading to bronchial or pleural bleb rupture and is more commonly seen in those with pre-existing lung disease or patients requiring high peak positive inspiratory pressure as is seen in ARDS.

Positioning patients for central venous cannulation would involve using a Trendelenberg position which in itself would increase the peak inspiratory pressures required when volume directed ventilation is being used. This positioning therefore may have precipitated a bronchial rupture. Apart from a pneumothorax, one would also want to consider as potential causes endobronchial intubation, lobar collapse, mucus plugging and pulmonary embolus.

A plain chest radiograph is performed on this patient and reported as normal. Does this exclude a pneumothorax as the cause of the deterioration?

Although plain chest radiographs are a useful first line investigation in excluding a large pneumothorax, they are not 100% sensitive and often miss small anterior pneumothoraces especially in supine patients. In patients with ARDS even such small insults can be sufficient to cause life-threatening hypoxia and therefore other modes of investigation should be used when clinical suspicion is high. Both the adhesions between pleural layers in chronic lung disease and the reduced lung compliance in ARDS can lead to unusual presentations of pneumothorax. Adhesions, for example, allow localised or loculated air collections, whilst due to poor lung compliance, a tension pneumothorax in patients with ARDS may show no signs of mediastinum shift. A lateral decubitus radiograph could be used although this is technically difficult on the intensive care unit and its sensitivity is also poor. With the advent of portable ultrasound, early use of this modality has been shown to be sensitive for diagnosis of small pneumothoraces in this patient population.

In addition, a site of drainage can be marked before intercostal drain insertion as the volumes in such pneumothoraces are often small. Finally, the gold standard for diagnosis would be a thoracic computerised tomography scan although the logistics in carrying out such an investigation would be challenging.

An intercostal drain was inserted in this patient but despite placement for 48 hours, the underwater drain is continuing to bubble. What is the most likely cause and how should it be managed?

As this is the Final FRCA be prepared to think around topics and incorporate the anaesthetic subspecialties, such as thoracic anaesthesia, into your answer.

There appears to be a communication between the bronchial tree and the pleural space, which has persisted for over 24 hours. This is known as a bronchopleural fistula. This can be a major problem for patients on the intensive care unit due to the inability to apply positive end-expiratory pressure, loss of tidal volumes, persistent lung collapse and prolonged duration of mechanical ventilation. In general, these patients are treated conservatively by continuing intercostal drainage with suction and attempting to minimise tidal volumes, PEEP, inspiratory times, peak pressures and respiratory rate. This will often lead to permissive hypercapnia being required. Ideally, rapid weaning to spontaneous ventilation is the ventilatory mode of choice although this is often not possible. Advanced ventilatory strategies are occasionally used including high-frequency ventilation and differential lung ventilation using a double-lumen tube. Small leaks can be sealed via a bronchoscope whilst larger leaks need formal surgical intervention.

Further Reading

The British Thoracic Society. Clinical information. http://www.brit-thoracic.org.uk/clinical-information.aspx.

1.8.2. Chronic obstructive pulmonary disease and asthma – Matthew P Morgan

This topic is most likely to appear as part of the SOE.

How would you assess a 70-year-old man with chronic obstructive pulmonary disease who presents for an emergency laparotomy?

This is a common situation that you will have often encountered. The examiner will want to see a well-structured approach demonstrating your competence at dealing with this important scenario.

The term *chronic obstructive pulmonary disease* (COPD) describes a wide spectrum of illness severity encompassing the clinical entity of chronic bronchitis and the pathological process of emphysema. Although these are two distinct entities, they frequently coexist. Pre-operatively I would focus on assessing disease severity and looking for related comorbidities such as smoking related ischaemic heart disease. Disease severity can be assessed clinically or by using investigations. Whilst taking a focussed history I would classify the patient's exercise tolerance according to the Medical Research Council's Dyspnoea Scale where a rating of 1 would describe no restriction of activity and a rating of 5 would describe breathlessness whilst undressing. Alternatively, I may quantify the distance a patient is able to walk on the flat or on an incline. I would ask about recent admissions to hospital with exacerbations of COPD including any previous intensive care admissions. I would actively seek evidence of current infection and quantify the amount of sputum produced. Finally, I would note the gentleman's regular oral and inhaled medications, including the use of steroids and home oxygen therapy.

Moving on from the history, a focussed clinical examination may show evidence of a barrel-shaped chest, nicotine staining, bronchospasm, active infection or cor pulmonale with an elevated jugular venous pressure and hepatomegaly. The patient's pattern of breathing, including the use of accessory muscles and posturing, may reveal dyspnoea at rest. In addition, the use of pursed lip breathing to provide a degree of positive end-expiratory pressure, therefore preventing premature airway collapse, may also be seen. Finally, the presence of a long expiratory phase would indicate long time constants of some alveoli with resultant air trapping.

What investigations may be useful?

Try to avoid the temptation to jump straight into a discussion of lung function tests, but be prepared to move on swiftly if the examiner accepts that you would look at common blood tests first.

A full blood count may reveal polycythaemia as evidence of chronic hypoxia and an elevated neutrophil count may suggest active inter-current infection. Arterial blood gas analysis may show evidence of hypoxia and compensated type two respiratory failure with a normal pH despite hypercarbia as a result of an elevated bicarbonate concentration. An electrocardiogram may show evidence of right ventricular hypertrophy, right axis deviation and right atrial enlargement.

Moving on to more specialist investigations, I would expect this patient's pulmonary function tests to show an obstructive defect with the FEV_1/FVC ratio being less than 70%, thus indicating small and medium sized airway obstruction. If an emphysematous disease

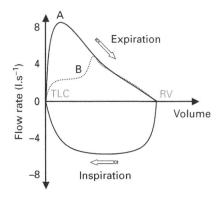

Figure 1.8.2a. Normal flow–volume loop. TLC, total lung capacity; RV, resting volume.

process is also present, the carbon monoxide transfer factor may be reduced. Although an absolute value of FEV_1 less than 1 litre is included in the British Thoracic Society guidelines for assessment for thoracic surgery, there is little evidence for its application in non-thoracic surgery. We can say however that an FEV_1 of more than 0.8 litres is required for an adequate cough and therefore values less than this would indicate a high chance of post-operative respiratory morbidity and mortality. In addition to these basic lung function tests, this patient may show evidence of reversibility with bronchodilators or steroids.

If flow/volume loops were obtained, they would show the characteristic "scooped-out" appearance to the initial expiratory phase (Figures 1.8.2a,b,c). This is because maximal expiratory flow rates during the latter two thirds of an expiratory manoeuvre are largely effort independent but vary directly with the elastic recoil of the lung and inversely with the airway resistance upstream of the equal pressure point. Lung compliance may be increased if emphysematous changes predominate or may be reduced if chronic bronchitis is the main pathology.

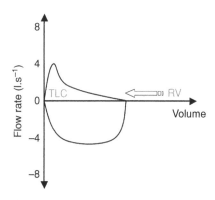

Obstructive disease reduces peak expiratory flow rate (PEFR) and increases RV via gas trapping. The TLC may also be higher although this is difficult to demonstrate without values on the *x* axis. The important point to demonstrate is reduced flow rates during all of expiration, with increased concavity of the expiratory limb owing to airway obstruction. The inspiratory limb is less affected and can be drawn as for the normal curve but with slightly lower flow rates.

Figure 1.8.2b. Obstructive disease flow–volume loop. TLC, total lung capacity; RV, resting volume.

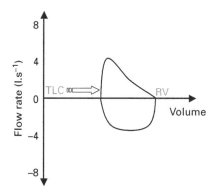

In contrast to obstructive disease, restrictive disease markedly reduces TLC while preserving RV. The PEFR is generally reduced. Demonstrate these points by drawing a curve that is similar in shape to the normal curve but in which the flow rates are reduced. In addition, the left-hand side of the curve is shifted to the right, demonstrating a fall in TLC.

Figure 1.8.2c. Restrictive disease flow–volume loop. TLC, total lung capacity; RV, resting volume.

An echocardiogram may show evidence of right ventricular failure as a result of chronic lung disease leading to elevated pulmonary artery pressures. Finally, cardiopulmonary exercise testing is now being increasingly used for risk stratification before major elective surgery. A VO_2 max of less than 15 ml/kg/min or an anaerobic threshold of less than 11 ml O_2/kg/min has been shown to significantly increase post-operative mortality.

Your history and investigations suggest that this man has severe COPD. In addition, he has been shown to have an active pneumonia with an elevated neutrophil count and a mild pyrexia. What role should a regional technique play when considering post-operative analgesia in this patient?

There is no right answer to whether an epidural should or should not be inserted in this case. Instead, the examiner wants to see your thought process balancing the risks against the benefits of such an intervention.

As well as the usual contraindications to central neuraxial blockade such as clotting abnormalities and anti-platelet agents, we need to balance the risks of epidural abscess against the benefits that a regional technique could bring to this patient with severe chronic lung disease. Although the MASTER trial showed no significant overall mortality benefit when comparing epidural analgesia to systemic opioids following major surgery, a subset of patients with severe lung disease did have marginal mortality benefits. Epidural abscess is a very rare complication of epidural use, occurring in around 1 in 200,000 episodes.

The recent third national audit project carried out by the Royal College of Anaesthetists was designed to look into the incidence and risk factors for such complications in the UK. The report found an incidence of epidural abscess following central neuraxial blockade of 1 in 24000. The incidence of permanent harm was 6 in 312450 (1 in 52000). Identified risk factors included compromised immunity, anti-thrombotic drug therapy, traumatic procedure (multiple epidural attempts), source of infection, failure of aseptic technique and duration of catheter placement. In this case, unless the patient shows signs of severe systemic sepsis, I would proceed with epidural analgesia as I feel the benefits of an improved cough, improved respiratory function and reduced thromboembolic events outweigh the risks of epidural use, including that of epidural abscess.

What mode of ventilation would you use intra-operatively?

Again, there is no right answer to this question and you could justify your answer either way.

The two basic modes of ventilation used are volume and pressure directed ventilation. The former uses a constant flow generator to deliver a set tidal volume whilst the latter uses a set pressure to deliver tidal volumes in accordance with the patient's total chest compliance. Both can be triggered either by time or by patient effort in the form of synchronised intermittent mandatory ventilation. The high peak pressures delivered when using constant flow generators have theoretical disadvantages for those patients with chronic lung disease. In addition, it is known that such patients have alveoli with a wide range of different time constants and therefore rates of inflation. Thus, using constant flow generators tends to over-expand some lung units whilst under-expanding others in accordance with Laplace's law. As this can result in a combination of barotrauma and atelectasis, it has been suggested that constant pressure ventilation may be of benefit.

What can be done post-operatively to help reduce the problems associated with chronic lung disease?

This man should be managed in a critical care environment. Good analgesia with a regional technique will help with coughing and therefore sputum clearance as well as avoid the need for systemic opioids, which may result in type 2 respiratory failure. Regular physiotherapy is essential and may include the use of incentive spirometry, percussion therapy and vital capacity breathing. Regular arterial blood gases and timely adjustment of the inspired oxygen concentration will help ensure that oxygenation is maintained whilst avoiding oxygen toxicity. Any supplemental oxygen used should be humidified to reduce drying of secretions. If the patient requires invasive ventilation post-operatively, there is controversy as to the role that an early tracheotomy may have in reducing ventilator days, and hence mortality. The Trachman study has yet to formally report the findings around the issue of the role of tracheotomies in ICU.

What causes asthma?

A broad summary of asthma and its aetiological factors is required here but try not to get fixated on one or another particular cause.

Asthma is characterised by episodes of breathlessness, chest tightness and wheeze as a result of airway narrowing. This in turn is due to a triad of smooth muscle spasm, mucosal oedema and increased secretions. It can generally be classified into atopic asthma, which occurs in early childhood in individuals with IgE hypersensitivity to common environmental allergens, and late onset asthma, which is not IgE related. The causes are multifactorial and controversial. There is evidence that environmental, genetic, infective and immunological factors all play a role in the pathogenesis of asthma although recently the so-called "clean hypothesis" has aroused particular interest. This describes how immunomodulation of eosinophils and the IgE system occurs due to modern living conditions reducing greatly the bacterial and parasite load that children are exposed to.

Can you classify the pharmacological strategies used in the management of asthma?

These can be divided into three main groups: drugs causing bronchodilation, reducing mucosal oedema or modulating the immune response. Bronchodilators are generally sympathomimetic or anti-cholinergic. The sympathomimetic drugs act as β2-adrenoreceptor agonists activating G proteins and therefore inducing bronchodilation. Examples include short-acting salbutamol, longer acting salmeterol and related drugs such as ephedrine, adrenaline and the S+ stereoisomer of ketamine. Anti-cholinergics commonly used include inhaled ipratropium. Beware that neostigmine, by increasing the concentration of acetylcholine, can precipitate bronchospasm by antagonising this mechanism. Other agents which act by decreasing bronchospasm via a G protein mechanism include volatile anaesthetic agents and phosphodiesterase inhibitors such as theophylline. A reduction in mucosal oedema is achieved primarily by using inhaled and oral corticosteroids and newer agents such as the monoclonal anti-IgE anti-body omalizumab manipulates the immune system to improve symptoms of asthma.

Should positive end-expiratory pressure be used when anaesthetising an asthmatic for a laparotomy?

Positive end-expiratory pressure (PEEP) is generally used during major intra-abdominal surgery to help minimise basal atelectasis and hence reduce ventilation/perfusion mismatch. However, asthmatic patients tend to have high levels of gas trapping and develop high levels of intrinsic or auto PEEP. In theory, applying additional levels of extrinsic PEEP may cause hyperinflation of the chest, reduce venous return and increase peak inspiratory pressures. This in turn leads to a patient who is difficult to ventilate and may precipitate a pneumothorax. However, there is controversy in the use of PEEP in the intensive care management of acute asthma with some sources arguing that it can be of benefit.

Would you use non-steroidal anti-inflammatory drugs in people with asthma?

Although non-steroidal anti-inflammatory drugs are a very effective adjunct in balanced analgesia, in around 10% of asthmatics they can precipitate bronchospasm. This is due to the biosynthesis of arachidonic acid derivatives being shifted towards leukotrienes and away from endoperoxides due to the inhibition of cyclo-oxygenase (COX) one and two. The groups most likely to be affected are those with atopic asthma, especially those with nasal polyps. Although a history of non-steroidal use is helpful in deciding whether they are safe to prescribe, different non-steroidal anti-inflammatory drugs have differing levels of COX inhibition and may therefore produce differing results. There are many other drugs used in anaesthesia that can precipitate bronchospasm including thiopentone, atracurium and suxamethonium.

Should steroid supplementation be given to an asthmatic on long-term inhaled fluticasone undergoing major surgery?

Classically, steroid supplements have been given to patients in order to avoid an Addisonian crisis precipitated by steroid withdrawal after long-term administration and a blunted stress response to surgery. Recent guidelines suggest that steroid supplementation is only necessary when patients have been taking greater than 10 mg equivalent of prednisolone daily or have stopped doing so less than three months previously. Inhaled steroids mainly exhibit a local effect although systemic effects can also be seen. They are therefore not included in these recommendations and generally supplementation is not required.

What is your approach to asthma in pregnancy?

Asthma affects around 1% of pregnancies with 10% of these requiring hospital admission either due to superimposed respiratory tract infection or worsened bronchospasm. Although asthma can improve, worsen or remain unchanged in pregnancy, these women should receive antenatal counselling and those with moderate to severe asthma should be encouraged to have early epidural analgesia. If operative interventions are required, a regional technique is the preferred method of choice. Regular medications should be continued during pregnancy and are overall thought to be safe. Salbutamol, for example, as a β2-agonist acts as a tocolytic and therefore has been used to prevent early labour. However, those taking high-dose inhaled or oral steroids may show evidence of big baby syndrome (macrosomia) and are more likely to develop gestational diabetes, now termed type 3 diabetes by the most recent classification system.

Further Reading

Bestall JC, Paul EA, Garrod R, et al. Usefulness of Medical Research Council (MRC) dyspnoea scale as a measure of disability in patients with chronic obstructive pulmonary disease. *Thorax*. 1999; **54**: 581–586.

Royal College of Anaesthetists. Third National Audit Project (NAP3) – National audit of major complications of central neuraxial block in the United Kingdom. Jan 2009. http://www.rcoa.ac.uk/index.asp?PageID=717.

1.8.3. Pneumonia – Matthew P Morgan

This topic would be well suited to the SOEs. As this is such a common and important disease, you should be able to answer the questions confidently, accurately and with recent guidelines or evidence-based medicine at the forefront of your mind.

What are the different types of pneumonia?

A structured approach is vital to ensure that you do not forget any of the key points and a brief summary will instill confidence in the examiners mind.

Pneumonia is an important and common clinical problem, responsible for around one quarter of all admissions to a general intensive care unit. Although we now have a range of anti-biotics to treat the causative organisms, mortality from pneumonia remains around 10% overall and as high as 40% for patients that develop severe sepsis. We can generally classify the disease into community acquired, nosocomial and aspiration pneumonia. This classification gives us information not only about the likely pathogens, but also the pattern of lung involvement and likely prognosis. Community acquired pneumonia can be further subdivided into primary, where no underlying lung disease is present, and secondary where lung disease is present. The most common causative organism found overall in community acquired pneumonia is the Gram-positive aerobic coccus *Streptococcus pneumoniae*. Other so-called atypical pneumonias also feature including mycoplasma, legionella and *Staphylococcus aureus*. Hospital-acquired or nosocomial pneumonia is of particular importance for anaesthetists for two main reasons. Firstly, the vast majority of post-operative pneumonias are nosocomial. Secondly, ventilator-associated pneumonia is also a type of nosocomial pneumonia. Here resistant organisms tend to be responsible including Gram-negative species, *Staphylococcus aureus*, methicillin resistant *Staphylococcus aureus* (MRSA), pseudomonas and *Klebsiella*. Finally, an aspiration pneumonia is normally precipitated by an event leading to poor bulbar or oesophageal function. Causative organisms tend to be anaerobic and the prognosis is particularly poor. Despite this microbiological knowledge, most pneumonias are termed culture negative and no single causative organism is identified. This does not mean that a causative organism is not present or responsible but rather the influence of early anti-biotic administration may affect its growth in culture. Patients should therefore be treated empirically according to clinical suspicion and their clinical condition and not simply on microbiological results. Where an organism is identified, therapy could thus be narrowed to a more specific agent.

What is the mechanism causing hypoxia in severe pneumonia?

Hypoxia in pneumonia results from a mismatch between oxygen supply and demand. Increased oxygen is required to sustain the systemic inflammatory response syndrome of tachycardia, pyrexia and high systemic inflammatory mediators. Supply is reduced due to ventilation/perfusion mismatch from bacteria and inflammatory cell parenchymal infiltration. Localised oedema also contributes which leads to overall reduced ventilation to affected lung areas. Hypoxic pulmonary vasoconstriction is less effective in these areas than during health due to the many inflammatory mediators released and hence there is an overall reduction in the ventilation/perfusion (VQ) ratio in these segments, also known as shunt.

What is ventilator-associated pneumonia?

Ventilator-associated pneumonia (VAP) is responsible for around 50% of all hospital acquired infections in the intensive care unit, prolongs mechanical ventilation and can lead to increased patient mortality. Although no formal diagnostic criteria exists, new or progressive pulmonary infiltrates with fever, leucocytosis, and purulent tracheobronchial secretions in patients ventilated for over 48 hours have been used to indicate the presence of VAP. Increasingly, evidence now suggests that directed or non-directed bronchiolavage should be included in this criteria. Although the pathogenesis is unknown, it is likely that aspiration of oropharyngeal contents is primarily responsible, therefore explaining why the causative organisms are mainly Gram-negative species as well as *Staphylococcus aureus* and MRSA. The main risk factors identified which increase the risks of a VAP occurring include nursing patients in a fully supine position, prolonged ventilation, heavy sedation, inadequate cuff pressures and possibly the use of H2 receptor antagonists, although this is controversial.

What are the correct cuff pressures, what cuffs are currently used and how do they contribute towards VAP?

Don't be put off by questions that are small print. The examiner is probing your knowledge and wants to see basic concepts applied to clinical practise.

The cuff of an endotracheal tube aims to minimise the passage of secretions from above to below the cuff. Obviously, greatly increasing the cuff pressure would form a more secure seal in the short-term but these benefits must be balanced against the trauma that this would cause from mucosal ischaemia after long-term use. Is it now thought that small folds appear in tracheal cuffs, which allow the passage of material from above to below therefore contributing towards the incidence of VAP. The use of high volume, low pressure cuffs has helped balance the benefits of a secure seal against the risks of mucosal oedema and the use of new soft flexible silicon cuffs is becoming increasingly popular. A pressure of between 15 and 40 mmHg is considered acceptable in these high volume cuffs and protection can be optimised by using an endotracheal tube of correct size.

What can be done to minimise the risk of post-operative pneumonia in a patient with chronic lung disease undergoing a laparotomy?

This is a bread and butter issue for anaesthetists and one that you should be able to talk at great length about. Unlike the previous small print question, performing poorly here would not be tolerated.

The two main important factors in preventing post-operative chest infection would include providing adequate analgesia and providing good quality respiratory after-care. Regional analgesia, such as a thoracic epidural, will allow good quality pain relief to be achieved without giving systemic opioids which may result in hypoventilation, basal atelectasis and hence nosocomial pneumonia. Good regional analgesia should allow deep breathing and coughing to occur, again helping to prevent sputum retention and basal atelectasis.

Respiratory after-care should include regular chest physiotherapy, humidified inspired oxygen and the continuation of a patient's usual respiratory medications such as bronchodilators. For ventilated patients, one should follow the "ventilator care bundle" as promoted by the Institute for Healthcare Improvement's Save 1000 Lives Campaign. This bundle consists of four main elements: ensuring prophylactic anti-thrombotic measures are taken, ensuring gastric ulcer protection, maintaining the bed at a 30 degree head up tilt and providing regular sedation breaks where appropriate. The latter two of these components have been shown to reduce ventilator-associated pneumonia. An early tracheotomy in patients that are anticipated to undergo prolonged mechanical ventilation may reduce post-operative chest infection, although this is controversial and the Trachman study looked into this issue and is yet to formally report.

You are asked to see a patient on the intensive care unit with community acquired pneumonia. He has been increasingly difficult to ventilate over the last 24 hours and now has an intermittent high-grade pyrexia. A plain chest radiograph shows evidence of a large pleural effusion. What are the possible causes of this effusion and how should it be managed?

The two main differential diagnoses in this patient would be an exudative pleural effusion and an empyema. Pleural effusions are defined as fluid between the visceral and parietal layers of pleura. For an effusion to be seen on plain chest radiography at least 400 ml of fluid must be present and so smaller effusions may be demonstrated by using computerised tomography. Effusions can be divided into transudates or exudates, where para-pneumonic effusions tend to be exudate in type. Although it is normally stated that a transudate will have less than 30 g/L of protein, this is dependent upon the plasma albumin level. As this is often reduced in critically ill patients, a level of protein in pleural fluid greater than one half of the plasma level is accepted to be sufficient to term an effusion an exudate. Alternatively this may be an empyema, a collection of bacteria and pus cells which normally has a pH less than 7.2. This would certainly account for the high pyrexias that the patient has been experiencing. If any effusion, regardless of type, is causing respiratory embarrassment, it should be drained by inserting an intercostal drain. If the effusion is exudative or an empyema, a large bore intercostal drain should be used using a surgical dissection method rather than the Seldinger approach used for smaller drains suited for the treatment of pneumothoraces. It is important the fluid from the effusion be sent for microscopy and culture in order to direct anti-microbial therapy.

Further Reading

Chastre J, Fagon J. State of the art: ventilator associated pneumonia. *American Journal of Respiratory and Critical Care Medicine*. 2002; **165**: 867–903.

Hunter JD, Corey PR. Ventilator-associated pneumonia. *British Journal of Anaesthesia. CEPD Reviews*. 2002; **2**(5): 148–150.

1.8.4. Lung cancer and pulmonary fibrosis – Matthew P Morgan

This is a topic that you may not have studied since medical school. It does have important implications for anaesthetists not only from a respiratory mechanics perspective but also from an endocrinology point of view.

What are the different types of lung cancer?

Although not a topic that you may be very familiar with, the final examiners will often find topics that lay on the boundary of knowledge and apply them to the practice of anaesthesia.

Lung cancer can be divided into small cell and non-small cell types. Small cell lung cancer is most closely associated with smoking and has often metastasised on presentation. Although termed small cell cancer, these tumours can grow very large and obstruct early generations of bronchi resulting in functional unit collapse, V/Q mismatch and secondary infection. Although more sensitive to chemotherapy than non-small cell cancer, overall their prognosis is worse and is associated with different types of para-neoplastic syndromes. Non-small cell cancers on the other hand, are further subdivided into squamous cell cancer and adenocarcinoma. Adenocarcinoma is sometimes seen in patients with no history of smoking whilst squamous cell cancers often cavitate.

How do you decide whether a patient would be suitable for tumour resection?

The two main considerations here are those related to the tumour and those related to the patient. The tumour should be a non-small cell cancer type with an absence of significant mediastinal spread or distant metastases. Depending upon the location of the tumour, surgical resection may not be possible if central airways are involved. Although these factors are important, as anaesthetists we tend to focus on those considerations related to the patient and their fitness to undergo surgery.

In this instance, the British Thoracic Society has published clear guidelines outlining the main strategy for patient assessment. These guidelines include assessing a patient's nutritional and performance status, their cardiovascular function and their respiratory function. Weight loss is often used as a surrogate for nutritional status and the American Heart Association classification of cardiovascular disease used to assess cardiovascular status. If we concentrate on assessment of respiratory function, the main important factors include interpretation of arterial blood gases, spirometry values and exercise capacity indices such as those gained from CEPEX testing. Generally, patients can safely undergo a pneumonectomy if they are shown to have an FEV_1 greater than 2 litres. Patients with values less than this should proceed to have predicted post-operative values quantified and, in some centres, CEPEX testing. In this case a VO_2 max of above 15 ml/kg/min would suggest that surgery can be performed all be it with caution.

What are the systemic effects of lung malignancy?

The most notable effects of systemic malignancy include weight loss and cachexia. Although the mechanism for these problems is poorly understood, it most likely results from a combination of poor nutritional intake and increased energy expenditure as a result of pro-inflammatory cytokines including TNF-α and interleukin-6.

Small cell lung cancer is also notable in producing a range of para-neoplastic syndromes. These include hypercalcaemia resulting from parathyroid related peptide release, Cushing's syndrome from ectopic ACTH release, muscle weakness from Lambert-Eaton's syndrome and hyponatraemia from SIADH. Finally, localised metastasis and compression can result in superior vena cava compression leading to headache, facial swelling and shortness of breath.

What is the pathophysiology of Lambert-Eaton's syndrome and how does it differ from other diseases of the neuromuscular junction?

This demonstrates that one should not mention topics in the answers to questions unless you can subsequently discuss them. In this case, the mention of Lambert-Eaton's syndrome in the previous answer had prompted the examiner to ask for further clarification.

Lambert-Eaton's syndrome is an example of a para-neoplastic syndrome most commonly seen with small cell lung cancer. It is an autoimmune disease affecting the pre-synaptic voltage gated calcium channels at both the neuromuscular junctions and autonomic ganglia. Preventing opening of these channels results in reduced acetylcholine release and ultimately muscle weakness. Unlike myasthenia gravis, weakness in Lambert-Eaton's syndrome tends not to affect the face or respiratory muscles but rather proximal muscle groups such as the hip extensors. In contrast to myasthenia gravis, improved muscle strength after repeated effort is characteristic and therefore fade is not a feature. Although treatment should initially focus on treating the underlying malignancy, other management strategies include the use of steroids, immunoglobulins or plasma exchange.

How would you approach pain management in patients with advanced lung cancer, local erosion and bone metastases?

I would start by assessing the patient's pain, concentrating especially on whether there were any neuropathic features. My pharmacological management would follow a stepwise progression through the analgesic ladder starting with simple analgesics such as paracetamol and adjuvants including non-steroidal anti-inflammatory drugs. Most patients in this scenario will need strong opioids as part of their analgesic regimen. Here we have a choice of using slow release oral opioids such as morphine sulphate with breakthrough short-acting oral opioids such as oromorph. Alternatively, lipophilic opioid patches can now be used to provide consistent background analgesia. If there are elements of neuropathic pain, drugs such as the N-type voltage gated calcium channel antagonist gabapentin and the anti convulsant carbamazepine have been shown to be of help. Furthermore, evidence is now emerging that steroids such as dexamethasone and bisphosphonates can be of benefit in treating patients with symptomatic bony metastases. Finally, if pain from local erosion is not adequately controlled, regional techniques can be used for short- or longer-term therapy. Here both thoracic epidural and paravertebral blocks may help alleviate distressing levels of pain and whilst such interventions would carry risks higher than those seen in the elective scenario, these risks may be outweighed by the benefits from a palliative perspective.

What patterns of abnormality would be seen on lung function testing in a patient with amiodarone-induced lung disease?

Amiodarone is a class III anti-arrhythmic and prolongs phase 3 of the cardiac action potential. Although a very useful drug, it has a range of common and occasionally serious side effects. Amiodarone initially can cause a mild pneumonitis after starting treatment. However, in those patients with co-existing lung disease, the elderly and people who undergo prolonged treatment, interstitial fibrotic lung disease can develop. Fibrotic lung disease in general shows a pattern of abnormalities on pulmonary function testing quite different from obstructive processes. Although the ratio of FEV_1 to FVC may be normal or even increased, due to the changes in lung architecture and compliance, the absolute volumes will be reduced.

In addition, if fibrosis occurs at the alveolar capillary membrane as is the case in amiodarone-induced pulmonary fibrosis, this will result in a decrease in both diffusing capacity (DLCO) and carbon monoxide uptake (KCO).

What are the other causes of fibrotic lung disease?

We can divide these causes into three main groups: iatrogenic, occupational and medical. Patients will often have a degree of iatrogenic restrictive lung disease following long courses of radiotherapy focussing on lung tissue. This may impact not only on their lung function and lung mechanics, but also on the external tissues of the head and neck and hence make positioning and intubation difficult. Occupational causes are concerned primarily with the so-called dust diseases including pneumoconiosis, silicosis and berylliosis. A careful occupation history will reveal those patients most at risk and examination of the chest radiograph in cases of pneumoconiosis may show evidence of pleural plaques and pleural thickening as well as the characteristic appearance of interstitial honeycombing common to fibrotic lung disease.

Finally, medical causes include extrinsic fibrosing alveolitis, which is an autoimmune disease process, and idiopathic fibrosis alveolitis. In addition, fibrosis can develop as part of a generalised autoimmune process seen in patients with rheumatoid arthritis. As discussed previously, certain drug groups including methotrexate, amiodarone and gold can also produce a drug-induced restrictive lung pattern of abnormality.

What are the physiological implications of fibrotic lung disease and how should you anaesthetise these patients?

Most of these patients will be hypoxic at rest due to a combination of poor diffusion capacity and V/Q mismatch. This is worsened by an increase in physiological dead-space. The changes in compliance will result in a downwards and rightwards shift in the pressure volume curve. Although respiratory failure is commonly a feature, many patients will decompensate and ultimately die from right heart failure. Therefore, this should be actively searched for and treated appropriately. Before embarking on a general anaesthetic, lung function tests, resting arterial blood gases, a plain chest radiograph and ideally a trans-thoracic echocardiogram should be available. When conducting anaesthesia, one should consider steroid cover if long-term steroids are being used. Due to the V/Q mismatch and diffusion capacity changes, a high inspired oxygen concentration should be used and an arterial line placed so that regular blood gas analysis can be undertaken. To match their respiratory mechanics, small tidal volumes with a rapid respiratory rate is often used with minimum peak pressures. In the presence of right heart failure, measures including minimising PEEP and avoiding α-agonists will help prevent large rises in pulmonary vascular resistance.

Further Reading

American Heart Association.
www.americanheart.org.

British Thoracic Society; and Society of Cardiothoracic Surgeons of Great Britain and Ireland Working Party. BTS guidelines: guidelines on the selection of patients with lung cancer for surgery. *Thorax.* 2001; **56**: 89–108.

Peyton PJ, Myles PS, Silbert BS, et al. Perioperative epidural analgesia and outcome after major abdominal surgery in high-risk patients. *Anaesthesia & Analgesia.* 2003; **96**: 548–554.

Renal

1.9.1. Chronic renal failure – Jessie R Welbourne

Acute renal failure is covered in Chapter 3.2.6. "Renal replacement therapies".

A 40-year-old woman presents for formation of an arterio-venous fistula to allow dialysis. She has established end-stage renal failure secondary to diabetes.

Describe your approach to the management of this patient

A structured approach is essential. Start off with an opening statement about the condition and then classify.

Patients with renal failure have a spectrum of problems affecting all of their organ systems. Their renal failure will also affect their drug handling.

A full pre-operative assessment must be made, with particular attention to co-morbidities and biochemical state. The pre-operative assessment and knowledge of the effects of renal failure may alter induction, maintenance of anaesthesia and post-operative care.

Can you expand on the effects of renal failure?

Yes, considering each system in turn:

- Cardiovascular: ischaemic heart disease, hypertension, congestive cardiac failure, peri-carditis and endocarditis
- Respiratory: pulmonary oedema and pneumonia
- Haematological: coagulopathy, specifically platelet dysfunction and prolonged bleeding time and anaemia due to iron deficiency and the reduction of erythropoietin production and red cell lifespan due to uraemia
- Endocrine: diabetes and parathyroid dysfunction which causes hypocalcaemia and hyperkalaemia
- Gastrointestinal: peptic ulceration and gastric reflux due to delayed emptying
- Immune: impaired immunity with a propensity for infection
- Nervous: neuropathy (motor, sensory and autonomic) and myopathy.

Dr. Podcast Scripts for the Final FRCA, ed. Rebecca A. Leslie, Emily K. Johnson, Gary Thomas and Alexander P. L. Goodwin.   Published by Cambridge University Press.
© R. A. Leslie, E. K. Johnson, G. Thomas and A. P. L. Goodwin 2011.

What are the main causes of chronic renal failure?

The main causes of chronic renal failure (CRF) are:

- Vascular diseases such as hypertension, embolic disease, autoimmune vasculitides and renal artery stenosis
- Glomerular diseases which can be primary, such as IgA nephropathy and focal and segmental glomerular sclerosis (FSGS), or secondary such as diabetes mellitus and SLE
- Tubulointerstitial diseases as a result of drugs, following infections or in patients with polycystic kidney disease
- Obstruction or post-renal failure which can be caused by benign prostatic hypertrophy, strictures and tumours.

How is chronic renal failure classified?

Renal failure can be classified by the cause or by functional deterioration.

The causes of renal failure may be classified into pre-renal, renal and post-renal. This classification is appropriate for both acute and chronic renal failure.

Pre-renal causes include:

- Hypovolaemia
- Inadequate renal blood flow
- Low cardiac output states.

Renal causes include:

- Acute tubular necrosis
- Glomerulonephritis.

Post-renal causes include:

- Mechanical obstructions such as prostatism, tumour and raised intra-abdominal pressure.

CRF is a functional diagnosis and is determined by the degree of reduction in glomerular filtration rate (GFR). Normal GFR is 120 ml/min. When it is reduced to 10% of normal, or less than 20 ml/min, a diagnosis of CRF is made. When GFR falls below 5% of normal, or less than 10 ml/min, a diagnosis of end-stage renal disease (ESRD) is made.

In 2002 the Kidney Disease Outcomes Quality Initiative (KDOQI) of the National Kidney Foundation (NKF) defined chronic kidney disease (CKD) as when GFR is less than 60 ml/min for 3 or more months. CKD is associated with an increased risk of CRF. CKD is further classified into five stages:

1. Kidney damage – GFR >90 ml/min and abnormalities in blood, urine or imaging to support the diagnosis
2. Mild reduction in GFR 60–89 ml/min and abnormalities in blood, urine or imaging to support the diagnosis
3. Moderate reduction in GFR 30–59 ml/min
4. Severe reduction in GFR 15–29 ml/min
5. Kidney failure GFR <15 ml/min or dialysis.

What are the surgical considerations specific to this patient?

Patients with renal failure frequently present for fistula formation or insertion of a peritoneal dialysis catheter. For fistula formation, it is important that blood pressure is kept as near normal as possible to maintain limb perfusion. The possibilities of a regional or local infiltration technique may avoid the risks of general anaesthesia while providing good analgesia and maintaining perfusion. However, the choice of anaesthetic technique may be influenced by surgical preference. There may be concern that a regional nerve block may mask the pain of an ischaemic limb following complications of fistula formation.

Wound healing is impaired and coagulation may also be affected by renal failure, with resulting surgical complications.

What examination findings are of particular importance?

Assessment of fluid status is important, by looking at heart rate, blood pressure, CVP or JVP, extent of oedema and weight trends. Fluid status should be assessed as fluid over-load, pulmonary oedema, and pleural effusions may be present and should be treated pre-operatively.

What investigations are important?

Here is a golden opportunity to show you are safe, which is an important fact to convey in any anaesthetic exam!

Of particular relevance in renal failure is the most recent potassium level. If there has been absent or inadequate dialysis and poor renal function, this is likely to be raised. This may result in significant arrhythmias peri-operatively. If the serum potassium is >6.0 mmol/L then surgery should be delayed as correcting the hyperkalaemia is the priority. Suxamethonium should ideally be avoided in these patients, as its use will result in a rise in serum potassium. A single dose of suxamethonium may increase the potassium by 0.5 to 1 mmol/L.

A full blood count may reveal a normochromic, normocytic anaemia. In chronic renal failure this is secondary to decreased erythropoietin secretion.

The 2,3-DPG concentration in the red cell is increased in chronic anaemia, so aiding the offloading of oxygen to the tissues. It is for this reason that some anaesthetists will proceed with surgery when the patient's haemoglobin concentration is as low as 6 g/L. However, the predicted operative blood loss, which may be affected by underlying coagulopathy and platelet dysfunction, will often dictate the need for a higher pre-operative haemoglobin concentration.

Platelet count and function may be impaired and there may be a coagulopathy secondary to uraemia. Significant disturbances should be corrected pre-operatively. It is important to note that the tests of coagulation and platelets may be normal, but it is often the bleeding time that is prolonged.

The severity of uraemia is important, and this has multi-system effects such as:

- Peri-carditis
- Encephalopathy
- Peripheral neuropathy
- GI effects: anorexia, nausea, delayed gastric emptying, vomition and diarrhoea
- Dermatological: dry skin, bruising, pruritis
- Restless leg syndrome
- Fatigue

- Coagulopathy secondary to platelet dysfunction
- Erectile dysfunction, amenorrhoea.

Magnesium levels may be high or low depending on the adequacy of filtration and this may predispose to cardiac arrhythmias.

Valvular dysfunction, effusions and ventricular dysfunction are common in patients with renal failure. Often patients will have had a series of echocardiography investigations over time, allowing the clinician to see a trend in the patient's cardiac function.

What other pre-operative details are of importance?

The timing of dialysis will particularly affect potassium and fluid status. Many centres favour 24 hours post-dialysis as the optimal time for surgery. A patient immediately post-dialysis may be fluid depleted, worsened by fasting for surgery, whereas fluid over-load is more likely if dialysis is overdue.

What are the practical factors that affect your choice of anaesthetic?

At this point, try to visualise this patient in your anaesthetic room and what your normal options include.

Depending on the site of surgery and surgical preference, regional anaesthesia may be offered to the patient. This reduces the risks associated with general anaesthesia such as haemodynamic instability.

Vascular access may be limited due to multiple previous access sites and a frail general condition.

Induction may need to be via a pre-existing permacath, with care taken to aspirate back the heparin in the line before injection of intra-venous drugs. The risks and benefits of intra-venous and inhalational techniques should be considered. A rapid sequence induction will reduce the risk of aspiration pneumonitis, however there is the risk of haemodynamic instability, which is less pronounced with an inhalational technique. Total intra-venous anaesthesia is favoured by some anaesthetists.

What factors affect your choice of drugs?

Drugs that are renally excreted will have a prolonged duration of action, for example morphine. Morphine is metabolised in the liver and excreted in urine or bile. The metabolites morphine glucuronide and morphine sulphate are renally excreted. Small single doses are safe but the dosing interval needs to be increased in renal failure. This may mean a reduced dose is administered rather than avoiding the drug altogether. Drugs that show significant protein binding will have an increased free fraction in the plasma in patients with renal failure.

Many muscle relaxants are renally excreted so the duration of action for these drugs is increased. The duration of action of atracurium is not affected by renal failure and so it is a common choice when muscle relaxation is required.

NSAIDs should be avoided as they inhibit prostaglandin mediated intrinsic renal vasodilatation.

Anaesthetic agents will cause decreased SVR and some depression of myocardial function. This results in reduced blood pressure, reduced renal blood flow and glomerular filtration rate. It is therefore important to administer intravenous anaesthetic agents cautiously to minimise these effects. Some inhalational agents with fluoride groups have been experimentally shown to be nephrotoxic, but the significance of this in practice is not thought to be significant.

Renal failure affects protein binding, increasing the free fraction of available drug, and also prolonging the duration of drug action. Low albumin and reduced levels of glycoproteins affect the free fraction due to reduced binding capacity.

Remifentanil undergoes ester-hydrolysis in the plasma and has a fixed context sensitive half-life. Its dosing and duration of action are therefore unaffected by renal dysfunction. It can provide predictable control over the onset and offset of anaesthesia.

The loading dose of a drug will be unchanged but maintenance doses are normally reduced.

Overall a balanced anaesthetic should be given, using a combination of short-acting and non-cumulative opioids, simple analgesia, local anaesthetics and cautious use of intra-venous and inhaled agents.

What complications may occur peri-operatively?

Cardiovascular instability is a common complication, particularly arrhythmias and hypotension. Particular care should be taken with anaesthetic agents as hypotension may result relating to depth of anaesthesia. Hypotension should be treated with low volume fluid challenges (100 ml). α-Agonists can produce vasoconstriction of the renal vasculature and so should be avoided. Ephedrine is better tolerated in renal failure, but should be used with caution as hypertensive surges may also occur.

Hypoxia should be rapidly corrected with increased FiO_2 and use of PEEP in the first instance. Other causes including reduced oxygen carriage due to anaemia should be assessed and corrected if needed.

What care will the patient need post-operatively?

The normal safety measures for post-operative care should be followed and a level 2 care environment should be considered. Monitoring should include pulse oximetry, non-invasive blood pressure, oxygen saturations, respiratory rate and estimation of fluid status. Bedside estimation of haemoglobin may be performed and there should be a low threshold for its use in recovery in view of the coagulopathy associated with renal failure and resultant blood loss. Post-operatively, serum electrolytes and routine biochemistry should be checked.

Analgesia should be provided with a balance of agents, including local anaesthetic, paracetamol and opioids. Caution is needed with opioids to ensure the dosing interval should be increased and the respiratory rate monitored.

Further Reading

Milner Q. Pathophysiology of chronic renal failure. *British Journal of Anaesthesia. CEPD Reviews.* 2003; **3**(5): 130–133.

National Kidney Foundation. The National Kidney Foundation Kidney Disease Outcomes Quality Initiative (KDOQI). http://www.kidney.org/professionals/kdoqi/.

Chapter

Cardiac/thoracic

2.1

2.1.1. Anaesthesia for cardiac surgery, cardiopulmonary bypass and cardioplegia – Jessie R Welbourne and Emily K Johnson

Don't panic if this topic comes up. Your examiners will either not be cardiac anaesthetists or are not allowed to use specialist knowledge in the exam, unless you are doing extremely well and have already achieved a good pass. This is a large subject, and you only need to demonstrate that you have a working knowledge of the normal principles and practice of cardiac anaesthesia.

A 68-year-old man presents for elective aortic valve replacement with coronary artery bypass grafting.

It is likely you will be questioned about the valvular defect first. The following questions give an idea how the structured oral exam may commence. (This topic is covered in Chapter 1.2.1. "Pre-operative assessment and management of patients with cardiac disease" and Chapter 1.2.7. "Valvular defects".)

What areas in the history are of particular relevance to your anaesthetic management plan?

How do we classify aortic stenosis?

What are the causes of aortic stenosis?

What are the signs and symptoms of aortic stenosis and why do they occur?

What investigations are of particular importance for this patient's anaesthetic management?

What are the principles underlying anaesthesia of a patient with aortic stenosis?

Dr. Podcast Scripts for the Final FRCA, ed. Rebecca A. Leslie, Emily K. Johnson, Gary Thomas and Alexander P. L. Goodwin.   Published by Cambridge University Press.

Would you offer a "pre-med" to a patient such as this?

A pre-operative sedative can be useful to reduce the cardiovascular effects of anxiety, including the effects of increased catecholamines. In our unit a pre-med is used routinely for all patients undergoing cardiac surgery.

Describe how you would induce anaesthesia in this patient

It pays to visualise what you do in practice and talk though it step by step. An examiner will not expect you to have had extensive first-hand experience of cardiac anaesthesia, but knowledge of the principles of managing patients with severe cardiac disease will be required.

All anaesthetic and resuscitation drugs, equipment and staff should be ready before the patient arrives in the anaesthetic room. Inotropes, vasopressors and vasodilators must be prepared in advance.

Prior to induction of anaesthesia continuous ECG using a CM5 configuration, oxygen saturations probe and invasive arterial monitoring should be established. It may be appropriate to monitor central venous pressure, insert a pulmonary artery catheter or use non-invasive methods of cardiac output monitoring at this stage.

At least one large-bore intra-venous cannula should be inserted whilst oxygen is administered, and the patient should be pre-oxygenated. If sedatives are administered as premedication on the ward, oxygen therapy should commence at this early stage.

The choice of anaesthetic agents is governed by the preference of the anaesthetist and the requirement for cardiovascular stability.

Intra-venous induction may be performed using a combination of high-dose opioid such as 10–15 μg/kg of fentanyl and a carefully titrated intra-venous induction agent such as propofol while carefully monitoring the arterial pressure. Midazolam may be used to reduce the requirement for propofol and improve haemodynamic stability. It is important to obtund the pressor response to endotracheal intubation, avoid myocardial depression and sudden decreases in systemic vascular resistance. Any adverse haemodynamic changes should be treated promptly.

A muscle relaxant is given after loss of consciousness and mask ventilation with oxygen performed with anaesthesia being maintained with a volatile agent such as sevoflurane, or an infusion of propofol, until neuromuscular blockade is adequate for intubation.

Once the airway has been secured with a tracheal tube, mandatory ventilation is continued whilst a central venous catheter is inserted to provide venous pressure monitoring and access for inotropic agents. Routine cannulation of the internal jugular vein with a large bore sheath to allow floatation of a pulmonary artery catheter introducer is advocated in many centres. Prior to surgery, the patient should have a urinary catheter and a nasopharyngeal temperature probe inserted. A temperature probe positioned to measure core temperature should also be used. Capnography should be used as per Association guidelines. Some centres advocate cerebral perfusion and processed EEG monitoring during cardiopulmonary bypass, as awareness during anaesthesia is a recognised risk. Trans-oesophageal echo is now used in most centres.

Maintenance of anaesthesia can be provided using a volatile agent or a total intra-venous technique with propofol and remifentanil. Increments of neuromuscular blockade and longer-acting analgesics will also be required. Nitrous oxide is best avoided because of cardiovascular depression, and there is a risk of expanding air bubbles within the circulation.

Which volatile agent would you use?

The volatile agent of choice is a subject of some debate, with isoflurane being implicated in coronary steal.

Coronary steal is when blood flow is directed away from ischaemic areas due to vasodilatation of healthy coronary arteries. However, this is not thought to be a major consideration clinically and isoflurane can be used. Desflurane may be best avoided as it can cause sympathetic stimulation and tachycardias.

What can you tell me about ischaemic pre-conditioning?

Don't panic if you don't know much on the subject, if you get asked this you are doing well!

Ischaemic preconditioning involves the induction of short ischaemic periods prior to a period of prolonged tissue ischaemia. The brief ischaemic periods have been shown to render the tissue more resistant to the adverse effects of prolonged ischaemia or reperfusion. The mechanism underlying this phenomenon is thought to involve reactive oxygen species triggering the release of endogenous agents such as:

- Adenosine
- Nitric oxide
- Heat shock protein
- Protein kinase C
- Mitochondrial ATP-dependent potassium channels.

Studies have shown that, in addition to brief ischaemic periods, pharmacological agents, particularly the volatile agents can be used peri-operatively to precondition the myocardium via similar pathways.

What is cardiopulmonary bypass, and what are its functions?

Cardiopulmonary bypass is an extracorporeal circulation that takes over the role of the heart and lungs to allow open-heart surgery to proceed. That is, it allows continued oxygenation and circulation of the blood.

The functions are to allow surgical access to a bloodless and motionless heart and provide the patient with oxygenated, non-pulsatile blood flow at a predetermined temperature and pressure. Carbon dioxide can also be removed by the bypass machine. Anaesthetic vapour and vasopressors or vasodilators may be added to this flow. The cardiopulmonary bypass machine can also enable rapid cooling or heating of blood whenever required, and temperatures between 15 and 37°C can be used.

Which operations require cardiopulmonary bypass?

Cardiopulmonary bypass is required for coronary artery bypass surgery, valve surgery, repair of large septal defects and congenital heart defects. It is also necessary for heart and lung transplants and repair of some aneurysms.

Newer techniques are evolving which avoid the use of cardiopulmonary bypass. These include minimally invasive direct coronary artery bypass surgery, robotic surgery or endovascular valve surgery. These techniques are referred to as "off pump" surgery.

What are the key steps in instituting cardiopulmonary bypass?

The skin is prepared and draped by the surgical team, and a median sternotomy is performed soon after skin incision. The surgical stimulation of this and perhaps concurrent harvesting of leg veins may result in a surge in blood pressure and pulse rate, which will need intervention without producing negative inotropy. A short-acting opioid is often used. Blood samples for measurement of baseline routine biochemical and haematological variables are sent prior to cardiopulmonary bypass. Before the arterial and venous bypass cannula are inserted, the patient will need to be fully anti-coagulated. Heparin should be administered via the central line at a dose of 3 mg or 300 IU/kg. An activated clotting time should be checked after 3 minutes to ensure adequate anti-coagulation. The ACT should be 4 times normal, which is 100–140 seconds, to allow bypass to proceed.

The addition of "pump-priming" solution to the extracorporeal circuit will result in a fall in haematocrit during bypass, which potentially improves microcirculatory blood flow. The solution can be crystalloid, such as Hartmann's, heparin and occasionally mannitol. The systolic pressure may need to be reduced to 80–100 mmHg to reduce the risk of aortic dissection at the time of aortic cross-clamping. Cardioplegia solution should be prepared and administered in a bubble-free pressurised circuit, if it is to be used.

Once the patient is on bypass, the ventilator can be turned off and an infusion of propofol started, or a volatile agent can be used by mounting the vapouriser on the bypass machine.

What are the key components of the cardiopulmonary bypass circuit?

Remember to keep it simple – it's just a circuit with tubes in and out, a pump, an oxygenator and a heat exchanger.

Venous cannulae from the superior and inferior vena cava or right atrium drain blood into a reservoir. Filtered blood from the suction can be added to the reservoir. The blood is passed through an oxygenator, normally a membrane oxygenator, and a heat exchanger, before being pumped through a filter into the arterial cannula, which is normally inserted into the ascending aorta distal to the cross-clamp, so returning blood to the patient's circulation.

What do you know about blood pumps?

The pumps used are either roller or centrifugal pumps and are required to deliver flow against resistance. They must avoid any areas of blood stasis potentially causing emboli or turbulence, which may cause haemolysis. The pumps deliver a flow of 2.4 L/min/m^2, to correspond with a normal cardiac index. In contrast to the physiological circulation, the flow delivered is non-pulsatile.

You mentioned membrane oxygenators, do you know any other types of oxygenators and their advantages and disadvantages?

Yes, I am aware of membrane and bubble oxygenators.

Membrane oxygenators are most commonly used. They contain hollow fibres giving a large surface area for gas exchange, which occurs down concentration gradients.

Bubble oxygenators are when the gases are bubbled through the blood, but this leads to increased risk of air embolism and is less commonly used.

What are the complications associated with cardiopulmonary bypass?

The complications of cardiopulmonary bypass (CPB) relate to the circuit and to perfusion. Circuit related complications include:

- Obstruction of the cannulae
- Failure of the oxygenator
- Inadequate anticoagulation causing embolism
- Aortic dissection
- Air embolism
- Haemorrhage – during the surgery or post-operatively.

Complications associated with perfusion include:

- Hypothermia: careful temperature management and active rewarming are essential prior to coming off bypass
- Fluid over-load
- Myocardial stunning
- Coagulopathy: occurs particularly with pump time greater than 2 hours
- SIRS: prolonged bypass can lead to release of cytokines
- Electrolyte and acid–base disturbances: should also be corrected prior to coming off bypass
- Cerebrovascular events: 1–5% of patients affected, ranges from a transient post-operative cognitive dysfunction to a major disabling stroke.

What do you understand by the term *myocardial preservation*?

Myocardial preservation or protection aims to preserve myocardial function and prevent cell death. Cardioplegic solutions are used to achieve this. They are administered to the myocardium to cause a diastolic electromechanical arrest. A cold solution can be used to reduce metabolic rate. Cardioplegia solution is stored at 4°C then injected into the coronary arteries or coronary sinus. Cooling is also achieved with cold cardioplegia put into the pericardium and chambers to achieve a uniformly cooled heart, ideally at between 10°C and 12°C. Further doses of cardioplegia are required every 20 minutes or when electrical activity returns. The core body temperature is allowed to fall to a target value of between 28°C and 32°C. Modifications of this technique are used in different centres.

What is the composition of cardioplegia solution?

There are a number of different formulations. These are crystalloid or blood-based solutions to which a number of ingredients are added. Ringer's lactate, dextrose and saline/dextrose solutions have all been used. Potassium is the agent used to induce cardiac arrest. It is added at a concentration of 20 mmol/L of potassium chloride to depolarise myocardial cells, with procaine as a membrane stabilising agent and magnesium may also be added. The cardioplegia solution is stored at 4°C and is rapidly infused under pressure, making sure no air bubbles enter the coronary circulation. There is some debate as to whether blood cardioplegia is superior to its crystalloid counterpart due to the theoretical advantage of oxygen carrying capacity.

What is the sequence of events when coming off bypass?

There must be clear communication between the surgeon, anaesthetist and perfusionist. The patient's temperature should be returned to 37°C, the potassium should be 4 to 5 mmol/L and the haematocrit should be greater than 24%. A sinus rate of 70 to 100 beats per minute is desirable, and if sinus rhythm does not return spontaneously DC cardioversion or an internal defibrillator or temporary and pacing wire may be needed. The venous pump is gradually restricted, so allowing venous return back into the right atrium. As cardiac activity in the heart returns blood begins to circulate into the pulmonary vasculature, and artificial ventilation with oxygen and the inhaled agent is recommenced. Once the ventricles are contracting well, the circulating volume is returned to the heart.

Protamine 1 mg per 100 units of heparin is administered by slow infusion to reverse the effects of heparin, but only when surgically indicated, and at this point the perfusionist must turn off the suction. Protamine may precipitate systemic hypotension, pulmonary vasoconstriction and anaphylaxis so must be given slowly and cautiously.

What investigations should be performed post-bypass?

Serum samples should be taken for an ACT, haematology, biochemistry and coagulation screen and an arterial blood gas should be taken to allow prompt correction of disturbances.

What are the important features of post-operative care?

The patient should be looked after in a critical care environment with invasive monitoring and appropriate experienced nursing and medical care.

The patient will usually require a period of sedation and ventilation post-operatively. The length of time will depend on which anaesthetic drugs and analgesic drugs are used and whether the patient is stable. "Fast-track" cardiac anaesthesia, meaning extubation within 8 hours after cardiac surgery, has been established as routine in many cardiac centres in the world.

The patient should be normothermic, haemodynamically stable and have any acid–base or electrolyte disturbances corrected prior to extubation. Most patients will require volume expansion as they "warm up," and a high urine output as a result of the filtration of the "pump prime" can lead to hypokalaemia. Bleeding from chest or the pericardial drains in the postoperative period may need investigating, necessitating the administration of blood, platelets, FFP or more protamine. If bleeding continues, then surgical exploration may be required.

Once extubated, analgesia can be maintained using patient-controlled opioid analgesia and regular paracetamol. High thoracic epidural anaesthesia provides good haemodynamic stability throughout surgery, superior analgesia facilitating respiratory movements, and adequate muscle tone, all necessary criteria for safe and early extubation. Centres using this technique claim that immediate extubation at the end of surgery is possible.

Extubation is not contraindicated if the patient is dependent on moderate doses of inotropes.

Further Reading

Jameel S, Colah S, Klein AA. Recent advances in cardiopulmonary bypass techniques. *Continuing Education in Anaesthesia, Critical Care & Pain.* 2010; **10**(1): 20–23.

Machin D, Allsager C. Principles of cardiopulmonary bypass. *Continuing Education in Anaesthesia, Critical Care & Pain.* 2006; **6**(5): 176–181.

2.1.2. Anaesthesia for patients with cardiac disease for non-cardiac surgery – Andrea C Binks

A 75-year-old man presents on the general surgical list for an AP resection for an invasive sigmoid tumour. He had an MI 2 years ago and has since had a coronary artery bypass graft. He gets angina on severe exertion, and a recent coronary angiogram showed a stenosis of one of the diagonal arteries, not amenable for stenting or surgical treatment. He is hypertensive for which he takes an ACE inhibitor. He is also in atrial fibrillation, which is rate controlled with digoxin, and he is taking warfarin.

What are the main issues that concern you with this gentleman?

You need to summarise the salient points from the history.

   This is an elderly gentleman with significant cardiac disease who needs a major laparotomy for a cancer. He has other co-morbidities that increase his peri-operative risk and is taking medications that will need to be managed in the peri-operative period.

What would be your anaesthetic plan?

I would start off with pre-op assessment, formulate an intra-operative management plan and then plan for appropriate post-operative care.

What would you look for in your pre-operative assessment?

This is asking about pre-operative assessment for any high-risk patient.

   My pre-operative assessment would be concerned with assessing the risk of anaesthesia and surgery for this particular patient, assessing if the patient's condition can be optimised prior to surgery, formulating a plan for intra-operative management to minimise the risk of an adverse outcome and planning for post-operative care.

   I would also take the opportunity to discuss the anaesthetic plan with the patient and inform him of the particular risks he is facing.

What factors are involved in this particular case that would put the patient at increased clinical risk?

Try and classify your answer here.

   Predictors for clinical risk can be divided into patient factors and surgical factors.
   Patient factors can be classified as major, intermediate and minor.
   Major factors are:

- Unstable coronary syndromes
- MI or coronary intervention within the past 6 weeks
- Unstable angina
- Decompensated congestive cardiac failure
- Symptomatic arrhythmias
- Severe valvular disease.

This patient does not have any major risk factors.

Intermediate factors are:

- Stable angina
- Previous MI
- Congestive cardiac failure
- Diabetes.

This patient has two intermediate factors, stable angina and a previous MI (based on history).

Minor factors are:

- Age of greater than 70 years
- Abnormal heart rhythm
- Hypertensive
- History of stroke
- Hyperlipidaemia
- Renal insufficiency
- Smoker.

This patient has three minor factors, age greater than 70, atrial fibrillation and he is hypertensive.

I would also make an assessment of his functional capacity, as reduced functional capacity is another minor risk factor.

The surgical factors are based on the type of surgery and again are divided into high-risk procedures with a complication rate of more than 5%, intermediate-risk procedures with a complication rate of 1 to 5% and low-risk procedures with a complication rate of less than 1%.

High-risk procedures are:

- Emergency procedures
- Aortic and major vascular procedures
- Long operations
- Operations producing large fluid shifts or haemodynamic instability.

Intermediate-risk procedures are:

- Minor vascular procedures
- Orthopaedic surgery
- Head and neck surgery
- Prostate surgery
- Intra-peritoneal surgery
- Intra-thoracic procedures.

Low-risk procedures are:

- Endoscopic procedures
- Superficial surgery
- Plastic and reconstructive surgery
- Breast surgery
- Eye surgery.

How would you assess his functional capacity?

Functional capacity is based on exercise tolerance and can be assessed by history. The patient's maximal oxygen consumption is estimated and expressed in metabolic equivalents or METs, where 1 MET is equal to approximately 3.0 ml of oxygen/kg/min.

Poor functional capacity would be between 1 and 4 METs, and the patient's activities would be limited to light housework, walking slowly on the flat and taking care of themselves, e.g., showering or dressing.

Moderate functional capacity is between 4 and 7 METs, and the kind of activities required to produce this are climbing a flight of stairs without stopping, walking briskly on the flat or light gardening.

More than 7 METs represents excellent functional capacity and this would include activities such as digging in the garden, lifting heavy furniture or more strenuous sporting activities.

Patients with poor functional capacity and patients who are limited by other conditions should have more detailed investigations prior to surgery.

Can you describe cardiopulmonary exercise testing?

The examiners want a basic description of the test and important findings.

Cardiopulmonary exercise testing is a non-invasive technique that allows maximal oxygen consumption to be calculated. The patients are asked to exercise on a treadmill or bicycle with continuous ECG monitoring and breath-to-breath determination of oxygen uptake and carbon dioxide consumption. This allows calculation of the anaerobic threshold, which is the amount of oxygen being consumed at the point where aerobic metabolism starts to be supplemented with anaerobic metabolism. An anaerobic threshold of 11 ml/kg/min or more tends to be associated with a good outcome following surgery.

How would you work this patient up for surgery?

Start with basic assessment and then think of more specific investigations.

Included in the pre-operative workup for this patient would be a full history and clinical examination, baseline investigations such as a 12-lead ECG, chest X-ray and blood tests including full blood count, urea and electrolytes and a clotting sample. More specialist investigations can be considered at this stage. This gentleman has a history of coronary artery disease and has had angiography recently that does not suggest any reversible lesion. His angiogram would also have an estimate of his left ventricular function, so further echo or angiographic studies are not warranted.

What advice would you give him regarding his medications?

His medications should be reviewed, and he should be advised to omit his ACE inhibitor for 24 hours prior to surgery. His warfarin will need to be stopped in sufficient time for the INR to return to 1. As he is taking warfarin for atrial fibrillation, he may not need heparin peri-operatively, but this should be discussed with his cardiologist.

Are there any other optimisation strategies that you are aware of?

This is testing your awareness of the literature and may provoke some debate as there are no right answers.

Other optimisation strategies have been discussed in the literature targeting tissue oxygen delivery. Patients are admitted to the intensive care unit pre-operatively, arterial and central lines are inserted and cardiac monitoring is instituted. Fluid therapy and dopexamine are titrated to achieve a tissue oxygen delivery of 600 ml/min/m^2 of body surface area. Unfortunately the studies to date have not shown a survival benefit from this strategy and it is costly in terms of resources.

There has also been some discussion in the literature about the use of β-blockers and statins in the peri-operative period.

The POISE study looked at the use of metoprolol 2 to 4 hours before surgery, continuing for 30 days afterwards, and they found that although the risk of cardiovascular complications was reduced, the risk of death, stroke and significant hypotension were increased. Until more studies are done looking at the types of β-blocker and duration of use, their routine use in high-risk patients cannot be recommended.

There is a growing body of evidence that suggests that patients who are taking statins prior to major surgery have better outcomes. There is also a suggestion that stopping statins in patients who are taking them can worsen outcome. There are no data however, on whether starting a statin in a patient in the peri-operative period will improve the outcome for that particular patient. There are also potentially serious side effects such as rhabdomyolysis associated with statin use, so their routine use in high-risk patients is not without risk. Until further evidence is available, patients on statins should continue them in the peri-operative period, but patients should not be started on statins de novo.

How would you manage this patient's anaesthetic?

Try and present this in a logical order, so monitoring, induction, maintenance etc.

I would ensure I had full AAGBI monitoring in place, including a five-lead ECG in order to detect myocardial ischaemia in the intra-operative period. I would put in an arterial line to monitor blood pressure and a central line and urinary catheter to guide fluid use. Ideally, I would have a trans-oesophageal echo available during the procedure to monitor fluid status and cardiac performance.

I would site a low thoracic epidural for pain relief both during the procedure and in the post-operative period. There may also be an attenuation of the stress response using an epidural. There is, however, a significant risk of hypotension so I would have a metaraminol infusion running in order to maintain coronary perfusion pressure.

I would induce the patient with propofol and a large dose of opiate to attenuate the hypertensive response to intubation, and I would maintain anaesthesia with a volatile anaesthetic agent.

If an epidural were impossible to site in this patient, I would run a remifentanil infusion intra-operatively, again to attenuate the stress response to surgery, and to maintain haemodynamic stability.

Are there any other considerations during surgery?

This is for bonus marks!

Other factors I would want to pay attention to are temperature control and glucose control. I would aim to maintain normothermia during the procedure, as there is a higher incidence of cardiac morbidity in patients who become hypothermic. I would keep the patient warm using warmed IV fluids, a warm air blanket and by wrapping the patient's head to minimise heat loss.

How would you manage the patient in the post-operative period?

Think about why, where and how to manage the patient.

The 72 hours following surgery is when most peri-operative myocardial infarcts occur as the period after surgery is associated with a hypercoagulable state and increased circulating catecholamine levels.

This patient would be best managed in a high-dependency area post-operatively. He should have humidified oxygen for 48 to 72 hours, and his analgesia well managed. He will need thromboprophylaxis, and anaemia should be avoided. His normal cardiac medications should be restarted as soon as possible.

Further Reading

Fleisher LA, Beckman JA, Brown KA, et al. ACC/AHA 2007 guidelines on perioperative cardiovascular evaluation and care for noncardiac surgery: a report of the American College of Cardiology/American Heart Association Task Force on Practice Guidelines (Writing Committee to Revise the 2002 Guidelines on Perioperative Cardiovascular Evaluation for Noncardiac Surgery) developed in collaboration with the American Society of Echocardiography, American Society of Nuclear Cardiology, Heart Rhythm Society, Society of Cardiovascular Anesthesiologists, Society for Cardiovascular Angiography and Interventions, Society for Vascular Medicine and Biology, and Society for Vascular Surgery. *Journal of the American College of Cardiology.* 2007; **50**: e159–e241.

Le Manach Y, Coriat P, Collard CD, Riedel B. Statin therapy within the perioperative period. *Anesthesiology.* 2008; **108**: 1141–1146.

POISE Study Group, Devereaux PJ, Yang H, Yusuf S, et al. Effects of extended-release metoprolol succinate in patients undergoing non-cardiac surgery (POISE trial): a randomised controlled trial. *Lancet.* 2008; **371**: 1839–1847.

Wilson J, Woods I, Fawcett J, et al. Reducing the risk of major elective surgery: randomised controlled trial of preoperative optimisation of oxygen delivery. *British Medical Journal.* 1999; **318**: 1099–1103.

2.1.3. Congenital heart disease – Richard LI Skone

Congenital heart disease (CHD) is a broad topic which can be categorised in very general terms. The number of children with congenital heart disease surviving to adulthood is increasing (there are now more adults with CHD than children). It is therefore a topic of increasing interest, even to those who do not intend to work in paediatric centres.

Should your SOE start with a general question or instruction it is important to have a clear structure prepared, as it is very easy to become confused while discussing CHD.

Tell me about congenital heart disease

Structural congenital heart disease occurs as a result of failure of normal heart or circulatory development. It occurs in approximately 1% of all live births (more frequently if one considers rhythm disturbances), and can present in childhood or adulthood. The mode of presentation varies depending on the structural abnormality and its severity.

Congenital heart disease can be an isolated phenomenon or be associated with syndromes that affect other systems. For instance Down's syndrome is associated with AVSDs and Fallot's tetralogy, while Turner's syndrome is associated with coarctation of the aorta.

In most cases the cause of CHD is unknown although factors that can increase the incidence include:

- Maternal health during pregnancy, e.g., diabetes, systemic lupus erythematosus (SLE) and other autoimmune disease
- Family history of CHD
- Drugs taken during pregnancy such as anti-epileptic medication, illegal drugs or alcohol.

About half of children born with CHD will have a minor defect and will not need any intervention. The other half will need surgical or medical treatment such as diuretics for heart failure or NSAIDs to close a patent ductus arteriosus. The treatment of complicated congenital heart disease can be either curative or palliative. Palliative treatment aims to achieve adequate physiological function, rather than normal anatomy.

The most common cardiac defects are:

- Ventriculo-septal defects (VSD), approximately 30% of all CHD
- Patent ductus arteriosus (PDA), approximately 9% of all cases
- Atrial septal defect (ASD), approximately 7.5% of cases.

How would you classify congenital heart disease?

Congenital heart defects can be classified as cyanotic or acyanotic.

Cyanotic heart disease occurs as a result of blood shunting from the "right" side of the heart to the "left". This blood by-passes the lungs and results in hypoxia and cyanosis.

Cyanotic heart conditions include:

- Tetralogy of Fallot
- Pulmonary atresia
- Transposition of the great arteries (TGA)
- Total anomalous pulmonary venous drainage (TAPVD).

In tetralogy of Fallot and pulmonary atresia physical obstruction of flow out of the right ventricle means that blood passes directly from the right ventricle to the left via a VSD.

The consequences of cyanotic heart disease include:

- Polycythaemia
- Heart failure
- Paradoxical emboli
- Cerebrovascular accidents
- Brain abscess
- Infective endocarditis
- Impaired growth and development.

Acyanotic heart disease occurs when there is left to right mixing of blood.

Conditions include:

- Atrial septal defects
- Ventricular septal defects
- Patent ductus arteriosus.

The movement of blood across these defects is usually driven by a pressure difference between the systemic and pulmonary systems.

One of the consequences of acyanotic heart disease is pulmonary overflow, which can subsequently lead to pulmonary oedema and pulmonary hypertension. Ultimately this can lead to right heart failure.

With disease progression in acyanotic heart disease the pressures in the right side of the heart can increase. When they exceed those of the left side of the heart then the blood flow across a defect can reverse (becoming a right to left shunt). This situation is called Eisenmenger's syndrome. This condition is cyanotic as venous blood bypasses the lungs.

This initial classification of CHD may satisfy the examiner if they are keen to press on with the management of CHD patients for anaesthesia. However, they may press for more information about the classification of CHD.

Do you know of any further ways of classifying congenital heart disease in babies?

CHD can also be classified as duct-dependent or non-duct-dependent circulations. They can then be further classified according to whether they are cyanotic or acyanotic.

What is meant by a duct-dependent circulation?

The ductus arteriosus (DA) forms a connection between the descending aorta and the left pulmonary artery. It usually closes during the first few days of life. Duct-dependent circulations require the DA to remain patent in order for the patient to survive. Because blood flow across the DA can occur in either direction (depending on the pressure gradient placed across it) a child might be dependent on blood crossing the duct to perfuse the lungs such as in pulmonary atresia, or to perfuse the systemic circulation such as in interrupted aortic arch or severe coarctation of the aorta.

This last point is very difficult to explain without drawing a basic diagram to show how the blood flowing in either direction along the DA can supply either the pulmonary or systemic circulation (Figures 2.1.3a,b,c).

How might a baby with a duct-dependent circulation present?

Babies in whom a duct-dependent circulation has not been diagnosed ante-natally may present in extremis when the DA closes. They may be cold, clammy, peripherally shut down and peri-arrest.

Is there anything you can do to prevent that happening, or even reverse it?

The duct can often be kept open temporarily by the use of prostaglandin E_1 or E_2 or radiologically guided stents. This allows time for further management of the child's condition to be instigated.

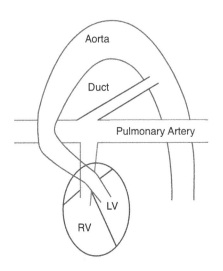

Figure 2.1.3a. Normal circulation at birth. LV, left ventricle; RV, right ventricle.

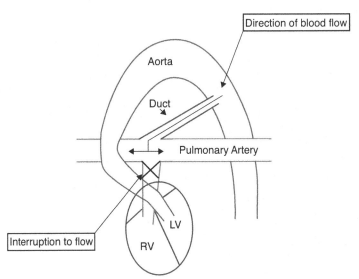

Figure 2.1.3b. Pulmonary atresia. Blood supply to lungs is via ductus arteriosus from the aorta. LV, left ventricle; RV, right ventricle.

It is unlikely that the examiner will press any further along this line in the management of a baby with CHD. They may however decide to quiz you about the management of an adult with CHD presenting for surgery. Don't forget that the basis of your answer still involves giving a SAFE and BALANCED anaesthetic.

Previous papers have discussed the anaesthetic management of patients with ASDs. The scenario has usually progressed to a patient who becomes cyanotic in spite of a high oxygen delivery. Remember that blood flows across ducts or defects along PRESSURE GRADIENTS. It is therefore possible for patients with abnormal left to right blood flow to reverse the direction of flow across a defect, i.e., becoming a right to left shunt if the systemic vascular resistance drops or the pulmonary vascular pressures increase.

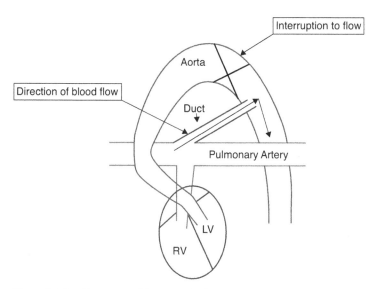

Figure 2.1.3c. Coarctation of the aorta. Blood supply to lower body is via ductus arteriosus from the pulmonary artery. LV, left ventricle; RV, right ventricle.

A right to left shunt will be refractory to oxygen therapy as the shunted blood will not pass through the lungs!

What considerations would you take into account when anaesthetising a patient who is known to have congenital heart disease?

The implications for anaesthesia in an adult patient with CHD will depend upon many factors. I would take a detailed history and examine the patient with specific questions in mind.

I would want to know what the nature of the disease is. For instance, do they have an ASD, a VSD or more complicated conditions such as a Fontan circulation.

If there is a shunt present I would like to know in which direction the abnormal flow passes.

I would like to establish the current anatomy of the patient's circulation, particularly if they have complicated congenital heart disease or have undergone surgery.

I would also like to know whether the patient has an isolated CHD problem or whether it is associated with other conditions/syndromes that might lead to problems, for example, learning difficulties or difficult airways.

I would then want to know about their current cardiac status. I would gauge this by taking a thorough history (paying particular attention to the patient's exercise tolerance), examination (looking for signs of heart failure) and organising relevant investigations (such as echocardiography).

I would also like to establish what is "normal" for that patient. For instance if they normally have oxygen saturation levels of around 90 to 92% I would not aim to try and achieve higher levels post-operatively.

Why would you worry about which direction the shunt flows?

If a shunt persists, the direction of the shunt will dictate the principle risks to the patient. For instance a right to left shunt increases the risks of paradoxical embolus. It also causes polycythaemia and low oxygen saturations, which may not be correctible with oxygen therapy.

If there is a left to right shunt then there is a significant risk of pulmonary hypertension and right heart failure.

I would also bear in mind that acyanotic heart conditions can become cyanotic if the shunt reverses as may occur if the systemic vascular resistance drops or the pulmonary vascular resistance rises.

You mentioned a Fontan circulation earlier. What is that?

The Fontan circulation is a palliative procedure that leads to patients having a uni-ventricular circulation. Blood flow returns directly from the vena cavae to the pulmonary artery. It only passes into the heart after passing through the lungs. The remaining ventricle then pumps blood around the body.

Are there any particular problems that a Fontan circulation poses for an anaesthetic?

The main considerations are:

- The need for adequate venous return. This is because the pre-load to the systemic ventricle depends on the passive return of blood. Therefore the patient needs to be adequately fluid resuscitated.
- Excessive increases in pulmonary vascular resistance should be avoided, or minimised. This is because blood flow across the lungs depends on a pressure gradient between the blood returning in the vena cavae and the single atrium (the transpulmonary gradient). As the blood flow is essentially passive, any increase in pulmonary vascular resistance will decrease flow. For a similar reason positive pressure ventilation should be avoided where possible.
- It is also important in a uni-ventricular system to work out which ventricle remains, as a morphological right ventricle pumping systemic blood may start to fail early in adulthood, posing further problems.

Because of these factors, regional anaesthesia should be considered where appropriate.

Further Reading

Burns J, Mellor J. Anaesthesia for non-cardiac surgery in patients with congenital heart disease. *British Journal of Anaesthesia. CEPD Reviews.* 2002; **2**(6): 165–169.

Nayak S, Booker PD. The Fontan Circulation. *Continuing Education in Anaesthesia, Critical Care & Pain.* 2008; **8**(1): 26–30.

2.1.4. Post-operative management of cardiac surgery patients – Catherina Hoyer

It is unlikely that this will be the only topic of a SOE, even though potentially there is a lot to cover.

What are your concerns when looking after a patient, having undergone on-pump coronary bypass grafting, on cardiac ICU?

It is best to stick to organ systems here, to keep things in a logical order. Try and start with an overview, the examiner will probably pick up on specific issues from there.

When looking after patients on cardiac ICU I would aim to prevent, or promptly diagnose and treat post-operative complications. In straightforward cases the main aims are rewarming, the correction of acid–base and electrolyte abnormalities and early extubation.

I would monitor patients for ongoing bleeding and keep a close eye on their fluid balance. Some patients may require inotropic support and can have problems with arrhythmias. Weaning off mechanical ventilation needs to be managed carefully and post-operative analgesia optimised.

Tell us a little bit more about problems with bleeding

During on-pump as well as during off-pump cardiac bypass surgery patients are given large doses of heparin, which is reversed with protamine at the end of the procedure. The use of cardiopulmonary bypass itself leads to haemodilution of all blood components. In addition, platelet numbers and function can be reduced.

The patients leave theatre with a number of chest drains in situ, which serve as monitors for ongoing bleeding. However, bleeding can also be concealed, and may present as pericardial or pleural effusions. My index of suspicion for bleeding would always be high in these patients. Close monitoring and communication with the surgical team is crucial in managing post-operative bleeding. Blood loss should be less than 200 ml/hr.

Bleeding may have surgical or haematological causes. I would check a full blood count, coagulation screen and a bleeding time. If any of the tests are abnormal, the patient may need blood products or a further dose of protamine. In the case of heavy bleeding, more than 400 ml/hr, surgical re-exploration may be necessary. In cases of most severe bleeding, this has to be undertaken immediately on the intensive care unit. Appropriate sedation and analgesia are crucial under these circumstances. Re-sternotomy carries increased in-hospital mortality.

How would you manage these patients' fluid balance?

Large fluid shifts take place during cardiopulmonary bypass. This leads to an increase in extra-cellular fluid due to the volume of priming solution given and capillary leakage. Haemodilution occurs. The extra-cellular fluid load increases with the duration of bypass. However, there may be coexistent relative intra-vascular hypovolaemia. This can be worsened by post-operative vasodilatation with rewarming, ongoing blood loss and a marked diuresis post-bypass.

Post-operative fluid replacement therapy is usually a combination of colloid and crystalloid fluids as well as blood products. I would be guided by urine output, blood pressure, heart rate and CVP trends as well as blood gas studies, whilst monitoring ongoing losses.

Otherwise healthy patients tend to tolerate haemoglobin levels down to 8 g/dl. The associated reduced viscosity has been shown to improve coronary perfusion as well as cardiac output by reducing left ventricular work.

Tell us about problems with electrolyte disturbances after cardiac surgery please

In post-operative cardiac patients I am mainly concerned about electrolytes like potassium and magnesium, since derangement of those can predispose patients to arrhythmias. Potassium tends to be low with increased renal excretion and pre-operative use of diuretics. Severe hypokalaemia may present as ECG changes, like ST depression, T inversion and U waves. Hypokalaemia can predispose to tachyarrhythmias. I would aim to keep serum potassium in the normal range between 4.5 and 5 mmol/L and replace it by infusing potassium chloride centrally.

Hyperkalaemia can also occur, and in severe cases presents as peaked T-waves, AV block and broadening QRS complexes. Treatment of severe hyperkalaemia is urgent, with calcium chloride 10 mmol intra-venously and 50 ml of 50% dextrose with 10 units of actrapid added.

Hypomagnesaemia is a common problem after cardiopulmonary bypass. It can lead to tachyarrhythmias, decreased cardiac output and prolonged ventilatory support. It should be replaced by slow intra-venous infusion of 2 g of magnesium sulphate.

How would you manage patients' acid–base balance?

Disturbances in acid–base balance are also common after cardiopulmonary bypass. Careful adjustment of mechanical ventilation is necessary to correct any respiratory component.

Metabolic disturbances need treating according to the underlying cause. A combination of fluid replacement therapy, inotropes and vasodilators is used to optimise tissue perfusion and cardiac output. Hyperglycaemia should be corrected and renal impairment managed appropriately. Careful monitoring for other causes, such as sepsis, is crucial.

How would you manage post-operative arrhythmias?

Arrhythmias are a common problem after cardiac surgery and require prompt and effective treatment. There is a multitude of possible underlying causes, which should be corrected before pharmacological treatment is commenced. Possible reasons for post-operative arrhythmias are:

- Myocardial ischaemia
- Hypoxia
- Hypercarbia
- Electrolyte imbalances
- Drugs
- Pre-existing arrhythmias
- Pacemaker failure
- Surgical damage to the conducting system.

Treatment of arrhythmias can be by physical or pharmacological methods.

Can you tell us more about physical methods

The physical method of DC cardioversion is used to convert SVTs, VT and AF back to sinus rhythm. A DC shock is applied via defibrillator paddles to the chest. The timing of shock application is synchronised with the R wave on the ECG. The shock energy delivered depends on the underlying rhythm and the type of defibrillator used.

Cardiac pacing is another physical method to control arrhythmias. It can be used in the treatment of bradyarrhythmias as well as tachyarrhythmias. Many patients will leave theatre with temporary pacing wires in situ to control transient post-operative rhythm problems. If possible, the sequential nature of atrial and ventricular contraction is maintained. That improves ventricular filling and can be achieved by atrial or sequential pacing.

What do you know about drug treatment of arrhythmias?

Pharmacological methods may sometimes involve the discontinuation of pro-arrhythmic agents, such as dopamine or adrenaline.

Thereafter anti-arrhythmic drugs can be considered.

In the treatment of tachyarrhythmias the clinical picture needs to be considered. DC cardioversion is the method of choice in supra-ventricular and ventricular tachycardias with haemodynamic compromise. In uncompromised patients amiodarone is the drug of choice for many tachyarrhythmias.

In atrial fibrillation and flutter the duration of the arrhythmia is also important. If it has been present for more than 48 hours, the patient should be fully anti-coagulated before any cardioversion is attempted. Digoxin or β-blockers can be used for rate control.

In supra-ventricular narrow complex tachycardias without compromise, vagal manoeuvres, such as carotid sinus massage, can sometimes be successful in terminating the abnormal rhythm. Failing that, adenosine can be used. Other effective drug treatments include amiodarone, calcium channel blockers or β-blockers.

Uncompromised ventricular tachycardias can be treated with amiodarone or lignocaine.

Bradyarrhythmias can be treated with cardiac pacing (internal or external), atropine or isoprenaline.

In complex or treatment-resistant arrhythmias, expert help from a cardiologist should be sought early.

How would you manage low cardiac output after cardiac surgery?

Cardiac output can be low because of pre-existing ischaemic damage or because of myocardial stunning after the use of cardiopulmonary bypass.

Firstly, I would have to ensure adequate filling, guided mainly by urine output and central venous pressures. If response to fluid therapy alone is unsatisfactory an estimate of afterload and cardiac performance would be required. This can be achieved by trans-oesophageal Doppler or PiCCO measurements. The use of more invasive pulmonary artery catheters is less common nowadays as there is no evidence they improve outcomes, and they have higher complication rates than other less invasive techniques.

I would then choose an appropriate inotropic or vasopressor agent to augment cardiac performance. Some patients may need intra-aortic balloon pumps or other assist devices.

Can you tell us more about inotropic agents?

Dopamine or dobutamine are often chosen as the first-line inotropic agents. Noradrenaline tends to be the first-line vasopressor agent.

Dopamine is a noradrenaline precursor and acts as an agonist at α-, β-, and dopaminergic receptors. It causes mesenteric and renal vasodilatation via dopaminergic receptors at lower doses. Its use at those doses for renal protection has been abandoned. At higher doses, sympathomimetic effects predominate with positive chronotrophy and inotropy via β-receptors. It also acts at α-receptors to produce vasoconstriction.

Dobutamine is a synthetic β-agonist with mainly β1-cardiac effects. It therefore causes positive inotropy but also a marked tachycardia, which can be a limiting factor in its use.

Noradrenaline tends to be the first line vasopressor because of its predominating α-effects. It also has limited inotropic activity via cardiac β1-receptors.

Adrenaline is a potent inotrope with both α- and β-adrenergic effects. β1-effects are responsible for an increase in heart rate and myocardial contractility. It also acts on α-receptors and thereby causes peripheral vasoconstriction. Bronchodilatation is caused via β2-effects.

What second line inotropes do you know about?

Phosphodiesterase III inhibitors, such as milrinone or enoximone, act via an increase in cyclic AMP. These agents decrease intra-cellular cAMP degradation via the PDE III enzyme. They therefore increase contractility whilst also causing peripheral vasodilatation.

Dopexamine is a dopamine analogue with effects on dopaminergic and β2-receptors but no α-effects. It is therefore an inodilator, which increases myocardial contractility but decreases SVR. It also dilates the splanchnic circulation.

Digoxin is also used for its inotropic properties and acts via an increase in calcium in the sarcoplasmatic reticulum.

How would you go about managing renal impairment after cardiac surgery?

Cardiopulmonary bypass decreases renal blood flow and glomerular filtration rate by about 30%. Renal failure is a major contributing factor in peri-operative morbidity and mortality and appropriate management of impaired renal function is crucial. In the first instance it is important to maintain renal perfusion pressure throughout the peri-operative period. Patients with co-morbidities such as pre-existing renal disease, hypertension or diabetes will need higher mean arterial pressures than those with no other medical problems.

Nephrotoxic drugs such as NSAIDs or aminoglycosides should be avoided if possible, or doses adjusted carefully according to plasma levels.

Fluid management is very important to eliminate any pre-renal component of renal impairment.

In established renal failure loop diuretics such as furosemide are often used to turn oliguric into polyuric failure, but this does not change the course of the disease. Renal replacement therapy is sometimes necessary to bridge the time until recovery of renal function. Continuous venovenous haemofiltration is usually the method of choice. This should be considered if there is prolonged anuria, fluid over-load, a significant metabolic acidosis or accumulation of electrolytes or metabolites.

What problems might you encounter when trying to wean the patient off mechanical ventilation?

Ideally, in straightforward cases, the period of mechanical ventilation post-operatively should be kept to a minimum. Sedation and ventilation after cardiac surgery allows for a period of stability. During that time physiological parameters such as temperature, acid–base and fluid balance and electrolytes are corrected, as well as significant ongoing bleeding excluded. Once all of these parameters are satisfactory, sedation and ventilation are weaned and the patient is allowed to wake up.

Problems with weaning may occur for a variety of reasons. It can be difficult in patients with pre-existing pulmonary disease, pneumonia, other sepsis or left ventricular failure. Surgical complications can also be responsible, for instance phrenic nerve damage, pneumothorax or pleural effusions. The use of cardiopulmonary bypass itself can also contribute to difficulties by causing neurological deficits or acute lung injury.

If ventilation is thought to be prolonged, many centres will opt for early elective tracheostomy to aid weaning.

Can you tell us more about acute lung injury after cardiopulmonary bypass?

Cardiopulmonary bypass invariably causes a degree of acute lung injury. This is usually mild and clinically insignificant. It is thought to be due to an inflammatory response caused by the exposure of circulating blood to the non-physiological surface of the bypass circuit.

About 2% of people will develop acute respiratory distress syndrome, which will significantly delay weaning and post-operative recovery. Management is as for ARDS from other causes, with pressure controlled ventilation at low tidal volumes of 6–8 ml/kg. Peak pressures should be limited to less than 35 cm H_2O. The use of PEEP is essential and FiO_2 should be kept to a minimal level required to achieve satisfactory oxygenation. Permissive hypercapnia may be tolerated with these ventilation strategies.

Mortality associated with cardiopulmonary bypass-related ARDS is significantly lower than that from sepsis or other major causes of ARDS.

Further Reading

Belisle S, Hardy JF. Haemorrhage and the use of blood products after adult cardiac operations: myths and realities. *Annals of Thoracic Surgery.* 1996; **62**: 1908–1917.

Gothard J, Kelleher A, Haxby E. *Cardiovascular and thoracic anaesthesia.* London: Butterworth Heinemann, 2003.

Hwang NC, Sinclair M (eds.). *Cardiac anaesthesia: a practical handbook.* Oxford: Oxford University Press, 1997.

Llopard T, Lombardi R, Forsello M, Andrade R. Acute renal failure in open heart surgery. *Renal Failure.* 1997; **19**: 319–323.

Myles PS, Daly DJ, Djaiani G, Lee A, Cheng DC. A systematic review of the safety and effectiveness of fast-track cardiac anaesthesia. *Anaesthesiology.* 2003; **99**: 982–987.

Shoemaker WC, Ayres SD, Grenvik A, Holbrook PR. *Textbook of critical care.* Philadelphia: WB Saunders, 2000.

Singh S, Hutton P. Cerebral effects of cardiopulmonary bypass in adults. *British Journal of Anaesthesia. CEPD Reviews* 2003; **3**: 115–119.

2.1.5. Anaesthesia for bronchoscopy – Neil J Rasburn

You have a 76-year-old man listed for rigid bronchoscopy. What information is important in the pre-operative assessment?

Patients listed for bronchoscopy fall into two categories:

1. Those having an isolated procedure for screening or sampling such as patients for thoracotomy have pre-operative bronchoscopy
2. Those having bronchoscopy for a therapeutic procedure such as tracheal dilatation or stent insertion.

It is therefore essential to evaluate the upper airway and assess for signs and symptoms of obstruction, such as stridor and breathlessness at rest. A cardiovascular history is also very important, as patients with lung cancer are often elderly smokers.

What investigations would you request?

Make sure you can justify each investigation and that you are familiar with them. Expect to be shown a flow/volume loop when discussing obstructive or restrictive pulmonary deficits. This is fundamental physiology that all anaesthetists should know well.

- CXR: mandatory to assess pulmonary pathology and to determine if the trachea is deviated
- CT and MRI may be indicated and should be reviewed pre-operatively
- Lung function tests are helpful in defining the degree of obstruction, particularly flow volume loops
- Routine bloods
- ECG
- Lateral neck X-rays should be sought in patients with a history of neck problems or rheumatoid arthritis as rigid bronchoscopy requires significant neck extension.

Does bronchoscopy always require a general anaesthetic?

No. Flexible bronchoscopy is usually carried out by respiratory physicians with topical local anaesthesia and sedation.

Make sure you have an appropriate management plan for topical anaesthesia of the airway, as this is important for awake fibre-optic intubation.

What anaesthetic technique would you use for this patient?

There is no one correct answer, think about what conditions you are aiming to achieve and what equipment you may have available. Simplify your answer to induction, maintenance and post-operative management.

The aims of bronchoscopy for an isolated procedure are to provide anaesthesia with abolished respiratory reflexes, muscular relaxation, safe ventilation and rapid emergence. I would use IV glycopyrrolate as an anti-sialogogue, if the airway is patent then intra-venous propofol is appropriate with a short-acting muscle relaxant such as suxamethonium or mivacurium.

Bronchoscopy can cause a profound vasopressor response and this must be controlled with short-acting opioids and short-acting β-blockers. Remifentanil infusions in combination with propofol or sevoflurane can provide good cardiovascular stability with rapid recovery. The vocal cords can be sprayed with lidocaine, 4 ml of 4%, to minimise post-operative laryngospasm.

The patient should be positioned with their head on a single pillow. I would take care to protect the eyes and teeth and monitor the degree of neck extension required as the bronchoscope is advanced.

What ventilator strategies can you use?

The most important thing to recognise is that the airway is shared in this procedure. I am aware that there are two ventilator strategies that can be employed, intermittent positive pressure ventilation (IPPV) via the ventilating arm of the bronchoscope or using injector devices such as the Sanders' or Manujet injector.

The difference between the Sanders' injector and the Manujet injector is that the Sanders' has no pressure control, so when the trigger is pressed, there is full pipeline pressure applied to the needle. Manujet has a variable pressure output and can thus be used for smaller patients.

Can you go into more detail about these differing techniques?

The injector uses a high-pressure oxygen supply to release a jet of oxygen from a needle at the operator end of the bronchoscope. This creates a Venturi effect, entraining atmospheric air and producing positive pressure at the distal end of the bronchoscope. Intermittent inflation/deflation provides satisfactory oxygenation and carbon dioxide clearance. It is essential that there is free passage of air from the upper airway to allow entrainment, and also passive expiration, thereby avoiding volutrauma. This method is usually preferred in adults.

When using an injector the needle size is important as it affects the amount of air entrained via the Venturi. If too large a needle is used, it can cause dangerous barotrauma.

The ventilating bronchoscope has a glass window or a rubber diaphragm to enable passage of instruments, and a side arm that can be connected to the anaesthetic circuit. This technique is most commonly used in infants and children using a T-piece and hand ventilation. There is minimal risk of barotrauma.

How would you maintain anaesthesia?

Demonstrate your awareness of complications of the different techniques.

When the ventilating bronchoscope is used, a volatile agent can be used. Rapid emergence is desirable, therefore, sevoflurane or desflurane are the desirable agents but I exercise caution with the latter agent as it can cause airway irritation.

The use of the Sanders' injector means an intra-venous technique must be employed. Propofol is the ideal agent due to its rapid offset, this can be used as intermittent bolus doses but I prefer a target controlled infusion as awareness is a potential and not uncommon complication.

Monitoring the depth of anaesthesia with, for example, the Bispectral Index (BIS) could be introduced at this point but is beyond the scope of this answer.

If your answers are progressing well, proceed to post-operative management without prompting.

Unless bronchoscopy is to be followed by a procedure, muscular relaxation should be reversed and rapid emergence is desirable. The patient should be nursed with an oxygen facemask and in the lateral position, with the diseased side down. Potential complications include teeth damage, aspiration of blood, awareness, pharyngeal rupture, airway rupture, cardiac arrhythmias, hypertension and myocardial ischaemia.

Be prepared to expand on the complications, for example airway rupture may present as a pneumothorax which could tension, tracheo-oesophageal fistula or surgical emphysema.

How do patients with inhaled foreign bodies present?

This problem occurs most frequently in children under the age of 3, but can occur at any age particularly in the obtunded. A specific history is often absent, and presentation is variable from acute upper airway obstruction to a more insidious onset with a chronic cough, recurrent chest infection that fails to improve following anti-biotic therapy and unilateral wheeze. Foreign bodies should always be removed as they can trigger an inflammatory response causing distal collapse and infection. This is particularly a problem with peanuts as they liberate an irritant oil.

Is a CXR indicated in this clinical scenario?

If there is a good history and the patient has acute upper airway obstruction there may not be time to perform a CXR. However, this is unusual. The CXR may be normal, it may show a radio-opaque foreign body and in the chronic case often shows non-specific changes of atelectasis and consolidation. Inspiratory and expiratory films may reveal hyperinflation with the foreign body acting as a ball-valve in the main bronchus.

How would you anaesthetise a patient with an inhaled foreign body?

This is a fairly open question and you must give a balanced account of the two schools of thought.

Good vascular access and routine monitoring are required. The traditional approach is an inhalational induction. This is the most common approach in children, the main advantage being that the airway can be safely maintained until bronchoscopy is performed. Anaesthesia can then be maintained with an inhalational agent and the patient spontaneously breathing. However, to avoid the use of a muscle relaxant the depth of anaesthesia has to be such that patients are usually rendered apnoeic with the current agents available.

(Halothane allowed very deep planes of anaesthesia in a spontaneously breathing patient. It also provided good relaxation, but is no longer in use in the United Kingdom.)

Therefore, a common approach is an inhalational induction with sevoflurane followed by muscle relaxation with suxamethonium. Ventilation is then gently taken over using the T-piece attached to the side arm of the ventilating bronchoscope. It is important to maintain a high concentration of oxygen. Incremental small doses of suxamethonium can be given if the procedure is likely to be quick, but it is important to manage the possible bradycardia with IV atropine.

IPPV was traditionally avoided as there is a concern that the foreign body could get blown more distally or may cause a ball-like effect resulting in distal air trapping. This argument is countered by the belief that any foreign body requiring removal is already impacted and unlikely to be displaced. If the obstruction is in the trachea, there are descriptions of the use of positive pressure to blow the foreign body distally to achieve some ventilation down either the right or left main bronchus.

In adults, the Venturi method of ventilation can be used safely. Intra-venous induction with propofol followed by suxamethonium provides a rapid and safe way to secure the airway.

For maintenance, incremental IV boluses of both an anaesthetic and analgesic, for example alfentanil and propofol, would be appropriate. More precise control can be obtained using a target controlled infusion (TCI) infusion. Propofol and remifentanil would be suitable.

What are the post-operative complications?

The main concern following repeated instrumentation of the airway is laryngeal stridor. This can be managed with nebulised adrenaline, 5 ml of 1:10 000, repeated every 2–4 hours and IV dexamethasone 600 µg/kg/day in four divided doses. Severe stridor may require reintubation and a smaller endotracheal tube should be available. Prolonged ventilation is occasionally required.

What other bronchoscopic interventions are you aware of?

In critical stenosis, a tracheo-bronchial stent can be sited, either as palliation or until definitive surgery can be undertaken.

Diathermy resection of tumours and laser therapy to debulk tumours are relatively common procedures.

What are the important anaesthetic considerations for these procedures?

If you get this far you are doing very well in your SOE.

Pre-oxygenation is essential, with cautious induction of anaesthesia as complete loss of the airway is possible. Intra-venous and inhalational induction both have advantages and disadvantages. The most important aspect is to have a skilled bronchoscopist on hand as this may be the only way to relieve the obstruction.

The routine precautions should always be adhered to when using lasers:

- A low concentration of inspired oxygen
- Avoiding nitrous oxide
- Using short burst of laser treatment.

Using a metal bronchoscope avoids the need for foil wrapped or metal endotracheal tube for tracheal and endobronchial tumour resection with a laser.

It is essential that good communication is maintained with the surgeon.

You mentioned earlier that flexible bronchoscopy is performed under local anaesthetic and sedation, do you ever come across this technique in your practice?

Yes, this technique is performed for awake fibre-optic intubation.

What are the indications for awake fibre-optic intubation?

- Known or anticipated difficult airway problem
- Unstable cervical spine injury or unstable neck, for example, rheumatoid arthritis with a risk of aspiration
- Obesity and obstructive sleep apnoea can also be considered.

Are there any contraindications?

Yes.

- Patient refusal
- Coagulopathy, particularly if the nasal route is to be used
- Periglottic masses: there is a risk of developing complete airway obstruction or laryngospasm
- Basal skull fracture or cerebrospinal fluid leak are contra-indications if the nasal route is to be used.

Is the nasal route best?

The nasal route is preferred, in my experience, as it is frequently easier in the group of patients with limited mouth opening, and the oral route gives a poor angle to approach the larynx.

And how would you anaesthetise the airway for the procedure?

It is important to emphasise that there are many ways to perform this procedure, explain that it can be done with or without sedation, although sedation is very common now. Describe a technique with which you are familiar.

1. I would give 0.3 mg of glycopyrrolate IV to minimise secretions, which helps to ensure topical anaesthesia is more effective.
2. I would position the patient at 45 degrees, apply full AABGI monitoring and give oxygen via a nasal catheter.
3. I would commence a low-dose target controlled remifentanil infusion (TCI) for the procedure with a starting dose of 3 μg ml^{-1}. The aim is to maintain verbal communication with the patient. The benefit of the remifentanil is its anti-tussive effects and cardiovascular stability. Propofol TCI or bolus doses of benzodiazepines are also well described in the literature.
4. If there were no contra-indications, I would spray the nostrils with 2 ml of 5% cocaine or Moffat's solution.
5. The patient can gargle 1.5 ml of 4% lidocaine, holding it in the oropharynx as long as possible, or this can be sprayed to the back of the pharynx using a nasal airway or atomiser. This should adequately anaesthetise the oropharynx and the posterior third of the tongue.
6. The nostrils are then dilated with nasal airways or gynaecological dilators lubricated with lidocaine jelly.

How would you anaesthetise the vocal cords?

1. One method is by delivering 3–4 ml of 4% lidocaine via a nebuliser with the patient sitting up. Alternatively 2 ml of 4% lidocaine can be injected down the suction port of the fibrescope with a further 2 ml being injected once the tip of the scope is through the cords.

2. A more invasive method is the cricothyroid membrane puncture. A 22-G cannula is used with the neck in extension, correct placement is confirmed by the aspiration of air. The 2 ml of 4% lidocaine is injected at end-expiration so the patient will breathe in, and the resultant cough from the patient gives appropriate spread to the local anaesthetic above and below the cords. It is important not to use a needle as this can snap when the patient coughs.

Are you aware of any specific nerve blocks that can be performed?

It is worth knowing a brief description of specific nerve blocks as they are a favourite of the examiners.

Superior laryngeal nerve blocks can be performed either by injecting local anaesthetic bilaterally, just above the thyroid cartilage at a point one third the distance between the midline and the superior cornu.

Alternatively pledgets soaked in local anaesthetic can be placed into each piriform fossa using forceps. I have never witnessed the use of these blocks in my clinical practice.

2.1.6. One-lung ventilation – Carl J Morris

This topic comes up frequently in SOEs.

What are the indications for one-lung anaesthesia?

You must have a structure to any question of this nature.

Indications for one-lung anaesthesia can be classified as absolute and relative. The absolute indications can be further classified:

Protection of the healthy lung from pathology in the contralateral lung, such as:

- Massive haemorrhage
- Infection
- Other fluid, such as lung lavage.

Preventing ventilation to one lung in the case of:

- Large broncho-pleural fistula
- Risk of rupture such as with a large bulla.

Some surgical procedures mandate one-lung ventilation, such as:

- Video-assisted thorascopy
- Surgery to proximal bronchial tree.

The relative indications are to improve surgical access (as opposed to lung retraction by the surgeon).

These are indicated by the surgical approach, and include:

- Pneumonectomy

- Lobectomy
- Thoracic aneurysm repair
- Oesophagectomy
- Spinal surgery.

How would you achieve one-lung ventilation?

If you have seen bronchial blockers being used, you can mention this, even if you would not use them yourself. The examiners want a sense of clinical experience as well as sound theoretical knowledge.

The most common method, and the one that I am familiar with, is the use of a double-lumen endobronchial tube. There are also techniques where single-lumen tubes are combined with bronchial blockers to achieve lung isolation. And in an emergency, deliberate endobronchial intubation with a long-single lumen tube has also been used.

Can you think of advantages and disadvantages to the use of bronchial blockers?

Hopefully this type of question means the SOE is going well and they are exploring your knowledge a little further.

Bronchial blockers are helpful when there is abnormal airway anatomy meaning it is difficult or impossible to pass a double-lumen tube. They can be used for lobar isolation. In patients already intubated with a single-lumen tube, the use of a bronchial blocker avoids the need to change the tube at the beginning or the end of the case. The disadvantages are that they give less reliable isolation, are more likely to become dislodged intra-operatively, and they don't give easy access to the deflated lung, for example for suctioning.

Would you have a preference between a left- or a right-sided double-lumen tube?

This is hopefully straightforward.

Unless a right-sided tube was essential, for example for surgery on the left main bronchus, I would always prefer to use a left-sided tube. This is because the adult distance from the carina to the left upper lobe bronchus is about 5 cm versus 2.5 cm on the right. So a left-side tube is much less likely to cause upper lobe obstruction.

What type of double-lumen endobronchial tube would you choose?

I have used the Mallinckrodt Bronchocath type.

If you know lots of others, feel free to list, but don't waste time.

And the size?

This would range from a 32-French gauge for a small woman, to a 41 for a large man.

How would you insert a double-lumen endobronchial tube?

Preparations would include assessing the patient and in particular reviewing the notes and any imaging for potential difficulties with intubation. I would carry out my standard pre-operative checks of drugs and equipment. In this case, the Y connector and 15-mm connectors should be connected correctly, particularly I would check they are connected the correct way up and that my trained assistant is familiar with the equipment. I would insert the stylet to curve the tube, making sure the tip of the stylet is not protruding from the distal end. Finally, I would make sure we had a working bronchoscope to check position, or assist with a difficult insertion.

After induction of anaesthesia and administration of neuromuscular blockade, I would insert the tube with the endobronchial section facing anteriorly to pass through the cords, withdraw the stylet and rotate the tube 90 degrees to the left and advance slowly until I felt resistance.

Then I would inflate the tracheal cuff and attempt to ventilate the patient's lungs and check for a satisfactory end-tidal carbon dioxide trace.

Do you know what depth to insert a double-lumen tube?

For adults 1.7 to 1.8 metres tall, the depth is usually 29 cm to the incisors. The depth is meant to increase or decrease by 1 cm for every 10-cm height difference.

And how would you confirm correct position

I would always use a bronchoscope for direct confirmation of tube position. I would also check the position after any change in the patient's position. I would look first through the tracheal lumen to make sure I could visualise the carina, and check that the endobronchial lumen is in the correct bronchus, with the blue cuff just visible below the carina.

Try to picture what you actually do.

I would also then check within the bronchial lumen that the upper lobe bronchus was patent. With a right-sided tube this would include checking the alignment of the tube's lateral slit with the upper lobe bronchus.

Why do you use a bronchoscope?

In various studies, critical malpositioning has occurred in around 25% of cases, and in the NCEPOD report, malpositioning of the double-lumen tube was associated with 30% of oesophagectomy deaths.

Could you talk me through the clinical checks

Hopefully asking this question after you've gone for the bronchoscope option means that things are going well, and you have plenty of time!

Use whatever technique you've been told, but don't get bogged down.

First I would check the tracheal cuff, as with any intubation, to confirm correct placement via auscultation and capnography, inflating the cuff until the leak at the mouth disappeared.

Next I would clamp the tracheal lumen at the catheter mount, and open the tracheal port, then I would ventilate through the bronchial lumen, with visual inspection and auscultation to confirm left-sided ventilation. I would then carefully inflate the bronchial cuff to a maximum of 3 ml of air, while listening for loss of the leak at the tracheal port.

Finally, I would also confirm with visual inspection and auscultation that I could ventilate both lungs with both cuffs inflated, and after clamping the bronchial lumen, that I could also isolate the contralateral lung.

What are the physiological consequences of one-lung ventilation?

One-lung ventilation usually takes place in the lateral decubitus position. The lower, dependent lung is ventilated. Gravity will aid perfusion, but may also lead to compression and pooling of secretions, causing hypoxaemia. The upper, non-dependent lung, which is either the surgical site, or facilitating surgical access, is not ventilated. Any blood flow to this lung, or to areas of alveolar collapse in the ventilated lung, lead to a shunt. The shunt fraction is estimated to be between 20 and 40%. Surgical retraction should help reduce any shunt by direct compression of vessels. Hypoxic pulmonary vasoconstriction should also reduce shunt, but only by 50%.

How would you deflate the non-dependent lung?

A surprisingly tricky question in the heat of a SOE, particularly if you are not familiar with doing it and sometimes even if you are!

I would clamp the catheter mount to the non-dependent lung, and open the port to the same lung. I would of course check with the surgeon that the lung was actually deflating.

How would you adjust ventilation when the non-dependent lung is deflated?

I would maintain an inspired oxygen fraction of at least 0.5, increasing this if necessary, though the effects of the shunt mean that increasing this is unlikely to have a major impact. I would keep the tidal volumes the same as for two-lung ventilation (up to a maximum of 10 ml/kg), while trying to maintain peak airway pressures below 30 cm of water. I would adjust the rate to try to maintain normocapnia.

How would you deal with hypoxaemia?

Depending on the severity, there are a variety of strategies, which can be grouped into those addressing the dependent or non-dependent lung.

Focussing on the dependent lung:

- Ventilation can be increased, while avoiding excessive pressures and volumes.
- Increasing the inspired oxygen concentration may be of use.
- Suctioning may help remove pooled secretions.
- Recheck the tube position with a bronchoscope, in particular to check the upper lobe bronchus is not occluded.
- Cautious application of positive end-expiratory pressure may improve oxygenation if atelectasis is the main problem, though it may cause a worsening of any shunt by increasing blood flow through the non-ventilated lung.

If ventilation appears adequate, there might be a problem with perfusion that is treatable with fluids, and/or vasopressors.

With the non-dependent lung, the strategy is to try to decrease the shunt. This could be via:

- Insufflation of oxygen through, for example, a suction catheter
- Application of CPAP
- Clamping the pulmonary artery
- Failing these measures, it may become necessary to ventilate the non-dependent lung.

What would you do if the patient became extremely hypoxic?

I would hand ventilate the patient with 100% oxygen and request immediate senior support. By hand ventilating I am able to simultaneously treat them, while assessing the adequacy of the circuit. Assuming that I found no major disconnection or obstruction to the oxygen supply, I would also be able to assess the patient's lung compliance before instituting the measures I've already discussed above.

Further Reading

Eastwood J, Mahajan R. One-lung anaesthesia. *British Journal of Anaesthesia. CEPD Reviews.* 2002; **2**(3): 83–87.

Grichnik KP, Shaw A. Update on one-lung ventilation: the use of continuous positive airway pressure ventilation and positive end-expiratory pressure ventilation–clinical application. *Current Opinion in Anaesthesiology.* 2009; **22**(1): 23–30.

Ng A, Swanevelder J. Hypoxaemia during one-lung anaesthesia. *Continuing Education in Anaesthesia, Critical Care & Pain.* 2010; **10**(4): 117–122.

2.1.7. Anaesthetic management of patients with transplanted organs, including heart, lungs and kidneys – Asim Iqbal

This topic is well suited to the clinical SOE, but the initial question may form part of a basic science SOE.

Can you draw a diagram of the sympathetic nervous system for me?

To avoid a long silence, explain to the examiner what you are drawing, whilst you are drawing it (Figure 2.1.7a). Draw a picture of a brain in sagittal section with the spinal cord extending caudally. Parallel to the spinal cord, draw another line and label this the sympathetic chain. Indicate that it starts at T1 and extends down to the L1/L2 level. If you wish, you can draw the organs and glands supplied by the nerves in a column next to the sympathetic chain (starting from top to bottom: the eye, the parotid gland, the heart, the lungs, the stomach, the liver, adrenal glands and the bladder).

Where does the sympathetic nerve supply of the heart originate?

The origin of the sympathetic chain of the heart arises from the T1 to T4 segments of the spinal cord.

What are these fibres called?

They are called the cardio-accelerator fibres.

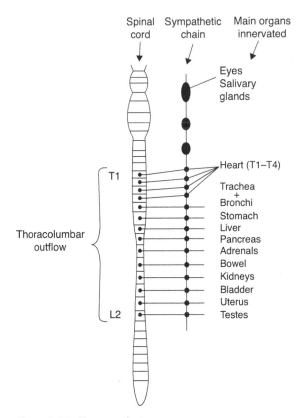

Figure 2.1.7. The sympathetic nervous system.

What can you tell me about the physiology of the transplanted heart?

The Frank-Starling relationship between end-diastolic volume and cardiac output is normal and the transplanted heart is said to be pre-load dependent. Maintenance of a high or normal pre-load is desirable in the management of these patients. Coronary autoregulation also remains intact after heart transplantation.

What about the other autonomic or sensory influences?

The transplanted heart has no parasympathetic, sympathetic or sensory innervation. All direct autonomic influences are absent. The loss of vagal tone produces a higher than normal resting heart rate, in the region of 90–110 bpm. The Valsalva manoeuvre and carotid sinus massage will not affect the heart rate. The baroreceptor reflex is also interrupted in the transplanted heart as the efferent limb (the vagus nerve) is denervated at the time of transplant. Other effects of cardiac denervation include the loss of the sympathetic response to laryngoscopy and endotracheal intubation. In terms of sensory changes, myocardial ischaemia and infarction may be silent due to the heart's denervated state. Patients usually undergo regular angiographic investigation for this complication. However, unpredictable re-innervation can occur after heart transplantation.

What about the response to circulating catecholamines?

Although the sympathetic fibres to the heart are also interrupted at the time of transplant, the response to circulating catecholamines remains normal or can even be enhanced secondary to denervation sensitivity. Catecholamine receptor density can be normal or increased. In a denervated heart, the catecholamine response is different from that in a normal heart because intact sympathetic nerves are necessary for the normal uptake and metabolism of catecholamines.

How does the transplanted heart respond to sympathomimetic drugs?

The transplanted heart responds well to directly acting sympathomimetics. Epinephrine and norepinephrine have an augmented inotropic effect in heart transplant recipients. Both drugs tend to have a higher β- to α-adrenoreceptor ratio. Isoprenaline and dobutamine have similar effects in both denervated and normal hearts, so both are effective inotropes in heart transplant recipients. They increase myocardial contractility more than dopamine, which acts predominantly by norepinephrine release. Dopamine is a less effective inotrope in the denervated heart, having predominantly α and dopaminergic effects.

What about indirectly acting drugs?

Directly acting agents are more effective than indirect ones, due to the lack of catecholamine stores in myocardial neurones. Indirectly acting drugs, such as ephedrine, have diminished responses on heart rate and blood pressure in heart transplant recipients. As vagolytic drugs will be ineffective in increasing heart rate, chronotropic drugs, such as isoprenaline, should be available. Neostigmine and other anti-cholinesterases do not cause bradycardias in denervated hearts.

Describe the anaesthetic management of a heart transplant recipient?

Be ready to divide you answer into the pre-operative, intra-operative and post-operative management of these patients.

The general considerations related to any transplant recipient should encompass the physiological and pharmacological problems of graft denervation, the potential for rejection, the adverse effects of immunosuppression, and to be cognisant of the risk or presence of infection. Along with taking a standard anaesthetic history, pre-operative assessment should focus on evaluation of the functional status of the organ and detecting complications of immunosuppressive therapy.

The highest incidence of rejection occurs within the first three months after the transplant. Rejection may be apparent from the history, with a decreased exercise tolerance as an indication of deteriorating myocardial function, or from biopsy results. Mild rejection does not usually compromise cardiac contractility, but severe rejection may cause significant systolic and diastolic dysfunction. Other clinical indicators of rejection include fatigue, congestive cardiac failure, accelerated atherosclerosis, evidence of myocardial infarction on the ECG and ventricular dysrhythmias.

Accelerated atherosclerosis in the graft is a serious and common problem. As both myocardial ischaemia and infarction are usually silent, the patient may have had a recent coronary angiogram.

A pre-operative 12-lead ECG may demonstrate two p-waves, one representing the recipient's sino-atrial (SA) node, which is usually left intact, and the other representing the donor's SA node. The patient may also have a permanent pacemaker in place.

What type of immunosuppressive therapy might the patient be receiving? Are there any particular problems associated with this?

Immunosuppressive therapy may be a combination of prednisolone, mycophenolate, cyclosporine, tacrolimus or azathioprine. Side effects of these drugs include steroid-related side effects, nephrotoxicity with renal impairment and subsequent hypertension, bone marrow suppression, hepatotoxicity and the development of opportunistic infections.

At therapeutic levels, tacrolimus and cyclosporine can cause a dose-related decrease in renal blood flow and glomerular filtration rate, secondary to renal vasoconstriction. Increased thromboxane A_2 and endothelin production are responsible for these altered renal haemodynamics.

Opportunistic infections secondary to immunosuppression may be bacterial, viral, fungal or protozoan. However, reducing the dose of immunosuppressive drugs in the peri-operative period may increase the risk of rejection. It is important to appreciate that the immunosuppressed patient may not present with the classical signs and symptoms of infection such as leucocytosis, fever and other physical signs.

Pre-operative blood tests may reveal thrombocytopenia and leucopenia secondary to azathioprine. Tacrolimus or cyclosporine therapy can additionally cause hypomagnesaemia and hyperkalaemia.

Are you aware of any interactions between immunosuppressant therapy and anaesthetic agents?

Immunosuppressive drugs can interact with and alter the pharmacological behaviour of many anaesthetic drugs. Cyclosporine and tacrolimus are metabolised in the liver through the cytochrome P 450 system. Therefore, many drugs administered during anaesthesia or peri-operatively can potentially affect cyclosporine or tacrolimus blood levels.

Cyclosporine enhances the effects of muscle relaxants and prolonged neuromuscular block has been described. Therefore, patients receiving this drug may require smaller doses of non-depolarising muscle relaxant.

Although reversal of neuromuscular blockade with anti-cholinesterase agents does not cause a bradycardia, it still requires concomitant administration of an anti-muscarinic agent to avoid the non-cardiac muscarinic effects.

How would you manage these patients intra-operatively?

There is no evidence to support one anaesthetic technique over another. Both regional and general anaesthesia have been successfully used for transplant recipients. However, the absence of reflex increases in heart rate can make the blood pressure particularly sensitive to rapid vasodilatation and therefore pre-load dependent. If an epidural or spinal technique is to be used, the platelet count and clotting studies should be normal. Thrombocytopenia as a result of immunosuppressive therapy increases the risks associated with central neural blockade.

How should these patients best be monitored during anaesthesia?

The choice of peri-operative monitoring techniques is determined by the type of surgery, the anaesthesia planned, and the equipment available. Central venous, intra-venous and arterial access may be difficult due to previous repeated use. Invasive monitoring requires strict aseptic precautions and should be evaluated in terms of the risk–benefit ratio to the patient. If a central venous line were required, it would be desirable to avoid the right internal jugular vein, as this is often accessed for cardiac biopsies. There may be a role for trans-oesophageal echocardiography.

How would you manage the patient's fluid balance intra-operatively?

Hypovolaemia is poorly tolerated due to the pre-load dependence, so maintenance of a high or normal pre-load is important. However, this must be balanced against clinically significant reductions of tacrolimus or cyclosporine serum levels, which can be caused by dilution with a large peri-operative fluid infusion.

How would you manage this patient post-operatively?

The pre-operative state of the patient and the nature of the surgery will define the most suitable post-operative environment for the patient, but I would have a low threshold for admitting them to a high dependency area.

Non-steroidal anti-inflammatory drugs should be avoided due to the risk of adverse drug interactions. They augment the nephrotoxicity of cyclosporine, as both drugs affect the renal microcirculation. Other interactions can result in gastrointestinal haemorrhage and hepatic dysfunction.

Immunosuppressive therapy should be continued during the peri-operative period and daily monitoring of cyclosporine or tacrolimus blood levels is recommended. The dose of immunosuppressive drugs should not be altered unless the route of administration needs to be changed from oral to IV. Supplemental "stress-coverage" doses of steroids are controversial, but are a relatively low-risk treatment and therefore are used frequently.

Strong consideration should be given to thromboprophylaxis in transplant recipients, especially if other risk factors are present.

This SOE will now progress to discuss the anaesthetic management of lung, liver and kidney transplant recipients. The general considerations related to any transplant recipient mentioned above (the physiological and pharmacological problems of allograft denervation, the potential for rejection, the side effects of immunosuppressant drugs and the risk or presence of infection) still apply. These questions in this section will focus on the specific problems encountered with these patients.

The anaesthetic management of a lung transplant recipient

How does denervation affect the lung?

The denervation of the lung(s) seems to have a minimal effect on the pattern of breathing, but it removes afferent sensation below the level of the tracheal anastomosis. Patients with a tracheal anastomosis lose their cough reflex and are therefore more prone to silent aspiration and retention of secretions. Bronchial hyperreactivity causing bronchoconstriction is a common occurrence. The ventilatory response to carbon dioxide remains normal.

How could rejection be detected pre-operatively?

Symptoms of rejection may be very similar to those of an upper respiratory tract infection and include fatigue, shortness of breath and fever. It can be difficult to differentiate between the two. Blood tests may reveal leucopenia, whilst an arterial blood gas may reveal hypoxaemia and an increased alveolar to arterial oxygen gradient. Rejection can also be detected with pulmonary functions tests. The forced expiratory volume, vital capacity and total lung capacity would be significantly reduced.

Obliterative bronchiolitis is caused by chronic rejection, and it usually presents after the third month post-transplantation. Chest radiography may reveal perihilar infiltrates or opacification of the graft. In this situation, pulmonary function testing would reveal an obstructive defect.

As transplanted lungs may have ongoing rejection that can adversely affect pulmonary function, patients should have pre-operative spirometry tests. A recent CT scan may be valuable in aiding anaesthetic management. If infection or graft rejection is evident, elective surgery should be postponed and appropriate investigations undertaken.

Do you have any concerns with ventilating these patients?

Single-lung transplant recipients may cause specific concern, especially if the native lung is emphysematous. The native lung may be highly compliant and the donor lung may have normal or reduced compliance, causing an imbalance. The majority of the pulmonary blood flow is usually to the allograft. With institution of positive pressure ventilation, dynamic hyperinflation of the emphysematous lung with haemodynamic instability and problems with gas exchange may develop. A double-lumen tube or independent lung ventilation techniques may be required, to reduce the airway pressure and minute ventilation in the native lung. Care should be taken when positioning tubes to avoid tracheal and bronchial anastomotic sites. A fibre-optic scope may be useful for this.

Would you have any preference for regional or general anaesthesia?

As lung transplant recipients lack a cough reflex below the tracheal anastomosis level, they cannot clear secretions unless they are awake. In view of this abolished cough reflex, the increased risk of chest infection, and the potential for bronchoconstriction, one can reason that a regional technique, if possible, may be preferable to one that requires insertion of an endotracheal tube.

Describe the fluid management of lung transplant recipients?

The lymphatic drainage in the transplanted lung is usually disrupted. This can predispose to interstitial fluid accumulation, particularly early on in the post-transplantation period. A careful and limited crystalloid infusion should be used peri-operatively. In combined heart–lung transplant recipients, however, fluid management can be particularly problematic. While the heart requires an adequate pre-load to maintain cardiac output, the lungs may have an increased propensity towards the development of pulmonary oedema. Invasive haemodynamic monitoring is often useful in this subset of patients.

The anaesthetic management of a liver transplant recipient

Describe what happens to liver function following transplantation?

Following a successful liver transplant, the tests of synthetic function of the liver should be normal. An initial significant increase in all liver enzyme levels gradually decreases to normal over the first two post-operative weeks as allograft function becomes normal. The recovery of the liver's capacity to metabolise drugs occurs almost immediately after reperfusion of the graft.

Liver transplantation reverses the hyperdynamic state that is characteristic of patients with end-stage liver disease and cardiac performance improves in the months after transplantation.

What relationships are you aware of between the lung and the liver? How might they change after transplantation?

Pulmonary dysfunction in patients with end-stage liver disease can result from:

1. Intra-pulmonary shunting caused by pulmonary vascular dilatation
2. Ventilation/perfusion mismatch (from pleural effusions, ascites and increased closing capacities)
3. Diffusion abnormalities caused by interstitial pneumonitis and/or pulmonary hypertension
4. Impaired hypoxic pulmonary vasoconstriction.

After successful liver transplantation, oxygenation does improve in most patients. The hypoxaemia caused by ventilation/perfusion mismatch often resolves within the first few post-operative months. Patients with pre-existing true shunts may require more time to achieve reversal of hypoxaemia, or it may not resolve at all.

How would you diagnose rejection in the transplanted liver?

The clinical signs of rejection include fever, malaise, hepatosplenomegaly, ascites and right upper quadrant pain. The most reliable indicators are an elevated bilirubin, AST and ALT.

Are there any other physiological and pharmacological considerations that may influence your management in somebody with a transplanted liver?

The normal physiological mechanisms that protect hepatic blood flow are diminished after liver transplantation. The liver functions as an important blood reservoir in hypovolaemic states by means of a vasoconstrictive response and this mechanism can be markedly impaired following liver transplantation. I would be happy to use the common inhalational anaesthetic agents in use today, as there is no evidence of increased risk of developing hepatitis after their administration. Renal impairment is common in liver transplant recipients and this has important pharmacological implications.

If the patient is returning to theatre in the immediate post-transplantation period and a blood transfusion is required, I would use blood products judiciously as hepatic arterial thrombosis has been retrospectively associated with overtransfusion of blood products and haemoconcentration. If this complication occurs, the mortality rate is high in this transplant population. These patients should have minimal blood viscosity (haematocrit approximately 28%) during the peri-operative period.

The anaesthetic management of a kidney transplant recipient

Describe the anaesthetic management of a patient who has had a renal transplant?

Although recipients with an adequately functioning kidney graft may have creatinine levels within the normal range, it is important to recognise that the glomerular filtration rate and effective renal plasma flow are likely to be significantly reduced. Hence, the activity of drugs that rely upon renal excretion may be prolonged and should be avoided.

During pre-operative assessment, it is important to recognise that there is an increase in the incidence and severity of cardiovascular disease in this population, especially due to the success of renal transplantation in elderly and diabetic patients. Hypertension is a frequent finding in this patient population and it is common for renal transplant recipients to be taking oral anti-hypertensive therapy for this. Both of these should be managed accordingly.

How would you detect rejection of the kidney graft?

Uraemia, proteinuria and hypertension may indicate chronic rejection of the graft. Patients with renal graft dysfunction may have also been recommenced upon haemodialysis.

Describe your intra-operative management?

If the patient has undergone recent haemodialysis, they may be hypovolaemic and/or hypokalaemic. Hypovolaemia leads to cardiovascular instability, and hypokalaemia causes cardiac arrhythmias and increased sensitivity to muscle relaxants. As the variables of renal function are likely to be abnormal in kidney transplant recipients, it is sensible to choose drugs that do not rely on the kidney for excretion, such as atracurium. Nephrotoxic drugs should be avoided. Diuretics should not be given without careful evaluation of the patient's volume status, and renal hypoperfusion from inadequate intra-vascular volume should be avoided.

Further Reading

Fabbroni D, Bellamy M. Anaesthesia for hepatic transplantation. *Continuing Education in Anaesthesia, Critical Care & Pain.* 2006; **6**(5): 171–175.

Morgan-Hughes N, Hood G. Anaesthesia for a patient with a cardiac transplant. *British Journal of Anaesthesia. CEPD Reviews.* 2002; **2**(3): 74–78.

Shaw I, Kirk AJB, Conacher ID. Anaesthesia for patients with transplanted hearts and lungs undergoing non-cardiac surgery. *British Journal of Anaesthesia.* 1991; **67**(6): 772–778.

Chapter

2.2

Day-case

2.2.1. Day-case selection criteria – Alison J Brewer

What are the advantages of day-case surgery?

There are many advantages of day-case surgery, and this is one of the reasons why the NHS plan has set a target of 75% of all elective surgery being performed on a day-case basis.

The advantages can be classified as:

Advantages for patients:

- Most patients prefer day-case rather than overnight stay
- In the elderly population it has been shown to decrease post-operative cognitive dysfunction
- Ideal for children and elderly patients, with minimal time away from a familiar environment so less psychological disturbance
- Reduced hospital acquired infection
- Early mobilisation reducing the DVT risk
- Reduced risk of cancellation due to emergencies on a designated day-case list.

Advantages to staff and the NHS:

- Staff are easier to obtain due to social hours
- Increased economic benefits to the trust as there can be an increased efficiency in a well-run day-case service
- Reduced waiting lists
- Increases availability of inpatient beds for major cases.

Are there any disadvantages that you can think of?

It is important to carefully assess and have robust guidelines for the selection of patients for day-case surgery. There is also inherently a limitation of some anaesthetic techniques, such as epidural or indwelling catheter techniques for analgesia post-operatively. There also has to be facility for admission of a proportion of patients due to intra- and post-operative complications.

Dr. Podcast Scripts for the Final FRCA, ed. Rebecca A. Leslie, Emily K. Johnson, Gary Thomas and Alexander P. L. Goodwin.   Published by Cambridge University Press.

What surgery can be performed as a day-case, and what are the important considerations?

There has to be consideration as to what surgery is appropriate to be performed as day-case. It is important to make sure that any surgery can be safely done as a day-case without compromising patient care. The complication rate should be low, with minimal blood loss. There must be adequate control of pain, nausea and vomiting. The patients must also be able to eat and drink and mobilise within a reasonable time frame after the surgery is complete. The Department of Health has produced guidelines on day-case surgery, with a list of the cases deemed suitable. Overall the principles stated apply to selection of appropriate day-cases.

How are you going to select which patients are appropriate to have day-case surgery?

There are social and medical factors that affect whether a patient can have day-case surgery or not.

Social factors include:

- Willingness on the patients' behalf
- Easy access to a phone in their home environment
- Transport back to the hospital to hand
- A responsible adult who can stay with the patient for at least the first 24 hours post-operatively
- Conditions at home should be compatible with post-operative care with adequate toilet and bathroom facilities
- No more than 60-minute travelling time back to the hospital should complications occur
- Patients should have a telephone number to contact in case of emergencies
- Patients should be discharged with an advice sheet explaining what to do in case of complications.

Medical factors are more difficult to quantify and in many circumstances clinical judgement needs to be employed. In general patients should be:

- Relatively fit (ASA 1 or 2) patients
- Mobile
- Not morbidly obese
- Patients should be selected according to their physiological status and not their chronological age.

Some who fall outside guidelines may particularly benefit and should be discussed on a case-by-case basis, for example stable diabetics. Obesity is not an absolute contraindication for day-case surgery, but there are problems with this population.

What are the problems with treating obese patients in a day-case setting?

There needs to be appropriate resources and facilities for the management of obese patients, and specialist equipment and staff may not be available in the day-case setting. There is an increased risk of respiratory compromise in the obese population and late complications may develop more frequently, therefore a longer hospital stay may be appropriate in some circumstances. Morbidly obese patients may also provide increased technical challenge to surgeons. BMI, though not the ideal tool for assessing these patients, does give pre-assessment nurses a guide for selection. Some day-case units have a BMI cut off of 35 for all procedures, however, in many units there is no specific limit set and cases can be assessed on an individual basis.

Are there any other factors you would consider in the patient selection process?

Other general factors to consider include:

- The presence of any previous problems with surgery or anaesthetic.
- The type of surgery, considering potential for significant bleeding and or prolonged and difficult surgery.
- Length of surgery, though techniques such as TIVA and desflurane, that allow rapid emergence, mean that surgery does not have to be time limited to be performed as day-case.
- Requirement for specialist services such as radiological intervention. There may be a logistical reason why day-case surgery may not be appropriate. In these cases surgery should be planned as an inpatient.

What patient-specific factors would prevent you selecting an individual for day-case surgery?

Classify or die – systems approach works best here; CVS, RS, metabolic, endocrine etc.

Cardiovascular history should be explored with particular attention being paid to exercise tolerance and reserve. If there are signs of heart failure, such as ankle oedema and dyspnoea then these patients are not appropriate for day-case surgery. Also uncontrolled angina or myocardial infarction in the past 6 months should be an exclusion. Valvular heart disease with symptoms should be excluded for further investigation and quantification. Hypertension is controversial and should be controlled pre-operatively in a day-case surgery setting for an elective procedure above 180/110 mmHg. A general practioner should be able to re-refer the patient directly to the clinic for treatment once this is controlled.

Significant respiratory disease should be searched for and optimised prior to day-case surgery. A history of corticosteroid use or intensive care admissions recently would make day-case surgery less appropriate.

Diabetics can generally be done if performed first on the list, allowing time for eating and drinking to be established post-procedure. A sliding scale should be able to be performed if required in the day-surgery unit.

Significant renal, hepatic or severe central nervous system disease should be sought. Epilepsy is not an absolute contraindication, unless there is poor control. Recent TIAs or cerebrovascular events in the past 6 months may exclude day-case surgery. This population group is also more likely to be anti-coagulated and every case should be assessed to see if this could be stopped for surgery. If unable to stop, the patient should be done as an inpatient, allowing for transfer to heparin infusion.

Other drugs that would make day-surgery potentially more complicated and inappropriate for day-case include monoamine oxidase inhibitors and corticosteroids. Excessive alcohol or drug abuse may also exclude day-surgery.

What are the important principles of anaesthetic management for day-case surgery?

It is important to perform safe and effective anaesthesia with rapid emergence and few complications. The patients need to recover rapidly, have no cardiovascular or respiratory effects and be awake, orientated and comfortable. They should not have nausea or vomiting and should be able to drink fluids. Anti-emetics and avoidance of nitrous oxide or volatile anaesthetic agents in many circumstances is advisable. Adequate analgesia is vital and opiate sparing techniques are important. Local anaesthetic techniques and NSAIDs should be used if appropriate.

When should patients be discharged and what criteria should they meet?

Prior to discharge the following criteria should be fulfilled:

- Cardiovascularly stable
- No excessive or continuing blood loss
- Saturations maintained on room air with normal respiratory parameters
- Pain, nausea and vomiting should be controlled
- Any motor block from regional technique should have worn off
- No impairment of bladder function
- Be mobilising independently.

As previously mentioned, the discharge environment must also be considered (adequate social care at home, including access to a phone, bathroom and a responsible adult to care for them for 24 hours). Patients must be informed of the actions to take in emergencies or if complications were to develop and given contact details and information leaflets to this effect.

What are the common reasons for overnight admission following day-case surgery?

There are many reasons why patients get admitted following day-surgery. There are surgical reasons, such as bleeding or more extensive procedure being performed. There are also anaesthetic reasons such as pain, cardiovascular or respiratory instability, nausea and vomiting. If any of the discharge criteria are not achieved, such as urinary retention, then the patient should also be admitted. The commonest reasons for admission are inadequate pain relief, nausea and vomiting.

Further Reading

Aylin P, Williams S, Jarman B, Bottle A. Trends in day surgery rates. *British Medical Journal*. 2005; **331**(7520): 803.

Department of Health. Day Surgery: Operational Guide. http://www.dh.gov.uk/ prod_consum_dh/groups/dh_digitalassets/@dh/@en/documents/digitalasset/dh_4060341.pdf.

NHS Evidence. Mini topic review: anaesthesia for day case surgery. http://www.library.nhs.uk/Theatres/ViewResource.aspx?resID=277694.

Chapter

2.3

ENT

2.3.1. Difficult intubation – Jonathan J Gatward

In your day-to-day practice, how do you attempt to predict a difficult tracheal intubation?

Remember to classify your answer. A great way to approach this question is "history, examination and investigations". There are a lot of different aspects to remember here – it may help to jot things down on a piece of paper, but do ask the examiner first, it is after all an oral exam.

There are many factors that might contribute to a difficult intubation. I therefore approach airway assessment in a systematic way. I take a full medical and anaesthetic history from the patient, paying particular attention to previous airway management. The patient may have been told that they are difficult to intubate and may even have been given a card, letter or medic alert bracelet. They may have medical conditions which are associated with difficult intubation, such as rheumatoid arthritis or ankylosing spondylitis. I check previous anaesthetic charts for airway difficulties and Cormack and Lehane grades, bearing in mind that these may have changed over time.

I then examine the patient. On general examination, findings that are associated with difficult intubation are:

- Obesity
- Pregnancy
- Large breasts
- A short, thick neck
- Goitre, haematoma or other mass in the neck
- Micro- or macrognathia
- Prominent upper incisors
- High arched palate
- Large tongue
- Limited mouth opening.

Dr. Podcast Scripts for the Final FRCA, ed. Rebecca A. Leslie, Emily K. Johnson,
Gary Thomas and Alexander P. L. Goodwin.   Published by Cambridge University Press.
© R. A. Leslie, E. K. Johnson, G. Thomas and A. P. L. Goodwin 2011.

Are there any more specific airway assessments that we use?

There are several bedside tests that can be performed. None of these is entirely reliable, but in combination they may predict a difficult intubation about 75% of the time. I regularly use the modified Mallampati test.

Can you tell me how you would perform this test?

This involves visually inspecting the pharyngeal structures with the patient sitting with mouth fully open, tongue protruded and without phonation. In a Class I view, the soft palate, uvula and tonsillar pillars are visible, in Class II, the soft palate and the base of the uvula, in Class III, the soft palate only and in Class IV, just the hard palate. This test yields many false-positive results and 50% false-negative results.

What other bedside assessments do you perform?

Another bedside test is the thyromental distance, which is the distance, in centimetres, from the notch of the thyroid cartilage to the chin (or mentum), with the head fully extended. A distance of less than 7 cm is associated with difficult intubation.

I also always assess mouth opening. Less than 3 cm is abnormal in an adult. Mouth opening can be affected by acute local pain and inflammation, so it is important to try to assess whether pain is the only limiting factor, in which case, mouth opening can often improve on induction of anaesthesia.

I also test jaw protrusion. The patient should be able to protrude the lower incisors in front of the upper incisors (Wilson classified this as a – lower in front of upper; b – equal; c – upper in front of lower).

I also assess neck extension at the atlanto-occipital joint. A range of movement of 35 degrees or more is normal. This may be limited by arthritis, ankylosing spondylitis, injury or surgery to the cervical spine, a rigid collar or the need for manual in-line stabilisation.

How specific and sensitive are these tests?

A combination of a modified Mallampati test Grade III or IV with a thyromental distance of less than 7 cm has been shown to be highly sensitive and specific for a Grade IV Cormack and Lehane view at laryngoscopy.

Do you know any scoring systems for predicting a difficult airway?

The Wilson Risk Score combines five patient factors: weight, head and neck movement, mouth and jaw movement, receding jaw and prominent incisors. These are scored from 0 to 2. A score of over 3 predicts 75% of difficult intubations, but has a false-positive rate of 12%.

Is there anything else we can do to investigate further?

There are several special airway investigations we can request. X-rays can be used to assess the amount of neck extension at the atlanto-occipital or atlanto-axial joints, or the relative length and depth of the mandible. We can get CT scans to look for soft tissue swelling or airway compression by extrinsic forces. We can also perform fibre-optic examination, usually by nasendoscopy to help to predict the view we might get at direct laryngoscopy.

You are due to anaesthetise a healthy adult patient for an elective operation requiring tracheal intubation. After your airway assessment, you conclude that intubation by direct laryngoscopy will be difficult or impossible. How will you proceed?

Remember, the exam is all about putting patient safety first. You are going to perform an awake fibre-optic intubation. There are many "recipes" for awake intubation, and you may have limited experience. Choose a recipe and learn it and be prepared to justify the method you use.

I would explain to the patient that they require awake intubation. I would describe the technique to them and run through exactly what they would experience. I would try to put the patient at ease and reassure them.

Can you outline a method for awake intubation?

I gain informed consent and ensure that standard monitoring is in place. The procedure requires a skilled assistant, and ideally a second anaesthetist. I secure intra-venous access and have an intra-venous infusion running. I give intra-venous glycopyrrolate 200 μg as an anti-sialogogue, and then spray both nostrils with a vasoconstrictor, usually xylometazoline spray. I have found a low-dose remifentanil infusion to be useful for its sedative and anti-tussive properties. I run this at a rate that results in a respiratory rate of 8 to 10 breaths per minute. There are many ways to provide local anaesthesia for the airway, but the method I prefer is to atomise 2% lidocaine with a three-way tap attached to a long 20 G cannula and oxygen tubing with oxygen running at 2 L·min^{-1} as the driving gas. I then atomise 1 ml of 2% lidocaine on inspiration every 1 to 2 minutes until there is an obvious change in the patient's voice.

What is the maximum dose of lidocaine that you would use?

I use a maximum dose of 8 mg·kg^{-1}, which is the maximum dose recommended in the British Thoracic Society guidelines for flexible bronchoscopy.

What can the anaesthetist do to prepare for the unanticipated failed intubation?

This question is designed to assess your safety as an anaesthetist. The examiner wants to establish that if this potentially life-threatening situation happens to you, you will approach it in a calm and measured way, with patient safety as your prime concern.

About half of difficult intubations are not predicted and so anaesthetists should prepare for all intubations as if failure could occur. On a basic level we should ensure that we are familiar with all the airway equipment and techniques that can be used during a difficult intubation. We should all know exactly what equipment is available on the difficult intubation trolley, and where it is. A trolley should be present in all operating theatre suites, intensive care units and emergency departments.

Difficult intubation is a rare occurrence, so we need to practise the rescue techniques, for example, on manikins or in simulators. We should also be familiar with a difficult intubation algorithm.

Which difficult intubation algorithm do you use?

I use the Difficult Airway Society guidelines. These are well-regarded, evidence-based consensus guidelines, which give separate structured approaches to difficult intubation during routine and rapid sequence induction. I always have a clear plan A and plan B, which I communicate to my assistant, before any intubation attempt. The guidelines emphasise optimisation of the initial intubation attempt, summoning senior anaesthetic help as soon as possible, avoiding repeated attempts at laryngoscopy and maintaining oxygenation above all else.

You perform a rapid sequence induction of anaesthesia in a patient in whom you had not predicted difficulty and obtain a Cormack and Lehane Grade IV view on laryngoscopy. How do you approach this situation?

You should have a difficult airway algorithm, such as the Difficult Airway Society guideline or the one used in your own hospital, committed to memory.

Firstly, I would ensure oxygenation at all times. If oxygen saturations start to fall I would abandon intubation attempts and ventilate the patient with a facemask and airway adjuncts.

Let us assume that the oxygen saturations are maintained in the first instance. How would you proceed?

Initially, I would attempt to optimise the initial view at laryngoscopy. I would ensure that the head was in the correct position and try external laryngeal manipulation, like backward, upward rightward pressure (the BURP manoeuvre). I may try an alternative laryngoscope blade, such as the McCoy or straight blade. If I obtained a view of any laryngeal structures, I would attempt to pass a gum-elastic-bougie, either under direct vision or blindly into the midline. If I was successful, I may feel clicks as the bougie passes down the trachea and "hold up" as the tip of the bougie reaches the carina.

Unfortunately, none of your manoeuvres allows you to intubate. What do you do next?

I would avoid repeated attempts at laryngoscopy and would not give a second dose of muscle relaxant. After three attempts at intubation, or if oxygen saturations began to fall, I would abandon attempts at intubation. I would call for senior help and concentrate all my efforts on oxygenating the patient. I would allow the patient to wake unless surgery is immediately life-threatening. Initially, I would attempt facemask ventilation, with airway adjuncts such as an oropharyngeal or nasopharyngeal airway, and a two-person technique if necessary. If oxygen saturations fall below 90% using these techniques, I would attempt to insert a laryngeal mask airway. This may involve reducing cricoid pressure, both for insertion and subsequent ventilation, but this is acceptable in the circumstances.

Despite your best efforts, you are unable to ventilate the patient with the bag-valve mask or the laryngeal mask airway. Your patient is cyanosed, with falling oxygen saturations. No senior help is available. Now what will you do?

Don't mess about here – you are all the way down to Plan D of the Difficult Airway Society guidelines – the "can't intubate, can't ventilate" scenario. You have to perform a cricothyroidotomy.

The patient requires a cricothyroidotomy, which I could either achieve with a cannula or surgical technique. I could use either a standard intra-venous cannula, or a specialised cricothyroidotomy cannula.

What oxygen supply can you connect these to?

These cannulae require high-pressure ventilation, which means wall oxygen at 400 kPa. This involves either connecting oxygen tubing to a wall flowmeter turned to 15 L·min^{-1} or using a specialised, high-pressure ventilator such as the Sanders injector or Manujet. The common gas outlet of the anaesthetic machine cannot be used as there is a pressure relief valve which will vent at 40 kPa, which is insufficient for high-pressure ventilation. I would need to allow a long time for expiration, which needs to occur through the upper airway, to avoid volutrauma.

What is the alternative to needle techniques?

The other option is a surgical technique, which I could perform with either a kit that employs a Seldinger technique or by incising the skin and cricothyroid membrane using a scalpel, then dilating the orifice in order to insert a standard endotracheal tube of approximate size 6-mm internal diameter.

You have saved the patient's life, well done

2.3.2. Performing a tracheostomy – Jonathan J Gatward

You are called down to the emergency department to see a rugby player who has been on the receiving end of a high tackle to his neck. He has neck pain, bruising over his anterior neck, stridor, haemoptysis and a hoarse voice.

What injury do you suspect, and how will you manage him?

This is an uncommon injury, but is an ENT surgical emergency. Remember to adopt the Advanced Trauma Life Support approach in all trauma scenarios.

I suspect he has a laryngeal injury. This is an ENT surgical emergency, as swelling of the injured larynx can lead to airway obstruction. I would approach his management as I would with all trauma patients – with an ABCDE approach. I would begin to assess his airway, ensuring that cervical spine precautions were in place as he is at risk of a cervical spine injury. I know he already has stridor and haemoptysis and I would be aware that his airway

may deteriorate at any point. With patient reassurance and explanation, I would administer oxygen at 15 L·min^{-1} via a non-rebreathing mask and then examine him for signs of
adequate ventilation – namely his colour, chest expansion, respiratory rate, breath sounds
and oxygen saturation. I would then assess his circulation, looking for signs of shock and
obtaining intra-venous access.

He is saturating well on oxygen and has a normal respiratory rate. He is haemodynamically normal. What will you do next?

He needs to be transferred to the operating theatre for an awake tracheostomy under local
anaesthetic. He may have a laryngeal fracture and so endotracheal intubation via direct laryngoscopy may be very difficult and there is a risk of losing the airway. I would call my anaesthetic consultant and the ENT surgeons to attend urgently and prepare my own equipment
for a potential difficult intubation should the patient deteriorate.

What equipment would you prepare?

I would get the difficult intubation trolley into theatre and make sure I had access to Macin-
tosh and McCoy laryngoscope blades, a gum elastic bougie, a laryngeal mask of the correct
size, a range of endotracheal tubes including a microlaryngoscopy tube and equipment for
cricothyroidotomy including the high-pressure ventilator. I would also ask for the fibre-optic
bronchoscope.

How do you plan to manage the patient's airway?

Ideally, the patient would be able to tolerate an awake tracheostomy under local anaesthesia.
I would call for senior help and stay with the patient throughout the procedure.

**Unfortunately, before the ENT surgeon arrives, the patient's condition deteriorates and
his oxygen saturations start to fall. On examination, he has very poor air entry.**

What will you do now?

I would assess the patient and seek to gain control of the airway. I would pre-oxygenate him
as much as possible with a tight-fitting bag-valve mask. I would ask for the cricothyroidotomy kit to be opened and then perform a rapid sequence induction of anaesthesia using an
induction agent and suxamethonium, with manual in-line stabilisation as there is a question
of neck injury. I would then attempt direct laryngoscopy and see whether it was possible to
visualise the glottis. If I saw the glottis, I would pass a gum elastic bougie and then railroad
an appropriately sized tracheal tube through the visible lumen.

**Unfortunately, on direct laryngoscopy, you can only see badly distorted swollen pha-
ryngeal and laryngeal structures and lots of blood. Even after suctioning, you see no glottic
opening and the patient's oxygen saturations are falling rapidly.**

What will you do now?

I now need to perform an emergency cricothyroidotomy. There are three available techniques: surgical, cannula and Seldinger techniques.

Good. Can you describe the technique you will use, paying particular attention to the anatomy of the neck?

You will probably only be asked to describe one of these techniques, and you are unlikely to have done any of them in anger. Make sure you know the anatomy. Try to learn a simple line diagram of the larynx, which you can reproduce quickly and reliably (see Figure 2.3.2). You will need to know all the steps involved in at least one technique for emergency cricothyroidotomy. We have included all three techniques here for completeness.

The larynx lies at the level of the fourth to sixth cervical vertebrae. It is made up of the thyroid, cricoid, arytenoid, cuneiform and corniculate cartilages. The only ones palpable at the front of the neck are the thyroid and cricoid cartilages. The thyroid cartilage is the most prominent laryngeal cartilage, and is usually palpated easily, especially in men. The cricoid lies inferior to this, at the level of C6. It is a signet ring shape, with the narrower band portion lying anteriorly. The cricothyroid membrane is a palpable groove between the lower border of the thyroid cartilage and the upper border of the cricoid cartilage. It is usually easy to palpate, though may not be in this case, as there is injury to the front of the neck.

To perform a surgical cricothyroidotomy, I would extend the patient's neck as much as possible. The patient is at risk of a cervical spine injury, but this is a life-saving intervention. I would then use the thumb and forefinger of my non-dominant hand to stabilise the cricothyroid membrane and to protect the lateral vascular structures from injury. I would make a transverse incision through the skin and cricothyroid membrane, being careful not to damage the cricoid cartilage. I would then leave the scalpel in position and insert a tracheal hook, a pair of forceps or a gum elastic bougie into the incision alongside the scalpel. I would enlarge the opening with whichever instrument I was using and leave it in situ. I would then insert a size 6-mm internal diameter endotracheal tube, either over the bougie

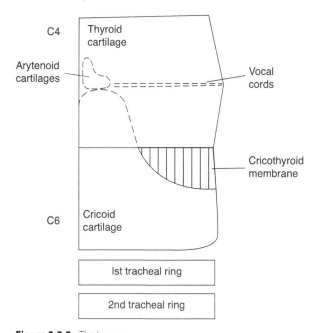

Figure 2.3.2. The larynx.

or alongside the forceps or tracheal hook. I would then connect a circuit and ventilate the patient with 100% oxygen, check that this is effective, then secure the tube to prevent dislodgement.

To perform a cannula cricothyroidotomy, I would attach a 14-gauge intra-venous cannula or a Ravussin cannula to a 5-ml syringe. The Ravussin cannula is a specially designed cannula for cricothyroidotomy. It is more resistant to kinking and has a flange to attach it to the neck. It has both Luer Lock and 15-mm connections. I would place a hand on the neck to identify and stabilise the cricothyroid membrane, and to protect the lateral vascular structures from injury from the needle, then insert the needle and cannula through the cricothyroid membrane at a 45-degree angle caudally, aspirating as I go. When I had successfully aspirated air, I would advance the cannula over the needle, being careful not to damage the posterior tracheal wall. I would then remove the needle, re-check that air can be aspirated from the cannula, and connect to a high-pressure oxygen supply.

What oxygen supply can you connect a cannula to?

Cannulae require high-pressure ventilation, which means wall oxygen at 400 kPa. This involves either connecting oxygen tubing to a wall flowmeter turned on full, or using a specialised, high-pressure ventilator such as the Sanders injector or Manujet. Ideally I would use a specialised ventilator to save having to make something out of oxygen tubing and a three-way tap. The common gas outlet of the anaesthetic machine cannot be used as there is a pressure relief valve which will vent at 40 kPa, which is insufficient for high-pressure ventilation. I would need to allow a long time for expiration, which needs to occur through the upper airway, to avoid volutrauma.

Good. Now, what is the third method of performing a cricothyroidotomy?

Many anaesthetists are used to performing percutaneous tracheostomies on the ICU using a Seldinger technique with either serial dilatation or a "rhino" dilator. They may therefore choose to use a Seldinger technique to perform an emergency cricothyroidotomy. There are now cuffed size 6-mm internal diameter emergency cricothyroidotomy kits available, and there is evidence that they can be inserted nearly as quickly as a surgical airway and may cause fewer complications. The kits contain a cannula, which I would insert just as for an emergency cannula cricothyroidotomy. I would then insert the guidewire through the cannula and make a horizontal incision in the skin either side of the wire. I would railroad the dilator and tube assembly over the wire, dilating the airway orifice and inserting the cricothyroidotomy tube in one movement. Finally, I would remove the dilator and guidewire, attach a breathing circuit and ventilate with 100% oxygen. It is important to observe the patient for chest movement and check the neck to exclude swelling from gas getting into surrounding tissues rather than the trachea.

What are the potential complications of cricothyroidotomy?

The immediate complications are malposition, the creation of a false passage, oesophageal perforation, surgical emphysema and haemorrhage. On trying to ventilate the patient, you can cause surgical emphysema, barotrauma and pneumothorax. Also, cannulae may kink or become displaced.

How does a percutaneous tracheostomy differ from a cricothyroidotomy?

Percutaneous tracheostomy is usually performed electively on ICU patients in the ICU itself, whereas cricothyroidotomy is an emergency airway rescue technique. The anatomy differs in that percutaneous tracheostomies are inserted through the anterior tracheal wall, below the cricoid cartilage, whereas cricothyroidotomy is performed via the cricothyroid membrane. Percutaneous tracheostomies are usually inserted between the second and third tracheal rings, as higher approaches may predispose to tracheal stenosis after decannulation. This risk is balanced by the fact that the thyroid isthmus lies between the second and fourth tracheal rings, so there is a risk of damage to this structure causing haemorrhage; however, the dilation technique will often tamponade any bleeding. In orally or nasally intubated patients, percutaneous tracheostomy is usually performed with a second operator observing the procedure from inside the trachea with the use of a fibre-optic bronchoscope down the tracheal tube, particularly ensuring the needle and wire enter the trachea in the mid-line.

What are the general indications for tracheostomy?

Remember, as always, to categorise if possible.

The indications can be subdivided into those for airway obstruction, those for airway protection and ICU uses.

- Airway obstruction may be caused by tumours, trauma, burns, anaphylaxis and infections, such as epiglottitis.
- Airway protection might be necessary during head and neck surgery involving the upper airway and larynx, in neurological or muscle diseases such as Guillain-Barré syndrome, bulbar palsies and head injury.
- In ICU, patients may require tracheostomy to aid sputum removal if they have a poor cough or are producing excessive secretions. Tracheostomies may also facilitate weaning from ventilation, as they decrease work of breathing compared to an oral or nasal tracheal tube, and allow for easier suctioning of secretions. Tracheostomies also allow the patient to be awake during a long wean therefore avoiding the complications of long-term sedation. Early tracheostomy has been found in a recent trial to decrease the number of ventilator days, though there was no significant difference in mortality.

You are asked to take an intubated ICU patient to theatre for a surgical tracheostomy. What are the potential pitfalls and how do you ensure that the airway is maintained throughout the operation?

ICU patients are often sick, physiologically unstable and their management complicated. I may not know the patient, so I would get a full handover and make sure I had read the notes, examined the patient and had seen recent blood gas and other blood results. I would also like to see a recent chest X-ray and make sure I knew the optimal depth of the tracheal tube for the patient. I would make sure I knew the patient's ventilatory requirements and what infusions they are on. I would make sure I had full monitoring for transfer and take a skilled assistant with me. I would have a transfer bag with all the relevant drugs and equipment for transfer.

Let's assume you have transferred the patient to the operating theatre and they are safely on the table. Talk me through the operation and your role in maintaining the airway

Patient positioning involves extending the neck, at which point the tube can become dislodged. I would stabilise the tube at this point. Once in position, I would administer 100% oxygen. The surgeons dissect down to the trachea, and then make a vertical incision through one of the second to fourth tracheal rings. They then make a flap or hole in the trachea, at which point the oral tracheal tube can be visualised. There is a risk of damage to the cuff during this process, so I would listen for a cuff leak and watch the oxygen saturations. When the surgeons are ready, they ask for the tracheal tube to be withdrawn. I do this slowly and leave some of it within the larynx in case it needs to be reinserted. The tracheostomy tube is inserted, which can be difficult. At this point, there will be limited ventilation due to the presence of the tracheostomy tube within the tracheal lumen. The tracheostomy tube cuff is then inflated and the breathing circuit is then swapped onto the tracheostomy tube. I would examine the patient for bilateral chest expansion; check the capnography trace and the oxygen saturations. At this point the responsibility for holding and securing the tracheostomy tube is transferred to the surgeons, who may place sutures or secure the tube by tying. I would only remove the oral tube when I was convinced the tracheostomy was sited correctly. If there was any doubt at all I would insert the fibre-optic bronchoscope to check, looking for positioning with respect to the carina.

Do you know what "stay sutures" are?

These are long sutures placed into the lateral walls of the tracheal orifice during tracheostomy, the ends of which are taped to the patients neck either side of the tracheostomy tube. They are used to help reinsertion of the tracheostomy tube should it require changing, fall out or become displaced. Pulling on them brings the tracheal orifice closer to the surface of the skin, so that the orifice can be visualised more easily.

2.3.3. Bleeding tonsil and foreign body – Caroline SG Janes

Part 1: The bleeding tonsil

This is a common scenario in the clinical structured oral exam, which you will be expected to know well – the examiners will not be sympathetic if you miss the key points.

You are called in the middle of the night by the ENT ST3 – he would like to take a 6-year-old girl to theatre who is bleeding 8 hours post-tonsillectomy. He would like to proceed immediately and says he is starting to make plans to transfer the patient. He says he will meet you in theatre.

What are the key issues with this case?

This case illustrates a number of anaesthetic challenges; it is a paediatric case involving a difficult airway, which will be shared with the surgeon. The child may be haemodynamically compromised and is at risk of pulmonary aspiration. These issues are further complicated by the likely presence of anxious parents.

The extent of blood loss will be difficult to quantify as the child may have swallowed it instead of spitting it out – signs of haemodynamic compromise should therefore be assessed and resuscitated promptly.

Laryngoscopy and intubation will be challenging as the airway may be compromised by oedema and blood. Children have smaller, more reactive airways, which tolerate manipulation less well. They also have a reduced functional residual capacity and can desaturate rapidly. The likelihood of a stomach full of blood further endangers the airway due to the risk of aspiration.

Other issues specific to paediatric anaesthesia include difficult intra-venous access, communication difficulties, anxious parents, temperature regulation and altered drug dosages.

How would you respond to the ENT doctor?

I would inform the ENT doctor that the patient should not leave the ward until I had reviewed her and done a thorough pre-operative assessment. In these cases there can be substantial occult blood loss and the child's haemodynamic status needs to be assessed carefully. Adequate fluid resuscitation should be carried out prior to induction as children compensate well despite considerable blood loss. I would also need to discuss this case with the duty consultant prior to proceeding and transferring the child to theatre.

What information would you look for during your pre-operative assessment?

The most important thing to determine is the haemodynamic status. I would assess this by thorough history, examination and investigations. I would ask the nurses and parents about excessive swallowing that would suggest occult bleeding or vomiting of blood. I would examine the child to assess capillary refill time, level of consciousness and signs of shock such as pallor and cool peripheries. I would review the ward charts for heart rate, blood pressure, respiratory rate and urine output. Hypotension and decreasing consciousness are late signs of hypovolaemic shock in children and would suggest decompensation. Intra-venous access should be present but this should not be assumed and it should be checked for. I would also request an urgent full blood count, clotting screen and crossmatch.

In addition I would carry out a routine anaesthetic history and review the initial anaesthetic chart and the drug chart. I would specifically look for the size of endotracheal tube used, recorded laryngeal view, analgesia administered and any difficulties encountered during the initial procedure.

The child's heart rate is 120 bpm, her respiratory rate is 30 bpm and her blood pressure is 80/40. Capillary refill time is 4 seconds, and her extremities are cool to touch. She is lethargic and complains faintly of feeling sick.

How would you resuscitate this child?

Given these vital signs it is clear that the child has suffered substantial blood loss and requires urgent resuscitation. I would discuss this case with the consultant on-call at the earliest opportunity as this case should be carried out by an experienced anaesthetist. The child should be given high-flow oxygen via a non-rebreathing face mask and intra-venous access should be obtained if this has not been done already. An initial bolus crystalloid of 20 ml/kg should be administered and further fluid resuscitation should be guided by clinical signs. The child should be moved to an area with appropriate monitoring – the most suitable place is often the anaesthetic room.

The bleeding needs to be stopped surgically as soon as possible; however, adequate resuscitation needs to have taken place prior to induction of anaesthesia to avoid cardiovascular collapse. Once the full blood count and clotting screen is known, the use of blood products should be considered. The child should be reassessed after each fluid bolus until she is considered stable enough to proceed with induction.

How would you anaesthetise this child?

I would anaesthetise the child in theatre with the help of an experienced assistant. I would want two suction circuits available in case one became blocked by a blood clot. I would prepare a selection of endotracheal tubes: – the same size as used previously and half a size smaller. I would have two of each available in case one became blocked with blood clots. The child should be fully monitored according to the AAGBI minimum standards of monitoring.

The two choices of anaesthetic for a bleeding tonsil are inhalational induction in the left lateral position and head down position or a rapid sequence induction.

The main advantage of an inhalational induction is that spontaneous ventilation is maintained. The head down position encourages blood in the airway to drain away from the laryngeal inlet. However this technique can be more challenging.

I am more familiar with a rapid sequence induction in the supine position using thiopentone and suxamethonium and it is usually the preferred option. This enables a more rapid procurement of a secure airway with a tracheal tube. Once the airway is secure, ventilation with the use of a non-depolarising muscle relaxant would facilitate a rapid emergence at the end of the procedure. Fluids can be titrated to response. At the end of surgery I would insert a wide-bore orogastric tube to empty the stomach of blood and then extubate the patient in the left lateral, head down position fully awake. Judicious use of analgesia peri-operatively may be topped up in the recovery room as required.

What post-operative care should the child receive?

The child should go to recovery for an extended stay with close monitoring. A full blood count and clotting screen should be sent post-operatively and any abnormalities corrected.

What is the difference between a primary and secondary tonsillar bleed?

The incidence of bleeding following a tonsillectomy is 0.5–2%, and it is usually caused by either venous or capillary ooze. A primary bleed occurs in the immediate post-operative period, usually within 24 hours of surgery, and is most commonly caused by poor haemostasis during surgery. A secondary bleed can occur up to 28 days post-tonsillectomy and is usually secondary to infection or less commonly caused by loosened vessel ties or sloughing off of dead tissue.

What is the blood supply to the tonsillar bed?

The tonsils are supplied by the external carotid artery and its branches. The superior pole is supplied by the tonsillar branches of the ascending pharyngeal artery and lesser palatine artery. The inferior pole is supplied by the ascending palatine artery, dorsal lingual artery and the facial artery branches.

Venous drainage of the tonsils goes to the lingual vein, the pharyngeal and tonsillar capsule plexuses.

What risk factors predispose to post-tonsillectomy bleeding?

The surgical technique is the most important determinant of risk of post-tonsillectomy bleeding. The use of diathermy carries three times the risk of post-operative bleeding compared to a more traditional technique using ties and packs. The latter, however, is accompanied by more intra-operative bleeding.

Other risk factors for post-tonsillectomy bleeding include increasing age and being male.

Part 2: Swallowed or inhaled foreign body

A 2-year-old boy presents on the emergency list for rigid bronchoscopy to remove an aspirated peanut.

What are the key considerations in this case?

The most important consideration is whether established or impending airway compromise is present. Other anaesthetic challenges include a shared airway and the risk of pulmonary aspiration, particularly if the patient is not starved.

Other considerations specific to paediatric anaesthesia include difficult intra-venous access, communication difficulties, anxious parents, temperature regulation and altered drug dosages.

How can you differentiate between upper and lower airway obstruction? And why is this important?

It is important to differentiate between upper and lower airway obstruction as they are managed differently.

Foreign bodies in the upper airway may present as emergencies requiring immediate attention. The child is more likely to present acutely with respiratory distress. They may have stridor and drooling, they may be using accessory muscles of respiration and have intercostal recession. In extreme cases they can even present with complete respiratory obstruction. The narrowest point of a paediatric airway is at the level of the cricoid ring and therefore foreign bodies can lodge at this point.

Foreign bodies that lodge more distally tend to present later and less acutely. The child may present with a persisting cough, bronchospasm and signs of infection. If they are pyrexial or have raised inflammatory markers they will require a course of anti-biotics. The oil from a peanut is especially irritant and can cause mucosal oedema and chemical pneumonitis.

In addition to a thorough history and examination, chest radiographs may help to determine the location of the foreign body. If the foreign body is radiolucent, areas of hyperinflation from air trapping may be present distal to the site of the foreign body.

What further information would you like about this case prior to proceeding with this case?

Firstly I would like to know whether the child is stable and whether there are signs of respiratory distress. If I suspected airway compromise I would attend to the child immediately and request senior help.

However, if the child is stable I would take a thorough pre-operative history and examine the child. I would review the CXR and discuss the case with ENT surgeons to determine the level at which the foreign body has become lodged.

Would you pre-medicate the child?

I would request topical local anaesthetic cream to be applied to both hands prior to intra-venous cannulation. I would also consider the use of an anti-cholinergic agent. This may be helpful in decreasing secretions and vagal tone thus aiding intubation and avoiding bradycardia during instrumentation of the airway. I would, however, avoid sedative pre-medication.

The child is stable when calmed by his mother. He has mild stridor when upset and is drooling. He has a heart rate of 130 beats per minute and a respiratory rate of 24 breaths per minute with an arterial saturation of 100% on air. Radiographically the obstruction is believed to be at the level of the cricoid cartilage.

How would you anaesthetise this child?

In this case there is sufficient airway compromise to proceed with anaesthesia without allowing time for fasting. I would contact the consultant-on-call and ask for them to come in. I would also request the help of an experienced anaesthetic assistant. Prior to induction of anaesthesia, I would ensure the ENT surgeons were immediately available and ready to proceed with the bronchoscopy, or help establish a surgical airway, if complete respiratory obstruction should ensue.

I would check all my equipment prior to induction and ensure all connections are compatible with the rigid bronchoscope. My preferred option for induction of anaesthesia is inhalation of sevoflurane in 100% oxygen with the child sitting on their parent's lap.

I would avoid neuromuscular blockers for two reasons. Firstly paralysis would cause loss of muscular tone, which can result in loss of the airway. Secondly positive pressure ventilation would be required which could push the foreign body down further causing complete occlusion, air trapping or in extreme cases a tension pneumothorax.

Following induction I would perform laryngoscopy and spray the cords with local anaesthetic to decrease stimulation during instrumentation. I would use sevoflurane in 100% oxygen for maintenance of anaesthesia, although halothane is sometimes preferred. This is due to its offset of action being slower than sevoflurane and therefore the patient is less likely to lighten during periods of breathholding and apnoea.

Retrieval of the foreign body can be attempted when a deep enough plane of anaesthesia is achieved. There are various anaesthetic options during retrieval of the foreign body. A T-piece can be connected to a Storz rigid ventilating bronchoscope, which allows delivery of volatile and oxygen to a spontaneously breathing patient. Intermittent positive pressure ventilation can be delivered with this system but as previously discussed is best avoided in this case.

Insufflation with a Sanders injector is not recommended for the same reasons. My preferred technique would be to allow the child to breath spontaneously and attach the T-piece to the bronchoscope during foreign body removal.

The child's vital signs should be continuously monitored and the chest continually observed. The most common problems encountered will be hypertension, tachycardia or ventricular ectopic beats, hypoxia, hypercarbia and coughing.

I would administer dexamethasone to decrease the incidence of airway oedema. With prior consent from the parents I would give rectal or intravenous paracetamol and rectal diclofenac if there are no contraindications. I would avoid opiates, as severe post-operative pain is uncommon.

Post-operatively the child should be extubated awake in the head down and left lateral position. They should then have a prolonged stay in recovery to observe for reactive oedema and monitor respiratory function.

Would the method of anaesthesia and post-operative care differ if there was a foreign body lodged in the lower airways?

With lower airway obstruction, the avoidance of bag mask ventilation and intermittent positive pressure ventilation is less critical, however the same mode of anaesthetic management may be used as for upper airway foreign bodies.

Cases of lower airway foreign body aspiration are less likely to present acutely with airway compromise and therefore there will be time to ensure the patient is adequately fasted. However, there may be signs of pneumonia or pneumonitis which may require treatment prior to surgery.

As in upper airway foreign body removal the child should have a prolonged stay in recovery to observe for reactive oedema and monitor respiratory function. The child may need a course of steroids and anti-biotics if the obstruction was prolonged. Chest physiotherapy and humidified oxygen may be beneficial. If the child shows signs of sepsis they should be monitored in a high-dependency environment until these resolve.

2.3.4. Obstructive sleep apnoea – Sarah F Bell

Sleep apnoea is a topic that comes up frequently in the SOE. You need to be confident with the definition, clinical presentation and anaesthetic management of the disease.

You are presented with a 56-year-old male obese smoker for an elective large inguinal hernia repair. He also says that he suffers from obstructive sleep apnoea, which was diagnosed 2 years ago. He currently uses a CPAP machine overnight.

How common is sleep apnoea?

About 3% of middle-aged adults have clinically significant sleep apnoea with the male:female ratio of 2:1.

What are the causes of sleep apnoea?

*Try and classify your answer since the examiner has not yet said **obstructive** sleep apnoea.*

Sleep apnoea can be caused by either obstructive or central factors. Obstructive sleep apnoea is characterised by persistent effort without airflow, whilst in central apnoea effort is absent.

Obstructive sleep apnoea is due to pharyngeal collapse that occurs during sleep. Vibration of the flaccid structures causes snoring which persists until sleep is interrupted and muscle tone restored. Obstructive sleep apnoea is associated with obesity, pharyngeal abnormalities and conditions such as hypothyroidism. Sedative drugs and alcohol can precipitate the condition.

Central sleep apnoea is due to reduced or absent respiratory effort due to disorders of ventilatory control or neuromuscular function. Patients have reduced ventilatory capacity that is sufficient when awake, but insufficient when asleep (as the respiratory drive decreases and compensatory mechanisms fail). Causes of central sleep apnoea include neuromuscular diseases such as polio or muscular dystrophy, central nervous system problems such as stroke, surgery and head injury, and finally, excessive respiratory load such as kyphoscoliosis.

What are the symptoms of sleep apnoea?

Try not to focus your answer solely on the respiratory symptoms.

The symptoms of sleep apnoea are heavy snoring with occasional wakening and excessive daytime somnolence. Poor memory, mood changes and headaches may be described. Gastro-oesophageal reflux disease, impotence and nocturnal epilepsy are associated with sleep apnoea. The patient's partner may describe witnessing apnoeas and sudden awakenings with choking. Children with sleep apnoea may have behavioural problems and frequent respiratory tract infections.

What are the signs of sleep apnoea?

The clinical signs of sleep apnoea may be divided into airway, respiratory, cardiac and other systems. The airway signs include maxillary hypoplasia, retrognathia, nasal obstruction, increased neck circumference (> 44 cm), changes to the soft tissues of the palate and decreased oropharyngeal dimensions. The respiratory signs include cyanosis, hypoxia, CO_2 tremor, bony and muscular chest wall abnormalities. The cardiac signs include hypertension, arrhythmias and right heart failure (raised JVP, pulsatile liver and peripheral oedema). Other systems that might indicate diseases associated with sleep apnoea are the neurological and endocrine systems, with diseases such as stroke, hypothyroidism or acromegaly possibly being present.

And what are the potential consequences of sleep apnoea?

As usual try and classify your answer!

The sequelae of sleep apnoea occur throughout the different physiological body systems.

Neurological – reduced memory and cognition, headaches, anxiety, depression and intra-cranial hypertension.

Cardiovascular – hypertension, ischaemic heart disease, cerebrovascular disease and right heart failure.

Respiratory – hypoxaemia, hypercapnia and pulmonary hypertension. Long-term sleep apnoea leads to desensitisation of respiratory centres with increased reliance on the hypoxic drive and eventually type two respiratory failure.

Haematological – polycythaemia

Endocrine – reductions in growth hormone and testosterone levels and predisposition to diabetes.

Gastrointestinal tract – Gastro-oesophageal reflux disease.

Sleep apnoea is also associated with poor wound healing.

How is obstructive sleep apnoea diagnosed?

The diagnosis of obstructive sleep apnoea is made after taking a full history and examining the patient. The gold standard of investigation is overnight polysomnography. This involves videoing a patient sleeping and recording measurements such as the EEG (to stage the sleep cycle), ECG, pulse oximetry, mouth and nasal airflow, chest and abdominal movement, snoring level and apnoeas. Apnoeic episodes are described as 10 seconds or more of total cessation of airflow despite continuation of respiratory effort against a closed glottis. More than five of these in an hour or thirty during a night are considered clinically significant.

What are the treatment options for obstructive sleep apnoea?

Treatment options are dependent on the severity of the condition and the preference of the patient. Initial measures include weight loss, reduction of alcohol or sedative consumption and cessation of smoking. CPAP is the treatment of choice for patients with moderate to severe sleep apnoea. It acts by splinting open the upper airway, reduces secondary complications and improves mortality rates. More severe cases may require BIPAP devices.

Some cases of obstructive sleep apnoea may require upper airway imaging to guide whether surgical intervention will be of benefit. Correction of nasal obstruction, tonsillectomy and even tracheostomy have all been performed for sleep apnoea patients.

What would be the general anaesthetic considerations for this man?

Sleep apnoea poses a number of challenges to the anaesthetist – firstly the altered respiratory drive, secondly the potential difficult ventilation and intubation and thirdly the multi-system effects of the sleep apnoea.

How would you assess the patient?

I would take a full history from the patient and his partner, paying particular attention to the sleep apnoea and any systemic effects that may have occurred. I would also want to discuss the inguinal hernia and the indications for the operation. My examination would focus on assessing the patient's airway, respiratory and cardiovascular systems. I would also want to see a recent full blood count and U&Es to assess for polycythaemia and possible effects of anti-hypertensive treatment on renal function. I would require an ECG, looking for evidence of right heart failure and ischaemic heart disease. An ECHO and sleep studies might be indicated depending on the severity of the patient's condition.

How would you anaesthetise this man?

Try and picture yourself actually seeing and anaesthetising this patient.

If local anaesthesia or regional anaesthesia are not options, I would proceed to general anaesthesia. I would avoid sedative premedication but would consider prescribing a pre-operative antacid.

If the inguinal hernia is large it is likely that the surgeons will require muscle relaxation. Given the increased risk of gastro-oesophageal reflux disease I would plan to intubate the patient. How I induced anaesthesia would depend on my findings at the pre-operative visit. If the airway appeared difficult I would consent the patient for an awake fibre-optic intubation; otherwise I would consider performing a rapid sequence induction due to the risks of gastro-oesophageal reflux disease. Patients with sleep apnoea can become harder to mask ventilate once the muscle relaxant has been administered, have a higher incidence of difficult intubation and airway complications such as laryngospasm. I would therefore request senior anaesthetic assistance for this case.

Considerations during maintenance of anaesthesia would include judicious use of opiates and any sedative medication, since this might lead to post-operative respiratory failure. I would use local anaesthetic techniques to provide analgesia wherever possible. I would aim to maintain normothermia, normocapnia, adequate oxygenation and hydration throughout the procedure.

What are your concerns for this patient in the post-operative period?

The patient will require his CPAP in the post-operative period. A high-dependency bed should be available. The patient should be nursed sitting (not supine) and care should be taken to monitor his oxygen saturations, respiratory rate and conscious level.

Patients with sleep apnoea are at higher risk of developing deep vein thrombosis and so I would consider starting clexane early with TED stockings and pneumatic foot pumps.

Further Reading

Williams J, Hanning C. Obstructive sleep apnoea. *British Journal of Anaesthesia. CEPD Reviews* 2003; **3**(3): 75–78.

2.3.5. Upper airway infections – Sarah F Bell

This topic would normally feature in the clinical structured oral exam. The examiners want to know that you are safe and have a structured approach to managing a potential airway emergency.

You are called to the resuscitation room in casualty to see a 3-year-old boy with stridor. His oxygen saturations are 92% on air, his respiratory rate is 40 and he has audible stridor.

Can you tell me what exactly is stridor?

The examiners might ask an unexpected question to start with. Try and stick to what you know and answer the question!

This is the harsh vibratory sound produced when the airway becomes partially obstructed. It is caused by turbulent flow within the respiratory system. The loudness of the stridor does not relate to the degree of airway narrowing.

Can you explain to me why children are more likely to develop stridor?

Paediatric patients have smaller diameter upper and lower airways. A small reduction in the airway causes a marked increased in resistance to flow as described by the Hagen Pouseille equation.

How would you assess this child with stridor?

Describe your assessment as though you are performing it in real life. This will reassure the examiner that you have seen or thought carefully about this type of situation before and that you appreciate the important considerations in this case.

I would take a history from the parents, examine the patient and initiate interventions as appropriate. The speed of my actions would depend on the severity of the respiratory compromise of the child. The key to assessment is to disturb the child as little as possible since crying or agitation may precipitate complete airway obstruction. I would allow the parents to comfort the child to minimise anxiety and stress.

My history would focus on the presenting complaint. Specifically I would want to know the duration and onset of symptoms, whether any previous treatment had been commenced and whether the child had had any previous episodes. Generally I would enquire about the past medical history, drug history, allergies and anaesthetic history. I would also want to know when the child last ate and drank.

In my examination I would assess the child by observing the airway and respiratory system. I would look to see that the airway was patent and listen to any airway sounds such as stridor, wheeze, grunting or gurgling. I would assess the work of breathing by looking at the respiratory rate, whether there was any head bobbing, nasal flaring, sub- or intercostal recession or tracheal tug. I would note the position of the child and whether it preferred a sitting position. I would not attempt to lay the child flat. If tolerated, I would attach a pulse oximeter.

What would be your initial actions?

Again, picture yourself in A&E actually in this situation.

I would attempt to give the child supplementary oxygen via facemask or tubing held near the child, depending on what was tolerated. I would manage the child in a quiet, calm environment with the parents. I would assess the severity of the respiratory compromise by observing the respiratory rate, oxygen saturations, respiratory effort of the child and its conscious level. Importantly I would be looking to see whether these parameters improved with my interventions. I would take a full history from the parents in order to try and formulate a possible diagnosis. I would administer nebulised adrenaline, if tolerated, and call for senior ENT and anaesthetic assistance. I would consider obtaining IV access and a baseline temperature reading, but this would depend on the individual child's temperament and the severity of the illness. It is crucial to avoid further upsetting the patient and worsening the respiratory compromise. I would aim to transfer the child to the theatre suite if no improvements were observed.

What would be in you differential diagnosis for a patient with stridor?

The patient may be suffering from an infection. This may be viral, in the case of croup, or bacterial, in the case of epiglottitis or diphtheria. The patient may have a pharyngeal or peritonsillar abscess. The problem may be due to trauma from burns, prior intubations or there may be a foreign body in the airway. Allergy including anaphylaxis and angioneurotic oedema may also cause stridor as may congenital larynogmalacia.

Can you tell me more about croup?

Croup is also known as laryngotracheobronchitis. It is the cause of 80% of child stridor and is due to parainfluenza virus, influenza, RSV or rhinovirus. The condition occurs in children of between 6 months and 3 years old. Only 1% of cases admitted each year require intubation. The infection causes subglottic and tracheal wall swelling which can progress to respiratory obstruction. It is typically seen a couple of days after an upper respiratory tract infection. The child may present with a barking cough, low grade fever and increased respiratory effort. There may also be superimposed bacterial infection.

How would you treat croup?

Try and describe treatment in terms of conservative and then surgical interventions.

The treatment is initially conservative. Depending on the progress of the condition definitive airway management is occasionally required. I would commence therapy with humidified oxygen, nebulised adrenaline (5 ml of 1 in 1000) and consider steroids. The child might need fluid rehydration, anti-pyretic medication and anti-biotics if superimposed bacterial infection is suspected.

If you needed to intubate a child with croup how would you go about it?

Again, think of yourself in the situation so that you don't forget anything.

Ideally I would intubate the child in theatre with an experienced anaesthetic team and an ENT surgeon present, since there is always the possibility of a "can't intubate, can't ventilate" scenario developing. The parents should ideally remain with the child until induction of anaesthesia. I would require a range of airway equipment including different sized tubes and bougies in preparation for a difficult intubation. I would have oxygen saturation monitoring and perform a gas induction with sevoflurane and oxygen.

Why would you use sevoflurane rather than halothane?

I have seen inductions using halothane, which is favoured by some anaesthetists, but since I have more practical experience using sevoflurane I would use this inhalation agent. Both agents have negligible pungency and minimal effects on airway reactivity making them favourable for gas induction. An induction with halothane will take longer but once the patient is deep the longer offset time of this agent gives potentially more time for airway manipulation before lightening of the plane of anaesthesia. A further consideration with halothane is its effect on the cardiovascular system with the potential for arrhythmias.

OK, let's go back to your gas induction that you were just about to start!

Induction may take longer than expected due to the reduced alveolar ventilation. I would maintain spontaneous ventilation throughout induction but give manual CPAP via the Jackson Rees modification of the Ayre's T-piece to help splint open the airways. Once the patient has lost consciousness I would ask the parents to leave and obtain IV access. When the patient has reached a deep plane of anaesthesia (with the pupils small and central) I would then wait a further few minutes before obtaining iv access (if this had not already been established) and then attempting to intubate with a smaller than predicted oral tracheal tube.

I would aim to keep the patient breathing spontaneously and sedated in a high care area, preferably a paediatric intensive care unit, until a leak developed around the endotracheal tube. Antibiotic therapy might be required depending on the clinical situation. Sometimes the oral tube is changed for a nasotracheal one if the patient spends a long time on the intensive care unit.

And where would you care for this child?

Ideally the child should be managed on a paediatric intensive care unit. If I were in a district general hospital I would contact the regional centre to arrange a transfer via a retrieval team.

Can you now tell me about epiglottitis?

Yes, epiglottitis is a bacterial infection caused predominantly by *Haemophilaus influenzae* B, but also by β-haemolytic streptococcus, staphylococcus and pneumococci. The disease has reduced in incidence since the introduction of the Hib vaccine. The bacteria infect the epiglottis, aryepiglottic folds and arytenoids. Epiglottitis tends to affect children aged 2 to 6 years.

How would a child present with epiglottitis?

Try and identify the key features that differentiate this from croup.

The child would have an abrupt onset of high fever and sore throat. They would look extremely unwell. Classically the child would have stridor and sit forward drooling. They might also have dysphagia and loss of a spontaneous cough with muffled speech. The condition might be transiently relieved by nebulised adrenaline.

How would you manage a child with epiglottitis?

Epiglottitis is an infective condition that may lead to rapid loss of the airway with coexisting septic shock. I would perform my initial assessment at the same time as starting initial treatments. I would also delegate a member of the team to contact the anaesthetic consultant on call and the ENT surgeon on call to alert them of the patient. My assessment would include a general history and specific to the presenting condition. I would also examine the child looking at the respiratory rate, oxygen saturation, respiratory effort and evidence of dehydration.

Depending on the severity of the child's condition the management can be either conservative or surgical. Initial conservative treatment would include oxygen via facemask and nebulised adrenaline if tolerated. Fluid resuscitation and anti-biotics are required but may not be initially administered since complete airway obstruction may occur if the child is stressed. The child should be nursed with its parents in an attempt to alleviate anxiety.

If no improvement with conservative measures then the patient should be transferred to theatre for intubation.

Now let's say you have transferred the child to theatre uneventfully. You are fully prepared for a gas induction and have a consultant anaesthetist and ENT surgeon with you in theatre.

What are the potential problems that might occur and how might these differ from the child with croup?

As with the croup patient, the induction of anaesthesia and intubation may be difficult with the risk of developing into a "can't intubate, can't ventilate" scenario. In epiglottitis the deterioration of the child may be more rapid. Furthermore on laryngoscopy a cherry red epiglottis may be seen and the glottic opening may be extremely difficult to visualise.

Asking an assistant to press on the chest and looking for bubbles may guide tracheal tube placement.

The child with epiglottitis may develop severe septic shock with cardiovascular instability requiring aggressive fluid resuscitation and even vasopressor or inotropic support. This is less likely in a child with croup, but co-existing bacterial infection can occur leading to similar complications.

What would be your further management once the airway was secured?

Blood cultures would need to be sent to confirm the organism and broad spectrum anti-biotic should be commenced as soon as possible. The child would need to be nursed in an intensive care environment until a leak around the tube indicated recovery. This would be expected to occur approximately 48 hours after starting anti-biotics. Fluid resuscitation may be required depending on the severity of the sepsis.

Can you tell me anything about bacterial tracheitis?

Bacterial tracheitis is usually caused by staphylococcus, *haemophylus*, streptococcus or neisseria. A preceding upper respiratory infection may occur. The patient would present with a rapid onset of serious illness characterised by fever and respiratory distress. Coughing produces copious tracheal secretions and retrosternal pain. The patient would not usually drool but stridor and a hoarse voice may be present. The treatment would be similar for epiglottitis but initial intubation may lead to complete obstruction due to pus in the endotracheal tube, forcing the clinician to change the tube. Regular suction will be required and possibly bronchoscopy to remove purulent debris from the trachea. The patient may require intubation for a significant length of time together with a prolonged course of anti-biotics such as cerfuroxime. Tracheal stenosis is a late complication of this condition.

Finally what do you know about retropharyngeal abscesses?

A retropharyngeal abscess is a collection of pus in the space between the posterior pharyngeal wall and prevertebral fascia from lymphatic spread of infection from the sinuses, teeth or middle ear. The infective organism is usually a staphylococcus or streptococcus. Children less than 6 years old tend to be affected but adults may also develop this condition.

What would be the clinical features, investigations and management?

The patient may complain of neck swelling, pain and reduced movement. They would have trismus, drooling and usually fever. A lateral neck X-ray may reveal retropharyngeal thickening. Surgical drainage is usually required but intubation may be extremely difficult. An ENT surgeon should be on standby during induction and I would be prepared for a difficult intubation. A gas induction may be suitable in a child or awake fibre-optic intubation in an adult patient. Care should be taken not to rupture the abscess during intubation since the patient is then at risk of aspirating pus. Anti-biotics will be needed along with fluids and anti-pyretics.

Chapter

Neurosurgery

2.4.1. Head injury and control of ICP – Justin C Mandeville

A 24-year-old motorcyclist is brought into the emergency room. You attend the trauma call. There is profuse bleeding from the nose and ears and his breathing is noisy. His best response to painful stimulation is to open his eyes, moan, and flex his arms.

What are the important points in the *immediate* management of this patient?

Think of your management of any major trauma patient.

Maintenance and protection of the airway with immobilisation of the cervical spine are my first concern.

The bleeding nose, noisy breathing and reduced Glasgow Coma Scale score means he will need tracheal intubation to secure his airway. This is complicated by the fact that he is at risk of cervical spine injury and will therefore need to be intubated with manual in-line stabilisation. Initially, I would give high flow oxygen, ensure that the cervical spine is immobilised, perform a careful jaw thrust and, if tolerated, insert a Guedel airway. I would like a senior anaesthetist and an anaesthetic assistant to be called. I would then proceed to perform tracheal intubation using a rapid sequence technique with manual in-line stabilisation of the cervical spine.

In assessing his ventilation I would examine the chest, particularly looking for signs of a haemothorax or pneumothorax that would need decompressing before positive pressure ventilation was attempted.

I would then assess the circulation by feeling the pulse, checking the capillary refill time and asking for monitoring to be attached. I would simultaneously be considering potential sources of haemorrhage.

I would ask for blood to be taken for full blood count, coagulation, biochemistry, glucose and crossmatching of blood.

Next I would make an assessment of neurological function using the Glasgow coma score which in this case is 2 for eyes, 2 for verbal and 4 for motor – that's 8 out of 15 in total.

I would ask that the head end of the bed be raised safely to 30 degrees if possible though this may be difficult to achieve if we are concerned about injury to the thoracic spine.

Dr. Podcast Scripts for the Final FRCA, ed. Rebecca A. Leslie, Emily K. Johnson, Gary Thomas and Alexander P. L. Goodwin. Published by Cambridge University Press.

To complete this systematic ACBDE approach, the patient should then be exposed and examined.

If possible, and if time allowed, I would try and obtain information from next of kin, GP or hospital notes about medical, surgical and anaesthetic histories, as well as details of current medication and allergies.

How do you categorise the severity of head injury?

You may know more than one way but this categorisation is widely used.

There are a number of scoring systems, but the most widely used involves the Glasgow coma score. The Glasgow coma score comprises tests of motor, verbal and eye responses.

The motor test is scored from 1 to 6. A score of 1 represents no motor response, 2 is extension to pain, 3 corresponds to abnormal flexion to pain, 4 is withdrawal from pain, 5 localises to pain, and a score of 6 represents a patient who is obeying commands.

The verbal component has a maximum score of 5. 1 correlates to no verbal response, 2 is incomprehensible sounds, a score of 3 is given if inappropriate words are used, 4 is for the confused patient and 5 represents an orientated patient.

The eye responses are scored from 1 to 4. A score of 1 is awarded if there is no eye opening, 2 for eye opening to pain, 3 for eye opening to voice, and 4 for spontaneous eye opening.

A GCS of 13 to 15 out of 15 on arrival at hospital indicates mild injury, 9 to 12 indicates moderate injury and 8 or below severe injury.

What features of a patient with a traumatic brain injury would make you consider intubation of the trachea and ventilation?

There are NICE and AAGBI Guidelines you may want to make reference to here.

Those patients whose airway and ventilation is compromised are the most worrying so I would consider intubation in anyone with a loss of protective airway reflexes, those with a GCS of 8 or less, and those whose GCS is significantly deteriorating (particularly if the motor score has fallen by 2 points or more). In addition mechanical ventilation is indicated for any patient who is hypoxic or hypercarbic and also those who are hyperventilating, especially if their $PaCO_2$ is less than 4.0 kPa.

Other conditions that indicate the need for intubation are those with bilateral mandibular fractures, oral or pharyngeal bleeding and seizures.

When ventilating, I would try to achieve a PaO_2 of more than 13 and a $PaCO_2$ of 4.5 to 5.0 kPa.

What is secondary brain injury?

Secondary brain injury is the additional neurological damage that happens after the primary injury. It occurs due to localised or generalised physiological upset. Particular causes are hypoxia and hypotension, however, hypercapnia, intracranial hypertension and cerebral artery spasm also play a role.

These problems result in ischaemia, disruption of the blood–brain barrier and loss of the autoregulation of cerebral blood flow.

At a cellular level it's thought that the generation of free radicals are probably responsible for cell death. This may be due to what's called "excitotoxicity"; a process in which the excessive release of excitatory neurotransmitters (for example glutamate) cause overstimulation of receptors leading to rising intra-cellular calcium. The calcium influx activates a number of enzymes, including proteases, phospholipases and endonucleases. These enzymes then go on to damage cell structures such as the cytoskeleton and DNA.

What can be done to prevent it?

In other words this is asking how you would avoid the causes you just mentioned.

In order to prevent secondary brain injury, I would ventilate the patient to achieve adequate oxygenation (PaO_2 of more than 13 kPa) and normocapnia ($PaCO_2$ of 4.5 to 5.0 kPa). I would take measures to avoid high intracranial pressure whilst maintaining a cerebral perfusion pressure of at least 60 mmHg.

Intracranial pressure should be measured in all patients with severe brain injury who have an abnormal CT. Ideally these patients should be managed at a specialist neurosurgical centre. If the intracranial pressure was unknown, I would assume that it is equal to 20 mmHg and try to keep the mean arterial pressure at 80 to 90 mmHg to ensure an adequate cerebral perfusion pressure.

It is also important to normalise other physiological parameters such as glucose levels and temperature. Some units routinely use mild hypothermia in the management of traumatic brain injury but, even if hypothermia is not used, hyperthermia must be avoided.

The avoidance of seizures is also very important. There is currently ongoing research into therapeutic agents to attenuate damage at the cellular level, these may play a role in the future.

Tell me about the Munro-Kellie hypothesis

Draw the elastance curve (Figure 2.4.1).

The Munro-Kellie hypothesis is an explanation of the pressure-volume relationship within the skull. The cranium is basically a rigid box that contains blood, brain tissue and CSF. This means that an increase in the volume of any of these components must be compensated for by the reduction in volume of another or the intracranial pressure will rise.

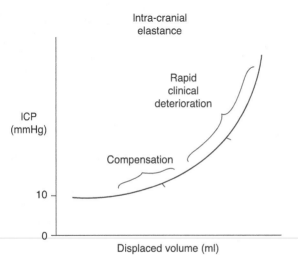

Figure 2.4.1. Intra-cranial elastance.

Compensation usually occurs due to a reduction in the volume of venous blood, from compression of the veins and by the movement of CSF out of the cranium into the spinal canal. This means that there's a period of tolerance during which the pressure rises very little in response to changes in volume. When the compensatory mechanisms are overcome the pressure begins to rise sharply, this corresponds to the inflexion point on the elastance curve.

This patient has surgery to relieve an intracranial haemorrhage. Post-operatively, in the intensive care unit, his intracranial pressure starts to rise. Briefly tell me of the options available to you for controlling his intracranial hypertension.

Include the options available to you and the surgeons.

I would first address the possibility that there may be further intra-cranial haemorrhage and in discussion with the neurosurgical team, consider CT imaging to check for this. I would try to control the intra-cranial pressure aiming to keep it below 20 mmHg, to achieve this I would use measures that decrease brain volume, decrease cerebral blood volume, or decrease CSF production or CSF volume.

So how could you decrease blood volume?

Think how you reduce obstruction to veins and how you reduce oxygen requirement and therefore blood-flow demand.

To decrease cerebral blood volume I would optimise venous drainage by sitting the patient up at 30 degrees and minimise jugular venous flow restriction. Moderate hyperventilation can be used to cause vasoconstriction and therefore reduce arterial blood volume.

A reduction in the cerebral metabolic rate will also reduce local vasodilatation and can be achieved using drugs such as thiopentone, midazolam, propofol, or more controversially by cooling the patient. It is also important to prevent rises in the cerebral metabolic demand for oxygen due to seizures or pyrexia – these must be treated urgently if they occur.

Blood in the form of a haematoma may need surgical intervention.

And how can you reduce brain volume?

A decrease in the brain volume is commonly attained with 0.5 g/kg of 20 % mannitol. This can be repeated as required to achieve the desired effect or to attain a plasma osmolarity of around 310 to 320 mOsm/L. Loop diuretics are thought to produce further benefit perhaps by working synergistically with mannitol.

Hypertonic saline is increasingly used in place of mannitol and there is mounting evidence of its benefits. It is important to avoid the use of hypotonic solutions in the resuscitation of these patients.

And to reduce CSF production?

There is little that can be done to decrease CSF production. It has been proposed that the effectiveness of mannitol in reducing intracranial pressure is partly due to its ability to reduce the production of CSF. Surgical intervention is generally required to reduce the volume of CSF; an external ventricular drain or lumbar drain may be appropriate.

Further Reading

National Health Service. NICE Guidelines on Head Injury Management. Head injury: triage, assessment, investigation and early management of head injury in infants, children and adults. http://guidance.nice.org.uk/CG56/Guidance.

The Association of Anaesthetists of Great Britain and Ireland (AAGBI) Guidelines. Recommendations for the safe transfer of patients with brain injury. 2006. http://www.aagbi.org/publications/guidelines.htm.

2.4.2. Anaesthesia for craniotomy – Timothy JB Wood

You have been asked to assess a 55-year-old gentleman who is scheduled for a craniotomy and debulking of a primary brain tumour.

What are the key considerations in the history when pre-assessing a neurosurgical patient?

A structured approach is vital, mentioning routine history first before focussing on the specific neurological history.

I would first of all focus on the general points of a history relevant to all patients and then concentrate on those factors that are specific to the neurosurgical condition. Eventually both the history and examination need to focus on the symptoms and signs of neurological deficit and whether the presenting features have been acute, chronic or fluctuating. The surgical condition may have resulted in clouding of consciousness or motor deficits and there may be signs or symptoms of raised intra-cranial pressure. It is important to establish a baseline neurological evaluation as anaesthesia and surgery may profoundly affect post-operative neurological status. Any new medication started recently, such as dexamethasone or osmotic diuretics to reduce cerebral oedema should be noted along with the duration of treatment and dose as they may cause hyperglycaemia, hypovolaemia and electrolyte imbalances. Anti-convulsants should be noted as they may affect the metabolism of drugs such as vecuronium by microsomal enzyme induction.

What investigations might you require for this patient?

An ECG to show any underlying cardiac abnormalities, arrhythmias or ischaemic changes. Urea and electrolytes should be measured in order to reveal any imbalance caused by diuretics or persistent vomiting. If the patient has been on anti-convulsants the liver function tests might be deranged. Full blood count and coagulation studies to ensure there are no coagulation problems or low platelets that might interfere with surgical haemostasis. I would expect imaging of the lesion to be available for the surgeons in the form of CT or MRI scans.

What premedication would you consider in this patient?

As with all areas of anaesthetic practice this needs to be individualised. The risk of an extremely anxious patient becoming hypertensive and raising their intra-cranial pressure has to be balanced against the risk of respiratory depression causing a rise in the $PaCO_2$ that may also result in an increase in the intra-cranial pressure. Benzodiazepines may be considered for anxiety, dexamethasone for cerebral oedema and anti-convulsants, if not already started, for seizure prophylaxis.

What would influence your choice of intra-venous induction agent for a neurosurgical patient?

The aims for patients with intra-cranial pathology are to avoid sudden changes in mean arterial pressure or sudden increases in intra-cranial pressure during the induction and maintenance of anaesthesia. Cerebral perfusion pressure should be maintained at all times.

Induction of anaesthesia may cause sudden falls in blood pressure and may require prompt correction with vasopressors and fluid. The intra-venous agents propofol and thiopentone are most commonly used because they decrease cerebral blood flow and the cerebral metabolic rate. Thiopentone's barbiturate structure makes it a particularly good induction agent in patients at risk of seizure activity. Etomidate also reduces the cerebral metabolic rate but it maintains the blood pressure, its use is limited because induction is less smooth and there are concerns surrounding its effects on steroid synthesis. Ketamine should be avoided as it causes a marked increase in cerebral metabolic rate and cerebral blood flow.

What volatile agents would you use for a neurosurgical patient?

Volatile anaesthetic agents decrease the cerebral metabolic rate by up to 40% but, in contrast to the intravenous agents, they cause dose related cerebral vasodilatation. The most potent cerebral vasodilators are halothane and enflurane and they are no longer used. Isoflurane and sevoflurane are the most commonly used volatile agents in current practice as they have the least effect on the cerebral blood flow. They, in effect, uncouple cerebral blood flow and cerebral metabolic rate.

There is probably no place for nitrous oxide in neuroanaesthetic practice as it has well-documented detrimental effects such as a significant increase in cerebral perfusion pressure in healthy subjects and diffusion into air filled spaces. However this is difficult to extrapolate into clinical practice, as other agents influence the effects of nitrous oxide making it difficult to demonstrate an adverse clinical outcome.

Do the neuromuscular blocking agents affect intra-cranial pressure?

Non-depolarising muscle relaxants do not directly affect the intra-cranial pressure. The benzylisoquinoliniums, such as atracurium, can cause a histamine release that can produce a reduction in the blood pressure. Also, all of the muscle relaxants have the potential to cause anaphylaxis that would have potentially catastrophic effects on the intra-cranial pressure.

The depolarising muscle relaxant suxamethonium can cause an increase in intra-cranial pressure, in one study a rise of 15–20 mmHg is quoted. However, this rise is limited by deep anaesthesia and suxamethonium is unequalled in its ability to achieve rapid total paralysis facilitating prompt airway control and reducing the risk of aspiration. Hypoxia and hypercarbia are more harmful to the brain than the transient elevation in intra-cranial pressure seen with suxamethonium.

What would be your preferred technique to maintain anaesthesia in this patient?

The aim is for a smooth induction avoiding coughing, hypoxia, hypercarbia and raised intra-cranial pressure.

Assuming that this patient does not require a rapid sequence induction and does not have any anticipated airway difficulties, my preferred technique would be total intra-venous anaesthesia (TIVA) using propofol and remifentanil and a non-depolarising neuromuscular blocker such as rocuronium. Remifentanil provides cardiovascular stability during times of intense stimulation, such as intubation and head-pin application, preventing a rise in mean arterial pressure and intra-cranial pressure. Propofol and remifentanil are both short-acting and allow for a rapid wake up and assessment of neurological status post-operatively. Also if neurophysiological monitoring is required for the surgery then further muscle relaxation can be avoided with adequate infusion doses of remifentanil.

If a candidate is not familiar with TIVA techniques for neurosurgery then a simple approach using a volatile agent and fentanyl would also be appropriate. Take care to explain what technique would be used to obtund the pressor responses at stimulating points in the procedure such as laryngoscopy, the insertion of pins into the head, surgical incision and closure. This could be achieved by deepening anaesthesia with supplemental IV induction agent or by the intra-venous administration of lignocaine 1.5 mg kg^{-1} or esmolol 1.5 mg kg^{-1}. It would also be worth mentioning that neuromuscular blockers should be given by an infusion.

What monitoring would you use for this neurosurgical patient?

Mandatory monitoring for any neuroanaesthetic procedure include ECG, pulse oximetry, NIBP, capnography, inspired oxygen concentration, expired volatile concentration depending on technique and peripheral nerve stimulator. In many procedures temperature and urine output monitoring is required. Invasive arterial blood pressure monitoring should be instituted for any craniotomy and central venous pressure monitoring will be required in patients at risk of air embolism, a precordial Doppler ultrasound may be used to aid detection of air embolism.

Intra-cranial pressure, sensory evoked potentials and jugular bulb oximetry can be used to gain further information.

Can you tell me more about sensory evoked potentials and why are they monitored?

They are principally used to monitor the integrity of the sensory pathways during anaesthesia particularly when they are at risk of damage due to the surgery. The electrical manifestation of the central nervous system's response to external stimuli is monitored. The low amplitude signal is difficult to distinguish from background EEG activity, therefore the activity following both a repetitive evoked and spontaneous sensory stimulus is averaged and the signal is then extracted by electronic summation and subtraction. Brainstem auditory evoked potentials are used for surgery near the auditory pathway or posterior fossa and brainstem surgery. Visual evoked potentials can be used in any lesion close to the optic pathway.

What positions are patients commonly placed in for neurosurgical operations? What are the implications and what special care should you take with each position?

Neurosurgical procedures tend to be relatively long operations therefore specific attention should be taken to safeguard the pressure areas. Pneumatic calf compression boots should be used where possible.

A supine position is commonly used and the important consideration here is that there is good venous drainage, a 10-degree reverse Trendelenburg tilt decreases the intra-cranial pressure and leaves the cerebral perfusion pressure unchanged. Tracheal tubes should be taped rather than tied to prevent obstruction to the flow of blood returning to the heart from the head.

The prone position is used for spinal cord and posterior fossa surgery. It is important with prone positioning to ensure that the patient is cardiovascularly stable prior to turning and that all intra-venous and monitoring lines are well secured. Care is required with respect to all the pressure areas: axillae, breasts, iliac crests, groin and knees. There must be adequate support of the chest and pelvis to allow free movement of the abdomen and diaphragm. Support of the head is imperative so that it is not over extended or flexed at the neck and there should be no pressure on the eyes that could cause retinal ischaemia and subsequent blindness.

Sitting is a controversial position used for surgery for tumours in the cerebello-pontine angle and in the posterior third-ventricular region. The advantages of this position are optimised surgical access, improved surgical field and reduced tumour vascularity. The disadvantages are increased risk of air embolism, haemodynamic instability causing profound hypotension, tension pneumocephalus and quadriplegia. It has been suggested that the risks are higher if there is poor patient selection and inexperienced teams making use of the position with inadequate monitoring. In dedicated neurosurgical departments it may still have a place, however, the patients should be evaluated with echocardiography searching for a patent foramen ovale and intra-operative monitoring should include a precordial Doppler probe.

The lateral or "Park Bench" position is commonly used for spinal cord and lateral posterior fossa surgery as it presents a lower risk of venous air embolism than the sitting position. Consideration should be given to all of the pressure areas particularly the arms, the lower due to pressure and the upper due to traction. Care is required that the patient is not moved after head fixation as this could cause considerable stress on the cervical spine and alter venous drainage.

Could this patient be operated on awake and what advantages or disadvantages would this create?

It is possible to perform an awake craniotomy on this patient providing they are not confused and there are no communication difficulties since absolute co-operation is required from the patient. Low occipital tumours requiring the prone position are an absolute contraindication and extreme anxiety is a relative contraindication. Patients would also be excluded if their lesions require significant dural resection, as this is potentially painful. Also excluded would be patients for whom physiological or anatomical factors, such as orthopnoea or joint pain, would prevent them from lying relatively flat and still for many hours. Ideally an experienced surgeon will keep the operative time to a minimum. The advantages of awake craniotomy are that, during surgery undertaken on lesions in or adjacent to eloquent areas of the cortex, continuous reassurance can be provided to the neurosurgeon that essential neurological function is not being compromised. It is also used in surgery for Parkinson's disease and epilepsy as it allows more accurate intra-operative localisation of the area requiring surgery. These advantages have to be balanced against the loss of control of ventilation and the assurance of immobility. There is also a risk of seizures developing in approximately 16–18% of patients most commonly during epilepsy surgery, and nausea and vomiting occurs in 8–50% of patients with the risk of pulmonary aspiration. Respiratory depression and airway obstruction may occur due to sedation and analgesic regimens. There is a 2–6% requirement for conversion to general anaesthetic.

How may vascular neurosurgical lesions present?

Subarachnoid haemorrhages may present with: severe, sudden onset headache, transient or prolonged loss of consciousness, vomiting and seizures. Focal neurological signs may occur due to pressure from haematoma or a large aneurysm. The presence of blood in the subarachnoid space may result in neck stiffness, reactive hypertension and pyrexia.

Arterio-venous malformations present with headache, seizures, focal neurological signs due to the mass effect, high output cardiac failure and subarachnoid or intra-cranial haemorrhage.

What definitive treatment is available for these vascular lesions and how would this affect your anaesthetic?

Intra-cranial aneurysms may either be surgically clipped via a craniotomy or occluded by an interventional radiologist using coils or balloons using minimally invasive techniques.

For surgical clipping, the goals of anaesthesia are to provide optimum operating conditions for the surgeon by preventing an increase in transmural pressure, that may rupture the aneurysm, and maintaining adequate cerebral perfusion pressure and cerebral oxygenation. Therefore, consideration needs to be given to preventing a rise in mean arterial pressure at times of stimulation such as intubation and head pin placement. Previously controlled hypotension was used to reduce transmural tension in the aneurysm prior to clipping. More recently most surgeons prefer to temporarily clip major feeding arteries at the time of aneurysm clipping. Routine monitoring should include ECG, pulse oximetry, capnography, intra-arterial blood pressure, central venous pressure, urine output and temperature. Intra-cranial pressure monitoring, brainstem evoked potentials and jugular venous bulb oximetry should be considered in patients at high risk of cerebral ischaemia.

For interventional radiology the same anaesthetic goals are important, however there is the caveat that these procedures are often performed in angiography suites that are at remote sites, away from main theatres and often cramped for space with reduced access to the patient once the procedure has started. Rupture of the lesion can be catastrophic so the anaesthetist should be prepared to reverse heparin anti-coagulation with protamine and take prompt measures to reduce the rises in intra-cranial pressure with hyperventilation and mannitol prior to surgery if appropriate.

What can you tell me about surgery in the posterior fossa?

Tumours in this region are considered critical lesions because of the limited space in the posterior fossa and the potential involvement of vital brainstem nuclei. Posterior fossa tumours are more common in children accounting for 50–70% of brain tumours in this group compared to 15–20% of brain tumours in adults. The clinical presentation depends on the site, biological behaviour and aggressiveness of the tumour and the rate of growth. The indications for surgery are to decompress the posterior fossa and release pressure on the brainstem to avoid the risk of herniation or to obtain a histopathological diagnosis allowing further management planning.

What specific complications are you aware of during and following surgery in the posterior fossa?

As with any surgical procedure there are the risks of infection, haemorrhage, chest infection, atelectasis, peripheral nerve injuries, deep venous thrombosis and pulmonary embolism. However, the specific complications that the anaesthetist needs to be aware of intra- and post-operatively often relate to the position that the patient is in during the operation. Complications related to posterior fossa surgery are venous air embolism, paradoxical air embolism, pneumocephalus, haemodynamic instability, macroglossia and quadriplegia.

The commonly used positions are prone and lateral or park bench. Occasionally the sitting position is used. The sitting position deserves special consideration as it carries the highest risk of specific complications, especially venous air embolism. Therefore, patients should be screened for intra-cardiac connections between the left and right side of the heart prior to surgery to identify those at risk of paradoxical air embolism. Methods to reduce this risk should be taken such as avoiding hypovolaemia, the use of compression stockings, and possibly application of PEEP but this does increase the risk of paradoxical air embolism. Despite these steps the incidence of venous air embolism is in the order of 30%. However, the risk of haemodynamically significant events is much lower and relates to the volume and rate of air entrainment along with the patients pre-anaesthetic cardiopulmonary reserve.

Hypotension is much more likely in the seated position due to the impairment of venous return to the heart. Venous pooling in the lower body, the effects of positive pressure ventilation, application of PEEP and the effects of the anaesthetic agents can all result in decreased venous return. The transition from the supine to the sitting position following the induction of anaesthesia must be gradual as sudden hypotension would be undesirable. Hypotension commonly requires treatment with fluids and vasopressor agents. Secondary cardiovascular responses by surgical stimulation of the brainstem may be sudden and can be masked with the use of anti-cholinergics or β-blockers.

Macroglossia is thought to be due to extreme flexion of the neck and a reduction in the oropharyngeal volume, which reduces lingual venous drainage or lymphatic drainage. Extreme flexion is also thought to be the cause of quadriplegia due to insufficient nutrient supply and drainage of the cervical spinal cord.

If there is a delay in emergence from anaesthesia post-operatively, then alongside the usual differential diagnoses, symptomatic tension pneumocephalus, cerebral ischaemia due to paradoxical air embolus and brain stem injury, haematoma or cerebral oedema need to be considered so that appropriate therapy can be instituted promptly. Post-operative respiratory compromise may be due to injury to brain stem respiratory centres, airway obstruction from macroglossia or injury to the lower cranial nerves; IX, X or XII.

How would you diagnose and manage a suspected venous air embolism?

To allow early diagnosis you need to be aware when a patient is at a high risk of a venous air embolism and maintain a high index of suspicion. The main methods for detecting them are precordial Doppler, trans-oesophageal echocardiogram or trans-thoracic echocardiogram. A drop in the end-tidal CO_2 is indicative but not specific.

Once a significant venous air embolism has been detected which is causing cardiovascular instability, management should incorporate prevention of further air entrainment by flooding the wound with saline, lowering the head and considering compression of the jugular vein, and respiratory and cardiovascular support in the form of 100% oxygen, fluid resuscitation and vasopressors or inotropes. Ideally a central venous catheter should be sited prior to the procedure and this should be used to aspirate any air from the right side of the heart.

How would you confirm the correct placement of this central venous pressure line?

There are three ways to confirm the correct placement of the catheter tip, which is just proximal to the cavo-atrial junction. Chest X-ray may be used however there are possible difficulties in interpreting the image. The pressure waveform from a pulmonary artery catheter will allow you to identify the correct placement. The last way involves the use of an IV-ECG that has an ECG electrode at the tip of the catheter and therefore allows you to identify the correct position when a bifid P-wave occurs; this technique has the additional risk of microshock. In all cases there is a high chance that the catheter tip will move when the patient's position is changed for surgery and therefore rechecking will be necessary, making the latter two techniques more appropriate.

Further Reading

Dinsmore J. Anaesthesia for elective neurosurgery. *British Journal of Anaesthesia.* 2007; **99**(1): 68–74.

Jones H, Smith M. Awake craniotomy. *Continuing Education in Anaesthesia,* *Critical Care & Pain.* 2004; **4**(6): 189–192.

Sutcliffe AJ. Subarachnoid haemorrhage due to cerebral aneurysm. *Continuing Education in Anaesthesia, Critical Care & Pain.* 2002; **2**(2): 45–48.

2.4.3. Management of subarachnoid haemorrhage – Justin C Mandeville

A 55-year-old woman presents with sudden onset of headache. She is drowsy and confused in the emergency department. CT reveals a subarachnoid haemorrhage likely to be from a left anterior cerebral artery aneurysm. You are asked to anaesthetise the patient for angiographic coiling 3 days after this presentation.

What are the important features of the pre-operative assessment for this patient?

Essentially normal neuroanaesthesia with potential for catastrophic problems!

This is a procedure generally done in a physiologically stable patient to prevent a more catastrophic second bleed. In contrast to the open approach to an aneurysmal bleed the cranium remains closed so that haemorrhage during the procedure is more dangerous.

At the pre-operative visit I would ensure that the patient is not hypovolaemic and that the systolic blood pressure is controlled and is between 120 and 150 mmHg. I would check for evidence of cardiac ischaemia by requesting an electrocardiogram and I'd examine the patient for signs of pulmonary oedema. Nimodipine should have been started as prophylaxis against cerebral vasospasm and I would check that this had been done. I would perform a neurological assessment to ensure both that the clinical grade of the haemorrhage had not deteriorated and that there were no signs of active vasospasm. Finally, I would want to identify any concurrent medical problems that may complicate the anaesthetic, particularly pre-existing hypertension, which is common in those with subarachnoid haemorrhage.

In what ways do you think giving this particular anaesthetic differs from most neuroanaesthesia?

Because the cranium is not open, a further bleed may cause a sudden rise in intra-cranial pressure that the operator cannot deal with directly. Most angiography suites are in a separate part of the hospital from main theatres resulting in remote site anaesthesia, and may produce problems with staffing and equipment. A senior anaesthetist familiar with the surroundings and the procedure should supervise this procedure. In addition, the procedure is not stimulating, which can cause problems with swings in blood pressure and in particular, hypotension.

How would you manage the induction and maintenance of anaesthesia in this case?

Talk about the way you would do it and give reasons for your choices.

I would make sure routine AAGBI monitoring was in place as well as invasive blood pressure monitoring. In addition some units would routinely measure central venous pressure. A naso-pharyngeal or oro-pharyngeal temperature probe should be used, and a urinary catheter should be inserted as the procedure can take several hours. I would make sure that the patient is positioned so that there is no obstruction to flow of jugular venous blood.

My choice would be total intra-venous anaesthesia as it's well-suited for induction and maintenance of anaesthesia. Blood pressure control at laryngoscopy is particularly important and in addition to the induction agents I would consider using lidocaine (1 to 1.5 mg kg^{-1}). I would use rocuronium for muscle relaxation and ensure adequate muscle relaxation throughout the procedure by using a nerve stimulator. I avoid nitrous oxide in these cases for a number of reasons; it may cause cerebral vasodilatation, it may enlarge bubbles that might be inadvertently introduced into the cerebral circulation, and it worsens excitotoxicity. I would have ventilator settings that minimise airway pressures and maintain an end-tidal carbon dioxide of 4.0–4.5 kPa.

Vasoactive drugs for control of blood pressure should be readily available. This is important throughout the operation as I may be requested to raise or lower the blood pressure by the operator. Anti-coagulation is often used so heparin and protamine should be readily available.

How would you manage this patient post-operatively?

How and where?

The important points in post-operative management are the maintenance of a systolic blood pressure between 140 and 160 mmHg and regular neurological assessment looking in particular for the occurrence of vasospasm. Some centres will monitor all patients on a neurosurgical high-dependency unit during the immediate post-operative period. I would be vigilant for the complications of subarachnoid haemorrhage.

Which complications would you be mindful of during the procedure?

And how might it affect your anaesthetic?

Intra-cranial haemorrhage is a possibility during the procedure and may be seen radiologically or may only be noticed when its physiological consequences are seen such as Cushing's sign (hypertension and bradycardia) or cardiac arrhythmias. If it does occur, a decision

Table 2.4.3. World Federation of Neurosurgeons classification of sub-arachnoid haemorrhage

Grade	GCS	Focal neurological deficit
1	15	Absent
2	13–14	Absent
3	13–14	Present
4	7–12	Present or absent
5	<7	Present or absent

needs to be made as to whether the procedure should be continued, whether the patient should be moved to the neurological intensive care or whether they need an urgent craniotomy. Ischaemia and thrombo-embolic phenomena can occur due to vessel obstruction by the catheter or injectate although there is unlikely to be any obvious sign of this until the patient is woken.

And what complications may occur after the procedure?

Re-bleeding after subarachnoid haemorrhage occurs in about 20 percent of patients within 2 weeks of presentation and 50% within 6 months, if the aneurysm has been secured this is dramatically reduced.

Raised intra-cranial pressure can occur in the absence of a further bleed and may be due to impairment of CSF flow or oedema in the tissue surrounding a haematoma.

Seizures are also a potential problem both at the time of the bleed and in the ensuing weeks and anti-epileptic medication may be needed lifelong.

Groin haematoma is another potential complication and can be worsened by the use of anti-coagulants. It may need surgical repair of the vessel defect.

Can you tell me about any scoring systems for subarachnoid haemorrhage?

Clinical and radiological.

There are a number of scoring systems, both clinical, including the Hunt and Hess score and the World Federation of Neurosurgeons score, and radiological, such as the Fisher score.

Pick one of them and outline it for me

The World Federation of Neurosurgeons score uses the Glasgow coma score and the presence or absence of a focal neurological deficit.

The score relates to mortality so that grade 1 patients have a mortality of only a few per cent whereas those with grade 5 have nearly 100% mortality.

What can you tell me about vasospasm?

It is a potential consequence of subarachnoid haemorrhage in which arterial vasoconstriction occurs as a result of irritation by subarachnoid blood. It is generally more likely to happen in those with higher grade haemorrhage and more blood in the subarachnoid space. It usually doesn't start until 3 days after the bleed and rarely starts more than 2 weeks afterwards. The consequences of vasospasm for the patient can include focal neurological deficit or a more generalised picture with a reduced level of consciousness.

How do you prevent it?

Any hypovolaemia should be corrected and hydration maintained. Nimodipine 60 mg should be started 4 hourly orally or if this is not possible, intravenously. Infusion should start slowly and be titrated to effect and blood pressure. Nimodipine should be continued for 3 weeks. The patient should be regularly checked for focal neurological deficits and if present then urgent imaging should be considered.

How do you treat it?

Again, you and the surgeons.

A decision should be made quickly as to whether it is amenable to angiographic treatment or whether medical management should be used first. On the neurosurgical intensive care most centres advocate "triple H" therapy as part of the medical management. This involves:

- Hypertension

  · Secured aneurysm: systolic blood pressure 160–200 mmHg
  · Unsecured aneurysm: systolic blood pressure 120–150 mmHg

- Haemodilution: Administration of fluid to achieve a haematocrit of 30%
- Hypervolaemia
- Fluids titrated to give a central venous pressure of 10 to 12 mmHg or a pulmonary capillary wedge pressure of 15 to 18 mmHg
- The nimodipine should be continued for 1 to 2 weeks once vasospasm has occurred.

2.4.4. Management of acute spinal cord injury – Carl J Morris

A 24-year-old male motorcyclist is brought into the Emergency Department after a high-speed traffic accident, with signs and symptoms compatible with a spinal cord injury around C5.

Describe your initial management of this patient.

Potentially, there's a lot that could be said here – including the entire ATLS approach. But clearly the spinal injury is going to be a focus of the structured oral exam. By structuring your answer, and signposting, you avoid wasting time. Your examiner can indicate if they require more details in any area.

I will divide my answer into two parts, firstly looking briefly at the management of serious trauma in general and then specifically looking at the cervical cord injury.

For any major trauma, I would facilitate, or lead a structured team approach seeking to identify and treat life-threatening injuries in a systematic manner. This would start with the airway (with cervical spine immobilisation to avoid exacerbating cord injury). A decreased level of consciousness, facial or laryngeal injuries might threaten his airway. Initially I would ensure delivery of a high concentration of oxygen via a face mask with a reservoir bag. If there were signs of airway compromise I would proceed to tracheal intubation using a rapid sequence induction with manual in-line stabilisation of the cervical spine.

You might assume these basics are obvious, but if you don't mention them, the examiner may assume you wouldn't do it.

I would then assess and treat injuries threatening ventilation such as pneumothoraces. Subsequently, I would move rapidly onto the circulation – securing large bore intravenous access, sending bloods for routine haematology, biochemistry and for cross-matching, assessing circulatory adequacy, identifying and where possible attempting to control any major source of haemorrhage, e.g., splinting the pelvis and reducing long bone fractures. Haemorrhage control may often require surgical intervention, for example in the case of intra-abdominal, or pelvic bleeding. This would be followed by a neurological assessment, including the Glasgow Coma score and an attempt to establish the level of any motor or sensory deficit.

With a well-organised team, these activities should happen concurrently, while gathering any relevant history of the event and any medical conditions.

Hopefully, that sort of answer is sufficient to demonstrate that you have experience of major trauma and an overview of the priorities.

To focus in on the spinal cord injury – almost certainly associated with a bony injury to the cervical spine, I will also look at the systems affected.

With any neck injury there is a risk of haematoma and airway compression. I would have a low threshold for early intubation, with manual immobilisation. I would be wary of profound bradycardia due to an unopposed vagal response to laryngoscopy. A complete transection of the cord at C5 should leave sufficient diaphragmatic function for the patient to breathe in the long term. However, with the loss of intercostals, as well as reduced diaphragmatic function, there will be a high risk of ventilatory compromise. It is possible that the phrenic nerve itself could have been directly injured.

This patient is at risk of neurogenic pulmonary oedema, due to either the spinal cord injury itself, or an associated head injury. I would monitor this clinically and with the use of arterial blood gases. Again, I would have a low threshold for intubation and ventilation. I would also bear in mind that with haematoma and cord oedema, the level of the lesion may move cranially.

Finally, this patient is very likely to require a CT scan. If there were any concerns about deterioration in his condition, I would consider elective tracheal intubation and ventilation. This may also be necessary if he were uncooperative due to intoxication, cerebral irritation, or the effects of his other injuries.

How would you intubate this patient if it became necessary?

This is likely to be a difficult intubation due to the combination of cervical immobilisation, and any associated facial or laryngeal injuries. As part of my standard preparations, I would ensure a variety of airway equipment were available, including different laryngoscopes, gum elastic bougies and the means to perform a cricothyroidotomy. My goal is to avoid secondary injury to the central nervous system by avoiding hypoxia, hyper- or hypocarbia and maintaining an adequate perfusion pressure. I would perform a rapid sequence induction, with skilled assistants providing two-handed cricoid pressure (to minimise displacement of the cervical spine at C6) and manual in-line immobilisation. I would have both vasopressors and atropine immediately available.

There are arguments that spinal injury is a contra-indication to cricoid pressure.

Would you have any concerns using suxamethonium?

No, not with a new spinal cord injury. I would be concerned from 48 to 72 hours post-injury though, due to the proliferation of acetylcholine receptors and the associated risk of hyperkalaemia.

With regards to the cardiovascular system, there is a risk of arrhythmias particularly at the time of the injury, with the massive sympathetic response and α-adrenergic receptor mediated hypertension. With this high spinal lesion, I would also be concerned about spinal shock.

What do you mean by spinal shock?

Sometimes this is called neurogenic shock in order to differentiate it from the flaccid paralysis and loss of motor reflexes initially seen after cord injury. In this case I mean the disruption of the sympathetic nervous system, leading to hypotension and bradycardia. In particular I would want to avoid over aggressive fluid therapy, this could lead to pulmonary oedema. In this situation I would elect to use vasopressors as required, to maintain sufficient blood pressure for cerebral and renal perfusion. I've mentioned the increased risk of bradycardias or even asystole with manoeuvres that provide vagal stimulation such as intubation or even suction of the tracheal tube.

With which level spinal cord injury are these problems associated?

Above T6 for hypotension and T1 for bradycardias. Spinal shock can persist for up to 8 weeks post-injury.

What other factors are important in the initial management of this patient?

In the assessment of disability, it is important to remember the high risk of an associated head injury, which in turn would affect airway and ventilatory management. There is likely to be an ileus following the injury and therefore a gastric tube should be inserted early. Temperature regulation will be affected so measures to maintain temperature or to re-warm patients should be instituted. Finally, I would suggest the trauma team liaise with a spinal injuries centre with regard to treatment with high-dose steroids.

What reasons are there for or against this?

There is evidence that high-dose steroids within eight hours of the injury can reduce the extent of impairment. But the effect is small and there are all the risks of steroid use, as well as the worsening of outcome in head injured patients as was shown in the CRASH trial.

Do you know which steroid was recommended and the initial dose?

Methylprednisolone initially at a dose of 30 mg kg^{-1}.

Are there any other specific problems you anticipate with this patient in the coming months?

As well as the issues already discussed, he will be at risk of gastro-intestinal stress ulceration, pressure sores, and in the first few months in particular, at risk of deep vein thrombosis and pulmonary embolism.

Your patient turns out to have an isolated unstable cervical spine injury with a complete transection of the cord. His spinal injury is stabilised in the following few days and he proceeds to rehabilitation.

Can you describe the clinical effects of incomplete transection of the spinal cord, for example anterior spinal cord damage?

The neurological sequelae will reflect the anatomy of the spinal cord and its neural tracts.

Damage to the anterior cord will result in paralysis, due to loss of motor pathways, but proprioception, touch and vibration sense, which are carried in the dorsal columns, will be preserved. This pattern may also be seen with ischaemic damage resulting from the loss of the anterior spinal artery supply to the anterior two thirds of the spinal cord.

In a posterior cord injury, the opposite is seen, with preserved motor power, but loss of touch, vibration and proprioception.

A central cord lesion, causes greater motor loss of the upper limbs than lower, with variable sensory loss and sometimes preservation of bladder and bowel control. This pattern may result from a hyperextension injury.

In a Brown-Sequard lesion – with a hemi-section of the cord – such as may result from a penetrating injury, there is ipsilateral paralysis with loss of proprioception touch and vibration sense and contralateral loss of pain and temperature sensation.

Further Reading

Bracken MB. Steroids for acute spinal cord injury. *Cochrane Database of Systematic Reviews*. 2002; Issue 2. Art. No.: CD001046. DOI: 10.1002/14651858.CD001046.

Bracken MB, Shepard MJ, Collins WF, et al. A randomized controlled trial of methylprednisolone or naloxone in the treatment of acute spinal-cord injury: results of the Second National Acute Spinal Cord Injury Study. *New England Journal of Medicine*. 1990; **322**: 1405–1411.

Bracken MB, Shepard MJ, Holford TR, et al. Administration of methylprednisolone for 24 or 48 hour tirilazad mesylate for 48 hours in the treatment of acute spinal cord injury. Results of the Third National Acute Spinal Cord Injury Randomized Controlled Trial. National Acute Spinal Cord Injury Study. *Journal of the American Medical Association*. 1997; **277**: 1597–1604.

Veale P, Lamb J. Anaesthesia and acute spinal cord injury. *British Journal of Anaesthesia. CEPD Reviews* 2002; **2**(5): 139–143.

2.4.5. Late management of patients with spinal cord injury – Carl J Morris

You are asked to anaesthetise a patient for debridement of an ischial tuberosity pressure sore, 7 months after complete transection of the cord at C5 level. He gives a history of significant reflux.

Please describe your anaesthetic management of the case

I will divide this into the pre-, peri- and post-operative phases.

The main anaesthetic issues specific to his spinal injury are the risk of hyperkalaemia with suxamethonium secondary to proliferation of acetylcholine receptors, and also the risks of sympathetic dysreflexia.

Most anaesthetists will not have direct experience of these patients. Therefore an awareness of the key issues should be sufficient for your answer. By structuring your answer, and flagging up the key points at the beginning, your examiner is able to relax, already confident in your approach. Also, if time is short you have already gained crucial marks.

What do you mean by the term "dys-" or "hyper-reflexia"?

This refers to a massive disordered autonomic response to stimuli below the level of the lesion. In the awake patient, there can be headache, sweating and other sympathetic signs such as Horner's syndrome. The most dangerous effect is hypertension, which may be severe and could lead to intra-cranial haemorrhage. It is more common with high spinal lesions, and seems to be caused by loss of descending inhibition and altered neuronal connections within the distal spinal cord. The most common triggers are from caudal root levels, in particular bladder distension. The patient may already be receiving prophylactic agents such as clonidine to try and minimise cardiovascular instability.

This is a difficult question. The pathophysiology of dysreflexia is tricky. It should be enough that you are aware of it.

Please go on with your anaesthetic management …

Pre-operatively, as well as the usual equipment and drug checks, I would clarify patient positioning with the surgeon – surgery may be conducted in the lateral or prone position. I would review the notes, looking for details surrounding the admission with the injury and any subsequent anaesthetics, in particular focussing on any airway difficulties, whether the patient required a tracheostomy at the time of his injury, ventilatory difficulties, including the need for post-operative non-invasive or invasive ventilation, and problems with dysreflexia. I would take a full anaesthetic history and examine the patient, again focussing on these areas. If he had spinal fixation he may have limited neck movement. Contractures may lead to difficulties with positioning, vascular access, or surgical access. In addition, I would ask him about muscular spasm, which could interfere with surgery.

You have mentioned he had a complete transection of the cord, so I would expect him to have no sensation or motor power below that level. I would clarify this with him and assess any requirement for analgesia. I would also ask him about the symptoms of gastro-oesophageal reflux. Most spinal cord injured patients have delayed gastric emptying, but this does not usually lead to reflux. I would prescribe antacid and prokinetic therapy.

With regards to the anaesthetic plan, after clarifying positioning and estimate of duration with the surgeon, I would discuss with the patient the anaesthetic options. These include sedation with or without analgesia, central neuraxial blockade and general anaesthesia. If there were no symptoms and signs of autonomic dysreflexia, and he had no sensation, then the simplest approach would be for him to remain awake for the procedure.

And what if there was a history of dysreflexia?

If there was a history, or if the risk was unknown, I would suggest central neuraxial blockade with a spinal anaesthetic to abolish the risk.

Your patient declines central neuraxial blockade and asks to "have a general"

In that case, I would first seek to clarify his concerns and any misconceptions about spinal anaesthesia, for example if he fears worsening of his lesion. Or whether he simply wishes to be "asleep" and light sedation might be sufficient. If he still insisted on general anaesthesia, I would seek senior anaesthetic advice and explain the increased risk of aspiration with all its consequences. If the consensus was that a general anaesthetic was reasonable, I would go ahead and prepare for that. Given his C5 lesion, unless there was good evidence of previous uneventful operations, without any respiratory complications, I would request a high-dependency bed for his post-operative care.

And how would you anaesthetise him?

I will consider induction, maintenance, monitoring and position.

Induction first. With trained assistance and all my usual checks, I would establish large bore intra-venous access, which may be difficult with atrophic skin and poor blood flow. I would connect a giving set with crystalloid. The patient may have a reduced blood volume, so I would consider a fluid pre-load. I would also have prepared an α-agonist such as metaraminol, anticipating exaggerated hypotension on induction of anaesthesia. As with any induction, I would have atropine in a pre-drawn syringe. If there were any concerns regarding his airway, I would consider an awake fibre-optic intubation. Otherwise I would carry out a modified rapid sequence induction with thiopentone and rocuronium as a rapid onset non-depolarising alternative to suxamethonium.

Why avoid suxamethonium?

As I have mentioned, in spinal cord injury there is a proliferation of acetylcholine receptors throughout the muscle, away from the motor endplate, presumably as a response to the sudden loss of efferent transmission. The use of suxamethonium can therefore lead to a massive depolarisation with subsequent hyperkalaemia and potentially arrhythmias and cardiac arrest.

Do you know how long the risk lasts?

I have read various estimates of the time period. Taking a cautious approach, I would avoid suxamethonium from 48 hours after the initial event, until 9 months later.

In all circumstances?

Every case would have to be assessed on a benefit/harm basis. The potential for a hyperkalaemic crisis within that time period is unquantifiable. Hyperkalaemia is also treatable with calcium, insulin and other measures. It is possible to imagine a situation where an airway crisis may lead to the need to use suxamethonium despite the risk. In an elective case, such as this, it should be avoidable.

These types of questions are more about awareness of the issues and a safety first approach, than any one technique.

You successfully intubate the patient and after a period of initial hypotension, the patient remains stable.

You've described induction, please continue

So on to maintenance. I would ensure adequate depth of anaesthesia with sevoflurane. I would use remifentanil to minimise the risk of muscular spasm or dysreflexia. Intermittent positive pressure ventilation should be used to avoid the increased risk of hypoxia or hypercapnia with his high cord lesion, while being alert for the exaggerated hypotension that may ensue.

The original question was "how would you anaesthetise". You don't have to go through all possible methods, just what you would do. Not everyone would use remifentanil for example. Alternatively, a total intra-venous anaesthetic is equally appropriate.

I would actively warm the patient, using a forced air warmer, and fluid warming, as he is likely to have altered thermoregulation. Although I would not anticipate major blood loss, I would frequently monitor the surgical site and replace any losses immediately as the patient will not have the normal cardiovascular compensatory mechanisms. I would also have a rapid-acting anti-hypertensive such as glycerine trinitrate immediately available for any episodes of dysreflexia. As with any patient, I would take care with positioning using padding to protect sites vulnerable to pressure damage. He is at increased risk of pressure damage as, as I have already mentioned, his skin is likely to be thin and relatively avascular. As well as standard monitoring as per Association of Anaesthetists' guidelines, I would consider using intra-arterial blood pressure monitoring.

Would you use it or not?

As I do not have experience with these patients, and given the concerns with both hypo- and hypertensive crises, I would use it.

In fact some centres with a large volume of surgery for these patients, don't routinely employ intra-arterial monitoring. Given you have already explained the risk of cardiovascular instability it is probably easier to justify its use than not.

Despite all your preventative measures, during surgery his blood pressure rapidly rises to 210/140 mmHg. What would you do?

This is almost certainly spinal dysreflexia. I would send for senior assistance, ensure the patient is adequately anaesthetised, inform the surgeons and ask them to stop. If withdrawing surgical stimulus did not reduce blood pressure, I would increase the depth of anaesthesia. If that failed to obviate the hypertensive crisis, I would administer intra-venous glycerine trinitrate if available, or via metered dose oral spray. I would also consider bladder distension as a cause and check if the urinary catheter was blocked.

Intra-venous GTN is faster acting and can be titrated to response. In high volume centres where central neuraxial blockade is routinely used to obviate dysreflexia, hypertensive crises are rarely encountered. A metered dose spray may be kept immediately available in theatre.

Why use glycerine trinitrate?

The hypertension is likely to be paroxysmal and therefore any agent must be rapid-acting and have a short duration of action. An alternative is the α-blocking agent phentolamine.

There is a large list of drugs in the literature that have been used to prevent or treat sympa-thetic dysreflexia including reserpine, doxazosin, nifedipine and clonidine (which treats spasm as well as hypertension). Knowing one should be enough.

Having treated that crisis, the patient once again stabilises. You are nearing the end of the case and the surgeon informs you he plans to infiltrate with some bupivacaine and adrenaline.

What do you think about this?

I would suggest he doesn't use it. I would explain that the patient has a complete lesion, and therefore will not require the analgesia. If there was some concern about sensation then I would insist that he use plain local anaesthetic. The patient has already had one hypertensive crisis and is likely to have increased sensitivity to catecholamines.

Catecholamine levels, especially levels of noradrenaline, increase during dysreflexic episodes. Despite this they remain lower than levels in normal, non-injured patients. This implies that an increased sensitivity is at least partly responsible for the crises.

Most anaesthetists should be able to answer questions about the acute management of the patient with a spinal cord injury – you would be expected to be confident and decisive in your answers. However, the management of late complications from spinal cord injury deals with a specific patient group many anaesthetists will never encounter. Don't worry if you don't know all of the details, especially the pathophysiology of autonomic dysreflexia. Most of the issues you can work out – for example the risk of respiratory compromise. An awareness of the issues surrounding suxamethonium and hypertensive crises should be sufficient.

Further Reading

Hambly PR, Martin B. Anaesthesia for chronic spinal cord lesions. *Anaesthesia*. 1998; **53**(3): 273–289.

Krassioukov A, Warburton DE, Teasell R, Eng JJ. A systematic review of the management of autonomic dysreflexia after spinal cord injury. *Archives of Physical Medicine and Rehabilitation*. 2009; **90**(4): 682–695.

2.4.6. Brainstem death testing – Susanna T Walker

This is a question that I was actually asked in my Final FRCA structured oral examination. It was asked as part of the anatomy structured oral examination. Guidelines have been adapted from the Academy of Medical Royal Colleges Code of Practice published in 2008.

What is brainstem death?

Brainstem death was defined formally at the conference of the Royal Colleges in 1976, and it is this definition that has since been used in the English law courts. It is defined as "irre-versible loss of the capacity for consciousness, combined with irreversible loss of the capacity to breathe".

Please could you talk me through the functions of all the cranial nerves and tell me which ones are tested when we perform brainstem death testing?

The first cranial nerve (CN I) is the "olfactory nerve". This gives us the sense of smell, which is not tested during brainstem testing.

The second cranial nerve (CN II) is the "optic nerve". This nerve innervates the eye and enables us to see. It is involved as the afferent limb of the pupillary light reflex. This nerve is tested in brainstem testing by shining a bright light directly into the eye. A normal response would lead to constriction of the pupil. If someone were brainstem dead, there would be no response to light.

The third cranial nerve (CN III) is the "oculomotor nerve". This nerve innervates all of the muscles of the eye except the superior oblique and lateral rectus, and is therefore involved in movement of the eye. This is not directly tested in brainstem testing. However, the third nerve is indirectly tested, as parasympathetic efferent fibres, which control pupillary constriction, travel with the third nerve and are therefore tested as the efferent limb of the pupillary light reflex.

The fourth cranial nerve (CN IV) is the "trochlear nerve". This innervates the superior oblique muscle of the eye enabling the eye to look medially and down. This is not directly tested during brainstem testing.

The fifth cranial nerve (CN V) is the "trigeminal nerve". This is a large nerve with sensory and motor components. It supplies sensation to the face and scalp including sensation to the cornea, and motor supply to the muscles of mastication. This therefore supplies an afferent limb for the corneal blink reflex. This is tested during brainstem testing by lightly touching a strand of cotton wool onto the cornea. A normal response would be to blink, which is absent if someone is brainstem dead.

The sixth cranial nerve (CN VI) is the "abducens nerve". This innervates the lateral rectus muscle of the eye enabling lateral movement of the eye. This is not directly tested during brainstem testing.

The seventh cranial nerve (CN VII) is the "facial nerve". This is predominantly a motor nerve supplying muscles of facial expression. This is the nerve that results in blinking, and is therefore the efferent limb of the corneal blink reflex, which is tested in conjunction with CN V.

The eighth cranial nerve (CN VIII) is the "auditory nerve". This has two main components; the cochlear and vestibular nerves, which are responsible for hearing and balance respectively. Damage to the vestibular nerve therefore causes problems with equilibrium and balance leading to vertigo. Often the most obvious clinical sign of this is nystagmus of the eyes. This nerve is tested in brainstem testing as part of the vestibulo-ocular or caloric reflex. It is important to check that the auditory canal is free from earwax prior to testing as this would affect the results. To perform the test the ear canal is irrigated with 50 ml of ice-cold water. Normally this would lead to eye deviation towards the side being tested and a nystagmus with the fast phase going away from the side being tested. In a brainstem dead patient there is no response. The afferent nerve for this reflex is the vestibular nerve, and the efferent limb indirectly tests the third, fourth and sixth cranial nerves (eye movements).

The ninth cranial nerve (CN IX) is the "glossopharyngeal nerve". This is predominantly a sensory nerve and supplies sensation to the posterior third of the tongue, and the pharynx. This is tested during brainstem testing as it forms the afferent limb of the gag reflex. Patients who are brainstem dead have no afferent portion to the gag reflex and therefore do not gag when a spatula is placed at the posterior pharyngeal wall.

The tenth cranial nerve (CN X) is the "vagus nerve". This is a large nerve supplying parasympathetic motor innervation to many organs in the body, and importantly motor innervation to most of the pharynx and larynx via the recurrent laryngeal and superior laryngeal nerves. This is tested during brainstem testing in two ways. Firstly, by placing a suction catheter down the endotracheal tube, normally this would elicit coughing, but there is no response in a brainstem dead patient. The vagus nerve is also involved in the gag test as it forms the efferent limb of the gag reflex.

The eleventh cranial nerve (CN XI) is the "accessory nerve". This innervates the sterno-cleidomastoid and trapezius muscles, and is not tested during brainstem testing.

The twelfth cranial nerve (CN XII) is the "hypoglossal nerve". This is the motor supply to the tongue and is not tested during brainstem testing.

Cranial nerves I, XI and XII are the only ones that are not tested in any way, as they do not contribute to a brainstem reflex arc.

What preconditions are required before performing brainstem death testing?

There are certain preconditions that should be met before brainstem testing is performed. Firstly, the patient should have an irrecoverable condition causing brain damage, which can lead to brainstem death. Conditions would include a severe head injury or a subarachnoid haemorrhage. The patient should also be in an apnoeic coma, requiring ventilation.

Do you know of any factors that might exclude patients from brainstem death testing?

There are several factors that might mean that it is inappropriate to perform brainstem death testing. These are all factors that could themselves lead to a change in cerebral function affecting the Glasgow coma score of a patient, and therefore could potentially lead to inaccurate testing suggesting a patient is brainstem dead when they are not.

To perform the tests, the patient should not be hypothermic. The latest Academy of Medical Royal Colleges guidelines recommend that the core temperature should be greater than 34°C. There should be no metabolic or endocrine disturbance, such as hypoglycaemia or hypothyroidism that could lead to a coma. However, it is well known that brainstem death itself may lead to metabolic and endocrine disturbances such as diabetes insipidus causing hypernatraemia. These may be as a result of rather than the cause of lack of brainstem function, and do not preclude brainstem death testing. There should be no evidence of depressant drugs causing the coma. Any sedation that may have been given on intensive care should have been switched off for an appropriate length of time to be certain that there is no chance of any residual effects of sedative medications. If any neuromuscular blocking drugs have been used, then a nerve stimulator should be used to demonstrate that there is no residual effect of these drugs. Testing cannot be performed on patients with a medical cause of paralysis such as Guillain-Barré syndrome.

How would you actually perform the tests?

When the relevant preconditions and exclusion criteria have been addressed, the tests can be performed. Two doctors should perform the tests; they should both have been registered for more than 5 years, and one of them should be a consultant. A complete set of the tests should be performed twice with the doctors acting together. There is no stipulation about how far apart the two sets of tests are performed, other than that baseline parameters should be restored before starting the second set of tests.

I have already described the nerve roots that are tested. However, in practice the tests are performed by, first testing for a pupillary light reflex in both eyes. Then test for the corneal reflex in both eyes. Next, check that both ear canals are clear and then test for the vestibulo-ocular reflexes bilaterally. Ensure that there is no facial movement in response to a central painful stimulus, such as supra-orbital pressure. It is important to note that spinal reflexes may persist, leading to movement of limbs. This may be distressing for relatives to see, but does not affect the outcome of brainstem testing. Then confirm that there is no gag or cough reflex.

Finally the apnoea test is performed. The patient should be pre-oxygenated with 100% oxygen for 10 minutes. This is often done whilst the earlier tests are performed. The ventilation rate should be reduced during this period to allow the end-tidal CO_2 to rise above 6.0 kPa prior to disconnecting the ventilator. An arterial blood gas sample should be performed at this stage to confirm the $PaCO_2$ is at least 6.0 kPa and that the pH is less than 7.4. The ventilator is then disconnected and the patient is oxygenated by insufflating oxygen at 5 L min^{-1} into the lungs via a suction catheter placed down the endotracheal tube. If after 5 minutes, the patient has shown no signs of respiratory effort a further blood gas sample is analysed to ensure that the $PaCO_2$ has risen from the starting level by more than 0.5 kPa. The $PaCO_2$ usually rises by 0.4–0.8 kPa min^{-1} depending on the metabolic rate. Patients with pre-existing lung disease may normally have a raised $PaCO_2$, therefore an appropriate starting $PaCO_2$ for this patient should be determined on the basis of a blood gas demonstrating a mild acidaemia with a pH less than 7.4. The patient should not be allowed to become hypoxic whilst these tests are being performed. CPAP may be used to maintain oxygenation if required. Occasionally apnoea testing may have to be abandoned as a result of oxygen desaturation.

What are "doll's eye movements"? Are these required as part of brainstem death testing?

Doll's eye movements describe the oculocephalic reflex. In an unconscious patient, if their head is turned to the side, the eyes rotate in the opposite direction, therefore keeping the eyes pointing in the original direction in relation to the surroundings – as is seen in a child's doll. This reflex requires an intact brainstem, and therefore in a brainstem dead patient, when the head is turned, the eyes move in the same direction as the head. This is not a test that is required in brainstem testing in the UK, although may be tested in other countries.

What clinical features may be seen that are associated with brainstem death?

An injury to the brain leads to swelling of the brain within the skull, raising intra-cranial pressure which will lead to a reduction in cerebral perfusion and therefore a reduction in oxygen supply to the brain. All of the subsequent clinical features are related to this brain swelling. The final result of the swelling if this continues is for the brainstem to be forced through the foramen magnum. This is known as "coning" and leads to brainstem death. There are various clinical signs that may be elicited at various stages as a result of the brain swelling. A third nerve lesion may be seen as a result of herniation of the uncus. A sixth nerve lesion may be seen as swelling stretches the nerve. The Cushing's reflex occurs as a desperate attempt to improve cerebral perfusion. This leads to significant hypertension associated with a bradycardia, which is the result of the baroreceptor reflex. Various arrhythmias may then subsequently occur. There are also several endocrine manifestations of brainstem swelling, such as a failure of thyroid hormone synthesis due to hypothalamic and pituitary failure. This further exacerbates cardiovascular changes and instability. There is also a lack of anti-diuretic hormone, which results in neurogenic diabetes insipidus, leading to large quantities of very dilute urine. Finally, there is a loss in thermoregulation, which usually leads to hypothermia.

Do you know of any additional tests that may be required in other countries to confirm brainstem death?

If you're being asked these questions you're doing well – keep going!

In the UK there is no legal requirement to perform any tests in addition to brainstem testing. However, in certain situations these may be considered if, for example, pre-existing lung disease makes it impossible to complete the apnoea test as a result of oxygen desaturation, or if it is not possible to test some of the cranial nerves as a result of craniofacial trauma. In some countries, such as the United States, extra tests are commonly performed. The tests that may be performed aim to elicit a complete lack of electrical activity and blood flow to the brain. The gold standard to demonstrate lack of blood supply to the brain is four-vessel angiography. A radio-opaque contrast medium can be injected into both internal carotid and both vertebral arteries. In brainstem death flow is obstructed due to raised intra-cranial pressure. More recent, and less invasive, techniques include CT angiogram and MR angiogram, both of which also demonstrate the lack of blood flow. Transcranial Doppler ultrasonography is also mentioned, where a characteristic change in the velocity waveform of the basal cerebral arteries is seen. This is the least invasive test and can be performed at the bedside in ITU.

An EEG may be performed to demonstrate a lack of electrical activity. There are some controversies regarding the EEG as it is technically very difficult to perform in the ITU setting due to the large amount of interference from surrounding equipment. It is also possible to perform auditory evoked potentials (AEPs) to demonstrate a lack of brain activity.

What is the legal time of death?

The legal time of death is the time at which the first set of tests has been completed. However, the patient isn't actually pronounced dead until after the second set of tests have been performed.

Why do we have a shortage of organ donors in the UK compared with the rest of Europe?

This is quite a topical subject that has been in the news a lot over the past couple of years. You should be able to say at least something about this as it is something I'm sure there will be many more debates about in the future.

The UK donation rate is one of the lowest in Europe with a recent study from 2006 showing only 12 per million of the population donate their organs for transplant, compared with 33 per million of the population in Spain. The rate of donation has actually fallen in the UK. It is not known why this is, but it is thought that one of the main reasons is that relatives and family members are reluctant to allow transplantation procedures. During the 2-year study, by the UK Transplant organisation, of the potential organ donors whose families were approached for donation 41% of the families denied consent. The main reasons for refusal were that they did not want surgery on the body, they were not sure if the patient would have agreed, or that the relatives were divided. The refusal rates were highest amongst families from ethnic minorities (70%) in comparison to those of white donors (35%). It should be noted that organ donation was only discussed in 94% of potential cases, meaning that 6% of cases were missed opportunities. Therefore, in a small part, the lack of organs is a result of clinicians not discussing donation with the next of kin. This is a difficult subject to broach, and therefore there may be some delay or reluctance on the part of the clinician. To address this issue there has been a drive to increase numbers of organ transplant coordinators. They provide an important service as they are specifically trained to broach this issue and are often based within the hospital and can therefore be called upon very quickly to talk to relatives and initiate the required procedures leading to organ donation. There is also the benefit that they can identify inappropriate patients quickly and therefore prevent an unnecessary discussion with the family, which avoids causing further distress. They also have an important role of increasing awareness of organ donation amongst the general population.

The shortage of organs can also be attributed to the state of brainstem death being uncommon in the UK. This is partly due to a decrease in deaths from road traffic accidents, improved trauma care and a decrease in cerebrovascular deaths.

How may this shortage in donor organs be addressed?

Currently in the UK we have an "opt-in" system, whereby members of the general population can choose to carry an organ donor card or join the official organ donor register. In 2006 the government set up a taskforce to identify barriers to organ donation and to make recommendations with the aim of increasing organ donation by 50% by 2013. Recently a debate was held regarding the proposal to change the current opt-in donation scheme to a presumed consent opt-out system, which has been so successful in other parts of Europe including Spain. This has been rejected for the time being; however, it seems inevitable that this is a debate that will continue for many years.

It is thought that by having implemented a donor register that can be accessed by all hospitals, the rate of organ donation will increase. Members of the public can choose to join the donor register. Therefore, if the time comes that organ donation is appropriate, this removes the burden of decision making from the legal next of kin. Many relatives are comforted by the thought that "this is what he/she would want".

There has been a suggestion of starting social incentive programmes. In this situation, an organ donor could opt to donate first to people on the transplant register in their social group. This may make the concept of organ donation more acceptable to some people. Finally, some have suggested that there should be a financial incentive to induce people to join the transplant register. This, however, is not something that has been seriously considered yet in the UK.

What criteria would suggest to you a brainstem dead patient may not be suitable as an organ donor?

The main criteria that can be applied to organ donation are firstly to prevent transmitting a transmittable disease such as infection or malignancy and secondly, to ensure acceptable function of the donor organ. Various absolute and relative contraindications to transplant have been suggested.

Absolute contraindications would include age over 80 years, active metastatic cancer, DIC and sickle cell anaemia. HIV infection is an absolute contraindication, although in some states in America transplants between patients infected with HIV have been allowed in certain circumstances. Prolonged hypotension or hypothermia is also an absolute contraindication, although a brief period of resuscitated cardiac arrest is considered acceptable when putting a patient forward for organ transplant. Ultimately, the transplant team makes the final decision – often in theatre – regarding the suitability of organs.

Relative contraindications would include malignancy that has been in remission for over 5 years, hypertension, diabetes mellitus, physiological age greater than 70, hepatitis B or C infection, and a history of smoking. Some heart, lung, liver and renal dysfunction may be acceptable if it was caused in the context of trauma leading to brainstem death. Brain tumours are not an absolute contraindication, although it must be certain that the brain tumour does not represent a metastasis from another primary source.

Further Reading

Academy of Medical Royal Colleges. A Code of Practice for the Diagnosis and Confirmation of Death. Academy of Medical Royal Colleges. Published October 2008. http://www.aomrc.org.uk/publications/reports-guidance.html.

Barber K, Falvey S, Hamilton C, Collett D, Rudge C. Potential for organ donation in the United Kingdom audit of intensive care records. *British Medical Journal.* 2006; **332**(7550): 1124–1128.

2.4.7. Anaesthesia for MRI scanning – Sarah F Bell

This topic might be part of a clinical or physics structured oral exam. An extensive, in depth understanding of the workings of the MRI is not required. The examiner is looking to see whether you have a basic grasp of the physical concepts and whether you are aware of the safety issues that exist.

Can you start by telling me how an MRI scanner works?

Try and avoid getting bogged down with complicated physical principles.

The MRI machine produces an extremely strong magnetic field. This causes the protons within the hydrogen atoms of water to become aligned, either in the same direction as the magnetic field or in the opposite direction. The high water content of the body makes these paramagnetic protons vital to the formation of a magnetic resonance image.

A pulse of electromagnetic radiation (in the form of radio waves) causes the hydrogen nuclei to rotate from their equilibrium position. When this pulse is then removed, the nuclei emit radio waves as they return to their original equilibrium position. This radio wave signal is detected by the coil in the MRI scanner and processed by the computer system to produce a visual display.

What are the components of an MRI scanner?

The MRI machine is composed of a primary magnet, gradient magnets, a coil and a computer system to analyse the data.

Can you tell me more about the primary magnet?

Ferromagnetic materials such as iron, cobalt or nickel produce magnetic fields. They may also be generated by passing a current through a wire. The primary magnet in an MRI scanner consists of a coil of wire through which a current is passed. The wire is made from a super-conducting material. This material has no electrical resistance below a certain temperature. It is therefore able to produce a very large magnetic field. The low temperature required is in the region of $-260°C$ (or just above absolute zero). To achieve this temperature the wire is kept in liquid nitrogen and helium.

What can you tell me about the gradient magnets and the coil?

There are three smaller magnets within an MRI machine called gradient magnets. These magnets are much weaker than the primary magnet. They allow precise alterations of the magnetic field. They are important in generating the final images.

The coil is the part of the MRI machine that emits and receives the electromagnetic radiation, in the form of radio waves.

How strong is the magnetic field produced?

The MRI scanner produces a magnetic field of 1.5 to 3 Tesla.

What does Tesla mean?

Tesla is the unit of magnetic flux density. This is a measure of the strength of a magnetic field. Another unit used is the Gauss. Ten thousand Gauss is equal to one Tesla. The earth's magnetic field is equal to between 0.5 and 1 Gauss.

What is the 50 Gauss line?

The magnetic field of 50 Gauss is marked around an MRI scanner with a line. This is the 50 Gauss line.

The images produced are called either T1 or T2 weighted images. What does this mean?

T1 and T2 are called the relaxation time constants. They are different measures of how the hydrogen nuclei relax back to their original alignment. Either T1 or T2 is used to provide extra contrast to an image. In T1, fluid is seen as dark, whereas in T2, fluid is white. This can be useful in deciding the type of tissue seen in an image.

What are the challenges of anaesthetising a patient in the MRI scanner?

This question is testing your ability to recognise the many problems that might occur. Try and give some broad categories before going into detail.

There are many potential problems associated with anaesthetising a patient in the MRI scanner. These can be divided into patient-associated problems, problems with administering an anaesthetic in a remote and unfamiliar site and MRI-specific problems. The MRI problems can be subdivided into monitoring, equipment and safety issues.

Can you tell me anything about the patient-associated problems?

Yes. The patient-related factors are mainly due to the populations that require anaesthetic intervention for the scan to take place. These are generally children or adults who would otherwise not stay still, or have refused to have the scan without some form of anaesthesia (either sedation or general anaesthesia). These patients may have multiple inherited or acquired conditions, learning difficulties, difficult intra-venous access and a potentially difficult airway. Furthermore, the size of the patient is important since obese patients may not actually fit into the scanner. It is important to perform a thorough pre-scan assessment of the patient to allow adequate planning and preparation of the anaesthetic.

Can you talk me through the monitoring and equipment problems?

The monitoring problems may be split into difficulties obtaining a reading and then complications with interpretation of a value.

All patients who require an anaesthetic should be monitored as per the AAGBI minimum monitoring standards. The MRI tube is narrow and it can be difficult to access the patient during the scan. The monitoring therefore needs to be secure. The scan may take a variable length of time, which can lead to hypothermia in some patients. It is therefore important to consider warming devices and the ambient room temperature in certain cases.

The 50 Gauss line is marked on the floor of the MRI. This is an important boundary. Ferromagnetic items such as iron or molybdenum steel that are within this line will move and potentially act as projectile objects. There are also other materials that can behave differently and unpredictably in a magnetic field. All monitoring devices need to be able to function reliably under these conditions.

The ECG electrodes are made of non-magnetic materials. The cables connecting the pulse oximeter and ECG are fibre-optic. Care should be taken to avoid looping of cables and to pad the skin underneath them. This is to reduce the chances of burns to the patient. Burns might occur if currents are induced in the cables causing an increase in their temperature.

Can you tell me about the problems with interpreting the monitoring?

With regards to interpreting the monitoring, MRI can have some important effects.

Firstly, the ECG. The magnetic field can generate currents within the aorta. This can result in artefact in the ST region of the ECG. Monitoring for myocardial ischaemia can therefore be unreliable.

Secondly, the capnography and gas analysis is affected. This is because of the length of sampling tubing required to bring the gases out of the MRI scanner to the analysing equipment. Delays of up to 20 seconds can occur.

Finally the MRI is extremely noisy. Acoustic protection is required and so audible alarms are useless. The monitoring therefore needs to have visible alarms. The anaesthetist needs to ensure that they have an unobstructed view of the screen at all times.

What is the difference between MRI safe and MRI compatible equipment?

"MRI safe" means that there will be no safety issues when the equipment is taken into the MRI. It does not guarantee that the equipment will function normally or not interfere with the correct operation of the MRI.

"MRI compatible" equipment is MRI safe and does not interfere with the operation of the MRI.

Is the anaesthetic machine used for MRI safe or compatible?

The anaesthetic machine used in the MRI room must be MRI compatible. This includes the vapourisers and the gas cylinders.

What about your infusion pumps?

These should be MRI compatible. Some pumps will fail if the field strength is greater than 100 Gauss.

What type of circuit do we commonly use in the MRI scanner?

A Bain circuit is frequently used in an MRI scanner. It can be up to 5.4 m in length whilst maintaining low dead-space and resistance.

What are the hazards posed to staff and patients when in the MRI?

Try and structure your answer so that the examiner is aware that you know there are many possible complications.

The hazards may be due to the magnetic field, the noise, the anaesthetic gases and the potential for MRI malfunction.

Magnetic field hazards may be further divided into projectile effects and burns.

The patient and staff need to be screened for implanted ferromagnetic objects since they can act as projectile objects. Ferromagnetic objects include pacemakers, aneurysm clips and metal foreign bodies in the eye. The staff and patient also need to remove any ferromagnetic jewellery, ID badges or credit cards etc.

The MRI can cause burns by inducing currents in the monitoring cables, which will then heat up.

The current maximum safe level for exposure to the intense magnetic field is 200 mT within an 8-hour period. MRI should be avoided during the first trimester of pregnancy.

A magnetic field of greater than 3 Tesla will increase the risk of current induction and potentially fatal arrhythmias. This field strength is not used in hospitals.

The MRI produces a large amount of acoustic noise and so protection should be worn. This may be in the form of ear plugs or ear defenders.

During administration of an anaesthetic, there is the risk of anaesthetic gas inhalation if the scavenging equipment is not as effective as that in theatre. There are MRI compatible systems produced that should be used whenever possible.

If the MRI malfunctions or needs to be shut down, there is a risk of hypoxia.

Why is this?

When the MRI is shut down the liquid helium and nitrogen that surrounds and cools the superconductor is allowed to rapidly evaporate and escape from inside the magnet. If there is inadequate ventilation of the area, a fall in the oxygen concentration will occur. This can lead to a hypoxic environment.

Given all the risks of the MRI, why do we not just use CT for all cases that require imaging?

The CT is also not without risk. The same challenges of remote site anaesthesia, patient and procedure related factors still occur. In addition the patient is being exposed to X-ray radiation that can predispose to malignancy. The radiation exposure for a CT chest is approximately 50 times that of a plain X-ray.

The images produced by CT and MRI are different. The techniques are therefore used to view and diagnose different conditions. MRI is particularly good at imaging the nervous system and for pelvic disease. CT is useful for imaging bony deformities.

Do both techniques use contrast medium?

Yes, in both techniques the radiologist may require contrast medium to be given. This can cause anaphylaxis.

The MRI contrast most commonly used is gadolinium DTPA, which can cause nausea, vomiting and pain on injection.

The CT contrast mediums often contain iodine. This can cause acute renal failure in susceptible patients. The patient should be well hydrated prior to administration of the medium. If the patient has renal impairment or diabetes then the contrast medium may be avoided.

Are you aware of any guidelines regarding anaesthetising patients in the radiology suite?

The AAGBI have produced online guidelines regarding the provision of anaesthetic services in the MRI scanner.

Further Reading

The Association of Anaesthetists of Great Britain and Ireland (AAGBI). Provision of Anaesthetic Services in Magnetic Resonance Units. 2002. http://www.aagbi.org/publications/guidelines/docs/mri02.pdf.

2.4.8. Depth of anaesthesia monitoring – Susanna T Walker

This is an important topic that you will be expected to know about.

What is awareness?

There are a few definitions that you should be able to recite to convince the examiners that you have an understanding of this subject.

Anaesthetic awareness is a serious complication, and one of the most feared complications, of general anaesthesia. Awareness can be classified into explicit memory, implicit memory and deliberate awareness.

Explicit memory can be defined as the intentional or conscious recollection of experiences. Anaesthetic awareness specifically refers to explicit memory of intra-operative events, which involves spontaneous or conscious recall. The explicit recall may occur with or without the sensation of pain and recollections may be vivid, such as operating room conversation, or vague, such as dreams, or unpleasant sensations associated with the operation.

Implicit memory is the perception of "something" without spontaneous recall of events. The patient initially denies remembering anything, but may subsequently remember "something" under hypnosis or with repeated questioning.

Deliberate awareness occurs when patients are awake for surgery performed using local or regional anaesthesia. It also occurs during some neurosurgical procedures when the patient is woken up to assess whether surgery has affected, or will affect, important areas. This is, however, less common since the introduction of devices to monitor evoked potentials intra-operatively.

Can you tell me the incidence of awareness?

The incidence of awareness varies significantly depending on the clinical situation and the type of anaesthetic given. Overall, the incidence of awareness with explicit recall of severe pain is commonly quoted as being approximately 1 in 3000 (0.03%). The incidence of awareness without recall of pain is commoner, and overall, between 1 and 2 per 1000 people are thought to experience some sort of awareness. However, it is important to note that some of these figures may be exaggerated by memories generated during awakening or in recovery. A large survey published in 2007 found an overall rate of awareness of 1 in 14 000 general anaesthetics. This can be broken down into:

- 1 in 42 000 for patients with no risk factors
- 1 in 100 for cardiac surgery
- 1 in 20 for trauma surgery
- 1 in 250 for emergency caesarean section under general anaesthesia.

Awareness is almost twice as likely when neuromuscular blockade is used.

What are the consequences of awareness for the patient?

Awareness may have serious psychological repercussions for the patient, including insomnia, depression, post-traumatic stress disorder and a fear of future surgery.

What are the causes and risk factors for awareness?

Try to classify the causes and risk factors into a way that you will easily remember. There are many ways to do this. One might be patient factors, anaesthetic factors and surgical factors.

Patient factors:

- Disease processes (e.g., sepsis, hyperthyroidism)
- Social factors (e.g., alcoholism, recreational drugs)
- Medications (e.g., β-blockers)
- Previous history of awareness.

Anaesthetic factors:

- Equipment malfunction
- TIVA technique
- Difficult intubation
- Use of neuromuscular blockade.

Surgical factors:

- Trauma surgery
- Cardiac surgery
- GA caesarean section.

Ultimately, awareness results from an inadequate anaesthetic dose. Light anaesthesia, especially when a patient has received a muscle relaxant, is associated with the highest risk of awareness. There are four main reasons why an anaesthetic may be too light.

Firstly, not giving a large enough dose of anaesthestic. This may occur when a volatile agent is accidentally not given, or started late; or when an anaesthetic dose is reduced in a hypotensive patient to preserve the blood pressure. It is important to remember when selecting a dose that patients vary in their requirements, and often the chosen dose is based on patient averages. Minimum alveolar concentration (MAC), for example, is a population average and varies with age, gender and race.

Secondly, some patients, such as those with hypermetabolic states (e.g., pyrexia or hyperthyroidism), may have an element of resistance to anaesthetic agents.

Thirdly, there may be a problem with the equipment used. Breathing circuits may become disconnected, vapourisers may become empty, and TIVA infusion pumps may fail. For these reasons, a pressure fail alarm should always be used when ventilating patients. Volatile agent monitors with high and low alarm settings are widely available for use.

Finally, clinical signs of awareness, which would normally lead the anaesthetist to increase the anaesthetic dose, may be hidden. For example, patients taking β-blockers are less capable of mounting a tachycardia.

When discussing causes and risk factors for awareness, it is important to mention the type of surgery and the type of anaesthetic being given.

Certain operations carry a much higher risk of awareness. These are generally situations where there is a risk of patient instability, so therefore an insufficient dose of anaesthetic agent may be given. These would include emergency GA caesarean section, high-risk cardiac surgery and acute trauma with hypovolaemia, where the incidence of awareness is quoted as being up to 5% depending on the severity of the trauma.

Patients with airway issues, including unexpected difficult intubation, or those undergoing rigid bronchoscopy are also at higher risk of awareness due to a failure to give any further anaesthetic agent during the period where it is difficult to intubate or ventilate the patient.

What methods are you aware of for monitoring the depth of anaesthesia?

Think of a way to classify these as there are many, and you will then be less likely to forget the main important ones.

These could be classified into:

- Simple techniques
- Techniques which use a form of EEG monitoring
- Other techniques.

Simple techniques include monitoring for clinical signs of tachycardia, hypertension, tachypnoea, sweating and lacrimation. End-tidal agent monitoring is a simple monitor that is routinely used in most anaesthetics given in the UK. Whilst this does not actually measure depth of anaesthesia it is a useful adjunct to ensure attainment of the desired concentration of anaesthetic agent. It does, however, have its limitations and should therefore only be used as a guide in conjunction with other clinical signs.

Techniques that use a form of EEG monitoring include pure EEG analysis, cerebral function monitors, frequency domain analysis, compressed spectral array, bispectral analysis and entropy. EEG monitoring uses 19 electrodes to create a trace of cerebral activity. It is therefore time-consuming, impractical to use during a standard anaesthetic, and complex to interpret, all of which limits its usefulness for monitoring the depth of anaesthesia. Different anaesthetic agents affect the EEG pattern in different ways and factors such as hypoxia, hypercarbia and hypotension can also lead to changes in the EEG. This makes interpretation of the EEG complex and impractical for use as routine monitoring. Cerebral function monitors, frequency domain analysis, and compressed spectral array are all monitors which process and modify the conventional EEG to simplify the information. Fourier analysis is used to process the raw EEG data into their component sine waves. These are then further analysed with respect to the frequency distribution, the power contained within a waveform, i.e., its amplitude, and the relationships between waves of different frequencies. The output is displayed in different ways, but overall leads to a trace that is easier to interpret than the raw EEG. None of these monitors are widely available for depth of anaesthesia monitoring.

Other techniques include the isolated forearm technique, lower oesophageal contractility, somatosensory evoked potentials and frontalis scalp EMG.

How useful is the monitor for lower oesophageal contractility?

There are two types of smooth muscle contraction that can be detected in the lower oesophagus – spontaneous contractions and provoked contractions. Both have a reduction in latency and amplitude with increasing depth of anaesthesia. The provoked contractions result from a sudden distension of the oesophagus, which can be achieved by rapidly inflating a balloon catheter placed in the lower oesophagus. A distal pressure transducer detects the elicited contraction. The evidence for using this as a depth of anaesthesia monitor is fairly limited and it is generally thought to not be reliable.

What do you know about the isolated forearm technique?

This is small-print information, so don't worry if you are being asked this!

This is a technique which is mainly historical and of interest for research. A tourniquet on the patient's upper arm is inflated above systolic blood pressure prior to giving muscle relaxants. Therefore the arm with the tourniquet applied theoretically receives no muscle relaxant. Prior to induction of anaesthesia the patient is informed to move their arm if they are awake. After 15–20 minutes the tourniquet has to be let down to prevent limb ischaemia and subsequent temporary limb paralysis. It can be re-inflated if further relaxant is required. Research has shown that movement of the arm may not necessarily indicate explicit awareness, as the patient may have no recollection of moving their arm intra-operatively. It has also been argued that a response to command, or spontaneous movement, during surgery is a late sign when attempting to prevent awareness, and therefore this technique is not very helpful as a method of monitoring depth of anaesthesia.

How useful are evoked potentials at estimating depth of anaesthesia?

Of all the "other techniques", this is the one to know something about. There is renewed research particularly into the use of auditory evoked potentials to monitor the depth of anaesthesia.

Evoked potential monitors measure the response, using a recording electrode, in specific areas of the brain when a supra-maximal sensory stimulation is applied to a peripheral nerve. An increase in latency and reduction in amplitude of these responses is seen with increasing depth of anaesthesia with most anaesthetic agents.

Visual evoked potentials are less reliable than auditory evoked potentials. When using auditory evoked potentials, a repetitive auditory stimulus at 6–10 hertz is played to the patient through headphones. A response waveform can then be plotted against time. Repeated stimulation enables the response signal to be identified against the background EEG. The waveform formed consists of three peaks. Firstly, the brainstem response; secondly the mid-cortical response; and thirdly the late cortical response. The brainstem and late cortical responses are not affected by depth of anaesthesia. However, the mid-cortical response is – the amplitude of the waves is decreased and the latency increased in a dose-dependent manner. By processing the raw waveform, the "auditory evoked potential" (AEP) index can be calculated, giving a number which might be more meaningful to interpret than the raw waveform. A value of greater than 80 indicates an awake patient and a value less than 50 indicates an anesthetised patient. There is a sudden increase in the AEP index when a patient changes from being unconscious to being awake. Therefore it can be easier to distinguish between an asleep patient and an awake patient than with other monitors, such as the BIS. However, there is inter-patient variability for the index value at which this change takes place. Therefore it is difficult to define a sensitive and specific cut-off value, whilst in an individual patient the pattern is very reproducible with awakening repeatedly occurring at the same index values.

What do you know about BIS monitoring? Are you aware of any recent studies into the use of BIS?

There are two or three reasonably important recent studies that you might be expected to have heard of even if you don't know the details well.

The BIS monitor obtains an EEG trace from fronto-temporal electrodes which is then processed into a number on a scale of 0–100; 100 represents normal brain activity, 0 represents complete absence of cerebral function, and a value of less than 60 is thought to represent a value below which there is a very low probability of post-operative recall. BIS values decrease with an increasing dose of anaesthetic agent, irrespective of whether this is inhalational or intra-venous. The one exception to this is when using ketamine, which increases cerebral function, therefore increasing the BIS value. Studies have shown that BIS values decrease when muscle relaxant drugs are given, suggesting that the patient is at a deeper level of anaesthesia. However, the values do not change when opiate drugs or nitrous oxide are given, suggesting no change in depth of anaesthesia. These findings are obviously conflicting with what we know from clinical experience and should therefore make the anaesthetist cautious if delivering an anaesthetic to a targeted number.

There are several limitations to BIS monitoring. Firstly, there is no gold standard to compare BIS to, and so it is difficult to evaluate its effectiveness. The values themselves tend to have significant inter-patient variability. Whilst one patient is asleep at a high BIS value such as 75, another may still be awake at a lower value of 70. The BIS values show a continuum from awake to asleep, and therefore there is no clear-cut point (unlike auditory evoked potentials) where transition is made from asleep to awake.

There are two major recent trials assessing the effectiveness of BIS monitoring. The first to mention is the "B-Aware Trial" published in the *Lancet* in 2004. This was a large prospective, randomised, double-blind multicentre trial. The patients in the trial group were at high risk of awareness undergoing a variety of procedures including cardiac, trauma and obstetric surgery. They were randomly assigned to receive standard general anaesthesia, or a general anaesthetic with BIS monitoring. The patients were blinded to the protocol they received, as were the observers who assessed them for awareness at 2–6 hours, 24–36 hours and 30 days. The overall outcome from the study suggested that BIS-guided anaesthesia reduced the incidence of awareness with recall by approximately 82%. They also incidentally reported that the use of BIS led to a reduction of administration of volatile gases. The group therefore concluded by recommending the use of BIS in high-risk patients. It was estimated that if we were to routinely use awareness monitoring for most patients in the United Kingdom it would cost approximately £30 million annually.

The other recent trial published was the "B-Unaware Trial" which was published in the *New England Journal of Medicine* in 2008. This trial was based in Washington, USA. Once again, all of the patients included were considered to be at high risk of awareness under anaesthesia. There were various inclusion criteria, which were based on factors such as previous history of awareness, history of difficult intubation, ASA class 4 or 5, aortic stenosis, or end-stage lung disease. The patients were due to have a general anaesthetic with a volatile agent with or without nitrous oxide. The patients were randomly split into two groups. The first used BIS monitors and targeted values of 40–60. The second group used end-tidal agent monitoring targeting a MAC of 0.7–1.3. Alarms were set to alert the clinician when values were outside these ranges. Awareness was assessed using questionnaires – a well-accepted method–at 24 hours, 72 hours and 30 days. Patients and investigators were unaware of the groups to which they had been assigned. There were two definite cases of awareness in each group. The trial did not reproduce the results of the previous B-Aware trial, and therefore did not show a reduction in the incidence of awareness with BIS monitoring. Also the use of BIS did not result in a reduction in administration of volatile anaesthetic agents. Therefore, findings do not support the use of BIS as part of monitoring in standard practice.

Can you tell me what entropy is?

Entropy can be defined as being a quantitative measurement of disorder in a system. Entropy monitoring for depth of anaesthesia relies on assessing the degree of irregularity in the EEG signals. The amount of irregularity decreases with increasing brain levels of anaesthetic drugs. The monitor itself is similar to a BIS monitor in that it consists of EEG electrodes placed on the patient's forehead. The monitor processes the data collected and produces two different numbers. These are the response entropy (RE) and state entropy (SE). The SE reflects the cortical state of the patient while the RE incorporates EMG waveforms in addition to EEG waveforms, and is thought to measure adequacy of analgesia since painful stimulus may increase EMG activity. The RE looks at higher frequency waves and this enables a faster response time from the monitor. Manufacturers recommend targeting a range of 40–60 for both parameters by administering anaesthetic or analgesia accordingly. Studies have confirmed that entropy scores do relate to depth of anaesthesia.

How does entropy measurement compare with BIS?

Various studies have been performed trying to compare entropy and BIS in the measurement of depth of anaesthesia. Overall, it seems that they both perform similarly and that there is concordance between both and clinically observed depth of anaesthesia. It is notable that both BIS scores and entropy scores are unchanged by nitrous oxide use.

What should you be doing in your day-to-day practice to reduce the risk of awareness in your patients?

The Royal College of Anaesthetists published recommendations in January 2006. They stated that "close vigilance of all aspects of the patient and anaesthetic equipment" together with "observations of changes to normal physiological variables" should remain the principal factors in monitoring of awareness.

Therefore we should strive to give a "good" anaesthetic by firstly, checking all equipment thoroughly. Then, select an appropriate anaesthetic dose and identify those patients with increased requirements. Then, monitor the MAC of the volatile agent throughout anaesthesia. We need to have an idea of what the MAC should be for that particular patient. It is important to remember that because MAC is a laboratory-derived average, it is only a guide and one should not strive to follow MAC numbers if clinical signs indicate otherwise. It has been suggested that a MAC of greater than 0.8 significantly reduces the risk of awareness. The risk of awareness can also be reduced by considering an awake regional technique, considering the use of benzodiazepines and avoiding neuromuscular blockade whenever possible.

Further Reading

Avidan MS, Zhang L, Burnside BA, et al. Anesthesia awareness and the bispectral index. *New England Journal of Medicine.* 2008; **358**: 1097–1108.

Bein B. Entropy: best practice & research. *Clinical Anaesthesiology.* 2006; **20**(1): 101–109.

Guidance on the provision of anaesthesia services for intra-operative care 2009. Royal College of Anaesthetists.

Myles PS, Leslie K, McNeil J, Forbes A, Chan MT. Bispectral index monitoring to prevent awareness during anaesthesia: the B-Aware randomised controlled trial. *Lancet* 2004; **363**: 1757–1763.

Pollard RJ, Coyle JP, Gilbert RL, Beck JE. Intraoperative awareness in a regional medical system: a review of 3 years' data. *Anaesthesiology.* 2007; **106**: 269–274.

Royal College of Anaesthetists. Patient information sheet. Section 8: awareness during general anaesthesia. www.rcoa.ac.uk/docs/Risk_8awareness.pdf.

Sebel PS, Bowdle TA, Ghoneim MM, et al. The incidence of awareness during anesthesia: a multicenter United States study. *Anesthesia and Analgesia.* 2004; **99**: 833–839.

2.4.9. Electroconvulsive therapy (ECT) and anti-psychotics – Mari H Roberts

This topic could come up in the science structured oral exam where they may concentrate on the physiological changes that occur during ECT or in the clinical structured oral exam, especially as a short case.

They may start with an introductory question.

What is ECT?

Do not let this unnerve you. A simple answer is all that is required.

ECT is a treatment for severe depression and other severe psychiatric conditions. It involves passing an electrical current across the skull to induce a grand mal seizure. It is an effective but controversial treatment.

They may ask for further details of the stimulation used.

Do you know any of the characteristics of the electric current used?

The current is an alternating current delivered as a pulsatile, square waveform. It has a current of 500 to 850 mA, which is applied through electrodes placed at specific locations on the head. The energy used is 30–45 Joules and it is given over 0.5–1.5 seconds.

Can you describe to me the physiological changes that occur during ECT?

These can be classified into systems to ensure you don't leave anything out. Thinking of the effects of a grand mal seizure can also help you remember.

The induction of a seizure causes physiological responses in a number of systems.

Firstly, the central nervous system. The grand mal convulsion starts with a short latent phase, which is followed by a tonic phase that lasts about 15 seconds. During this tonic phase there is general skeletal muscle contraction. This is followed by a clonic phase, which lasts 30–60 seconds. The EEG seizure activity continues beyond the motor seizure activity, which is 30% shorter. There may also be a post-ictal phase with confusion and agitation. Other CNS changes include an increase in cerebral blood flow and an increase in both intra-cranial pressure and intra-ocular pressure. The cerebral oxygen consumption also increases by up to a factor of four.

Secondly, there may be significant cardiovascular changes. Initially there may be a parasympathetic discharge following the passage of the current. This may be intense and can cause bradycardia, hypotension or even asystole. Atropine should always be readily available. This is followed by a sympathetic discharge, which starts as the clonic phase of the seizure begins. Adrenaline levels may rise 15 times higher than baseline and noradrenaline levels three times higher, potentially causing tachycardia, hypertension and arrhythmias. The myocardial oxygen consumption also increases.

Good. What other systems are involved?

There are gastrointestinal changes associated with ECT. These include an increase in intra-gastric pressure, increased salivation and nausea and vomiting.

The musculoskeletal system is also affected by ECT. Uncontrolled muscular contractions may cause bony and musculoskeletal injury, for example vertebral fractures and joint dislocations. The jaw muscles are stimulated directly by the passage of current causing clenching of the jaw and possible injury to teeth, tongue or other structures in the oral cavity.

You have been allocated to administer anaesthesia for the electroconvulsive therapy (ECT) list. Describe your pre-operative assessment

Again a structure to your answer is important and a systems approach works well. Start by reassuring the examiner that you would take a thorough history and examination as for any anaesthetic but he or she wants you to concentrate on those points that are of particular relevance to ECT.

The pre-operative assessment should include a detailed history and examination. There are some specific considerations in relation to ECT. The patient population is often elderly with numerous co-morbidities.

A history of any cardiovascular disease should be sought. ECT should not be used in patients who have suffered a myocardial event within 3 months. The severity of any ischaemic heart disease should be evaluated by assessing exercise tolerance and frequency of chest pains. Severe ischaemic heart disease is a relative contraindication to ECT and therefore, if there are any concerns, should be investigated prior to starting on a course of ECT. A resting 12-lead ECG should be taken and a referral for further assessment and investigations by a cardiologist may be needed.

In relation to the CNS, a history of any intra-cranial pathology is also important. ECT should not be administered to a patient who has had a cerebrovascular event within 3 months or who has raised intra-cranial pressure or a CNS mass lesion.

With regards to the musculoskeletal system, a history of osteoporosis or any other bone disease that increases the likelihood of fractures should be identified. ECT should probably be avoided in patients who have a high risk of fractures but this needs to be discussed with the psychiatrist and the physician involved in the patient's care.

As with any patient a careful assessment of fasting status and risk of aspiration, for example a hiatus hernia, should be made.

Finally, glaucoma is a relative contraindication to ECT and the treatment should be discussed with an ophthalmologist if there are any concerns.

During the pre-operative assessment, it is important to remember that these patients are often unreliable historians, making the assessment difficult. It is often worth talking to nursing staff and other care givers for information and it is important to get hold of medical notes to help identify and quantify any coexisting disease. It is worth remembering that these patients will often be having a course of ECT and will therefore receive a number of general anaesthetics in close succession, which may be a problem for frail patients.

Are there any specific drugs that the patients may be taking that may be of concern to us as anaesthetists?

Yes and a detailed drug history should be taken. Firstly, all anti-convulsants should be withheld prior to ECT. Secondly, the patients are often taking psychiatric drugs that may interact with drugs given during anaesthesia. In particular, anti-depressants such as monoamine oxidase inhibitors, tricyclic anti-depressants and selective serotonin reuptake inhibitors.

Can you explain how monoamine oxidase inhibitors work?

There are two monoamine oxidase enzymes that these drugs inhibit; MAO-A and MAO-B. MAO-A is mainly intra-neuronal and degrades dopamine, noradrenaline and serotonin. Increased levels of these amine neurotransmitters are thought to elevate mood. MAO–B is extra-cellular and degrades other amines such as tyramine, tryptamine and phenylethylamine.

The older MAO inhibitors such as phenelzine are irreversible and block both MAO-A and -B. Newer drugs such as moclobemide are reversible and selective for MAO-A.

Why are they of concern to us as anaesthetists?

Monoamine oxidase inhibitors potentiate the actions of any indirectly acting sympathomimetics such as ephedrine and metaraminol. This can cause an exaggerated hypertensive response. Co-administration should therefore be avoided. Directly acting drugs such as noradrenaline and adrenaline should be used in small amounts if needed.

MAOIs also interact with piperidine derived opiates such as pethidine. This interaction may result in agitation, tachycardia, hyperpyrexia, muscle rigidity, hypertension and even coma. It is thought that this is due to excessive serotonin activity.

The newer drugs that are selective for MAO-A, cause less potentiation of amines. However, the drugs mentioned should still be avoided. Ideally, if elective surgery is planned, these drugs should be stopped two to three weeks beforehand. This should be done only after discussion with the patient's psychiatrist due to the risk of worsening depression.

Why are the other anti-depressant drugs of concern to us?

Tricyclic anti-depressants such as amitriptyline, and selective serotonin reuptake inhibitors such as fluoxetine may cause an exaggerated response to sympathomimetic drugs and increase anaesthetic requirements.

Anaesthesia for ECT is often given in remote, isolated locations. What are the concerns with anaesthetising patients in such areas?

In these remote locations help and backup may not be readily available. There may not be critical care facilities close by and there may not be adequate equipment available to deal with an unforeseen event. The patients should therefore be assessed with special consideration made to their suitability for anaesthesia in a remote site. In general ASA grade 1 and 2 patients can be anaesthetised in remote sites. Patients graded ASA 3 or more should be discussed with a Consultant Anaesthetist on a case by case basis. However, unexpected problems can also occur in ASA 1 and 2 patients. Resuscitation equipment should be available as well as a trained assistant and recovery facilities.

Describe how you would anaesthetise a patient for ECT

It is a good idea to classify your answer into pre-operative, peri-operative and post-operative management. If the examiner only wants you to discuss the peri-operative management, he or she will guide you towards this.

Pre-operatively I would take a detailed history and examination as I've already discussed. Any co-existing disease should be optimised. Sedative premedication should be avoided, in particular benzodiazepines, which increase the seizure threshold. Anticholinergics may be given to decrease the risk of bradycardias and salivation.

Resuscitation equipment should be available. Minimal mandatory monitoring should be used including pulse oximetry, ECG, non-invasive blood pressure, FiO_2 and ET CO_2. I would also ensure that I had a trained assistant.

If there were no concerns regarding the airway or risk of aspiration, I would pre-oxygenate the patient before inducing anaesthesia with a single minimal sleep dose of propofol. I would then maintain the airway with a facemask and a 100% O_2, hand ventilating as required. I would give a 0.3 to 0.5 mg kg^{-1} dose of suxamethonium to cause incomplete muscular paralysis and then insert a bite block, making sure that it is correctly placed, before allowing the psychiatrist to administer the stimulus. The doses of induction agent and suxamethonium should be recorded, as should the patient's response to them, this will allow the dose to be adjusted next time if needed. If I had any concerns regarding risk of aspiration, I would perform a rapid sequence induction using a 1 mg kg^{-1} dose of suxamethonium.

I would observe the patient for signs of a fit and carefully monitor his or her cardiovascular response, treating any bradycardias with atropine or glycopyrolate if required. I would continue to ventilate the patient until spontaneous ventilation returns.

Post-operatively, the patient should be recovered as normal until fully alert. Headaches are common post-operatively and should be treated with simple analgesics.

Good. We discussed the anti-depressant drugs that patients undergoing ECT may be taking. What other mood altering drugs do you know of?

Although you may mention drugs such as the anti-psychotics, the examiner is likely to want you to discuss lithium, which has clinical implications in anaesthesia and intensive care.

Lithium is used to control mood in bipolar manic depression.

Tell me about lithium

Lithium imitates the action of sodium and enters cells via fast, voltage gated channels. However, it cannot be pumped out by the sodium–potassium ATPase pump and accumulates in the cytoplasm. It is then thought to interfere with cyclic-AMP and inositol triphosphate second messenger systems. Lithium has a very narrow therapeutic index therefore plasma levels should be measured regularly to ensure effective plasma levels of 0.5 to 1.0 mmol L^{-1} and avoid toxicity.

What are the adverse effects of lithium?

Lithium has a number of adverse effects including diarrhoea, vomiting, hypothyroidism and renal impairment. Inhibition of ADH may cause polydipsia and polyuria.

What signs and symptoms might make you suspicious of lithium toxicity?

Acute toxicity may present as ataxia, confusion, convulsions, arrhythmias or as a coma.

What are the important considerations when anaesthetising a patient on lithium?

The two main considerations are lithium toxicity and potential drug interactions. To prevent toxicity, plasma levels should be measured pre-operatively as well as urea and electrolytes. Dehydration, the use of diuretics and hyponatraemia can potentiate toxicity. Therefore, it is important to maintain hydration and ensure electrolytes are normal prior to surgery.

The main drug interaction that is of concern to us as anaesthetists is that it prolongs the effect of all muscle relaxants. Care should also be taken when using NSAIDs as they may reduce lithium clearance and increase plasma levels.

2.4.10. Epilepsy – Imran Mohammad

A 28-year-old female presents to the Emergency Department with generalised tonic–clonic seizures for the past 30 minutes. You have been called to provide assistance. What is your approach?

Epilepsy is important to the anaesthetist in clinical practice and therefore is likely to be covered in the Final FRCA. Epilepsy is a common co-morbidity in our surgical patients, and we need to be aware of medication and drug interactions, the effects of our anaesthetic technique on post-operative seizures, and the intensive care management of status epilepticus.

This is a case of status epilepticus. It is a medical emergency. The immediate management involves protecting the airway, ensuring adequate breathing, obtaining intravenous access and supporting the circulation.

The first line anti-epileptic is lorazepam 0.1 mg kg^{-1} (4 mg in most adults). In the face of continued seizures, phenytoin 15 mg kg^{-1} (1 g in a 70-kg adult), it should be given at a rate of less than 50 mg min^{-1}, i.e., over 20 minutes with BP and ECG monitoring. An alternative at this stage would be fosphenytoin 15 mg kg^{-1} at a rate of 100–150 mg min^{-1}. Continued seizures may prompt general anaesthesia with thiopentone, requiring intubation and ventilation.

Further management includes: ECG, BP, pulse oximetry and fluids to maintain cerebral perfusion pressure. Venous blood should be taken for FBC, U&Es, glucose, toxicology, drug levels and an arterial blood gas should be performed. EEG monitoring is useful if available.

What are the complications of status epilepticus?

The complications can be split up into the systems of the body. Beginning with the central nervous system; cerebral hypoxia, oedema, haemorrhage and venous thrombosis can occur.

In the cardiovascular system, there may be hyper- or hypotension, myocardial infarction, arrhythmias, cardiogenic shock and cardiac arrest.

In the respiratory system, complications include apnoea, respiratory failure, pulmonary oedema, aspiration and pneumonia.

Metabolic complications include hyponatraemia, hypoglycaemia, hyperkalaemia, metabolic acidosis, acute tubular necrosis, acute hepatic necrosis and acute pancreatitis.

Other complications include DIC, rhabdomyolysis, fractures and dislocations.

What is the differential diagnosis of epileptic seizures?

The differential diagnosis is broad and includes pseudoseizures, arrhythmias, drug-induced seizures, hypoglycaemia, head injury, syncope, transient ischaemic attacks, narcolepsy and cataplexy.

Can you classify epileptic seizures?

Define and classify.

Epilepsy is defined as recurrent (two or more) epileptic seizures unprovoked by any immediately identifiable cause. A seizure can be defined as the clinical manifestation of an abnormal and excessive discharge of neurones, which is seen as alteration of consciousness, motor, sensory or autonomic events. Seizures are classified based upon their clinical presentation and the electroencephalographic (EEG) picture. They can be divided up into generalised and partial seizures.

Generalised seizures are characterised by diffuse symmetric brain involvement and can be further broken down into inhibitory and excitatory. Inhibitory generalised seizures can be absence, petit mal or atonic. Excitatory seizures are the classic tonic, clonic and myoclonic variations.

In partial seizures, there is seizure activity restricted to discrete areas of the cerebral hemispheres. Consciousness is preserved in simple partial seizures whereas it is impaired in complex partial seizures.

What drugs are used in preventing epileptic seizures?

Commonly used drugs include phenytoin, sodium valproate, carbamazepine and lamotrigine. Other anti-epileptics include levatiracetam and gabapentin. Clonazepam is used for absences and atonic seizures.

Tell me about phenytoin

If asked about a drug, use a template for breaking down the information into easily memorable chunks. This also gives the impression of comprehensive knowledge about a drug. A convenient template is to use the headings presented in Sasada and Smith's Drugs in Anaesthesia and Intensive Care. These headings are Uses, Chemical, Presentation, Main Actions, Mode of Action, Routes of Administration/Doses, Pharmacodynamics which is divided into the relevant body systems such as CNS, CVS, Metabolic, etc, Toxicity/Side Effects, Pharmacokinetics split up into Absorption, Distribution, Metabolism, Excretion, and any other special points.

Phenytoin is used for prevention and treatment of generalised tonic–clonic seizures. It is also used as an anti-arrhythmic and neuropathic pain-modulating agent. The chemical class is a hydantoin derivative. In its intra-venous form it is presented as a clear, colourless solution of 50 mg ml^{-1} of phenytoin sodium. The main actions are anti-convulsant and anti-arrhythmic. Phenytoin works by inhibiting sodium and calcium influx during depolarisation, thereby exerting a membrane-stabilising effect.

The intra-venous loading dose for the management of epilepsy is a slow bolus of 10–15 mg kg^{-1}. It is highly lipid-soluble and peak brain levels are achieved within 15 minutes. The maintenance dose is 100 mg 8 hourly.

Phenytoin has an anti-convulsant effect on the CNS, stabilising the neuronal membrane and preventing the spread of seizure activity. It exhibits class I anti-arrhythmic properties but may cause hypotension and arrhythmias itself. Metabolic effects include hyperglycaemia, hypocalcaemia, alterations in liver function tests and inhibition of ADH secretion. The side effects include gum hyperplasia, megaloblastic anaemia, nausea and vomiting, tremor and ataxia.

Phenytoin is 95% protein bound. It is metabolised in the liver, exhibiting zero order kinetics just above its therapeutic range. It is excreted as inactive metabolites by the kidney. It is a potent enzyme inducer increasing the metabolism of many drugs including carbamazepine, benzodiazepines and warfarin. Importantly phenytoin toxicity can be precipitated by metronidazole and isoniazid co-administration.

What specific features would you look for during pre-operative assessment of an epileptic patient scheduled for elective surgery?

I would perform a full routine pre-operative anaesthetic assessment. In the history I would focus on seizure frequency and complications, and a full drug history of anti-epileptics and compliance. Airway assessment may reveal gingival hyperplasia and poor dentition caused by phenytoin. ECG may reveal dysrhythmias caused by carbamazepine or phenytoin. Full blood count may identify anaemia, thrombocytopaenia or leucopenia – again caused by anticonvulsants. Electrolyte abnormalities include hyponatraemia, hypocalcaemia and hyperglycaemia. A number of anti-convulsants cause hepatocellular dysfunction and cholestatic jaundice. Anti-convulsant drug levels may be relevant where poor compliance or toxicity is suspected.

Which anaesthetic drugs are pro-convulsant?

Etomidate and ketamine can precipitate generalised tonic–clonic seizures in epileptic patients. Toxic doses of local anaesthetics can also cause seizures. Tramadol lowers the seizure threshold and high doses of other opioids can induce seizure activity. The metabolites of pethidine and atracurium are epileptogenic. Enflurane is pro-convulsant at 2 MAC.

Which anaesthetic drugs are anti-convulsant?

Benzodiazepines are potent anti-convulsants at sub-anaesthetic doses. Thiopentone effectively terminates seizures in therapeutic doses. Propofol is anti-convulsant but may cause myoclonic jerks, which mimic seizures. The inhalational anaesthetic agents (barring enflurane) are anti-convulsant.

Obstetrics

2.5.1. Physiological and anatomical changes of pregnancy – Sarah F Bell

What can you tell me about the physiological and anatomical changes of pregnancy?

A structured approach is vital to ensure that you do not forget any of the key points. It may be worth making an opening statement explaining the reason for all of these changes!

The physiological changes of pregnancy are aimed at supplying oxygen and nutrients to the increased demand of the utero-placental unit and foetus. The adaptions are also key in preparing the mother for delivery. The changes may be divided into the body systems.

Firstly the cardiovascular system. From the first trimester there is an expansion of plasma volume by about 50%. Red cell volume also increases, but due to the relatively greater increase in plasma volume a dilutional anaemia develops. Cardiac output increases by 40% from the tenth week of gestation, with an increase in both heart rate and stroke volume. The systemic vascular resistance falls by 15%. This is due to the development of the intervillous space (which is a low resistance vascular bed) and the vasodilator effects of the pregnancy hormones. The blood pressure falls during pregnancy. Diastolic blood pressure decreases more than systolic by mid-gestation but both parameters then return to normal levels at term. Due to volume expansion, cardiac dilatation and hypertrophy, ECG changes of left axis deviation and ST segment changes may occur. A further important effect is that of aortocaval compression. The gravid uterus compresses the inferior vena cava, reducing venous return. It can reduce aortic blood flow, particularly when the parturient is in the supine position. This effect can have severe implications for the uteroplacental unit which does not have a system of autoregulation but relies on perfusion pressure to maintain adequate blood flow. In order to minimise the effects of aorto-caval compression a left lateral tilt or wedge posture is assumed when the pregnant woman is supine.

Dr. Podcast Scripts for the Final FRCA, ed. Rebecca A. Leslie, Emily K. Johnson, Gary Thomas and Alexander P. L. Goodwin.   Published by Cambridge University Press.
© R. A. Leslie, E. K. Johnson, G. Thomas and A. P. L. Goodwin 2011.

How much weight would you expect a woman to gain during a normal pregnancy?

The examiner may interrupt if he feels you are performing well and he wants to probe your depth of knowledge further.

The weight gain varies tremendously but average values are approximately 12 kg. This is due to the combination of increase in tissue mass of the breasts, placenta, uterus and foetus. There is also an increase in the volume of both plasma and interstitial fluid.

Can you now describe the changes to the respiratory system?

There are a number of important changes so try and remember as much as you can of this important topic. If the examiner allows you to continue you should indicate the anaesthetic implications.

The oxygen consumption of a pregnant woman increases by 30–40% at term. The minute ventilation increases by 45% to meet this increased demand. This is achieved predominately by an increase in tidal volume rather than respiratory rate and it is thought to be caused by the stimulatory effects of progesterone on the central respiratory neurones. A mild respiratory alkalosis is observed which shifts the oxy-haemoglobin dissociation curve to the left, but the coinciding increase in maternal 2,3-DPG offsets this potential deleterious effect. The upward displacement of the diaphragm by the uterus causes a decrease in the functional residual capacity (FRC) of up to 25%. The combination of reduced FRC and increased oxygen consumption leads to an increased risk of hypoxemia. Tracheal intubation of a pregnant woman can be more challenging due to upper airway capillary engorgement and oedema, breast enlargement and possible laryngeal distortion from cricoid pressure (when the woman is in the left lateral position). The incidence of a difficult airway in the pregnant state is eight times higher than in the non-pregnant population or about 1 in 250–300 patients.

Can you tell me how pregnancy alters the gastrointestinal system?

The anatomical effects of the gravid uterus lead to both an increase intra-gastric pressure and under the influence of progesterone, a decrease in the lower oesophageal sphincter tone. This leads to a fall in the barrier pressure (the difference between the lower oesophageal sphincter tone and the gastric pressure). Whilst gastric motility is normal during pregnancy it can be significantly reduced during labour, especially when opioid analgesia is administered.

What effects do these changes have?

Up to 70% of women suffer from gastro-oesophageal reflux during pregnancy due to reduced barrier pressure leading to an increased risk of pulmonary aspiration.

What are the anaesthetic implications?

Women should receive antacid prophylaxis during labour if there is an increased risk of caesarean section. A prokinetic may also be given. The 30 ml of 0.3 M sodium citrate is given prior to induction of general anaesthesia to neutralise acidic gastric contents. Furthermore a rapid sequence induction technique is employed to reduce the chance of airway soiling by gastric contents.

How does pregnancy alter renal function?

The enlargement of the uterus leads to dilation of the ureters and calyces with reduced bladder capacity. Due to increased renal plasma flow, the glomerular filtration rate increases and creatinine and urea levels fall. Glycosuria is commonly observed.

What haematological changes occur during normal pregnancy?

Increases in blood volume and an increase in iron requirements by the mother and foetus lead to iron deficiency anaemia.

Patients become relatively hyper-coagulable during pregnancy, a possible adaptive process to prevent post-partum haemorrhage. This is achieved by an increase in the concentration of the coagulation factors VII, VIII, IX, X, XII and fibrinogen. Enhanced platelet turnover occurs and thrombocytopenia is seen in approximately 1% of pregnant women.

How does this affect your management of a woman after a caesarean section?

Any woman who has a caesarean section should be prescribed thrombo-embolic prophylaxis.

How does the white cell count (WCC) change during pregnancy and why is this important?

The leucocyte count increases slightly during pregnancy and then further increases during labour with levels reaching about $15-20 \times 10^9$/L. This is important to consider when using the WCC as a marker for sepsis (e.g., when deciding whether to perform an epidural) as it may be unreliable.

Do the plasma proteins change during pregnancy?

Yes, the concentration of albumin falls, but globulin and fibrinogen increase. The overall total protein level falls leading to a reduction in colloid osmotic pressure. Drug binding is altered and free drug concentrations may increase if normally bound to albumin. Plasma concentration of pseudocholinesterase may be reduced by up to 20% and prolong the action of suxamethonium.

Do you know of any endocrine changes of pregnancy?

The thyroid gland increases in size but the mother usually remains euthyroid. Plasma corticosteroid levels increase 3–5 times and ACTH secretion is increased. The pituitary gland becomes enlarged, predominantly due to the increased activity of the prolactin secreting lactotrophs, thus making it more susceptible to falls in perfusion due to its portal blood supply.

During the first trimester of pregnancy, women are relatively insulin sensitive; resistance may then ensue with the development of gestational diabetes.

How is the musculoskeletal system affected?

The effects of progesterone and relaxin act to increase ligamentous laxity and increase the lumbar lordosis. It is therefore important to take care when positioning the patient.

Can you describe to me any of the central nervous system effects of pregnancy?

The pregnancy hormones, progesterone, and the β-endorphins released during labour may act to reduce minimal alveolar concentration (MAC) by as much as 25%. They also increase sensitivity to both sedatives and hypnotics.

Venocaval compression caused by the uterus results in distension of the epidural venous plexus. This can lead to an increased risk of both intra-vascular injection or "bloody tap" during regional anaesthesia. The spread of local anaesthesia due to the reduced capacity of the epidural space itself may also be enhanced. The sympathetic nervous system activity is increased during pregnancy in order to produce lower limb vasoconstriction and counteract the effects of aortocaval compression.

Can you describe the innervations of the bladder, uterus, vagina and cervix?

The bladder has sympathetic innervation derived from roots T11 to L2 and parasympathetic innervation from S2 to 4. The uterus is innervated via sympathetic pathways in cervical tissue and the broad ligament from roots T10 to L1. The vagina and cervix are innervated via the pudendal, genitofemoral, illioinguinal and sacral nerves from roots S2 to 4.

What level sensory block do you therefore need for a caesarean section using central neuraxial blockade?

The sensory block should be at or above T6 for light touch and T5 for cold sensation.

What are the effects of maternal pain on the foetus and the mother?

Pain will cause sympathetic nervous system stimulation. This can lead to diversion of blood flow from the uteroplacental unit. Since there is no autoregulation in this organ, the effects of pain will directly affect the foetal blood supply. Pain can also cause a metabolic acidosis and an increase in plasma cortisol and endorphins.

2.5.2. Anaesthesia in early pregnancy – Sarah F Bell

You may be asked about anaesthesia in early pregnancy within a number of different clinical scenarios. The examiner will want to know that you recognise the key differences that occur in pregnant patients compared to the non-pregnant population.

You are asked to anaesthetise a 35-year-old woman who is 24 weeks pregnant. The surgical team are keen to take her to theatre as soon as possible because she has the signs and symptoms of acute appendicitis.

She is previously fit and well and has not had any complications during the pregnancy so far. She was admitted yesterday with abdominal pain, fever and a leucocytosis on her full blood count.

Can you tell me what would be your differential diagnosis for this woman's abdominal pain?

The abdominal pain may be obstetric or non-obstetric.

Obstetric causes would include pre-eclampsia and liver capsule pain, placental abruption, intra-uterine infection and rarely uterine rupture or torsion.

Non-obstetric causes can be further divided into the systems.

The gastrointestinal system may be affected by appendicitis, Crohn's disease, diverticulitis, cholecystitis or ascending cholangitis, hepatitis, pancreatitis, peptic ulcer disease, gastro-oesophageal reflux disease, intestinal obstruction and perforation.

Renal conditions such as pyelonephritis, urinary tract infections or renal stones may have caused the discomfort. Gynaecological complications include salpingitis, fibroid torsion, ovarian torsion, cyst, haemorrhage or rupture, and even ectopic pregnancy (although the woman should have had an antenatal scan which would have excluded this possibility).

Respiratory problems such as pulmonary embolism and pneumonia can cause abdominal pain, as can cardiovascular disease such as a myocardial infarction. Haematological causes of abdominal pain included sickle cell crisis and finally metabolic conditions such as diabetic ketoacidosis and porphyria may present with an acute abdomen.

Can you briefly summarise the main issues to the anaesthetist regarding this case?

The main issues are that the woman has an acute abdomen requiring urgent surgery and that she is in the second trimester of pregnancy.

So what further information would you obtain at the pre-operative visit?

I would want to take a full history, examine the patient and review the investigations performed. I would be looking to ascertain whether the patient was dehydrated, septic and in shock. I would also be looking to confirm the diagnosis.

In taking the history, I would pay particular attention to the presenting complaint. I would want to know how and when the pain had started, where it was located, whether it radiated, its severity and character, whether there were any exacerbating, relieving or associated factors. I would enquire about the patient's ability to eat and drink recently and whether she had had any vomiting or diarrhoea. I would also ask about fever and whether the patient had experienced any of these symptoms previously. I would enquire about the patient's past anaesthetic and medical history and take a full systems history. I would then ask about medications, allergies and dentition. Regarding the pregnancy I would enquire about any complications so far such as gestational diabetes, hypertension or cholecystitis of pregnancy.

What would you look for in your examination of this woman?

On examination I would again be looking to assess the degree of dehydration, confirm the diagnosis and decide whether the patient was septic and or in shock. I would therefore look at the observation chart to review the respiratory rate, heart rate, blood pressure, temperature, urinary output and pain score. I would then examine the cardio-respiratory system and the abdomen. Whilst talking to the woman I would assess her conscious level and pain score. I would check whether the obstetricians had performed a vaginal examination and look in the notes to see their examination findings.

What investigations would you want to review before taking this woman to theatre?

I would want to have confirmation of the pregnancy, either by urine, blood test or by ultrasound scan. I would check the urinalysis results and review the full blood count, urea and electrolytes, liver enzymes, amylase and glucose level. I would also ensure that a blood sample had been sent for group and save. Depending on the clinical picture an ECG, arterial blood gas and blood cultures might be required.

How would you manage this patient prior to theatre, assuming that she has acute appendicitis?

Prior to taking this woman to theatre I would want to pre-optimise her condition as much as possible. This would require large bore intra-venous access followed by fluid resuscitation, anti-biotics and analgesia. Depending on the severity of her condition this might need to be done in recovery or the high-dependency unit. Invasive arterial and central venous pressure monitoring might be required if the patient were in septic shock. The duration of time taken to pre-optimise that patient needs to be balanced against the need to take the patient to theatre to remove the source of sepsis.

I would also want to inform both the obstetricians and the neonatologists of the patient and her condition because there is a risk that she might develop premature labour either due to the sepsis or the operation. In addition, I would inform the consultant anaesthetist on call of the patient's condition.

Premedication would be indicated in this case. I would administer ranitidine 50 mg intra-venously, metoclopramide 10 mg intra-venously and sodium citrate 30 ml of 0.3 molar solution orally in order to reduce the volume and acidity of the gastric contents. I would ensure that an experienced surgeon was available to perform the procedure since this may be technically challenging. I would also ask my assistant to have available the difficult airway equipment.

Why might intubation be more difficult in this patient?

Pregnant women have increased breast size, chest wall diameter, nasal engorgement and possibly laryngeal oedema which can all make intubation more challenging. They need to be positioned in a left lateral tilt to avoid aorto-caval compression. This should be considered by the anaesthetic assistant performing cricoid pressure so that the view at laryngoscopy is not distorted. Furthermore from 6 weeks gestation the increase in oxygen consumption and fall in oxygen reserve leads to a faster onset of hypoxia.

Why is the oxygen reserve lower?

The upward displacement of the diaphragm causes a reduction in the functional residual capacity (FRC). Closing capacity can then encroach on the FRC particularly in the supine position. The oxygen reserve is therefore reduced, even after careful de-nitrogenation.

What are the effects of progesterone on the respiratory system? Would they affect your general anaesthetic?

The hormone progesterone mediates tracheal and bronchial smooth muscle relaxation and so causes an increase in dead-space. Progesterone also sensitises the respiratory centre to changes in the partial pressure of carbon dioxide. This, coupled with the increase in carbon dioxide production occurring during pregnancy leads to an increase in the minute volume (mainly by increases in tidal volume). The pregnant woman develops a respiratory alkalosis due to the increase in minute volume. During an anaesthetic this normal physiological adaption should be maintained.

What might be the cardiovascular effects of pregnancy on this woman? How might they affect your general anaesthetic?

In addition to the effects of aorto-caval compression, the 24-week parturient will have a significantly raised plasma volume and cardiac output. Her diastolic blood pressure will be lower than pre-pregnant levels. This should be taken into consideration during the operation and resuscitation since her observation parameters will be different from the non-pregnant population. Any fall in blood pressure should be treated aggressively.

How might the pregnancy alter the effects of the induction agents, volatile agents and suxamethonium?

Pregnancy is associated with lower anaesthetic requirements. The exact mechanism is unknown. The minimum alveolar concentration for the volatile agents is reduced by 30% by 12-weeks gestation. The dose of intra-venous induction agents is also reduced. In contrast, the effects of suxamethonium can be prolonged by the reduced concentration of plasma pseudocholinesterase but in reality this is offset by the increase in volume of distribution so minimal change in duration of action is usually observed.

What are the effects of pregnancy on the renal system?

The increase in glomerular filtration rate leads to lower plasma concentrations of urea and creatinine. This should be considered when reviewing the patient's renal function with regard to dehydration and sepsis.

How would you anaesthetise this woman?

I would prepare all my emergency equipment, drugs and check my machine prior to the patient entering the anaesthetic room. I would ensure that I had suction available and a trained assistant who is able to perform cricoid pressure. I would then establish mandatory monitoring as stated by the AAGBI guidelines. I would ensure that the woman was placed in a left lateral tilt position. I would pre-oxygenate the woman with 100% oxygen for 3 minutes with a tight fitting facemask. I would then ask my assistant to apply cricoid pressure and induce anaesthesia with thiopentone 5 mg/kg and suxamethonium 2 mg/kg. After 30 seconds and the cessation of muscle twitches I would intubate the patient with an appropriately sized cuffed oral tracheal tube. I would confirm correct positioning of the tube visually, by auscultation and by capnography. Then I would maintain anaesthesia using sevoflurane, oxygen and air, bearing in mind the reduction in minimum alveolar concentration associated with pregnancy. I would use a nerve stimulator to monitor neuromuscular function, since plasma cholinesterase enzyme activity may be impaired and cause prolonged effects of suxamethonium. With regard to analgesia, I would give IV paracetamol and increments of morphine. I would also ask the surgeons to infiltrate the wound with levo-bupivicaine. Non-steroidal anti-inflammatory drugs (NSAIDs) should be carefully considered due to the risk of premature closure of the ductus arteriosus in the foetus and so I would avoid their use in this case.

What would be you post-operative plan for this patient and where would you manage her?

I would ensure that the patient was comfortable, conscious and that her observations were stable prior to discharge from the recovery room. Depending on the extent of the surgery, a morphine PCA might be required for post-operative analgesia in addition to regular paracetamol. I would contact the obstetric team to review the patient and ensure the wellbeing of the foetus. I would also discuss thrombo-prophylaxis with the surgical team

The patient should be managed on the high-dependency unit if there are concerns regarding her fluid balance or cardio-respiratory stability. If she were stable she could be nursed on an obstetric ward provided the nursing staff had some surgical experience or vice versa on a surgical ward. She would need to be regularly reviewed by both the obstetric and surgical teams.

Finally, can you tell me when anaesthetic drugs are most likely to have teratogenic effects?

Between the days 15 and 56 of gestation are when the foetus is most vulnerable. Whenever possible, surgery should be delayed until the second trimester. Elective surgery should not be performed.

2.5.3. Complications of pregnancy – Sarah F Bell

You are the anaesthetist present at an elective caesarean section for a healthy primigravida diagnosed with a breech presentation. She had an uneventful spinal anaesthetic and delivery. The obstetricians are suturing the uterus when she becomes acutely short of breath. What potential differential diagnoses would you consider in this case?

This is a clinical question that is initially testing your ability to cover all the potential problems. Use a structured approach to try and remember as many possibilities as you can, whilst recognising the important conditions particular to this situation!

There are a number of potential causes of dyspnoea in a woman undergoing an elective caesarean section under spinal anaesthesia. These may be divided into respiratory, cardiovascular or drug-related problems. The respiratory complications may be due to bronchospasm. This may be associated with asthma, hyperreactive airways in a smoker, anaphylaxis or aspiration. Further potential respiratory causes are hypoxia secondary to atelectasis, pulmonary oedema, pulmonary embolism (which might be amniotic fluid or blood clot) or even a pneumothorax. Cardiovascular complications such as acute haemorrhage or decompensation from pre-existing valve or cardiac disease may have caused the dyspnoea. Finally there may be a drug related problem such as a high spinal, anaphylaxis or drug reaction such as carboprost induced bronchospasm.

How common is amniotic fluid embolism?

Amniotic fluid embolism is uncommon. Its incidence varies from 1 in 8000 to 1 in 80000 pregnancies. It accounts for 0.8 maternal deaths per 100000 deliveries. The disease process occurs most frequently during labour.

Factors associated with an increased risk of developing amniotic fluid embolism may be divided into maternal, foetal and uterine or placental. Maternal factors include multiparous, older mothers and women with a history of atopy. Foetal factors include intra-uterine death, meconium stained liquor and microsomia. Uterine or placental factors include polyhydramnious, chorioamnionitis, strong or tetanic uterine contractions, uterine rupture and placenta accreta.

Can you describe the pathophysiology of amniotic fluid embolism?

Amniotic fluid enters the maternal circulation (via ruptured membranes or uterine vessels) down a pressure gradient. The foetal antigens in the fluid stimulate the release of a cascade of biochemical mediators. Initially these cause pulmonary artery vasospasm followed by acute elevation of right ventricular pressures and right ventricular dysfunction. This in turn leads to hypoxemia, hypotension and myocardial damage. The patient may consequently develop left ventricular failure and pulmonary oedema. Disseminated intra-vascular coagulopathy (DIC) is also a feature of this condition.

What are the features of amniotic fluid embolism?

The symptoms of amniotic fluid embolism range from dyspnoea, cough and wheeze to headache and chest pain. Signs include foetal distress, hypoxia, tachypnoea, bronchospasm, hypocapnia (if intubated due to reduced cardiac output), tachycardia, hypotension, seizures, uterine atony, haemorrhage and coagulopathy.

Is there any specific management for suspected amniotic fluid embolism?

No. The management is supportive and preventative. Resuscitation of the pregnant woman should always be performed in the left lateral position until the baby is delivered, with aggressive treatment of hypoxia, cardiovascular failure and coagulopathy.

Let's move onto some pharmacology. What are tocolytic agents? What are they used for? Give me some examples and their mechanism of action

Tocolytics are drugs that are used to inhibit uterine contraction. They may be indicated to inhibit premature labour or to reduce uterine contractions in cases of uterine inversion or cord prolapse. Drugs that are used can be classified according to their mode of action. Drugs may act as oxytocin receptor antagonists, calcium channel antagonists, B_2 adrenoceptor agonists or act via nitric oxide. Atosiban is a specific oxytocin receptor antagonist. Calcium channel antagonists such as nifedipine, magnesium sulphate and the volatile agents may be used.

Drugs acting on B_2 receptors include salbutamol, terbutaline and ritodrine (although this particular medication is no longer recommended because of its poor side-effect profile). GTN may be used sublingually to relax uterine smooth muscle, acting as a nitric oxide donor.

What about the drugs that stimulate the uterus? What drugs do we use to augment uterine contraction?

The uterus contains a number of receptors that can be stimulated to cause contraction of its smooth muscle. These include oxytocin receptors, α_1-adrenoceptors, serotonergic and prostaglandin receptors. Syntocinon is a synthetic oxytocin analogue that acts to increase both the frequency and force of uterine muscle contractions. It does cause peripheral vasodilatation and so can induce hypotension and a reflex tachycardia. Ergometrine is an ergot alkaloid that acts via adreno- and serotonergic receptors to stimulate uterine contraction. Side effects include hypertension, coronary artery vasospasm and it is a potent emetic. Finally prostaglandin analogues are used to stimulate uterine contraction. These include prostaglandin ($F_2\alpha$), or carboprost. The side effects of carboprost include bronchospasm, pyrexia, flushing and hypotension. It is contraindicated in patients with asthma. The prostaglandin E_1 analogue, misoprostol can also be considered. This can be given orally, rectally or by direct myometrial injection. Side effects include shivering, nausea, vomiting, diarrhoea and pyrexia.

All of these drugs are used in a systematic manner when treating severe post-partum haemorrhage, in conjunction with surgical interventions.

How do you define massive obstetric haemorrhage?

A massive obstetric haemorrhage may be described as greater than one and a half litres of blood loss, a fall in haemoglobin of more than 4 g/dl or a transfusion of more that four units of blood. Obstetric haemorrhage can also be split into ante-partum and post-partum haemorrhage. An ante-partum bleed can occur between 24 weeks gestation and delivery. Post-partum haemorrhage occurs after delivery and may be further split into primary (within 24 hours), or secondary (within 6 weeks of delivery).

What proportion of the cardiac output passes to the uterus and why is this important?

Uterine blood flow increases from <5% to 10% of cardiac output at term, or 1 L/min. Haemorrhage can be brisk and potentially fatal.

What clinical signs may be evident in a woman who is bleeding post-partum?

The respiratory rate will increase initially and then a tachycardia will develop. This may be the only sign until 30–40% blood loss since maternal blood volume has already expanded prior to delivery. Aortocaval compression will compound haemodynamic instability. Hypotension, reduced urine output and changes in conscious level will occur if bleeding continues.

What might be the first sign in a woman with ante-partum haemorrhage?

The bleeding may be concealed and so foetal distress may be first sign.

What are the causes of obstetric haemorrhage?

The causes vary depending on the timing of the bleeding. Early pregnancy bleeding may be due to incomplete or septic abortion or a ruptured ectopic. Ante-partum haemorrhage may be due to placenta praevia, abruption, uterine rupture or trauma. A primary or secondary coagulopathy may also need to be considered.

Can you tell me any risk factors for abruption?

Yes, maternal hypertension, uterine over-distension, previous abruption, smoking and trauma.

And what about uterine rupture?

Previous caesarean section is the most common risk factor.

Tell me about the causes of post-partum haemorrhage

Post-partum haemorrhage is most commonly due to uterine atony. Additional causes include retained products, genital tract trauma, abnormally adherent placenta, clotting defects or uterine inversion.

So what are the risk factors for uterine atony?

These include prolonged or augmented labour, uterine over-distension, abnormalities or multiple gestation, placenta praevia, increased parity and increased maternal age.

And why might a pregnant or post-partum woman develop a clotting abnormality?

Intra-uterine death can lead to a coagulopathy as does amniotic fluid embolism, sepsis, pre-eclampsia, abruption and acute haemorrhage. Thrombocytopenia of pregnancy may also occur.

You are called to the obstetric ward urgently to a woman who has just had a vaginal delivery but is now bleeding significantly. What is your immediate management?

I would ask a member of staff to call for senior help and alert the haematology and portering services. It is vital to work as part of a team with the midwives and obstetricians. Having established a brief history from the midwifery staff, the patient's notes and the obsetricians, I would need to establish how much blood had been lost, how much fluid had already been given and assess the current haemodynamic status. I would give 100% oxygen, ensure the airway was patent and establish verbal communication with the patient. The blood pressure, pulse rate, oxygen saturation and capillary refill time would need to be assessed and large bore intra-venous cannulae inserted for further volume resuscitation. I would take blood for FBC, U&ES, coagulation studies and crossmatch 6 units of blood. I would initially resuscitate the woman with up to two litres of intra-venous crystalloid and then consider using blood. Ideally I would use warmed fluids. I would be in constant communication with the rest of the team to ascertain the extent of the bleeding and the planned treatment. This might include manual stimulation of an atonic uterus, placement of a urinary catheter and drug therapy with syntocinon, ergometrine and carboprost.

The obstetricians diagnose uterine atony and retained products of conception. They are keen to move to theatre and surgically intervene. The woman continues to bleed. What are your concerns?

I would appreciate the urgency of the situation and attempt to move the woman quickly. I would want to continue fluid resuscitation, consider invasive monitoring and have the woman catheterised in theatre. It might be necessary to transfuse fresh frozen plasma, cryo-precipitate and platelets depending on the blood transfusion requirements. Cell salvage and attention to normothermia would also be considerations. In order to provide anaesthesia for removal of the products of conception the options are a general or regional anaesthetic technique. My choice would depend on the urgency, haemodynamic stability of the patient and potential for coagulopathy.

What surgical interventions might be considered?

The obstetricians might only need to manually remove the placenta. Bimanual compression and massage of the uterus may be required to induce contraction. If this fails, further options include uterine tamponade with a balloon or pack, uterine and internal iliac artery ligation, B-Lynch suture and finally a hysterectomy. In some units radiological embolisation of pelvic vessels may be available.

On your post-natal ward round you identify a woman who complains of a headache. She had an epidural for labour and an uneventful vaginal delivery 24 hours ago. What are the possible causes of her headache and how might you differentiate between them?

This question is testing your ability to produce a relevant differential diagnosis.

There are many causes for a post-natal headache. It is important to take a thorough history, examine the patient and order appropriate investigations in order to ascertain the possible diagnosis.

The headache might be due to a neurological condition, a generalised condition or secondary to an anaesthetic intervention. Neurological conditions include simple headache, migraine, meningitis, encephalitis, benign intra-cranial hypertension, cortical vein thrombosis, intra-cranial bleed and tumour. Generalised conditions include pre-eclampsia, dehydration and stress. With regards to anaesthetic intervention, the woman may have developed a post-dural puncture headache.

What are the features of a post-dural puncture headache (PDPH)?

The classical features of a PDPH include an onset within 72 hours of neuraxial blockade with a severe frontal or occipital headache. This is worse when sitting, moving suddenly, coughing and straining and is relieved when supine. Neck stiffness and photophobia may occur. Rarely cranial nerve palsies and even subdural or intra-cranial haemorrhage have been reported.

How would you treat a suspected post-dural puncture headache?

I would discuss the possible diagnosis with the woman and advise that she should try and remain well hydrated and take oral analgesia as tolerated. I would screen for some of the serological markers of sepsis such as a raised white cell count and CRP and would also monitor the patient's temperature. If the headache persisted I would consider performing an epidural blood patch. The optimal timing for a blood patch is contentious. I would aim to perform the technique within 1 to 2 days of the headache's onset if conservative measures had failed. Prophylactic blood patching for patients with recognised dural tap is controversial as it may be unnecessary, less effective and poses an infection risk.

What is the success rate with an epidural blood patch?

Most patients will recover completely after an epidural blood patch with a success rate of up to 80% rising to 90% after a second blood patch.

The most recent CEMACH (2003–2005) report identified six maternal deaths in which anaesthesia directly contributed. Can you describe these?

The CEMACH report is published regularly so this discussion may now be out of date. Please read the most up to date version.

Three patients were obese with post-operative respiratory complications. Of these patients, one had an emergency removal of ectopic pregnancy and respiratory distress following extubation with failed re-intubation; one received a second dose of opiate prior to extubation and had respiratory failure in recovery; and the third had a fatal asthma attack after a caesarean section performed under regional anaesthesia.

The fourth patient received an overdose of intra-venous bupivacaine. The fifth patient developed a haemothorax after attempted central line insertion for pre-eclampsia and HELLP syndrome. Finally the sixth patient died two weeks after childbirth whilst having a general anaesthetic to have a septic focus drained from a kidney. The exact cause of her death was unknown.

What lessons can be learned from these cases?

The CEMACH report highlighted the need for trained, experienced recovery staff and anaesthetists being readily available at all times for this group of patients. There were some issues regarding the experience of trainees and the accessibility of senior support. The report reminded clinicians to consider the respiratory implications of a pes excavatum but accepted that the use of ultrasound might not avoid all complications of central line insertion. Finally the report identified factors that may contribute to the inadvertent intra-venous infusion of local anaesthetic drugs, such as the location of storage of these drugs in relation to standard infusion bags. Staff should also be aware of where the intra-lipid 20% is located for the treatment of severe local anaesthetic toxicity.

Did the report make any suggestions regarding the 31 deaths in which anaesthesia contributed?

Yes, the report identified a failure to recognise serious illness and poor management of haemorrhage, sepsis, pre-eclampsia and obese women.

What did the report say about the challenges now facing obstetrics?

The CEMACH report acknowledged the increasing migrant population as a challenge, since women are presenting late with complicated pregnancies, serious underlying medical conditions and poor general health. Furthermore, vulnerable women with socially complex lives are less likely to seek antenatal care and stay in contact with maternity services. More than 15% of all women who died from direct or indirect causes were morbidly obese. Finally as older mothers are now presenting, they have more chronic health problems.

What were the principle direct causes of death?

These included thrombo-embolism, amniotic fluid embolism, sepsis, pre-eclampsia, haemorrhage, anaesthesia and direct uterine trauma.

The CEMACH report suggested an national early warning score for identifying women who are unwell. What indices did they suggest might be measured?

The report suggested both general and specific indices. The obstetric-specific indices were lochia, proteinuria and liquor; whilst the general indices included respiratory rate, oxygen saturation, temperature, heart rate, blood pressure, urine output, conscious level and pain score.

Further Reading

Davis S. Amniotic fluid embolism: a review of the literature. *Canadian Journal of Anaesthesia*. 2001; **48**: 88–98.

Lewis, G. (ed.) The Confidential Enquiry into Maternal and Child Health (CEMACH). Saving mothers' lives: reviewing maternal deaths to make motherhood safer- 2003–2005. The Seventh Report on Confidential Enquiries into Maternal Deaths in the United Kingdom. London: CEMACH, 2007. http://www.cemach.org.uk/ Publications-Press-Releases/Report-Publications/Maternal-Mortality.aspx.

2.5.4. Pre-eclampsia – Sarah F Bell

The topics will probably come as part of a case-based discussion and so try to keep your answer relevant to the particular case to gain maximum marks.

You are asked to review a 28-year-old primigravida who is 36 weeks pregnant. She has been recently admitted to the labour ward for an induction of labour and is known to have hypertension.

What are the important issues that you would like to explore in her history?

The examiner is looking to see that you have had plenty of obstetric experience and that you can imagine yourself in this situation. A structured approach is vital.

When taking a history I would introduce myself to the patient and discuss a number of case-specific and more general issues. Specifically I would enquire about: why and how she is being induced; what her most recent blood pressures have been and whether she had hypertension prior to her pregnancy. I would want to know what anti-hypertensive agents she is taking and whether she has any other symptoms or signs of pre-eclamptic toxaemia (or PET).

In general I would want to know: how her pregnancy has progressed and whether there have been any complications; whether she has had any previous pregnancies; what is her past medical history, past anaesthetic history and drug history. Does she have any allergies; when did she last eat or drink; what is her dentition and is there a family history of problems with an anaesthetic.

How do you diagnose pre-eclampsia?

Pre-eclampsia is a multi-system disease with a number of manifestations that occur after the twentieth week of pregnancy. The main features are the triad of hypertension, oedema and proteinuria. The hypertension is diagnosed as a systolic greater than 140 mmHg, diastolic greater than 90 mmHg or a mean greater than 105 mmHg. Alternatively it is described as an increase in systolic or diastolic pressure of more than 30 mmHg or 15 mmHg respectively. The proteinuria is greater than 0.3 g/L in 24 hours.

How common is pre-eclampsia?

Pre-eclampsia occurs in approximately 2–3% of pregnancies but pregnancy-induced hypertension, without other features of pre-eclampsia, is more common and has an incidence of about 10%.

Why does pre-eclampsia develop?

Try not to get too bogged down in this answer since it is complicated and not yet fully understood.

The exact cause of pre-eclampsia is unknown. Patients may be genetically susceptible and there is thought to be an autoimmune reaction against the placenta. Failure of the normal vasodilatation of blood vessels within the placental bed leads to placental ischaemia and release of vasoconstrictor substances. This alters the thromboxane/prostacyclin ratio causing widespread organ system effects including vasoconstriction and altered capillary permeability.

What are the features of pre-eclampsia?

Try and use your systems approach to keep structure to your answer.

The symptoms and signs of pre-eclampsia may be split into the different organ systems. In the cardiovascular system the systemic vascular resistance is raised and hypertension is a feature. The plasma volume is reduced when compared to the expansion normally seen in pregnancy. Changes in capillary permeability and reduced plasma oncotic pressure lead to peripheral oedema. Furthermore, the combination of raised pulmonary artery pressure, low plasma oncotic pressure and altered capillary permeability in the lungs make these patients particularly susceptible to pulmonary oedema. With regards to the kidneys, a reduction in renal blood flow, glomerular filtration rate and urine output may be observed. Proteinuria and renal failure may develop. The haematological system may be affected with a fall in fibrinogen and platelet levels. The HELLP syndrome of haemolysis, elevated liver enzymes and low platelets is a recognised associated condition. In patients with severe pre-eclampsia disseminated intravascular coagulation may ensue. The gastrointestinal system may be involved as part of HELLP and the patient may experience abdominal pain due to oedema and enlargement of the liver capsule. Finally with regards to the neurological system the patient may describe visual disturbance and headaches. Hyperexcitability, hyperreflexia and papilloedema may be demonstrated and the patient may develop seizures.

How might pre-eclampsia affect the foetus?

The reduced placental perfusion may be compounded by ischaemia and infarction. This can lead to intra-uterine growth retardation. The incidence of placental abruption and preterm labour is also increased.

Are there any risk factors for pre-eclampsia?

Yes, these include women who have diabetes, multiple pregnancy, positive family history, pre-existing hypertensive disease, increasing maternal age and obesity.

What is the treatment for pre-eclampsia?

There is no specific answer to this question. The examiners are looking to see that you have an understanding of the general issues involved.

The treatment for pre-eclampsia is delivery of the baby, but this must be balanced against the gestational age of the foetus and the potential risks associated with uncontrolled hypertension. In many cases anti-hypertensive treatment will be commenced in order to regain control of blood pressure prior to delivery; but this does not prevent the disease progression. Close monitoring of observational parameters, haematological and neurological indices is indicated in these patients both before and after delivery.

What anti-hypertensive treatment might this woman be taking?

Try and think back to a case you have seen.

Methyl dopa, labetalol, hydralazine and nifedipine have all been used. Labetalol can be taken orally or intra-venously by infusion or as boluses. Methyldopa is taken orally, hydralazine intra-venously and nifedipine may be administered by either route.

What is the role of magnesium in pre-eclampsia and eclampsia? Can you tell me anything about the MAGPIE Trial?

The MAGPIE Trial was a large international study evaluating the effects of magnesium sulphate given to women with pre-eclampsia. Magnesium sulphate more than halved the risk of eclampsia. Currently magnesium sulphate is used to treat pre- and post-partum seizure activity. A loading dose of 4 g is given over 10 minutes followed by an infusion of 1 g/hr. Recurrent seizures are treated with further 2-g boluses of magnesium.

What clinical assessments would you perform on this woman and what would you be looking for?

I would examine the cardio-respiratory, neurological and gastrointestinal systems looking for any signs of pre-eclampsia. These might include hypertension, peripheral oedema, respiratory compromise, hyperreflexia, clonus, abdominal discomfort and right upper quadrant tenderness. I would also assess the patient's airway looking for factors that might predispose to a difficult intubation.

What would you consider necessary investigations?

Urine dipstick will indicate proteinuria. Twenty-four-hour urine collection will quantify this further.

I would request the results of a full blood count, urea and electrolytes, liver function tests, coagulation studies and ensure that a sample of blood had been sent for a group and save. I would be looking for anaemia, thrombocytopenia, renal failure, hepatic derangement and clotting abnormalities.

What advice would you give this woman regarding an epidural?

This question is assessing whether you have appreciated the role of epidural analgesia in women with pre-eclampsia.

A good working epidural placed early during labour has the potential to reduce the catecholamine release associated with pain. This should improve placental blood flow, thus benefitting both mother and foetus. It may also be rapidly topped up for instrumental or emergency caesarean section. I would discuss these benefits with the patient; but also explain the risks of epidural placement. I would list the complications with the level of risk as published by the Obstetric Anaesthetists' Association.

These are: failure or patchy epidural, nausea and vomiting, hypotension (the risk is 1 in 50), headache (the risk is 1 in 100), nerve damage (the risk is 1 in 1000 for temporary nerve damage and 1 in 13 000 for permanent nerve damage), and an increased risk of instrumental delivery (the incidence increases from 7 to 14% with an epidural).

What haematological parameters would you consider it safe for performing an epidural in this case?

I would need to review a full blood count and a clotting screen prior to the insertion of a spinal or epidural needle. I would consider a platelet count below 100×10^9/L a relative contraindication for an epidural. An abnormal clotting screen with platelet counts above 100×10^9/L would also be of concern. I would also review the white cell count. A leucocytosis of 25×10^9/L or more can be normal in labour. If the white cell count were raised I would check the patient's temperature and look for a source of sepsis prior to considering inserting an epidural. The risk of epidural infection needs to be weighed against the potential benefits of epidural placement and discussed with the patient and the consultant on call.

What about the platelet count considered safe for performing a spinal?

In my department the criteria are slightly different for spinal anaesthesia and a platelet count above 70×10^9/L with normal clotting is acceptable for a spinal anaesthetic.

How would you manage this patient's fluid balance?

Try and think of what your unit's protocol says!

Management of fluid balance in patients with pre-eclampsia can be extremely challenging. It is important to carefully monitor the input and output, usually with a urinary catheter in situ. Renal function blood tests should be regularly checked. Oliguria is common in pre-eclampsia and does not necessarily imply volume depletion. Overhydration may contribute to the development of pulmonary oedema, but over-enthusiastic fluid restriction or additional blood loss may also lead to renal failure.

One example is a fluid restriction regimen of 85 ml/hr of crystalloid, with a target urine output of 0.5 ml/kg/hr. If the urine output falls then 250-ml judicious boluses of colloid are considered, up to 500 ml. If this fails, two 20-mg furosemide boluses may be given. If this is still ineffective then central venous pressure monitoring may be required.

Once the epidural is sited and the test dose has been administered the patient has a tonic–clonic seizure. What are the possible causes for this?

The seizure may be due to an obstetric or non-obstetric condition. This classification can be further split into neurological, non-neurological or anaesthetic-related causes.

Neurological obstetric conditions might include eclampsia, subarachnoid haemorrhage or intra-cranial haemorrhage. Non-obstetric neurological conditions such as pre-existing epilepsy, intra-cranial mass or infection may have precipitated the seizure.

Respiratory conditions that cause significant hypoxia or hypercapnia can initiate seizures. These might be related to the pregnancy such as the amniotic fluid embolism or pulmonary embolism or be due to pre-existing conditions.

Metabolic conditions causing seizures include hypoglycaemia and hyponatraemia. These may be related to the pregnancy (for example, a gestational diabetic who is starved and has received insulin) or due to a pre-existing condition.

Finally, with regard to anaesthetic interventions, the epidural catheter may be in the intra-thecal space leading to a high spinal or the epidural solution may have been injected into a vein leading to local anaesthetic toxicity.

What would be your initial management of this scenario?

Try and picture yourself in this situation and describe how you would manage it.

This is an obstetric medical emergency that needs prompt management. I would delegate a member of staff to call the labour ward resuscitation team including senior anaesthetic help and an ODP. I would also request the emergency eclampsia box and have this available. I would start by assessing the airway, give 100% oxygen via a facemask and ensure that the patient was in left lateral tilt. I would then quickly examine the respiratory system and check the oxygen saturation level. The blood pressure, heart rate and any obvious blood loss would need to be assessed. The patient already has IV access but I would send blood samples to the laboratory for FBC, U&ES, LFT, glucose, coagulation studies and crossmatch if not already done. The obstetric team should examine the abdomen and uterus. I would give a bolus of 4 g of magnesium sulphate IV in an attempt to halt the seizure. Depending on whether the seizure stopped and the mother regained consciousness, I would consider intubating the mother at this stage. Further pharmacological treatment with anti-hypertensive drugs, magnesium sulphate infusion and benzodiazepines may be required. The baby may need to be delivered by emergency caesarean section. If possible a neurological assessment of the patient should be performed.

The seizure subsides and the woman partially regains consciousness but the obstetricians are keen to proceed to a Category 1 emergency caesarean section due to foetal distress. There is not time to top up the epidural and you are required to perform a general anaesthetic.

How would you perform this?

Having informed my senior support of the situation and asked for their assistance, I would prepare for a general anaesthetic. I would ensure that I had at least one skilled assistant, a tilting table, suction and a checked anaesthetic machine. I would administer 30 ml of 0.3 M sodium citrate. I would preoxygenate the woman for at least 3 minutes in a left lateral tilt position. During preoxygenation I would expect the obstetricians to be scrubbed and preparing the abdomen so that they are ready to start. I would prefer to have an arterial line in situ to closely monitor blood pressure but should not delay the induction of anaesthesia unnecessarily. I would induce anaesthesia using a rapid sequence induction with thiopentone 3–5 mg, suxamethonium 2 mg/kg and alfentanil 10–20 μg/kg. I would inform the paediatrician of the use of an opiate to obtund the pressor response to laryngoscopy. I would secure the airway with an endotracheal tube and confirm correct positioning prior to allowing the commencement of surgery. I would maintain anaesthesia using a 50:50 nitrous oxygen mix and 2% isoflurane for about 3 minutes, then reducing the isoflurane to 1% and maintaining levels about 0.6%. I would aim to achieve a mild respiratory alkalosis to maintain this physiologically normal adaption of pregnancy. Once the suxamethonium had worn off, I would administer a non-depolarising muscle relaxant such as atracurium, reducing the dose as magnesium sulphate had been given. After delivery I would give syntocinon 5 IU as a slow bolus. During the operation I would administer cautious fluid therapy. If necessary I would insert a central line to monitor central venous pressures and help guide fluid resuscitation.

With regards to post-operative analgesia, I would consider bilateral ilioinguinal nerve blocks or use the epidural to administer morphine or fentanyl. I would prescribe regular paracetamol and consider a NSAID such as diclofenac; although in this particular case I would not give this drug due to the risk of worsening the patient's renal function.

What potential problems might you anticipate during and after the operation?

The problems may be divided into cardiovascular and haematological, respiratory, neurological and renal. Cardiovascular instability may occur at any stage. Dramatic swings in blood pressure may require prompt treatment. Hypertensive crises may lead to intra-cranial haemorrhage and bleeding at the operative site. This may be complicated further by a coagulopathy. Fluid balance will be difficult to manage and so the measurement of urine output and central venous pressure will be helpful. With regards to the respiratory system, the intubation may be difficult due to airway oedema and the patient may be difficult to ventilate due to pulmonary oedema.

Post-operatively the patient may have further seizures and she may require admission to a critical care unit for respiratory, neurological, haematological or renal support.

Further Reading

Altman D, Carroli G, Duley L, et al., Magpie Trial Collaborative Group. Do women with pre-eclampsia, and their babies, benefit from magnesium sulphate? The Magpie Trial: a randomised placebo-controlled trial. *Lancet* 2002; **359**: 1877–1890.

Joint Formulary Committee. *British National Formulary*. 58th edition. London: British Medical Association and Royal Pharmaceutical Society of Great Britain, 2009.

Obstetric Anaesthetists' Association. Pain Relief in Labour, 3rd Edition. 2009. http://www.oaa-anaes.ac.uk/content.asp?ContentID=115.

Ophthalmic

2.6.1. Orbital anatomy – Poonam M Bopanna

Describe the anatomy of the orbit

The orbit is a bony cavity containing the globe, nerves, muscles and blood vessels that are necessary for the eye to function. The orbit can be thought of as a pyramid whose apex is directed inwards and upwards.

The borders of the orbit:

- The roof: frontal bone and the greater wing of the sphenoid
- The floor: maxilla and the zygoma
- The medial wall: maxilla, lacrimal bone, sphenoid and the ethmoid bone
- The lateral wall: greater wing of sphenoid and the zygoma.

The superior, inferior, medial and lateral recti muscles form a cone. The apex of this cone is a fibrotendinous ring surrounding the optic canal and the medial part of the superior orbital fissure. Anteriorly, these muscles insert onto the sclera.

The extraconal muscles are:

- Superior oblique
- Inferior oblique
- Levator palpebrae superioris
- Orbicularis oculi.

The following structures pass through the superior orbital fissure (see Figure 2.6.1a):

- Superior ophthalmic vein
- Oculomotor nerve
- Abducens nerve
- Trochlear nerve
- Lacrimal, frontal and nasociliary nerves.

The inferior orbital fissure transmits the following:

- Inferior ophthalmic vein

Dr. Podcast Scripts for the Final FRCA, ed. Rebecca A. Leslie, Emily K. Johnson, Gary Thomas and Alexander P. L. Goodwin.   Published by Cambridge University Press.
© R. A. Leslie, E. K. Johnson, G. Thomas and A. P. L. Goodwin 2011.

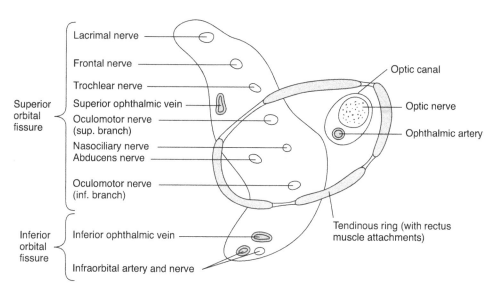

Figure 2.6.1a. Structures passing through the orbital fissures. Reproduced with permission from Smith, T., Pinnock, C. and Lin, T. 2009. *Fundamentals of Anaesthesia.* Cambridge: Cambridge University Press. © Cambridge University Press 2009.

- Infra-orbital artery
- Infra-orbital nerve

The ophthalmic artery and optic nerve pass through the optic canal.

Describe the nerve supply to the orbit

The oculomotor nerve supplies all the extraocular muscles except the superior oblique and lateral rectus. The superior oblique muscle is supplied by the trochlear nerve, whilst the lateral rectus is supplied by the abducens nerve.

The orbicularis oculi is innervated by the facial nerve and the levator palpebrae superioris has a sympathetic innervation.

The sensory nerve supply to the periorbital skin is via the supra-orbital, supra-trochlear, infra-orbital and lacrimal nerves, which are branches of the trigeminal nerve. These nerves, in addition to the long ciliary nerve, also supply the conjunctiva.

The cornea and sclera are predominantly supplied by the long and short ciliary nerves that are branches of the nasociliary branch of the ophthalmic division of the trigeminal nerve.

The sympathetic fibres come from the first thoracic ganglion and synapse in the superior cervical ganglion before travelling with the long and short ciliary nerves.

The parasympathetic fibres travel from the Edinger-Westphal nucleus, and accompanies the oculomotor nerve before synapsing with the short ciliary nerves in the ciliary ganglion.

Describe the anatomy of the globe?

The globe is a spherical structure which is asymmetrical and has an axial length between 20 and 25 mm in an adult and a volume of 6–6.5 ml.

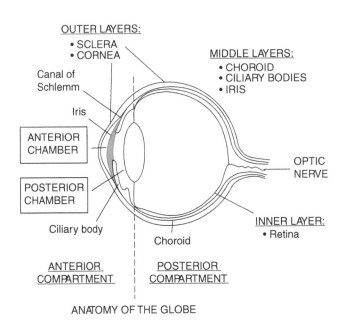

Figure 2.6.1b. Anatomy of the globe.

OUTER LAYERS:
• SCLERA
• CORNEA

MIDDLE LAYERS:
• CHOROID
• CILIARY BODIES
• IRIS

Canal of Schlemm

Iris

ANTERIOR CHAMBER

POSTERIOR CHAMBER

Ciliary body

Choroid

OPTIC NERVE

INNER LAYER:
• Retina

ANTERIOR COMPARTMENT

POSTERIOR COMPARTMENT

ANATOMY OF THE GLOBE

The globe can be divided into an anterior and a posterior compartment. The anterior compartment includes everything anterior to the lens and can be divided further into the anterior and posterior chamber. The anterior chamber is used to describe all structures anterior to the iris, whilst the posterior chamber describes those posterior to the iris but anterior to the lens (see Figure 2.6.1b). Both the anterior and posterior chambers of the anterior compartment are filled with aqueous humour. This is responsible for maintaining normal intra-ocular pressure. It is secreted by the ciliary body and is reabsorbed through a network of trabeculae into the canal of Schlemm. The posterior compartment contains the vitreous humour which is a gel like substance.

The globe has three layers:

• Outer layers: sclera and cornea
• Middle layers: choroid, ciliary bodies and the iris
• Inner layer: retina

The retina is made up of neural tissue the axons of which eventually form the optic nerve. The macula is a small portion of the retina that is responsible for distinct vision.

Describe the pre-operative assessment of a patient presenting for ophthalmic regional anaesthesia?

The majority of the patients presenting for eye surgery are elderly and will have pre-existing medical problems. A significant number of patients are pre-assessed in clinics by trained nurses.

Even if the patient is not having a general anaesthetic I would conduct a full pre-operative assessment, including co-morbidities, anaesthetic history, medications, allergies and social history. Importantly, patients with significant cardiorespiratory disease may be unable to lie flat for the duration of the procedure. Also angina and ECG changes can be induced due to the stress of having a regional technique so a thorough history is essential.

Orbital regional anaesthesia alone does not warrant fasting unless general anaesthesia is being considered.

Ophthalmic history and examination is mandatory to assess the suitability for a regional technique. Check the axial length of the globe (this is normally around 23 mm). If the axial length is >26 mm or patients are long-standing myopics they might have a pathological thinning of the sclera, choroids and retina causing an out pouching of the globe, called a staphyloma. This tends to occur inferior to the posterior pole. Damage to the globe from the needle is significantly higher in these patients if an inferotemporal approach is used, however subtenon and medial canthus blocks are safe.

Patients having trabeculectomy, vitrectomy, limbal relaxation procedures or difficult lenses are likely to have long and difficult surgery. This will have implications for the type of regional block used and the ability of the patient to lie supine for a long time.

It is always necessary to consider a general anaesthetic in patients with previous problems with a regional technique, patients with uncontrolled movement disorders, patients who are deaf or have learning difficulties, suffer from dementia and in children.

Examine the eye looking for any variations that might make regional techniques more difficult. These include narrow palpebral fissure, nystamus and evidence of previous eye surgery. If there is enophthalmos there is an increased risk of needle damage to the globe via the inferotemporal approach.

How would you perform a sub-tenon block?

As for all regional techniques it is a good idea to have a general introduction which covers pre-operative assessment, ruling out any contraindications, obtaining verbal consent, preparing the anaesthetic room with equipment and emergency drugs, gaining IV access and establishing routine monitoring.

I would start by applying a few drops of topical local anaesthetic, such as proxymetacaine or oxybuprocaine, to the conjunctiva. The 1:10 000 adrenaline can be added to minimise subconjuctival bleeding.

I would then clean the eye with a few drops of iodine. Remember never to do this before the eye has been topically anaesthetised as it is very painful in a non-anaesthetised eye.

I would then apply a lid speculum to keep the eyes open and ask the patient to look upwards and outwards. Using a Moorfields forceps I would take a small a bite of the conjunctiva and tenon's capsule in the inferonasal quadrant of the eye. Using a Westacott scissors I would make a small opening about 2 mm in length. I would then pass a 19-gauge, 25-mm sub-tenons cannula with a syringe containing local anaesthetic attached into the opening, advancing gently keeping the tip very close to the sclera. The syringe should be vertical and at a depth of 15–20 mm before injection is delivered. I would aspirate before injection to avoid intravenous injection. I would then remove the needle and close the eye and gently massage to facilitate the spread of local anaesthetic. Either 2% lignocaine or 0.5% chirocaine can be used. Hyaluronidase can be used as an additive.

Describe the peribulbar technique?

Follow the initial introduction as for the subtenon block.

The patient should be looking straight ahead. An injection is made inferotemporally, lateral to the lateral limbus either through the conjunctiva or percutaneously. The needle is directed parallel to the floor of the orbit and vertically backwards. The aim is to keep the tip of the needle extraconal. The 5–10 ml of local anaesthetic is injected after negative aspiration. This block may be supplemented by superonasal or medial canthus injections if required after checking muscle movements.

What are the complications of regional anaesthesia?

Globe penetration is more likely in patients with longer axial length and will lead to pain on injection, deviation of the globe and retinal detachment. Retrobulbar haemorrhage can occur. This increases the intraocular pressure and compromises retinal blood flow. Optic nerve damage, local anaesthetic toxicity, muscle palsies and corneal abrasion can occur but are relatively rare. Chemosis can occur and is quite common and subsides over 24–48 hours.

What are the contraindications to eye blocks?

These can be divided into absolute and relative contraindications.

Absolute contraindications are patient refusal, local anaesthetic allergies and localised infection of the globe.

Relative contraindications are patients who are unable to lie flat, patients with movement disorders, inappropriately high INR, bleeding diathesis and those with previous eye surgery for example sclera buckling.

Further Reading

Gordon HL. Preoperative assessment in ophthalmic regional anaesthesia. *Continuing* *Education in Anaesthesia, Critical Care & Pain.* 2006; **6**(5): 203–206.

2.6.2. Control of intra-ocular pressure – Corinna J Hughes

This is a common topic since understanding of IOP has implications for ophthalmic anaesthesia, in particular penetrating eye injury.

What is a normal IOP?

Define what they are asking for and then give a range of normal values.

Intra-ocular pressure is the tissue pressure of the globe contents on the sclera. The normal range is 10–20 mmHg.

What determines intra-ocular pressure?

As ever classify your answer.

IOP is determined by the contents of the globe, scleral rigidity and external pressure.

The globe contents are determined by aqueous humour production and drainage, blood volume (both arterial and venous) and vitreous humour. The vitreous humour volume is relatively fixed so does not normally affect IOP. Other factors may increase intra-ocular pressure form within the globe, such as tumour, haemorrhage or a foreign body.

The sclera becomes more rigid with age, and is therefore less compliant to changes in globe contents.

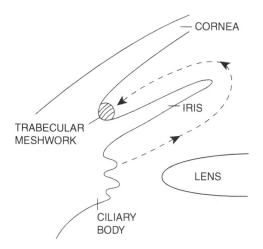

Figure 2.6.2. Drainage of aqueous humour.

The extra-global factors include extra-global muscle tone, retrobulbar haematoma, abscess, tumour or anaesthetic block. There may also be external pressure from face masks, position (for example prone or lateral positioning) or from direct pressure form the surgeon.

How is intra-ocular pressure normally regulated?

It would be worth drawing a diagram to show the drainage of aqueous humour (Figure 2.6.2).

IOP is normally regulated by aqueous humour volume. The aqueous humour is produced in the ciliary bodies. This is mainly by active secretion which is fairly constant. There is also some ultrafiltration which will be reduced if intra-ocular pressure is high. The fluid then flows from the posterior chamber, through the iris into the anterior chamber. It's then reabsorbed through the canal of Schlemm which is in the angle between the iris and cornea. This canal drains into the episcleral veins. If intra-ocular pressure rises, the rate of absorption will increase. If the reabsorption is blocked, or episcleral venous pressure is increased, then intra-ocular pressure will increase. There is a secondary, minor, uveal tract route.

Why do anaesthetists need to know about intra-ocular pressure?

Remember it is not only about penetrating eye injury.

It is important because in penetrating eye injuries an increase in intra-ocular pressure can cause expulsion of globe contents. It is also important to anaesthetists because patients with acute or chronically raised intra-ocular pressure may present for non-ophthalmic surgery, and anaesthetic drugs and procedures have effects on intra-ocular pressure.

Tell me how the blood volume affects IOP?

Examiners like to see you applying basic physiology to clinical applications. Don't wait to be asked.

The most important factor is venous pressure. The choroidal venous plexus drains into the episcleral veins. The pressure within these episcleral veins is determined by central venous pressure. If the CVP is high, draining is reduced and intra-ocular blood volume and pressure will increase. If trying to control IOP then a head up tilt, avoidance of neck ties, head in the neutral position and avoidance of coughing and straining will help.

Arterial blood flow is determined in the same way as cerebral blood flow, it increases linearly with arterial carbon dioxide tension, increases in hypoxia and high blood pressure.

How do anaesthetic drugs affect IOP?

Try to not come out with a random selection, one way to classify them is in the order that you use them.

All the induction agents except ketamine reduce intra-ocular pressure. Propofol has the greatest effect on reducing intraoccular pressure.

Non-depolarising muscular blockers decrease extraocular muscle tone and decrease IOP. Suxamethonium transiently increases IOP, this was initially thought to be due to extraocular muscle fasciculation, however it has been found to occur even if these muscles have been detached. Suxamethonium provides the best and quickest intubating conditions for rapid sequence induction in penetrating eye injury. It is normally given after an induction agent which decreases IOP, and prevents coughing which may accompany early intubation after a non-depolarising blocker and may increase IOP to an even greater extent. Therefore suxamethonium may be appropriate when given for rapid sequence induction for penetrating eye injury despite its direct effect on IOP.

What about volatile agents?

All the volatile anaesthetic agents decrease IOP.

What about nitrous oxide?

Nitrous oxide has little direct effect on IOP, however it should be avoided if other gases are being injected into the eye by the ophthalmic surgeons. For example sulphur hexafluoride may be injected in retinal detachment surgery, if nitrous oxide is used it will diffuse in more easily than nitrogen diffuses out, making the gas bubble bigger. Subsequently on stopping anaesthesia the nitrous oxide will diffuse out more quickly than nitrogen diffuses in, and the retina may again become detached.

What about opioids?

Opioids have little direct effect on IOP, but can decrease the hypertensive response to intubation, along with lidocaine, β-blockers and clonidine.

What can be done to reduce IOP acutely, for example if the surgeon says there is protrusion of the orbital contents?

Make sure you emphasise that you know this is an emergency. Don't go straight for mannitol, remember ABC.

This is an emergency. First, I need to ensure there are normal physiological variables, the patient is well oxygenated, is normocapnic and is normotensive.

I would ensure that venous pressure is not raised by making sure there are no ties around the neck impeding venous drainage and that the head is in the neutral position. I would also ensure that the patient is not coughing or straining with adequate depth of anaesthesia and paralysing the patient.

In the emergency situation, IV propofol can be given to reduce the intra-occular pressure. Propofol is also useful whilst waiting for other agents or techniques to work. Other drugs used in the management of intra-ocular pressure include mannitol and acetazolamide. It is important to remember the rebound side effects that mannitol may have on the circulation post-operatively, and the electrolyte derangements which may occur with acetazolamide, especially in the elderly. Regular electrolytes will need to be done if acetazolamide is given.

2.6.3. Penetrating eye injury – Sarah F Bell

This is a topic that has come up many times. It is a question that can be used to test a number of different areas including: your physiological and pharmacological knowledge; your ability to weigh up the pros and cons of immediate surgical intervention vs. the risk of aspiration; and your appreciation of the importance of communication with the rest of the surgical team. It is vital to indicate to the examiner that you have a solid knowledge base and appreciation of all of these problems.

You are the anaesthetic registrar on-call and have been called to the accident and emergency department to see a 20-year-old male patient. He has been brought in by ambulance having sustained significant facial injuries after being involved in a fight outside a pub.

What would be your initial actions?

Remember to try and picture yourself in this situation. There may be more going on than just the facial trauma. It may be worth making an initial statement to show the examiner that you appreciate this.

I would attempt to assess and start treatments in parallel. My assessment would follow a structured airway, breathing, circulation approach. If there were other members of the emergency department available I would ask them to assist me in obtaining baseline observations and obtaining intravenous access. Given the history I would be considering the possibility of airway and breathing complications; circulatory compromise due to haemorrhage; neurological change due to possible head injury, alcohol or drugs and hypothermia. It is important to remember that there may be more injuries than just the obvious facial trauma.

My assessment of the airway would involve trying to talk to the patient and then listening for sounds of airway obstruction or compromise. If the patient were experiencing difficulties I would consider further interventions including suction, airway adjuncts and intubation. I would apply oxygen to the patient. Next I would examine the respiratory system looking at the respiratory rate, oxygen saturations, observing and ascultating the chest. My circulation assessment would include measurement of the heart rate and blood pressure. I would attempt to identify any major sources of bleeding (which might be facial in this patient) and try and reduce haemorrhage where appropriate. I would examine the abdomen and long bones. My neurological assessment would include the Glasgow Coma Scale and a brief general assessment of the peripheral neurology. If possible I would assess the response of the pupils to light. Depending on the state of the patient I would then check the glucose and temperature and consider a secondary survey.

You find that there are numerous bleeding facial lacerations. The patient's left eye has been damaged by a glass bottle. You cannot find any other injuries and the patient is fully conscious and cooperative.

What would be your next steps?

My priorities would still be the airway, breathing and circulation. From your description the airway and breathing are stable at present and so I would concentrate on the circulation and attempting to halt the bleeding. I would ask one of the accident and emergency staff to exert pressure to the wounds and possibly suture the lacerations or bleeding points. I would obtain intra-venous access and send off baseline bloods. Analgesia, tetanus and anti-biotics may be required. I would contact the ophthalmologist on call to come and urgently review the eye injury. Depending on the extent of the facial lacerations, I may also need to contact a plastic, general or maxillofacial surgeon, although it may be possible to simply suture them in the accident and emergency department.

The ophthalmology registrar attends promptly and is extremely keen to take the patient to theatre urgently because he has a penetrating eye injury.

What further information would you want to know from the patient before proceeding to theatre?

I would need to ensure that the patient was haemodynamically stable and that their airway and breathing did not require assistance.

I would also want to take a full history from the patient. Specifically I would want to know the details surrounding the incident, whether a head injury could still be a possibility, whether the patient had consumed any alcohol or other substance and whether they had sustained any other injuries. I would also want to take a general history of the patient's past medical conditions, drug history, allergies, starvation history and dentition. I would want to assess the airway for intubation.

Finally I would discuss the case with the surgeon and then the Consultant Anaesthetist on call. I would want to know the planned operative procedure, the indication for emergency surgical intervention and whether this outweighed the aspiration risk posed by the patient with a potentially full stomach.

The ophthalmologist wants to take the patient to theatre to remove a piece of glass that is lodged in the patient's left eye. The maxillofacial surgeon is happy to then proceed to suture the facial lacerations and is confident that there are no facial fractures present.

Is there anything else you might consider before theatre?

I would discuss whether a CT head might be required to assess whether the glass had migrated intra-cranially.

Furthermore I would want to premedicate the patient with a prokinetic (such as 10 mg of metoclopramide given intra-venously), a drug to reduce the gastric acidity (such as 50 mg of ranitidine IV) and an acid neutralising medication (such as 30 ml of 0.3 M sodium citrate taken orally).

Let's think about some of the physiological considerations in this case. Can you tell me the normal range for intra-ocular pressure?

Yes, this is 10 to 20 mmHg.

What determines intra-ocular pressure?

The globe is basically a non-compliant sphere within a rigid bony box. The intra-ocular pressure will therefore change if pressure is exerted on the eyeball itself or if the volume of the contents of the orbit changes.

How is intra-ocular pressure normally regulated?

The main regulation is from the volume of aqueous humour in the anterior chamber. The vitreous humour in the posterior chamber has a relatively fixed volume and so plays a minimal role in regulation of intra-ocular pressure.

How is aqueous humour produced and where does it get reabsorbed?

Aqueous humour is produced by the ciliary body to supply glucose and oxygen to the lens and cornea. It flows from the posterior chamber to the lens and iris and is then reabsorbed in the anterior chamber, through the trabecular network and the canal of Schlemm (in the angle between the iris and the cornea). The fluid then flows into the episcleral veins. Drainage is dependent on the pressure gradient between the chamber and the veins.

How is intra-ocular pressure increased?

Intra-ocular pressure may be affected by aqueous humour drainage the arterial blood supply to the eye and certain drugs.

Intra-ocular pressure is increased if drainage of aqueous humour is reduced, either by a reduction in the drainage system (for example, glaucoma) or an increase in venous pressure.

Choroidal arteries differ to retinal arteries in that they do not have myogenic autoregulation. They will dilate in response to increased perfusion pressure, hypercarbia or hypoxia. Straining, vomiting and coughing will increase blood pressure and thus perfusion pressure. All of these factors will therefore cause an increase in intra-ocular pressure.

Drugs such as ketamine and suxamethonium are known to transiently increase the intra-ocular pressure, although this is only for 15 to 20 minutes duration.

Why is it important to avoid increases in intra-ocular pressure in this patient?

An increase in intra-ocular pressure may lead to expulsion of the global contents via the traumatic opening. This will cause further injury to the eye. It is therefore important to understand the mechanisms for increased ocular pressure so that they can be avoided.

Let's now return to our case history. You have agreed to anaesthetise this man for an emergency ophthalmic operation. His facial lacerations have been temporarily dressed and have stopped bleeding. He is in the anaesthetic room and has had premedication as discussed.

Can you describe to me how you would induce anaesthesia and the potential pitfalls that might be encountered?

The ideal induction would avoid hypoxia, hypercarbia, hypertension, coughing, vomiting and straining as these will all increase intra-ocular pressure. The risk of aspiration needs to be considered as does the need for endotracheal intubation, since laryngoscopy may also increase intra-ocular pressure.

The patient potentially has a full stomach. Their gastric emptying time may also be delayed by the effects of pain and opioid analgesia. I would therefore use a rapid sequence technique and secure the airway with an endotracheal tube. Prior to inducing anaesthesia I would ensure that I had resuscitation equipment and drugs available, a trained assistant, I would check the anaesthetic machine as per the AAGBI guidelines and I would have a tilting table. I would preoxygenate the patient for 3 minutes with a tight fitting facemask. I would have suction and difficult airway equipment available. Once my assistant had placed cricoid pressure I would induce anaesthesia with thiopentone 5 mg/kg and suxamethonium 1–2 mg/kg. I would expect the reduction in cardiac output due to the induction agent to off-set the increase in intra-ocular pressure caused by the suxamethonium. I would therefore aim to maintain a normal intra-ocular pressure during induction. I would not use ketamine because it would increase intra-ocular pressure.

Could you use a total intra-venous technique for induction and maintenance of anaesthesia?

Yes, you could use an intra-venous propofol infusion to induce and/or maintain anaesthesia. This might be advantageous due its anti-emetic properties. I would still use cricoid pressure and suxamethonium as part of a modified rapid sequence with this technique.

What drugs might you consider to reduce the increase in intra-ocular pressure during induction?

The increase in intra-ocular pressure might be reduced by a β-blocker or short-acting opioid such as alfentanil. Rapid reduction of intra-ocular pressure might be achieved by acetazo-lamide, which reduces aqueous humour production, or mannitol which acts as an osmotic diuretic.

How would you manage the patient intra-operatively?

I would aim to maintain normal oxygen and carbon dioxide levels. I would keep the blood pressure and temperature within normal limits. I would administer a combination of anti-emetics such as ondansetron and dexamethasone in order to try and reduce the risk of nausea and vomiting post-operatively. I would also administer analgesics titrated to the expected pain caused by the operation. I would position the patient supine or slightly head up and avoid tight neck ties to optimise venous drainage.

How would you extubate the patient?

The extubation poses further risk of raising intra-ocular pressure due to coughing, straining or vomiting. This may not be a problem if the eye wound has been repaired; unless the insult has the potential to cause elevated pressures post-operatively. The effect of an elevation in intra-ocular pressure needs to be balanced against the potential risk of aspiration.

I would aim to achieve a smooth emergence with no coughing, straining or vomiting. This might be performed by extubating the patient deep or exchanging the endotracheal tube for a laryngeal mask airway (also whilst deep). Alternatively β-blockers or lidocaine could be given intra-venously to reduce the hypertensive response. Personally, I would extubate the patient wide awake in a semi-recumbent position if I considered the aspiration risk to be significant.

Would a local anaesthetic technique be possible for this operation?

Penetrating eye injuries are almost never suitable to be done under local anaesthesia. This is due to the nature and duration of the surgery. Furthermore, local anaesthetic techniques can cause additional rises in intra-ocular pressure and the actual spread of the solution might be unreliable. A potential advantage of a local anaesthetic technique is that it would considerably reduce the risk of aspiration.

2.6.4. Cataracts and retinal detachments – Joy M Sanders

Each of these topics could be encountered in the clinical short cases or potentially as a prelude to discussing eye blocks in the case of cataract or vitreoretinal surgery. It is important to know the nuances of each type of surgery and the relevance to us as anaesthetists.

What are the main factors to consider in the anaesthetic management of an 80-year-old man presenting for cataract surgery?

There are many different approaches to answering this question. One would be to categorise the answer into pre-operative, intra-operative and post-operative factors.

This type of surgery is generally performed on a day-case basis, and all the usual day-case criteria should be met before embarking on surgery.

Pre-operative factors:

- It is important to take a brief but focussed history.
- The population that presents for this type of surgery are usually elderly with a high incidence of co-morbid disease, particularly cardiovascular and respiratory disease.
- Such patients may be taking warfarin for atrial fibrillation or artificial heart valves, and it is important to discuss with the surgeons the INR level at which they are happy to proceed with surgery.
- It is also important to elicit whether the patient has heart failure, chronic obstructive pulmonary disease, Parkinson's disease, dementia, musculoskeletal problems or any other reason why they may be unable to lie flat or still for the duration of surgery. Back and neck problems can be helped by placing a pillow under the knees, having a slightly flexed neck and if necessary using table tilt to get the eye horizontal under the microscope. Some surgeons can perform "face to face" surgery in the sitting patient, if the microscope is suitable.
- Patients are often diabetic and their usual regimen should be maintained on the day of surgery. This is possible because fasting is not usually required for cataract extraction under local anaesthesia.
- Before performing a peribulbar block, it is important to check the axial length of the eye, which should be less than 26 mm to reduce the risk of accidental globe perforation due to the presence of staphylomata. If the axial length is greater than this, a sub-Tenon's block is preferable, or, in older patients, a topical intra-cameral injection

(where local anaesthetic is injected into the anterior chamber of the eye) can be done intra-operatively.

- Ascertain whether the patient has had previous cataract surgery, the method of anaesthesia used and any problems encountered.
- Premedication is not normally used, to avoid the potential for movement on sudden waking, but may be necessary in small titrated boluses of intravenous midazolam. However, extreme caution should be exercised because the elderly can become disorientated on even tiny doses.

Intra-operative factors:
These depend on the anaesthetic technique employed.

- Cataract extraction is usually performed using a local technique but in some circumstances, a general anaesthetic may be required. Reasons for this might include patient refusal for local anaesthesia, allergy to local anaesthetics, clotting abnormalities, severe myopia, orbital pathology or young age.
- If performed using a local technique, communication should be maintained throughout, supplemental oxygen should be provided and oxygen saturation and heart rate should be monitored. Atropine should be available in case of bradycardia. If necessary, the surgeon can supplement the block with topical or sub-Tenon's injection.

Post-operative factors:

- Simple oral analgesics are usually all that is required, especially if a block has been used.

What are the local techniques that you have mentioned and describe one technique with which you are familiar?

It will be helpful in this answer if you have done a few of the blocks that you describe so that you can convey confidence in your technique.

The most commonly employed techniques include topical anaesthesia, sub-Tenon's and peribulbar blocks. Other techniques used include subconjunctival and retrobulbar blocks.

Sub-Tenon's block

My preferred technique is the sub-Tenon's block, which is a safe and effective alternative to retrobulbar and peribulbar blocks.

Tenon's capsule is a connective tissue layer surrounding the eye and extraocular muscles. Injection of local anaesthetic in the sub-Tenon's space between the capsule and the sclera effectively blocks the ciliary ganglion, long and short ciliary nerves. Usually enough local anaesthetic diffuses into the muscle cone to produce complete akinesia.

Before embarking on any regional block it is essential to obtain consent for the block, check the side of surgery, ensure resuscitation drugs and equipment are available and institute full monitoring of the patient. Although controversial, the joint Royal Colleges guidelines suggest that it is not mandatory to insert an intra-venous cannula for a sub-Tenon's block, however this is up to the discretion of the anaesthetist.

Firstly, topical anaesthetic is applied to the conjunctiva, for example, proxymetacaine 0.5%. A lid speculum is then inserted to retract both eyelids and the patient asked to look up and out. With Moorfield's forceps, the conjunctiva and anterior Tenon's capsule are lifted up approximately 7 mm inferomedial to the limbus.

A small incision is then made in the conjunctiva with Westcott's spring scissors and blunt dissection performed inferonasally in a plane underneath Tenon's capsule. Usually only 3 mm of dissection is required to access the desired plane.

An alternative technique is using hydrodissection to separate the Tenon's capsule from the sclera. The advancing "ball" of local anaesthetic renders the area ahead insensitive quite quickly.

A special curved and blunt ended cannula can then be passed into this space, aiming backwards towards the equator and 3.5–4 ml of local anaesthetic is slowly injected. The space itself holds only around 0.75–1 ml and the rest spreads along the muscle sheaths. Alternatively, a plastic intra-venous cannula can be used, which is cheaper and may be even less traumatic.

Gentle external pressure is then applied to the eye. However, oculopression should be used with caution in glaucoma patients and is best avoided if the intra-ocular pressure is very high. The Honan's balloon is a device designed for this purpose and can measure the applied pressure, which should not be more than 30 mmHg.

What solution of local anaesthetic do you use?

I use a mixture of 2% lignocaine and 15 U/ml hyaluronidase. This should last 30–40 minutes.

In complicated cataracts, phaco-trabeculectomies, or vitreoretinal surgery, it is advantageous to use a longer acting agent or lignocaine mixed with the longer acting agent. For example, 50:50 mix of lignocaine 2% and L-bupivacaine 0.75% would be suitable.

What is the purpose of the hyaluronidase?

Hyaluronidase promotes spread of the local anaesthetic and reduces intraocular pressure. A disadvantage of its use is that it is expensive and can rarely cause allergic reactions. The optimum dose is unknown but is probably between 5 and 50 U/ml. In the UK we commonly use 15 U/ml but many anaesthetists in the U.S. use only 1–5 U/ml.

What are the complications of the block that you have described?

Common complications include:

- Mild chemosis and superficial haemorrhage which although are cosmetically undesirable will resolve completely in a matter of days.
- Major conjunctival haematoma occurs in less than 0.5% of blocks and can be treated easily by cautery.
- Central nervous system spread of local anaesthetic is almost unheard of except with retrobulbar blocks. Peribulbar blocks with needles of less than 25 mm in length, such as those of 13 or 16 mm, do not risk entering the cone.

Major complications include:

- The oculocardiac reflex and angina, which are not infrequent.

Let's move on to a new clinical scenario.

A 65-year-old lady presents with retinal detachment, and the surgeons would like to proceed with surgery as soon as possible.

What are the important issues here?

Retinal detachments are not usually so urgent that they have to be done immediately on presentation and it is usually reasonable to wait for an adequate period of starvation.

The surgery is often prolonged and performed largely in darkness so the anaesthetist should ensure that there is sufficient lighting to perform anaesthesia safely.

Scleral buckling for retinal detachment can be extremely uncomfortable and is often performed under general anaesthesia, although local anaesthesia is increasingly being used. Controlled ventilation is usually preferable due to the duration of surgery and a wish to avoid hypercarbia which is said to increase IOP. The use of either armoured laryngeal masks or RAE endotracheal tubes are acceptable. Laryngeal mask airways however are useful as they avoid the pressor response to intubation and reduce the incidence of coughing on extubation.

Vagolytic agents must be available should the oculocardiac reflex occur during surgical manipulation of the globe.

Towards the end of the procedure, the surgeons may want to introduce a bubble of sulphur hexafluoride or perfluoropropane gas between the vitreous and retina to tamponade the retina. It is important not to use nitrous oxide for maintenance in these instances.

What is the reason for this?

Nitrous oxide is highly insoluble in blood and can diffuse and expand into closed gas-filled spaces because it is 40 times more soluble than nitrogen. It would therefore increase the volume of the gas bubble injected. Whilst this is acceptable during surgery, it will diffuse out during the post-operative period, reducing the volume of the bubble and therefore reducing the tamponade effect. If the patient subsequently requires non-ophthalmic surgery and nitrous oxide is used, the bubble is at risk of expanding. Nitrous oxide use should therefore be avoided in the 3 months immediately following surgery using intra-ocular gas. It is also important for patients not to fly with gas tamponade, because even a pressurised aircraft cabin is at a "pressure altitude" of about 8000 feet, so the gas bubble will expand.

Are local anaesthetic blocks suitable for this type of surgery?

Retinal detachment surgery can be painful post-operatively, particularly revision surgery, and so a local anaesthetic block should be routine. A sub-Tenon's blocks is ideal in combination with general anaesthesia as it improves intra-operative stability, reduces the need for opioids and reduces post-operative pain. This can be performed after induction of anaesthesia or by the surgeon during or at the end of surgery. If a supplementary block is not used, remifentanil can be a good alternative as scleral indentation is often very stimulating. In these cases supplemental analgesia must be given at the end, for example 0.1mg/kg intra-venous morphine, unless the patient is old and frail. Intra-venous paracetamol should be used routinely, and in the post-operative period, oral morphine with a non-steroidal anti-inflammatory and paracetamol are usually adequate.

If the patient is presenting for re-do retinal detachment surgery having previously had a scleral buckle, it may be difficult to get circumferential spread of local anaesthetic with a sub-Tenon's block. Injections are required in more than one quadrant, so in this instance, a peribulbar block is preferred. However, a sub-Tenon's top-up can be given after the Tenon's capsule is dissected off and opened for the surgery.

2.6.5. Strabismus – Joy M Sanders

You have been asked to anaesthetise a 4-year-old child for correction of a squint.

What factors should be considered in the pre-operative assessment?

In addition to the general assessment of the child it is important to consider whether this is an isolated strabismus or whether it is secondary to a muscular disorder. Squints are associated with rare conditions such as Cruzon's and Apert's syndromes and also with malignant hyperthermia, so it is important to elicit whether there is a family history of this condition. Muscle disorders associated with malignant hyperthermia include central core disease, myotonia congenita and Duchenne's muscular dystrophy. It is also important to establish whether there are any other congenital abnormalities or whether the child has learning difficulties.

General considerations for paediatric anaesthesia include a history of medical conditions such as asthma, recent respiratory tract infections, epilepsy or a history of prematurity. Other factors to consider include previous anaesthetic history, family history of anaesthetic problems, medications, allergies and period of starvation.

The child and parents must be prepared for the conduct of anaesthesia, involving the child where appropriate. The presence of a parent in the anaesthetic room and afterwards in recovery should be discussed. Consent should be taken for suppositories and a topical local anaesthetic such as Ametop should be applied. Pharmacological premedication such as oral midazolam, should be considered if difficulties with induction are anticipated. The parents should be warned of the risk of post-operative vomiting, which is high in strabismus surgery, but it should be explained that measures will be taken to attempt to reduce this risk, although it cannot be entirely eliminated.

So how would you anaesthetise this child?

If this is a short case scenario, it is unlikely that the examiners will expect you to go into any great detail regarding drug doses and equipment type and sizes, but it is worth mentioning that you would ascertain the child's weight and calculate drug doses accordingly. Be prepared to provide this information if asked.

Full monitoring to minimum standards and preparation of all drugs and equipment is essential, based on the child's age and weight. I would have 20 μg/kg of atropine drawn up and immediately available due to the high incidence of the oculocardiac reflex. A prophylactic dose of glycopyrrolate 5 μg/kg can be given to children under 2 years of age, however routine prophylaxis is not now recommended.

Induction may be inhalational or intra-venous, depending on the cooperation of the child.

The choice of whether to use an armoured LMA or to intubate the patient with a RAE tube depends on several factors, and there are advantages and disadvantages of each. It may be advisable to intubate children less than 1 year of age; however, using laryngeal masks in older children is perfectly acceptable. The pressor response to intubation and coughing on extubation are not usually a problem in squint surgery as it is not an intra-ocular procedure. If an LMA is used, it is essential that it is correctly seated as access to the airway during surgery will be restricted.

It is acceptable to use spontaneous or controlled ventilation, but my preference would be to use controlled ventilation because avoiding hypercapnia is thought to decrease the incidence of the oculocardiac reflex. In addition, many "squint" surgeons request complete muscle relaxation because of the requirement for a "forced duction test", whereby the eye is moved to assess any mechanical restriction in movement as distinct from that attributable to muscle tone. For this reason it is preferable to give a muscle relaxant at least to cover the period of the forced duction test. If bilateral surgery is planned, both eyes should be assessed at the same time. If the surgeon is repairing the squint with an adjustable suture, it is important that the effects of the muscle relaxant have worn off before the suture is adjusted. I would avoid suxamethonium due to its tonic contraction effects on extraocular muscles and its potential trigger for malignant hyperthermia.

I would use a mixture of oxygen and air or nitrous oxide with a volatile agent for maintenance. The depth of anaesthesia with volatile agents should be sufficient to ensure neutral gaze. This can sometimes be difficult to achieve with modern agents, especially sevoflurane, unlike halothane. The eyes may remain rolled up in to the head, which is known as Bell's sign.

Propofol infusion is being increasingly used for children over 6 years of age, where vomiting starts to become troublesome, as it is less emetogenic compared to volatile agents. TCI using Kataria's formula at 4–5 μg/ml target is appropriate.

Botulinum toxin is occasionally used in the treatment of strabismus and blepharospasm. Ketamine is a useful anaesthetic agent in this instance as it does not reduce muscle tone, which the surgeon tests intra-operatively. However, ketamine has well known side effects, which may deter its use.

You mentioned the oculocardiac reflex. Can you tell me more about this reflex, in particular the afferent and efferent pathways?

This reflex occurs frequently during strabismus surgery, in as many as 60% of cases. It is caused by traction on the extraocular muscles (particularly medial rectus) or pressure on the globe and reverts almost immediately when the stimulus is removed. It usually manifests as bradydysrhythmias with ectopics although very occasionally sinus arrest or major dysrhythmias may occur.

Afferent pathways run from the long and short ciliary nerves, via the ciliary ganglion, to the ophthalmic division of the trigeminal nerve. They are then transmitted to the Gasserian ganglion and finally to the main sensory nucleus of the trigeminal nerve in the floor of the fourth ventricle.

The efferent pathway starts in the nucleus of the vagus cardiac depressor nerve in the cardioinhibitory centre of the medulla and runs to the heart via the vagus nerve. Increased stimulation leads to decreased output of the sino-atrial node.

OK, so let's imagine that half way through the operation you notice that the heart rate has dropped to 50 beats per minute. What would you do?

Having quickly confirmed the rate, I would promptly inform the surgeons and ask them to remove the stimulus. This is usually all that is required because the reflex fatigues and is not as powerful the next time. However, if the heart rate does not improve, I would call for senior help and administer 10 μg/kg of atropine. This dose of atropine can be repeated if it has little effect. If cardiac output is lost I would commence cardiopulmonary resuscitation.

Fine. What would you use for intra-operative and post-operative analgesia for squint surgery?

This type of surgery is not particularly painful and opioids should be avoided to decrease the risk of post-operative nausea and vomiting. A combination of fentanyl or alfentanil with a diclofenac suppository 1mg/kg and intra-venous paracetamol 15 mg/kg is usually adequate. Supplemental local anaesthesia should also be used and subconjunctival local anaesthetic has a longer lasting effect than topical eye drops. Some surgeons also apply diclofenac 0.5% eye drops on the muscle insertions before closing the conjunctiva. Peribulbar blocks, whilst producing effective analgesia and reducing the incidence of the oculocardiac reflex are inadvisable in children due to the risk of globe perforation and retrobulbar haemorrhage.

The patients should be given regular ibuprofen 5mg/kg and paracetamol 15 mg/kg to be taken four times a day for 3 days post-operatively.

You mentioned post-operative nausea and vomiting, is this usually a problem?

Yes, it can be. Untreated, the incidence of post-operative vomiting in squint surgery is very high, and can be greater than 50%. It is not as high as that with resection/recession and is closer to 25–30%. It is much higher with the Faden operation, which involves the placement of a posterior fixation suture, however this is no longer performed in the United Kingdom. Post-operative nausea and vomiting is also worse with bilateral operations. Its precise mechanism is unknown but may be due to an oculo-emetic reflex involving the ophthalmic division of the trigeminal nerve and the vomiting centre in the medulla. It can be prevented by prophylaxis with intra-venous ondansetron 0.15 mg/kg and dexamethasone 0.15 mg/kg, a combination which is recommended by the APA guideline in 2009 on the prevention of post-operative vomiting in high-risk children. Maintaining adequate hydration is also important, and all children should receive 20 ml/kg of intra-venous fluids. It is possible to reduce the incidence of vomiting to less than 10% when a multi-modal approach is used. Also of note is that the predisposition to nausea and vomiting persists for 48 hours post-operatively. Motion sickness can be a particular problem so care should be taken to avoid violent cornering, sudden acceleration/deceleration and fairground rides.

Further Reading

Carr AS, Cortman S, Holtby H. Guidelines on the prevention of post-operative vomiting in children. The Association of Paediatric Anaesthetists of Great Britain and Irelend. Spring 2009. www.apagbi.org.uk/sites/apagbi.org.uk/files/APA_Guidelines_on_the_Prevention_of_Postoperative_Vomiting_in_ Children.pdf.

Orthopaedic

2.7.1. Procedures under tourniquet, reperfusion injury and antioxidants – Katherine A Holmes

You are asked to anaesthetise for an elective orthopaedic list. Your first patient is a 78-year-old woman for a right total knee replacement.

What are the primary issues you would want to consider?

As you have not been given much in the way of specific information for this patient, give a brief list of the likely main concerns in a case such as this, then move on to the rest of your normal anaesthetic history.

This is an elderly lady who is to undergo major elective orthopaedic surgery. My main concerns would be that of significant co-morbidities, possibly masked by pain-related reduced exercise tolerance and also the potential effects of undergoing joint replacement surgery. These would include blood loss and/or tourniquet and cement use, fluid balance and adequate pain and temperature control.

As part of my anaesthetic history I would enquire as to previous anaesthetics, as she may have had an arthritic joint replaced before, also about illnesses and medications, allergies and smoking, alcohol intake, reflux and fasting status. Airway assessment should be conducted with history and examination and there may be useful information in old anaesthetic charts. The presence of rheumatoid arthritis would also be significant because of the risk of reduced neck and temporo-mandibular joint mobility.

Specifically, I would seek evidence of cardio-respiratory disease, bearing in mind that she may have asymptomatic ischaemic heart disease if she cannot walk far. I would also seek contraindications to planned surgical or anaesthetic techniques. Examples of this include neuraxial or peripheral nerve blockade and anti-coagulation medication, or tourniquet use, sickle cell anaemia or profound peripheral vascular disease.

Another major concern after this type of procedure can be the risk of deep venous thrombosis and pulmonary embolism so a previous history of this or additional risk factors should be sought.

Dr. Podcast Scripts for the Final FRCA, ed. Rebecca A. Leslie, Emily K. Johnson, Gary Thomas and Alexander P. L. Goodwin. Published by Cambridge University Press.
© R. A. Leslie, E. K. Johnson, G. Thomas and A. P. L. Goodwin 2011.

Your surgeon tells you he routinely uses a tourniquet for knee replacements. In your experience, in which situations are tourniquets generally used?

Limb tourniquets are used to reduce bleeding and improve operating conditions in mainly orthopaedic or plastic surgery but are also used in intra-venous regional anaesthesia for procedures such as manipulation of Colles fractures. As the tourniquet occludes the blood supply to the limb, the use is limited by time.

What general concerns might you have with tourniquet use?

These could be divided into pre-operative, intra-operative and post-operative.

Pre-operative considerations include sickle cell disease, poorly controlled or unstable cardiac failure, critical peripheral vascular ischaemia and the presence of deep venous thrombosis that could be dislodged to become pulmonary emboli. Patients with uncontrolled hypertension may have exaggerated responses to tourniquet-related haemodynamic changes.

Intra-operatively, the application of the tourniquet requires limb exsanguination which could precipitate ventricular over-load and pulmonary oedema. Padding is needed under the tourniquet to preserve skin integrity and prevent pressure injury but skin preparation can cause chemical burns if it soaks into the padding. There may be a hypertensive response to prolonged tourniquet inflation even under general anaesthesia. A dull aching tourniquet pain may be felt if the patient is awake, despite peripheral blockade. The total tourniquet inflation time should be limited to an absolute maximum of 2 hours to prevent permanent ischaemic damage.

Post-operatively, there is a haemodynamic and metabolic response when the tourniquet is deflated at the end of surgery and this, coupled with blood loss, may cause profound hypotension in the elderly. There is also the risk of tourniquet-related nerve injury from compression or shearing forces, hence pressures and times should not be excessive. This is usually temporary and it is often blamed on regional nerve blockade. The metabolic insult from the ischaemic limb may worsen already poor cardiac or renal function. Of most concern is the rare risk of irreversible ischaemia and limb loss. In very high-risk patients it may be appropriate to consider surgery without using a tourniquet and some surgeons routinely operate like this.

How is the tourniquet inflated?

Just describe what happens in theatre.

Before the tourniquet is inflated it is padded and the limb has to be exsanguinated by elevation or application of a rubber Esmarch bandage. This is not done in the presence of infection or tumour. The inflation pressure varies; an example is systolic blood pressure plus 50–100 mmHg for the arm and double the systolic pressure up to a maximum of 250 mmHg for the leg, but it should be adjusted according to the size and weight of the patients. For intravenous regional anaesthesia, it is about 100 mmHg above systolic pressure with a maximum of 250–300 mmHg.

What are the physiological effects of tourniquet inflation?

Exsanguination and inflation expands the central venous blood volume and increases the peripheral vascular resistance which causes a rise in central venous and arterial pressure. A rise in pulmonary artery pressure can be seen in people with extensive varicose veins or poor ventricular compliance. There is a temperature reduction in the non-perfused limb and the production of anaerobic metabolites after just a few minutes. From about an hour after inflation there is a rising blood pressure and a tachycardia that is usually resistant to treatment such as deepening of anaesthesia. This may be because of cellular ischaemia so vasodilators or clonidine can sometimes moderate the response.

What is tourniquet pain?

This can be felt by patients as an aching or burning pain in the distal limb about an hour after tourniquet inflation. Intra-venous analgesia does not always work and the only really effective method is to deflate the tourniquet temporarily. It may be related to the intensity of the block.

You choose to anaesthetise this patient using a spinal block with sedation. Things proceed well but it becomes a teaching case for the new orthopaedic registrar so surgery is prolonged. Shortly after the tourniquet is deflated and the sedation turned off, the patient becomes distressed and tachypnoeic.

What could be happening?

Consider differential diagnoses as well as relating your information to this specific case.

The respiratory distress is likely to be related to the release of the tourniquet given the timing. It may be that she has an exacerbation of a pre-existing condition such as cardiac failure or precipitation of a myocardial ischaemic event which could be contributed to by reperfusion effects. It could also be an embolic event such as a fat or pulmonary embolus. It is possible that a reaction to the cement has been delayed by having had a tourniquet inflated.

What do you know about tourniquet release and reperfusion syndrome?

Reperfusion injury syndrome is a paradoxical tissue injury after blood flow is restored after a period of ischaemia. Deflation leads to the limb being reperfused and so reversal of the effects seen with inflation. Therefore there is a drop in systemic vascular resistance, blood pressure, central venous pressure and heart rate. This hypotension is exacerbated by vasodilatation secondary to the anaerobic metabolites and increased carbon dioxide from the limb. End-tidal CO_2 increases, there is a reduced oxygen tension in blood from the limb and subsequently an increased oxygen consumption. The patient's core temperature falls and they develop a mixed acidosis. There is also an increase in intra-cellular calcium and extra-cellular potassium, cell swelling and free radicals and the limb becomes red which is due to a reactive hyperperfusion.

Hypoxia and hypotension may be possibly worsened by delayed cement implantation effects.

Does this matter?

Fit and healthy patients can tolerate this well but in the elderly who have a poor cardio-respiratory reserve, such as in this case, can suffer a depressant effect on myocardial contractility, producing ischaemia, hypoxia and hypotension.

Can the reperfusion effects be reduced or prevented?

This can be answered with common sense.

Use of a regional technique, with or without a general anaesthetic, may ease the metabolic effects. The use of total intra-venous anaesthesia rather than an inhalational anaesthetic might scavenge free radicals. Limiting the time that the tourniquet is inflated and using limits for inflation pressures should help minimise anaerobic metabolism. Maintaining physiological normality as much as possible (for instance blood pressure, temperature and hydration) puts the patient in the best position to recover. Hyperventilation, if ventilation is being controlled, can be used after tourniquet release to reduce end-tidal CO_2 and acidosis.

Do you know anything about free radicals and anti-oxidants in this situation?

You could extrapolate information from reperfusion injury to other tissues, e.g., myocardial injury.

Free radicals are produced as part of reperfusion injury. They are molecules with unpaired electrons and act as intermediaries in biological reactions, reducing oxygen to oxide ions. They are normally part of the body's defence system but in ischaemia the production overwhelms normal controls and causes cell damage such as oxidation of cell membrane lipids.

The free radicals are usually controlled by anti-oxidants like vitamin E or glutathione, which act as scavengers, or by superoxide dismutase. It has been suggested that administration of anti-oxidants may help to limit tissue injury in ischaemia, but this has mainly only been demonstrated in experimental models.

Are you aware of any clinical studies of this?

You may not be. Don't worry.

There has been a study suggesting that propofol administration may inhibit lipid peroxidation and restore anti-oxidant enzyme levels in extremity surgery that requires tourniquet application. Another looked at acetylcysteine and ischaemic preconditioning and found they do not decrease rhabdomyolysis related to the use of a pneumatic tourniquet and do not improve the post-operative muscle recovery. But they seemed to show a significant reduction in post-operative morphine consumption.

Are there any specific concerns to consider once your patient has been moved to the recovery room?

Relate these to the case to answer the question but also include relevant general post-operative considerations.

Specific to operations like this, when a tourniquet is deflated at the very end of surgery; I would be concerned that any reperfusion effects could potentially occur in the recovery room.

Another particular concern would be that of blood loss which may begin once the tourniquet has been deflated. It can be significant, particularly in the frail elderly. There could also be hidden loss in the tissues.

Other concerns relate to temperature control and pain management. Patients often get cold in orthopaedic theatres despite the use of warming devices. Patients' temperature must be monitored regularly and forced air warmers and fluid warmers used for all operations lasting longer than 30 minutes. Patients must be actively warmed in recovery if their temperature is less than 36°C, to avoid increased oxygen consumption from shivering and coagulation abnormalities.

Pain must also be well managed; however in this case the spinal block should still be in effect.

Further Reading

Deloughry JL, Griffiths R. Arterial tourniquets. *Continuing Education in Anaesthesia, Critical Care & Pain*. 2009; 9(2): 56–60. http://ceaccp.oxfordjournals.org/cgi/reprint/9/2/56?maxtoshow=&hits=10&RESULTFORMAT=&fulltext=tourniquets&searchid=1&FIRSTINDEX=0&resourcetype=HWCIT.

Kahraman S, Kilinc K, Dal D, Erdem K. Propofol attenuates formation of lipid peroxides in tourniquet-induced ischaemia-reperfusion injury. *British Journal of Anaesthesia*. 1997; 78(3): 279–281.

Orban JC, Levraut J, Gindre S, et al. Effects of acetylcysteine and ischaemic preconditioning on muscular function and postoperative pain after orthopaedic surgery using a pneumatic tourniquet. *European Journal of Anaesthesiology*. 2006; 23(12): 1025–1030.

Paediatric

2.8.1. Principles of neonatal physiology – Helen L Jewitt

This subject would lend itself well to a clinical science physiology structured oral exam or could be approached via a specific case scenario in the clinical structured oral exam. Don't be put off if you have little or no experience of anaesthetising neonates, a good understanding of the main principles and their relevance to anaesthetic practice will impress.

How does neonatal physiology differ from that of the adult?

Begin by discussing normal physiology in the term neonate. An opening statement is very useful to show that you understand the question and have a clear idea of how your answer will be subdivided. This question is best approached with a systems classification, ensuring the important physiological differences between neonates and older patients are presented in an organised way.

A neonate is defined as a child within 28 days of birth. There are many important physiological differences between neonates and older patients which have a significant impact on anaesthetic practice. These will be dealt with by a systems-based approach.

Start with the cardiovascular system as some of the most important factors of relevance to anaesthetic practice are found here.

Neonates have a higher heart rate and lower blood pressure in comparison to adults. An average heart rate of 120–180 bpm and average systolic blood pressure of 50–90 mmHg would be expected in a healthy neonate. The neonatal cardiovascular system is subject to increased demand and has a limited ability to respond to change as compared to an adult. The increased demand is a consequence of the neonate's need to maintain a stable body temperature via production of heat energy. This results in an oxygen consumption of 7 ml/kg/min which is twice that of an adult. Cardiovascular compensation is limited by the neonate's relatively fixed stroke volume. An increase in cardiac output is brought about largely by an increase in heart rate. Parasympathetic tone predominates and bradycardia is common, most importantly as a reflex response to hypoxia as well as vagal stimulation such as tracheal suction.

Dr. Podcast Scripts for the Final FRCA, ed. Rebecca A. Leslie, Emily K. Johnson, Gary Thomas and Alexander P. L. Goodwin.   Published by Cambridge University Press.
© R. A. Leslie, E. K. Johnson, G. Thomas and A. P. L. Goodwin 2011.

What is the circulating volume in a neonate, and what is the significance of this?

A circulating volume at birth of 90 ml/kg corresponds to a total blood volume of 300–400 ml in an average neonate. Intra-operative bleeding of apparently small volumes can rapidly lead to loss of a significant proportion of this total volume.

What is a "transitional circulation"?

This question tests your knowledge of the changes which take place around the time of delivery to convert the foetal circulation into neonatal circulation.

At birth massive cardiovascular changes take place. There are rapid changes in both systemic and pulmonary vascular resistance. During foetal life systemic vascular resistance is low due to the presence of the low resistance foeto-placental unit. Following clamping of the umbilical cord the systemic vascular resistance increases markedly. In contrast pulmonary vascular resistance is very high in the foetus and falls as the first breaths are taken. The foramen ovale closes under the influence of the pressure effect of increased venous return to the left atrium from the pulmonary circulation. The ductus arteriosus closes under the influence of the increased partial pressure of oxygen in the blood in the pulmonary artery. Closure of both ducts is initially functional only and is potentially reversible.

It is possible for a normal neonate to revert to a foetal pattern circulation in certain pathological circumstances. Hypoxia, hypercarbia and acidosis can cause constriction of the pulmonary vasculature, raising pulmonary vascular resistance. This can result in opening of the foramen ovale and ductus arteriosus with right to left shunting. This can lead to a self-perpetuating cycle of worsening hypoxia and worsening shunt. This is known as a transitional circulation or persistent foetal circulation.

What are the important factors to be considered in the respiratory system?

In the neonatal respiratory system there is incomplete development of the alveoli, fatiguable intercostal and accessory muscles and a compliant chest wall. The functional residual capacity is small because the compliant chest wall is pulled inwards by the elastic recoil of the lungs. Tidal volume lies close to or within the closing range and airway collapse readily occurs producing intra-pulmonary shunt and hypoxaemia. This can be reduced with the application of continuous positive airway pressure (CPAP). The horizontal alignment of the ribs in the neonate means they are unable to generate the "bucket handle" movement seen in inspiration in adults. Breathing is predominantly diaphragmatic and the diaphragm is prone to fatigue given the reduced number of type 1 "fatigue-resistant" muscle fibres. Raised abdominal pressures can splint the diaphragm and precipitate respiratory failure. Resting respiratory rate is high and increases further if respiratory compensation is required. The capacity for an increase in tidal volume is limited.

The ventilatory response to hypercapnia is poorly developed and not well sustained.

Neonates are obligate nose breathers therefore nasal obstruction of any cause can precipitate respiratory failure. This is seen in the congenital condition choanal atresia where there is membranous or bony obstruction of the posterior nasal cavity or in respiratory tract infections where the nasal passages are blocked with secretions.

How does the central nervous system of a neonate differ?

In the central nervous system development is incomplete at birth. Myelination begins prior to full gestation and continues throughout the first year of life.

Normal intra-cranial pressure is lower than that of adults at 2–4 mmHg. The skull is less rigid than that of an adult due the presence of unfused sutures and fontanelles. An increase in intra-cranial pressure can be compensated for to an extent by expansion of sutures and bulging of fontanelles.

Cerebral blood flow in neonates is higher than that in adults with autoregulation occurring at lower mean arterial pressure. In premature neonates autoregulation is absent and cerebral perfusion is pressure dependent.

The blood–brain barrier is more permeable leading to increased sensitivity to sedative agents such as opioids, barbiturates and benzodiazepines.

It was previously thought that the relative immaturity of the nervous system meant that neonates did not experience the sensation of pain. This has now been demonstrated to be incorrect with characteristic behavioural and physiological responses recognised in neonatal patients experiencing pain. These include tachycardia, hypertension, grimacing, crying and restlessness.

How is temperature regulation achieved in the neonate?

Neonates have very different mechanisms for maintenance of a stable body temperature. They lose heat readily due to a high surface area to weight ratio and are unable to shiver. Heat is produced by the metabolism of brown fat in a process known as non-shivering thermogenesis. Brown fat constitutes 5–6% of the body weight of a neonate and is located around the scapulae, kidneys and mediastinum. The metabolism of brown fat is sympathetically mediated and is a significant contributor to the high oxygen demand placed on the neonatal cardiorespiratory system. Thermogenesis by this mechanism is ablated by β-blockade.

Can you think of any issues of relevance to the renal system?

In common with the lungs and central nervous system, the kidneys continue to develop after birth. In the neonatal period there is a reduced glomerular filtration rate, reduced capacity to concentrate urine and reduced tubular function compared to adults. This results in a limited ability to either conserve water in the event of dehydration or to cope with excessive solute or solvent administration. Fluid balance must be carefully calculated based on weight, insensible and observed fluid losses and maintenance requirements.

The afferent arteriole in a neonate is sensitive to prostaglandins therefore NSAIDs are avoided as they produce vasoconstriction and decreased renal blood flow.

Are you aware of any adaptations required to drug doses in neonatal patients?

Total body water is proportionally increased in neonates compared to adults. Water-soluble drugs have a greater volume of distribution and higher doses may be needed to achieve the same clinical effect. An example of this is suxamethonium which has a dose of 2 mg/kg in neonates compared to 1 mg/kg in adults. Suxamethonium can have an effect on the muscarinic acetylcholine receptors at the sino-atrial node producing profound bradycardia and even asystole. This can be opposed by giving intra-venous atropine before the suxamethonium.

Enzyme pathways in the liver are not fully developed and this combined with renal immaturity can lead to delayed metabolism and excretion of drugs. This is reflected in a considerable prolongation of the half life of morphine due to a reduced ability to produce glucuronide conjugates.

Circulating levels of plasma proteins such as albumin and α-acid glycoprotein are reduced leading to a higher free fraction of some drugs such as local anaesthetics.

The neuromuscular junction in neonates is more susceptible to the effects of non-depolarising blocking agents suggesting that reduced doses may be needed. However the large extracellular volume increases the volume of distribution of these agents and the required dose is unchanged.

Further Reading

Gormley S, Crean P. Basic principles of anaesthesia for neonates and infants. *Continuing Education in Anaesthesia, Critical Care & Pain.* 2001; **1**(5): 130–133.

Desborough JP. The stress response to trauma and surgery. *British Journal of Anaesthesia.* 2000; **85**: 109–117.

2.8.2. Neonatal resuscitation and the effects of prematurity – Helen L Jewitt

How do you identify a newborn baby requiring resuscitation?

A newborn baby that is blue, pale or floppy with a heart rate of less than 100 bpm and poor or absent respiratory effort requires resuscitation.

Can you think of some factors that make a neonate more likely to require resuscitation following delivery?

In some situations the potential need for neonatal resuscitation can be anticipated. These include preterm births, delivery following foetal distress, meconium stained liquor and complications at the time of delivery such as shoulder dystocia or cord compression. Administration of general anaesthesia or opioid analgesia to the mother is also a risk factor. Rarely there may be an antenatal diagnosis of a congenital abnormality.

What are the steps in resuscitation of a neonate?

Neonatal resuscitation follows an airway, breathing, circulation approach in the same way as resuscitation of older children and adults. Although it is something that many anaesthetists will not have carried out in practice, a sound understanding of the Neonatal Resuscitation Guidelines will be expected.

The first step is to dry the baby and wrap it in warm dry towels. At the same time a rapid assessment of the baby can be made looking at colour, tone, respiratory effort and heart rate.

If the child is blue or has poor tone, inadequate respiratory effort or a slow heart rate, the next step is to open the airway. The child's head should remain in a neutral position with a jaw thrust to optimise the patency of the airway. The neck should not be extended as this can obstruct the airway.

Five inflation breaths should then be supplied. Resuscitation can be commenced with air but oxygen should be immediately available in the event that the infant does not rapidly respond. The guidelines state that each breath should be maintained for 2–3 seconds at a pressure of 30 cmH$_2$O.

You can anticipate the next question … how will you know what the pressure is? How would you be able to estimate it?

N.B. Pop-off valve on neonatal self-inflating bag will release pressure at roughly 20 cmH$_2$O so you may need to hold the valve closed initially.

If the infant is being resuscitated on a resuscitaire there is a pressure gauge to measure the pressure applied with each inflation breath. In practice ensure that sufficient pressure is applied to inflate the infant's chest. In preterm infants there is a deficiency of surfactant in the lungs and a greater pressure will initially be required to overcome surface tension forces at first. When the lungs have expanded and the FRC has been established, less pressure will be required subsequently.

After this step, reassessment of colour, tone, respiratory effort and heart rate should take place.

If the finding is of a heart rate of greater than 100 bpm but absent respiratory effort mask ventilation at a rate of 30–40 per minute should continue until the baby is breathing effectively. If there is chest expansion with the inflation breaths but the heart rate fails to recover to more than 60 bpm then chest compressions should be commenced. These are best delivered with two hands encircling the neonate's chest and compressions delivered with two thumbs. The ratio of compressions to breaths is 3:1.

Heart rate should be reassessed at 30-second intervals. If there is no improvement in the situation it is vital to ensure that effective breaths are being delivered by checking that there is obvious chest expansion.

If the neonate remains unresponsive despite the above steps consideration should be given to drugs and intubation.

What would be an appropriate size endotracheal tube in a term neonate?

For an average sized neonate an endotracheal tube with an internal diameter of 3.5 mm would be appropriate.

It is important to be alert for profound bradycardia due to vagal stimulation during laryngoscopy. Atropine at a dose of 10–20 mcg/kg should be immediately available for intravenous administration.

How can you obtain intravascular access in a neonate?

IV access may be achieved via an umbilical vein, but this requires a catheter in situ, as it needs a catheter long enough to reach central circulation. In this situation, immediate intra-osseous access would be preferable.

What rhythm would you expect to see on the monitor in a neonatal cardio-respiratory arrest?

During this type of scenario it is extremely rare that the cardiac rhythm is anything other than asystole resulting from hypoxia. An exception to this is in infants with congenital heart disease. In this event shockable rhythms may rarely be encountered. In this event 4.5-cm diameter pads should be applied to the infant in anterior and posterior positions. Energy of 4 J/kg is appropriate.

A 10-week-old male infant presents for inguinal herniotomy. He was delivered prematurely at 32 weeks gestation. What are the anaesthetic implications of prematurity?

It is not expected that all candidates will have direct experience of anaesthetising preterm infants but the examiner will look for a good theoretical understanding of neonatal anaesthesia and the specific problems of anaesthetising premature infants.

An opening statement shows that you have organised your thoughts.

This case raises the general problems common to anaesthetising neonates in addition to the issues specific to preterm infants.

Use a systems approach to tackle the general issues of neonatal anaesthesia.

The cardiovascular system of a neonate has limited capability to increase cardiac output as stroke volume is relatively fixed. Compensation is achieved by an increase in heart rate. Neonatal oxygen consumption is twice that of an adult largely because of the energy required to generate heat and maintain a constant body temperature. The functional residual capacity is small and is exceeded by closing capacity. The combination of high oxygen demand and a limited reservoir in the FRC means that rapid desaturation takes place. Neonates are unable to significantly increase their tidal volume and an increase in minute volume is produced by increasing respiratory rate. Inspiration is predominantly driven by the diaphragm, with weak intercostal and accessory muscles. Abdominal distension due to bag and mask ventilation or intra-abdominal pathology can severely impair respiration.

The kidneys of a neonate are not fully developed and they show impaired concentrating ability and tubular function. For this reason both dehydration and excessive fluid loads are poorly tolerated.

Hepatic enzymatic pathways are not fully active at birth therefore the metabolism of some drugs may be prolonged.

Neonates are very susceptible to the effects of sedative drugs such as benzodiazepines, barbiturates and opioids. This is due to an immature blood–brain barrier and delayed hepatic inactivation of the drug.

Now move on to the problems specific to anaesthetising a preterm infant.

In addition to these general issues there are a number of additional concerns relevant in infants born prematurely.

A full history must be obtained from the parents of the infant and review of the medical notes. Particularly important information includes post-conceptual age at delivery, current post-conceptual age and complications since delivery such as the need for intubation, CPAP or supplemental oxygen.

Preterm infants have thin skin and limited subcutaneous fat stores and are very vulnerable to losing heat. They should be minimally exposed for the duration of the procedure, with the use of active warming methods such as overhead radiant heaters.

Hepatic immaturity in preterm infants means that glycogen stores are limited and hypoglycaemia can readily occur. Pre-operative fasting times should be minimised and intravenous fluids should contain dextrose as well as electrolytes.

Post-operative apnoea is common in infants of less than 60 weeks post-conceptual age. These infants should be monitored in a neonatal unit or high-dependency area where continuous apnoea monitoring can be used.

What do you know about retinopathy of prematurity? How can the risk be minimised?

Retinopathy of prematurity is due to abnormal development of blood vessels in the neonatal retina. These vessels can invade the vitreous humour and are prone to haemorrhage causing scarring and detachment of the retina. Prematurity is the greatest risk factor for this problem but it is exacerbated by the administration of high levels of oxygen. For this reason oxygen saturations should be maintained around 90% for the duration of the procedure.

Remember it is PO_2 rather than SpO_2 that is important. Pulse oximetry cannot detect hyperoxia. Neonates have foetal haemoglobin and saturations of 90% are quite safe.

Serial "arterialised" capillary blood samples (taken from warm, well-perfused skin on, for example, the heel) can be used to track PO_2. Use a purpose-made lancet to prick the skin, not a hypodermic needle.

Further Reading

Gormley S, Crean P. Basic principles of anaesthesia for neonates and infants. *Continuing Education in Anaesthesia, Critical Care & Pain.* 2001; 1(5): 130–133.

2.8.3. Development in infancy and childhood – Sarah F Bell

The developmental changes that occur during infancy and childhood have significant implications to the anesthetist. They are regularly examined in the clinical and science structured oral exam. A good understanding of the anatomical and physiological changes is vital.

Let's start by classifying the different ages of paediatric patients. Can you tell me how we decide when a neonate has become an infant or child?

Yes. A neonate is a baby within 44 weeks from the date of conception. This description therefore includes premature babies and full-term babies up to 1 month old. An infant is described as being over 44 weeks post-conceptual age and up to 12 months. A child is aged 1 to 12 years, an adolescent is 13 to 16 and an adult is over 16.

Good. That will help us to further describe the changes that occur during development. How might you classify these changes?

The changes may be divided into physiological and anatomical alterations. They may be further subdivided into the body systems.

Can you talk me through the anatomical differences between a paediatric and adult patient that occur in the respiratory system? Why are these important to the anaesthetist?

It might help to remember everything by starting at the head and then working your way down the respiratory system.

The infant has a large head with a prominent occiput. The neck is short and the mandible relatively small. The tongue and epiglottis are large, which can predispose to airway obstruction.

The larynx is at the level of the third or fourth cervical vertebrae in infants. This is high when compared to the adult level of the fifth or sixth cervical vertebrae. The higher position of the larynx and shape of the epiglottis mean that it may be easier to intubate an infant with a straight laryngoscope blade rather than a curved blade.

The narrowest part of the paediatric airway is the cricoid cartilage, rather than the vocal cords as in the adult. This has led to the use of uncuffed tubes for children less than 10 years old, since the cricoid acts as a cuff. Uncuffed tubes are thought to reduce the risk of barotrauma to the tracheal lumen. The size of tracheal tube for a neonate is approximately 3–3.5 mm, although this may vary. A small leak should always be present to ensure minimal risk of trauma to the tracheal lining. The formula for guiding tracheal tube size is age divided by 4, plus 4.

The trachea may be less than 4 cm in length in the neonate. This can lead to endobronchial intubation if the anesthetist is not meticulous when positioning and securing the endo-tracheal tube. The formula for the length of an oral tracheal tube is age divided by 2 plus 12. This gives the length at the lips. For nasal tubes the number to add is 15 rather than 12.

The carina branches at the same angle on both sides of the chest in infants. The airways are also much smaller in diameter than in adults. Any additional narrowing will lead to a marked increase in resistance to air flow.

In infants, the intercostal muscles and diaphragm are weaker, with fewer type I fibres. They therefore fatigue faster than adults. The diaphragm is the main muscle responsible for respiration and so anything that compromises its efficiency (such as abdominal distension) will cause breathing difficulties. The chest wall is also more compliant and so recession is a marker of respiratory effort.

What about the physiological changes that occur in the respiratory system?

Paediatric patients have higher oxygen consumption than adults. A neonate has an oxygen consumption of 6–9 ml/kg/min when compared to the adult 2–3 ml/kg/min. The alveolar minute volume is increased in order to meet this increased demand. Since the tidal volume of approximately 7 ml/kg is similar for paediatric and adult patients the increase is achieved by changes in respiratory rate. A neonate's respiratory rate ranges from 40 to 60 breaths/min, a child's 20–30 and the adult range is 12 to 24 breaths/min.

The significant difference in oxygen consumption means that neonates will desaturate faster than adults.

Can you talk me through the changes in functional residual capacity and closing capacity?

The functional residual capacity is similar for paediatric and adult patients. The value is about 30 ml/kg. In infants, neonates and young children closing capacity encroaches on the functional residual capacity, leading to airway closure at end-expiration. In order to counteract this, partial adduction of the cords occurs during expiration, producing physiological CPAP. When anaesthetising an infant or young child using a spontaneously breathing technique,

CPAP will aid oxygenation and reduce the work of breathing. When a paediatric patient is fully ventilated, the respiratory rate and tidal volume should be set appropriately. PEEP can be used to avoid airway closure and improve oxygenation.

What can you tell me about the control of respiration in a neonate or young infant?

The neonatal respiratory control is immature. The peripheral chemoreceptor response to hypoxia and the central chemoreceptor response to carbon dioxide are both weak and blunted. Apnoeas may occur up to 60 weeks post-gestational age. Patients under this age need to be monitored post-operatively with an apnoea monitor.

Now, let's move on to the cardiovascular system. Can you briefly summarise the changes that occur at birth?

This topic has been discussed in the neonatal physiology section, so we have only covered it briefly here. Try and talk through the changes as they occur so that the examiner knows that you have a strong grasp of the basics.

At birth the site of gas transfer switches from the placenta to the lungs. As the first breath is taken the lungs expand and the pulmonary vascular resistance falls by 80%. Pulmonary blood flow increases dramatically. The systemic vascular resistance increases due to the exclusion of the large, low-resistance placental vascular bed when the umbilical cord is clamped. The foramen ovale closes because of the reversal of the pressure gradient between the left and right ventricles. Blood flow through the ductus arteriosus is reversed due to the reduction in pulmonary resistance and increase in systemic vascular resistance. The increase in the partial pressure of oxygen and reduction in prostaglandin E2 stimulates closure of the ductus arteriosus.

Over what time period do the foramen ovale and ductus arteriosus close?

The foramen ovale closes as soon as the pressures reverse within the heart but it can reopen within the next five years of life. The ductus arteriosus contracts in the first few days of life and then fibroses within a month.

Can you tell me about the anatomical and physiological changes that occur in the cardiovascular system during child development?

The neonatal heart has non-compliant, stiff ventricles. At birth the right and left ventricles are similar in size.

The cardiac output is high to meet the high oxygen consumption. In a neonate cardiac output is 200–250 ml/kg/min compared to 80 ml/kg/min in an adult. Stroke volume is relatively fixed and so the only way to increase the cardiac output is by increasing the heart rate. The average heart rate in the neonate is 120 beats/min, falling to 100 in childhood and 75 as an adult.

The blood pressure is lower in the paediatric population. A neonate would have a systolic pressure of 50 to 90 mmHg and a child a systolic pressure of between 95 and 110 mmHg.

Bradycardias are tolerated poorly in paediatric patients due to the concomitant fall in cardiac output.

What about the hematological system?

The blood volume is greater in a neonate than an adult. The neonate value is approximately 90 ml/kg, falling to 80 ml/kg in a child and then 70 ml/kg in an adult.

Extra-cellular fluid is greater in the neonate: 40% of body water is extra-cellular in the neonate compared to about 20% in the adult. By the age of 2 this difference has disappeared. The greater metabolic rate results in a faster turnover of extra-cellular fluid in the neonate and infant. Interruptions in normal intake can lead to the rapid onset of dehydration.

How would you approach fluid management in a child?

I would consider fluids in terms of maintenance, replacement and deficit.

With regards to maintenance fluids I would use the 4, 2, 1 rule. This means for the first 10 kg weight the child will require 4 ml/kg/hr, for the next 10 kg 2 ml/kg/hr and for every subsequent 10 kg 1 ml/kg/hr.

Replacement fluid includes all ongoing losses. These losses should be closely monitored, for example weighing swabs and measuring suction fluid. For abdominal surgery approximately 10 ml/kg/hr is lost.

Calculation of the fluid deficit requires clinical assessment of the child. A 5% loss might present as dry skin and muous membranes. A 10% loss would lead to cool peripheries, depressed fontanelle and oliguria. A 15% loss would lead to changes in conscious level and hypotension. Replacement is calculated as 10 ml/kg multiplied by the percentage deficit. This should be given over 24 hours.

What fluids might not be appropriate for children?

This question is testing to see whether you are aware of any changes in practice due to safety alerts.

Hypotonic fluids, such as 0.18% sodium chloride with 4% glucose, are no longer recommended for paediatric patients. This report highlighted the link between hyponatraemia and serious injury or death in patients receiving these solutions. Surgery, pain and dehydration all stimulate ADH release which increases water reuptake and worsens the risk of fatal hyponatraemia.

Despite this advice, dextrose solutions do need to be given to neonates or children below the third centile for weight, since they are at risk of severe hypoglycaemia. Close monitoring of blood glucose and sodium levels are required in these cases.

Can you tell me anything about haemoglobin in neonates?

The foetal oxyhaemoglobin curve is shifted to the left due to a reduction in 2,3-DPG. It is therefore better suited to take up oxygen at the lower partial pressures present in the placenta (but oxygen is also less readily released). In order to maintain oxygenation to the tissues the neonate has a high hemoglobin concentration of about 17 g/dl, the blood volume is increased and the cardiac output is high.

A physiological anaemia occurs at about 3 months when foetal haemoglobin is replaced by adult HbA.

When might you consider transfusing a bleeding infant?

Generally I would give blood if the haematocrit fell to less than 25%, or the estimated blood loss was greater than 20% of the blood volume.

What about changes that occur to clotting factors and platelets?

The vitamin K dependent clotting factors 2, 7, 9 and 10 are deficient in the first few months. Therefore vitamin K is given to newborn babies. Platelet function is also reduced.

Why are neonates and infants at risk of hypothermia?

The paediatric patient is at risk of hypothermia due to increased heat loss and poor compensatory mechanisms. Heat is lost by thermal conduction from thin skin and lower levels of body fat. A high body surface area to weight ratio and increased minute ventilation further contribute to the loss. Infants less than three months old undergo non-shivering thermogenesis. Production of heat from brown fat is inefficient and actually increases oxygen consumption. In older infants and children, shivering is ineffective due to limited muscle mass. Vasoconstriction is also poor.

Why is this important to the anaesthetist?

This question could also lead onto the effects of hypothermia. This is covered in the hypothermia section, and only a brief summary given in the following answer.

It is vital to pay careful attention to temperature and warming since hypothermia can cause large increases in oxygen consumption and detrimental effects on cardiac output, nervous and hematological systems. As anaesthetists we can avoid this by monitoring body temperature and considering: covering, avoiding exposure, increasing ambient temperatures, heating covers, warming fluids, HMEs and circle breathing systems.

Can you tell me about any changes that occur in the central nervous system?

In neonates and infants the anterior fontanelle may be used to assess the intracranial pressure. This ossifies by about 18 months.

The cerebral blood flow is lower in a neonate (about 50 ml/100 g/min). It then rises significantly in childhood (to about 100 ml/100 g/min) before returning to the lower levels during adulthood. Cerebral oxygen consumption is also much higher during childhood reaching values of 5.8 ml/100 g/min compared to adult levels of 3.5 ml/100 g/min.

The blood–brain barrier is incomplete at birth. The volume of CSF, is proportionally larger in infants than adults (4 rather than 2 ml/kg). At term, the spinal cord terminates at L3. It then recedes to L1/2 by adolescence. The sacral hiatus is large and not ossified, making it an attractive location for caudal anaesthesia.

Myelination is incomplete until 1–3 years. The sympathetic nervous system is not fully developed until 6 years and so bradycardias are relatively common.

How do the actions of general anaesthetic agents differ in the paediatric patient?

With regards to the inhalation agents, both induction and emergence are more rapid due to the greater alveolar ventilation. MAC is reduced in neonates, whilst in infants and children it increases by up to 30% of that of adults.

In neonates the immature blood-brain barrier and reduced metabolism leads to increased sensitivity to barbiturates and opioids. Reduced doses are therefore required. In older children higher doses are needed.

Propofol infusions are not licensed for children below 3 years due to reports of neuro, cardiac, renal and hepatic impairment.

Do the muscle relaxants also have different effects?

Neonates and infants have increased sensitivity to muscle relaxants at the neuro-muscular junction. A similar loading dose to adults needs to be given due to dilution of the drug by the larger volume of distribution. The reduced GFR, clearance and increased sensitivity leads to prolonged effects.

What can you tell me about the changes to the renal system?

The glomerular filtration rate and renal blood flow are low at birth and gradually increase. The kidney initially has limited concentrating ability and mechanisms to maintain fluid, electrolyte and acid–base homeostasis. Values reach adult by about 12 months. Infants cannot handle large water or sodium loads. Urine output is normally 1–2 ml/kg/hr.

And what about the liver?

At birth the vitamin K dependent clotting factors are low as are glucose storage levels.

Physiological jaundice may occur in the neonate due to increased red blood cell breakdown with limited ability to metabolise unconjugated bilirubin.

Phase 1 and 2 reactions take 2–3 months to reach full activity.

Can you give me some guidelines for fasting for the paediatric patient?

The current guidelines in my hospital are that no food should be consumed for 6 hours preceding the operation, including formula and cow's milk. No breast milk should be taken for 4 hours and no clear liquid for 2 hours.

Finally, what psychological changes might occur and how might they affect the anaesthetist?

In infants less than 6 months no separation anxiety occurs. From 6 months to 4 years behaviour is unpredictable and separation anxiety is seen. It is important to try and keep the carer with the patient as much as possible. School children are upset by the thought of the surgical procedure, its mutilating effects and pain. We need to bear this in mind when explaining the induction, operation and post-operative analgesia.

With regards to adolescents they find the loss of control and thought of pain upsetting. Their reliance on a carer is varied.

It is important to use the pre-operative visit as an opportunity to assess the child and take time to build up a rapport with both them and their carers.

Further Reading

National Patient Safety Agency. Reducing the risk of hyponatraemia when administering intra-venous infusions to children. *NPSA* 2007; **22**. http://www.nrls.npsa.nhs.uk/resources/?entryid45=59809.

2.8.4. Pyloric stenosis – Sarah F Bell and Caroline SG Janes

This would generally form part of a clinical structured oral exam. The biochemical abnormalities are frequently asked, so make sure that you can explain them thoroughly.

What is congenital hypertrophic pyloric stenosis?

Pyloric stenosis is a congenital narrowing of the gastric outflow tract caused by hypertrophy of the circular pyloric muscle. The cause is unknown but there is a genetic predisposition.

The condition occurs in 1 in 500 births. It is the most frequent cause of intestinal obstruction in infancy and the commonest small baby condition treated outside a specialist centre. Boys are affected much more than girls, with a ratio of 4 to 1. A total of 40% to 60% of cases occur in first-born children. The condition is also more common in the white population.

Pyloric stenosis can also be acquired in adults as a result of gastric carcinoma or chronic peptic ulceration. These conditions will not be discussed in this podcast.

How does pyloric stenosis present?

The patient usually presents at 4 to 6 weeks of age with worsening symptoms of persistent, projectile, non-bilious vomiting. The infant typically feeds well but then vomits after each feed. The infant will be hungry and may have lost weight.

On examination a hard mass may be palpable. This is classically 1–2 cm in diameter and located in the right upper quadrant at the lateral edge of rectus abdominus muscle. The infant is often dehydrated.

What might arterial blood gas and urinalysis show?

Arterial blood gas will demonstrate a marked metabolic alkalosis with hypokalaemia and hypochloraemia.

Urinalysis will show acidic urine with high levels of potassium.

How can the blood gas results be explained?

This is complicated. Try and keep your explanation simple. By talking through the gastrointestinal changes followed by the renal compensation and then the respiratory alterations you will be able to remember all the key facts.

The blood gas results are due to a combination of gastrointestinal, renal and respiratory changes.

With regards to the gastrointestinal system, it is important to know the components of the gastric and small bowel secretions and the differences between normal vomiting and vomiting in pyloric stenosis. Gastric fluid is rich in hydrogen chloride. This is neutralised by the bicarbonate ions secreted by the small bowel. In normal vomiting there is mixing of gastric and small bowel fluid. There is therefore no change in the plasma pH but fluid and electrolyte loss will lead to dehydration. In pyloric stenosis the vomit does not contain bicarbonate due to pyloric obstruction preventing mixing. There is therefore only hydrogen and chloride ion loss.

Due to these biochemical changes, the kidney is presented with a large bicarbonate load. This exceeds the absorptive threshold and so alkaline urine is initially seen.

Prolonged vomiting leads to hypovolaemia and dehydration. This causes activation of the renin-angiotensin-aldosterone axis in an attempt to restore circulating volume. The aldosterone acts on the kidney to retain sodium at the expense of potassium and hydrogen ions. This leads to the production of paradoxical acid urine and worsening hypokalaemia and metabolic alkalosis.

The infant may attempt to compensate for the metabolic alkalosis by using the respiratory system. They may hypoventilate to produce hypercapnia, but this will never be sufficient to correct the alkalosis as the hypoxic drive will be triggered.

What other biochemical or haematological changes might be seen?

Hypoglycaemia, haemoconcentration, mild uraemia and unconjugated hyperbilirubinaemia may be seen.

A 5-week-old infant is brought into your hospital and diagnosed with pyloric stenosis. He is moderately dehydrated. Arterial blood gases demonstrate a pH 7.6, chloride of 80 mmol/L and potassium of 3.0 mmol/L. The bicarbonate ion concentration is 32 mmol/L. The child was born at term by normal vaginal delivery. There are no other cases on the emergency list and the surgeon is keen to proceed as soon as possible.

What are the issues with this case?

There are a number of issues with this case. These can be divided into problems specific to the pyloric stenosis and the general problems with anaesthetising a young infant.

With regards to the issues relating specifically to the condition these include: the markedly deranged acid–base status, the effects of dehydration and the increased risk of regurgitation due to the obstruction. Pyloric stenosis correction is not an emergency. The infant should be fully resuscitated and the electrolyte abnormalities corrected prior to surgical intervention.

The challenges of anaesthetising a small infant include the altered anatomy and physiology, the presence of anxious parents, difficultly obtaining intra-venous access and the altered drug dosages.

This case should be undertaken with the support of a Consultant Anaesthetist experienced in paediatric anaesthesia.

How would you go about resuscitating this infant?

The infant needs to be resuscitated in an area where the nursing staff are trained in the management of these complex cases. This might be a paediatric surgical ward or high-dependency unit. The parents should be with the infant whenever possible.

I would assess the degree of dehydration and obtain intravenous access. A full blood count, renal function tests, liver function tests and group and hold should be sent, along with blood gases. These will aid the resuscitation and help to decide on the required potassium supplementation. Regular blood gases will help to ascertain the success of resuscitation.

A nasogastric tube should be placed to remove the gastric residue and four hourly washouts performed.

Regular observations need to be taken. These include respiratory rate, oxygen saturations, heart rate, blood pressure, conscious level, urine output and ongoing gastric losses.

How would you assess the degree of dehydration in this infant?

Assessment can be divided into history and examination. In my history I would ask the parents how much the infant had been vomiting and how much he had been taking orally. I would ask about any diarrhoea and whether the infant had been febrile. I would also enquire about whether the parents had noticed a change in how often the infant was wetting his nappy and whether they had observed any change in the infant's alertness or conscious level.

I would examine the infant looking for dry muous membranes, a sunken fontanelle and eyes, tachycardia, hypotension, decreased conscious level and prolonged capillary refill time. As an estimate, 5% dehydration might present as dry skin and muous membranes; 10% loss would lead to cool peripheries, depressed fontanelle and oliguria; 15% loss would lead to changes in conscious level and hypotension.

How would you approach fluid management in this case?

Fluid management can be divided into resuscitation fluids, maintenance fluids and ongoing losses.

Resuscitation fluids should be calculated by assessing the degree of dehydration. The volume of fluid required to replace this can then be calculated by multiplying the percentage dehydration by the weight of the infant multiplied by ten. Hartmanns' solution or 0.9% N saline are both appropriate fluids. Half of the fluid deficit should be corrected within the first 24 hours followed by half over the second 24 hours.

In addition to this, maintenance fluids are given. This may also be Hartmann's solution or 0.45% saline with 5% dextrose. The four – two – one rule can be used to decide the amount of fluid to give per hour to a paediatric patient. Four millilitres per kilogram is given for the first 10 kg of body weight of the infant, followed by 2 ml/kg for the second 10 kg body weight and then 1 ml/kg for each following 10 kg.

What is this regimen based on?

This regimen is based on the amount of water required to give formula feed orally, on the assumption that the required calorie intake is 100 kcal per kg per day. The water supplied is in excess of actual maintenance requirements. The calculation relies on good renal function to excrete the excess water. Outside the neonatal period, hypoglycaemia is rare but water load can be a problem. It may be preferable to use 0.9% N saline with added glucose of 5 or 10%, checking frequently for hyperglycaemia.

Do you know how much potassium you would expect to add to the maintenance fluids?

The 3 mmol/kg/24 hour of potassium should be added to the maintenance fluids, as guided by regular blood gas analysis.

When would you be happy to proceed with anaesthesia?

I would want the infant to be normovolaemic and so I would be satisfied once the infant had had two wet nappies. If the infant had been catheterised I would aim for a urine output of 1–2 ml/kg/hr.

Blood chloride concentration should be above 95 mmol/L. The alkalosis will not be totally corrected until chloride exceeds 105 mmol/L and so I would accept a pH less than 7.5 with a base excess less than 6 mmol/L. I would want the bicarbonate concentration to be below 30 mmol/L and the potassium concentration to be within the normal range.

How long does a pyloromyotomy take and how is it performed?

This procedure tends to take about 30 minutes to an hour. It may be performed open or laparoscopically. Laparoscopic surgery on infants is generally only performed in specialist centres.

How would you anaesthetise this infant?

A senior, experienced, paediatric anaesthetist should be present.

Prior to induction I would aspirate the nasogastric tube, attempting to suction all four quadrants of the stomach by moving the infant.

Both inhalational and rapid sequence inductions with and without cricoid pressure have been described. An adequate dose of muscle relaxant should be given.

I would secure the airway with an appropriately sized, uncuffed, endotracheal tube. A size 3.5-mm tube would probably be adequate for this infant, but I would have a 3-mm and 4-mm sizes available. I would then hand ventilate the infant, before connecting to a either an Ayre's T-piece or paediatric circle system using pressure-controlled ventilation.

Paracetamol, local anaesthetic infiltration and opioids can be given for analgesia.

The paracetamol can be given intra-venously at a dose of 7.5 mg/kg every 4–6 hours to a maximum of 30 mg/kg in 24 hours. Suppositories are available and the dose is 30 mg/kg loading followed by 20mg/kg every 8 hours, to a maximum of 60 mg in 24 hours. The smallest suppository is 60 mg then 125 mg and 250 mg. The infant would therefore need to be at least 2 kg to be able to receive the smallest rectal dose of paracetamol (you cannot cut the suppository because the active drug may not be distributed evenly throughout the wax).

The dose of local anaesthetic needs to be calculated depending on the size of the infant. If bupivicaine is used, the dose is 2 mg/kg. Local infiltration can be performed by the surgeons.

Morphine can be given intra-venously at a dose of 200 µg/kg, but this is not often required.

The nasogastric tube can be removed at the end of surgery and the infant should be extubated in the left lateral position.

What would be your post-op instructions for the infant?

Due to the potential risk of post-operative apnoeas up to 60 weeks post-gestational age, the infant should be monitored with an apnoea alarm and oxygen saturation probe.

Feeding can be started about six hours after the operation, unless the bowel mucosa has been breached. Intra-venous maintenance fluids should be continued until feeding is established. The first feed should be clear fluid.

I would prescribe regular paracetamol for analgesia.

How can you assess pain in paediatric patients?

Pain assessment can be difficult in children due to communication and behavioural challenges. Specific pain assessment tools have therefore been developed for paediatric patients.

Assessment should be performed regularly with the support of the parents. Since pain is a subjective experience, it is important to seek the child's self-report of pain whenever possible.

Neonatal assessment uses a combination of physiological and behavioural markers including: facial expression, body and limb movements, cry, sleeplessness, cardiovascular and respiratory changes. Examples of tools available are the Neonatal and Infant Pain Scale (NIPS) and the Neonatal Pain Agitation and Sedation Score (N-PASS).

Infant assessment is also purely observational. Behavioural pain indicators include: facial expression, irritability, unusual posture, screaming, sobbing or whimpering, reluctance to move, increased clinginess, loss of appetite and disturbed sleep pattern. Examples of tools available are the Face, Legs, Activity, Cry and Consolatility scale (FLACC) and the Objective Pain Score (OPS).

Pre-school children may be able to self-report pain when given appropriate tools; for example, "Faces" is a face-based scale with happy to crying faces to represent the pain scale.

School children can usually communicate pain severity and location. They understand numerical concepts and so may use numerical rating scales. Other tools include faces, colour based scales and visual analogue scales.

Finally, adolescents can communicate pain severity, location and intensity and can use visual analogue scales or numerical rating scales

2.8.5. Intussusception – Sarah F Bell and Caroline SG Janes

What is intussusception?

Intussusception is caused by the small bowel telescoping, as if it were swallowing itself. This usually occurs at the ileocaecal junction. Intussusception can lead to venous congestion, bowel oedema and intestinal obstruction.

What age group tend to present with this condition?

Intussusception occurs predominantly in infants and young children. Fifty per cent of cases occur in infants and only 10% of cases occur in children older than five.

Is intussusception seen more in boys or girls?

The condition is seen more often in boys.

What are the causes of intussusception?

Ninety per cent of cases are idiopathic. Intussusception is the most common cause of intestinal obstruction in the first year of life. In children over one, intussusception may be the first presentation for a number of pathologies such as Meckel's diverticulum, intestinal polyp, lymphoma, haemolytic uraemic syndrome, Henoch scholein purpura or Peutz Jegher's syndrome.

Can intussusception recur?

Yes, the recurrence rate is 5%.

Now let's review a case. An 8-month-old boy has been admitted to your hospital. His mother says that he has been intermittently crying and pulling his legs up to his chest for the past 2 days. She found a redcurrant jelly-like stool in his last nappy. He has vomited occasionally, and she has noticed that his nappies have not been wet the last few times she changed them.

Your examination reveals a quiet, pale baby. His heart rate is 150 beats per minute and capillary refill time is 4 seconds. His abdomen appears distended and the infant cries when you examine him.

How might an infant with intussusception present?

The classical features are of paroxysmal abdominal pain and blood and mucus in the stool. This is sometimes described as having a "red currant jelly" appearance. The infant has episodes of inconsolable crying and drawing up its legs. Vomiting and dehydration may be evident, potentially leading to shock. Abdominal distension can cause respiratory compromise. Infection, bowel infarction, bleeding and perforation may all occur.

On examination, a sausage-shaped mass may be palpable in the right side of the abdomen. The abdomen may be distended with guarding or rigidity. The child may be profoundly shocked.

What would be your differential diagnosis for this history?

The infant is most likely to be suffering from a gastrointestinal condition. Intussusception with dehydration and possible sepsis would be my main diagnosis. I would also consider gastroenteritis.

How do you diagnose intussusception?

Diagnosis is made from the history and examination and then investigations. The investigation of choice is an abdominal ultrasound. An air enema can be diagnostic as well as curative in up to 70% of cases. This intervention is contraindicated if a patient is in shock, has peritonitis or has perforated.

An abdominal X-ray may aid the confirmation of bowel obstruction and possible perforation.

How would you treat intussusception if air enema has failed?

The patient will need either a laparotomy or laparoscopy. Any necrotic bowel found will need to be resected.

Would you advise air enema or surgical intervention in this case?

This infant has evidence of shock because he has tachycardia, increased capillary refill time, reduced urine output and conscious level. The infant should be resuscitated as a matter of urgency and an emergency laparotomy should then be performed.

How would you resuscitate this infant and prepare them for theatre?

Try and describe the resuscitation as you would actually do it. This will hopefully help you remember everything!

Resuscitation should either be performed in a high-dependency unit or in the anaesthetic room or recovery area prior to theatre. I would obtain intra-venous access and send bloods for full blood count, urea and electrolytes, liver function tests and crossmatch. I would regularly monitor the vital signs of the infant including the respiratory rate, oxygen saturations, heart rate, blood pressure, capillary refill, urine output and conscious level.

Fluid resuscitation is vital. I would give fluid boluses of 0.9% N saline, 20 ml/kg body weight to restore the circulating volume. After each bolus I would reassess the infant to see whether further fluid was required. My reassessment would consist of reviewing the observations of the infant and looking at the capillary refill and conscious level. The blood pressure might be maintained due to tachycardia and co-existing pain.

In addition to resuscitation fluids, I would give maintenance fluids calculated from the weight of the patient. Hartmann's solution can be used to provide this. If the blood results revealed any severe abnormalities in the urea and electrolytes then I would start correcting these prior to theatre.

I would place a NG tube, aspirate the stomach contents and then place the tube on free drainage.

If the infant's respiration were inadequate due to either the diaphragmatic splinting from abdominal distension or the effects of severe shock, I would consider intubating and ventilating the infant. This could be done in theatre.

How would you induce anaesthesia in this infant?

I would anaesthetise this infant with the support of a Consultant paediatric anaesthetist. A general anaesthetic with endotracheal intubation and ventilation is required.

Prior to induction I would ensure that the infant had been adequately resuscitated. I would suction the NG tube and preoxygenate the infant. I would obtain monitoring as per the AAGBI standards and have all my drugs for resuscitation and induction available.

The options for induction of general anaesthesia are a gas or intra-venous induction. I would prefer a rapid sequence induction with cricoid pressure. I would use thiopentone to induce the infant and then give muscle relaxant. This could be either suxamethonium or an adequate dose of non-depolarising muscle relaxant such as rocuronium 1 mg/kg. I would then intubate the infant with a straight blade and pass an uncuffed endotracheal tube. I would check the position of the tube by auscultating the chest, observing the capnography trace and checking the length at the lips. Provided the tube was inserted easily and not too tight I would not require a leak around the tube. I would then allow cricoid pressure to be released and secure the tube.

What about maintenance?

I would maintain anaesthesia using an inhalational agent. Personally I would use sevoflurane. I would then hand ventilate the infant, before connecting to a either an Ayre's T-piece or paediatric circle system using pressure-controlled ventilation. Hand ventilation throughout the operation would not be ideal as it is difficult to maintain regular ventilation with stable blood gases and capnography is unreliable.

What would you give for pain relief?

I would give a combination of paracetamol, local anaesthetic techniques and opioids for analgesia.

Paracetamol can be given intra-venously and rectally. The doses for an infant under 10 kg are 7.5 mg per kg 4 to 6 hourly up to 30 mg/kg/day intra-venously; or 40 mg/kg loading followed by 20 mg/kg 4 to 6 hourly to a maximum of 90 mg/kg/day rectally. Oral paracetamol 20 mg/kg 6 hourly may be commenced once oral fluids are tolerated.

Non-steroidal anti-inflammatories may be an option provided the infant is adequately hydrated with good renal perfusion and no evidence of sepsis. The dose of oral ibuprofen is 10 mg/kg 3 times a day. Diclofenac may be given orally or rectally at a dose of 1 mg/kg 3 times daily to a maximum of 150 mg/day.

Opioids can be used intra- and post-operatively. Morphine can be used in judicious boluses or by infusion. It is preferable to fentanyl due to its greater water solubility. It is less lipid soluble and so less cumulative and more predictable. Due to the risk of post-operative respiratory depression the infant should be carefully monitored. Local anaesthetic techniques such as wound infiltration, epidural or spinal may be used. Wound infiltration is effective and often used. The dose of bupivicaine is 2 mg/kg. I would also consider a regional technique. Epidural or spinal blockade may be performed, but they may be difficult to insert and require expertise in their post-operative management on the ward (both nursing and anaesthetic). A spinal would also be relatively short acting. Contraindications to regional techniques include sepsis and coagulopathy.

What would be your concerns during the operation?

My main concerns during the operation can be divided into specific concerns regarding the laparotomy and general considerations for paediatric patients. Specifically I would be vigilant of any surgical complications or haemorrhage. I would aim to maintain good communication with the surgeon.

Generally I would want to closely monitor the infant and avoid excessive heat loss, give adequate doses of analgesics and anaesthetic agents and give appropriate fluids, taking into account the fluid losses during surgery.

I would aim to maintain the oxygen saturation, end-tidal carbon dioxide, heart rate, blood pressure, temperature and urine output all within normal levels throughout the operation. I would also check the blood sugar levels of the infant to avoid hypoglycaemia.

The infant is at risk of hypothermia during the operation due to heat loss from the skin (aided by peripheral vasodilatation) and the surgical site. I would aim to increase the ambient temperature of the operating and anaesthetic rooms prior to and during surgery. I would use a heated mattress, Bair Hugger and cover the infant's head in order to avoid further heat loss from the skin. Bubble wrap and plastic drapes can also be used. I would warm the fluids given to the infant and use a HME to reduce the heat loss from the respiratory system. Use of a circle system also provides warm, fully saturated gas and is therefore superior to a T-piece system.

How would you approach intra-operative fluid management?

I would try and consider fluids in terms of pre-existing deficits, maintenance requirements and on-going losses.

I would resuscitate the infant prior to induction of anaesthesia, thus addressing the pre-existing deficit.

With regards to maintenance fluids I would calculate this from the weight of the infant. Four ml per kilogram is given for the first 10 kg of body weight of the infant, followed by

2 ml/kg for the second 10 kg of body weight and then 1 ml/kg for each following 10 kg. I would use Hartmann's solution as a continuous infusion, although this may need to be changed depending on the blood results. A glucose solution may also be required depending on the blood sugar measurements.

The ongoing losses would be mainly due to the operation. Blood loss should be closely monitored. As a general guide, approximately 10 ml/kg/hr fluid will be required to compensate for evaporation during a laparotomy. This can be replaced as 0.9% N saline or Hartmann's solution. Colloid may also be required during fluid therapy due to capillary leak. If the infant is septic boluses totalling 40 mg/kg are not unusual. If significant blood loss occurs, then I would give blood and consider the need for clotting factors or FFP.

What would be your post-operative plan for this patient?

If the infant requires ongoing ventilation due to respiratory compromise, septic shock, blood loss or surgical complications then they will need to be nursed in a paediatric intensive care unit. Otherwise, I would want the patient to be nursed on a high dependency unit, in order to closely monitor the vital signs and pain levels of the infant. Respiratory depression may occur due to the effects of opioid analgesics.

Regular blood tests will be necessary to check the full blood count and urea and electrolytes. Intra-venous fluids should be continued until the infant is able to feed. Blood transfusion may also be required.

2.8.6. Oesophageal atresia, diaphragmatic hernia and exomphalos – Helen L Jewitt

These are paediatric surgical problems, which many final FRCA candidates may not have encountered in their training. You are unlikely to encounter questions on more than one of these problems within a structured oral exam. A structured understanding of each problem and the main anaesthetic considerations relating to it will ensure you tackle a potentially difficult question well.

You are on call for paediatric emergencies and are asked to assess a term neonate with oesophageal atresia.

What do you understand about this condition?

Oesophageal atresia (OA) and tracheo-oesophageal fistula (TOF) are part of a spectrum of conditions where there is defective embryological development of the trachea and oesophagus. The incidence is approximately 1 in 3500 live births and many cases are diagnosed antenatally.

Can you describe the anatomical abnormality in more detail?

There are several patterns of abnormal anatomy (see Figure 2.8.6).

It is worth being able to sketch these as it makes remembering and explaining the differences easier.

The most common type involves a blind ending upper oesophagus with a fistula between the distal portion of the oesophagus and the trachea. This occurs in over 80% of cases.

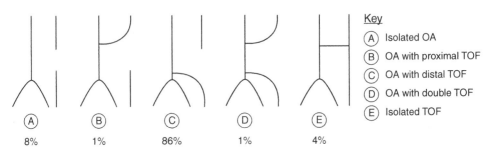

Figure 2.8.6. Types of tracheo-oesophageal fistula.

What would you look for in your pre-operative assessment of this infant?

It is important to look for other congenital abnormalities because 50% of infants with a TOF will have associated problems. It is particularly important to look for evidence of congenital cardiac problems. The baby may have been born prematurely, raising the possibility of lung disease, retinal problems and impaired blood sugar regulation.

What is the VACTERL association?

If you are doing particularly well up to this point this may be asked.

This is an acronym used to describe a group of congenital problems which can occur together. An affected infant has vertebral, anorectal, cardiac, tracheo-oesophageal, renal and limb abnormalities.

How does tracheo-oesophageal fistula present?

The baby may have repeated episodes of coughing, choking and cyanosis. This is exacerbated by attempts at feeding. There is resistance to passage of an orogastric tube.

How should the infant be managed pre-operatively?

The child cannot take oral fluids or nutrition so intra-venous fluids should be administered taking care to avoid hypoglycaemia. A specialised suction tube called a Replogle tube can be used to prevent pooling of secretions in the upper part of the oesophagus. This works by letting air in to avoid high negative pressures sucking the oesophageal mucosa into the catheter.

What is the optimum timing of corrective surgery after birth?

In an otherwise uncomplicated case of TOF or OA surgery should be carried out within 24 hours of delivery because accumulation of fluid in the upper oesophagus leads to a risk of aspiration.

How would you induce anaesthesia in this patient?

The tube in the upper pouch should be suctioned following attachment of a saturation probe. Inhalational induction with sevoflurane is carried out. Following an appropriate dose of a non-depolarising muscle relaxant the trachea is intubated with a size 3.0- or 3.5-mm tube.

Vigorous bag and mask ventilation is avoided because this can force air through the fistula from the trachea to the distal oesophagus and stomach. This can splint the diaphragm and impair ventilation. The infant is allowed to begin to breathe spontaneously on the tube at which point the tube can be removed to permit examination of the airway with a rigid bronchoscope. The exact anatomy of the TOF can be established. The endotracheal tube can then be replaced and positioned so that the TOF is occluded. In this way the escape of gas from the trachea to the distal oesophagus and stomach during positive pressure ventilation is minimised. Once the tube position is correct, a neuromuscular blocking agent can be administered and then gentle hand ventilation commenced.

What are the intra-operative concerns?

These relate to positioning, monitoring, temperature regulation and maintenance of reliable intra-venous access. The infant is usually positioned right lateral and strict attention must be paid to pressure areas. Invasive monitoring with arterial and central venous lines is appropriate. Active warming methods must be used.

How will you manage the child post-operatively?

Most infants remain ventilated post-operatively and are cared for on the neonatal or paediatric intensive care unit. Appropriate sedation and analgesia should be ensured.

What can you tell me about congenital diaphragmatic hernia?

Congenital diaphragmatic hernia occurs in approximately 1 in every 3000–4000 live births. The diaphragmatic defect is most commonly left sided and associated with a variable degree of lung hypoplasia. A total of 40% of patients have significant associated congenital abnormalities, of which cardiac anomalies are most common. Experimental data suggest that abnormal lung development begins at an early stage of embryonic development, before the diaphragm begins to form. Subsequent diaphragmatic development is disturbed leading to the observed anatomical defect. Herniation of abdominal contents through the defect in the later stages of foetal development exerts a pressure effect, further impairing lung development. The affected lung has poorly developed airways, reduced numbers of type II pneumocytes and abnormal, highly reactive pulmonary vasculature. All affected infants have some degree of pulmonary hypertension.

Is surgical correction of the defect an emergency procedure?

No, the condition of the child should be optimised prior to considering a surgical procedure. Surgery does not improve gas exchange because of the associated pulmonary hypertension and lung hypoplasia.

How should the patient be optimised prior to theatre?

Delivery should take place as close to term as possible to maximise lung development. Bag and mask ventilation should be minimised to prevent distension of the intra-thoracic bowel. Intubation and ventilation with close attention to avoiding barotrauma should follow. The bowel lying within the chest cavity can be decompressed with an orogastric tube. The child should be transferred to a paediatric critical care area for invasive monitoring and further stabilisation. Appropriate investigations include arterial blood gases, chest X-ray and echocardiogram.

The principles of ventilating the infant are to achieve adequate gas exchange whilst preventing iatrogenic injury to the lung. Inspiratory pressures are limited and permissive hypercapnia is used. Inhaled nitric oxide may be trialled in patients with significant pulmonary hypertension although the evidence of an improved outcome in this condition is so far lacking.

Surgery is generally delayed for 24–48 hours to allow a fall in pulmonary resistance.

What is exomphalos?

Exomphalos is a congenital defect of the abdominal wall. There is herniation of abdominal contents with a covering sac through a midline defect. It is caused by failure of the gut to migrate into the abdominal cavity during foetal development.

How does gastroschisis differ?

Gastroschisis is also an anterior abdominal wall defect allowing herniation of intra-abdominal contents. It does not occur in the midline and there is no covering sac over the exposed bowel.

Exomphalos is commonly associated with other congenital problems, particularly cardiac defects whilst gastroschisis is usually an isolated problem.

What are the problems associated with the two conditions?

There is significant loss of heat and moisture by evaporation from the exposed abdominal contents. The bowel can be damaged by the drying effect and is a potential route for the entry of infection.

What is the management?

The exposed bowel should be initially covered with a non-porous material such as cling film. Strict attention should be given to estimating and replacing fluid losses and to maintenance of normothermia.

Primary surgical closure is attempted once the infant is adequately resuscitated. Staged closure may be necessary if the abdominal contents cannot be reduced without compromising respiratory function.

Further Reading

Al Rawi O, Booker P. Oesophageal atresia and tracheo-oesophageal fistula. *Continuing Education in Anaesthesia, Critical Care & Pain.* 2007; 7(1): 15–19.

King H, Booker P. Congenital diaphragmatic hernia in the neonate. *Continuing Education in Anaesthesia, Critical Care & Pain.* 2005; 5(5): 171–174.

Poddar R, Hartley L. Exomphalos and gastroschisis. *Continuing Education in Anaesthesia, Critical Care & Pain.* 2009; 9(2): 48–51.

Vascular

2.9.1. Abdominal aortic aneurysm repair – Emily K Johnson and Jessie R Welbourne

Anaesthesia for abdominal aortic aneurysm is a big topic and may be a question in an SAQ or SOE. It is important you understand the physiological consequences of aortic cross clamping and the likely complications of the surgery, whether it be emergency or elective.

A man presents to the emergency department with collapse, back pain and confusion. He has a history of hypertension and is a life-long smoker. He has a heart rate of 100 bpm and a systolic blood pressure of 90 mmHg. There is a pulsatile expanding mass palpable in his epigastrium.

What is an abdominal aortic aneurysm?

An aortic aneurysm is a dilatation in the wall of the aorta greater than 3 cm in diameter. They develop as a result of disruption and degeneration of elastin and collagen fibres in the aortic wall over time, chronic inflammation of the vessel wall or smooth muscle cell loss. The commonest cause is atherosclerosis but they also occur in patients with Marfan's syndrome, TB, salmonella and Takayasu's disease.

The aneurysms are usually asymptomatic when they are small, but expand over time and the risk of spontaneous rupture increases exponentially with increasing diameter.

What are the risk factors for developing an aortic aneurysm?

Aneurysms most commonly occur in males, over 65 years and cigarette smokers. Smokers are four times more likely to have an aneurysm than non-smokers. A positive family history of aneurysms is also a risk factor.

Abdominal aortic aneurysms (AAAs) occur in 10% of all men over 65 and in 3% of women over 65.

What are the treatment options available?

Treatment can be medical or surgical management.

Medical management is aimed at preventing the expansion of the aneurysm. Drugs such as statins, indomethacin and tetracyclines prevent expansion in animals, however none have been shown to be effective in humans and surgical management is the definitive treatment.

Elective surgery has much lower morbidity and mortality than emergency surgery for a ruptured aneurysm. Evidence has shown a screening programme is cost effective in males over 65 years. Elective surgery is performed when aneurysm diameter exceeds 5.5 cm. The mortality of having an elective aortic aneurysm repair is 7%, however if it ruptures the mortality drastically increases and the operative mortality for an emergency AAA repair is 36–50%.

Elective repairs may be performed by an open procedure or by endovascular stenting.

Conservative management for ruptured aneurysms is an option if the patient is unlikely to survive a general anaesthetic or does not wish to proceed with an operation. Symptom control and family liaison are crucial in such cases.

What co-morbidities would you expect in patients presenting with an AAA?

These patients are commonly arteriopaths, suffering from coronary artery disease, hypertension, peripheral vascular disease and possible cerebrovascular disease. There is a high chance that they are smokers and have chronic obstructive pulmonary disease (COPD). They may have diabetes and suffer from renal impairment.

Exercise tolerance should be recorded, if the patient can walk up one flight of stairs without symptoms this demonstrates an exercise capacity equal to or greater than 4 metabolic equivalents (METs). Patients achieving 4 METs or more have improved outcomes, as METs can be used to provide an indication of an individual's functional capacity which is more formally measured by VO_2 max. An anaerobic threshold or VO_2 max of less than 11 ml/kg/min when measured during cardiopulmonary exercise (CPX) testing predicts high peri-operative risk, although this is not routinely tested in most centres.

Do you know any scoring systems for risk assessment?

General scoring systems such as APACHE II and POSSUM scoring can be employed to estimate risk but are not accurate at predicting outcome in ruptured AAA patients.

Goldman and Detsky analysis both look at cardiac risk factors and provide a score equating to relative risk of major adverse cardiac events in patients having non-cardiac surgery.

The Hardmann index for ruptured aneurysms has a score of 0–5 with one point being awarded for age greater than 76 years, creatinine over 190 µg/L, haemoglobin less than 9 g/dl, ischaemic ECG and history of loss of conciousness. A score of 2 or more gives a predicted mortality of 80%.

There is also the Glasgow aneurysm score that can be applied to both elective and emergency aneurysm repairs. The Glasgow aneurysm score adds age in years to other variables with allocated scores. These include shock, myocardial disease, cerebrovascular disease and renal disease. Scores of 84 or above indicate a mortality of 65%.

However, all scoring systems have limitations and need to be used as a tool to supplement clinical decisions.

What are the important points to anaesthetising a patient for an emergency AAA repair?

Classify your answer into pre-operative management, anaesthetic management and post-operative management. A good way of starting your answer is to identify the commonly encountered problems with ruptured aortic aneurysms. You are likely to be dealing with a highly unstable patient with co-morbidities and it is a surgical emergency. By stating these facts you let the examiner know you are aware of the key issues and give you time to think of a structured answer. It is also worth mentioning you would seek skilled assistance in the form of another senior anaesthetist and experienced ODP.

The management of a patient with a ruptured AAA requiring emergency surgery falls into pre-op, intra-op and post-op management.

Pre-operatively you are likely to encounter a number of difficulties. A ruptured AAA is a surgical emergency and the patient may be profoundly shocked. In addition they are likely to be elderly and have serious co-morbidities.

Your aims at this time are to make this high-risk patient as stable as possible. I would assess the patient using an ABC approach, administering oxygen and proceeding to obtain good IV access in the form of large bore peripheral cannula. Bloods for FBC, U&ES, clotting screen and crossmatch 10 units of blood plus fresh frozen plasma and cryoprecipitate should be sent urgently.

Cautious resuscitation should be commenced, it is important to avoid hypertension, straining or coughing as this may cause further bleeding by dislodging thrombus. In addition, large volumes of fluid may contribute to further bleeding by dilution of clotting products. Adequate analgesia should be given, usually IV morphine titrated to effect. A targeted assessment of the patient's history should be made with a succinct examination, including airway assessment.

Theatres need to be informed and senior anaesthetic assistance should be sought. The patient should be transferred to theatre without delay.

What other equipment would you need available before anaesthetising this patient?

Ideally you would want a rapid fluid infuser, a cell salvage system, and access to the HaemoCue. You may also consider cardiac output monitoring.

An example of a rapid fluid infuser device is a "level one" infuser. This allows warmed fluid to be infused under pressure from an automated pressure chamber, while simultaneously preparing a second bag for infusion. The giving sets are wide bore and unite into one set which passes through a heater that quickly warms the fluid to an appropriate temperature. The advantage of this device is that fluid may be rapidly pressurised and administered, with no interruption during bag changes. It allows the highest flow rate for intra-venous fluid administration.

The cell saver should be used from the start of the procedure to maximise the volume of autologous blood that may be returned to the patient. The salvaged blood is spun down, washed and resuspended in normal saline, then returned to the patient (although never under pressure as this may cause haemolysis) so reducing the need for donor blood transfusions. It is important to remember that call salvaged blood contains red blood cells only, and in cases of massive blood loss fresh frozen plasma, platelets and cryoprecipitate should be administered as appropriate.

Assuming the theatre is prepared and ready, how are you going to anaesthetise this patient?

It is important to state confidently exactly what you would do, giving details. Your answer needs to demonstrate you have done this and are confident and safe. There are a number of different approaches to most anaesthetics and in this situation no one method is associated with significantly improved outcomes, so state confidently what you would do and be prepared to give your reasons.

My goals in anaesthetising this patient are to attempt to maintain cardiovascular stability and normothermia.

I would proceed with a rapid sequence induction using thiopentone carefully titrated to effect and suxamethonium 1–2 mg/kg. I would use a high-dose opiate, such as fentanyl or alfentanil, to suppress the pressor response to intubation and reduce the dose of induction agent required. Ketamine could be used as an alternative induction agent.

This should be done in the operating theatre, with the patient prepped and draped and the surgeons scrubbed ready to start. I would also like the blood to be ready, checked in theatre and a second experienced anaesthetist present. I would have drawn up inotropes in advance and ideally have established invasive arterial monitoring, a CVP line and inserted a urinary catheter prior to induction. However, often the central venous line or even the arterial line can wait until after cross clamping has occurred. Both arms can be abducted on boards to allow vascular access.

I would actively warm the patient using warm fluids and blood and a forced air warmer. I would apply the warmer to the upper body and head but not the lower limbs after cross clamping as it may worsen ischaemic injury.

For maintanence of anaesthesia I would use a volatile agent in oxygen and air, opioids and neuromuscular blockade.

What are the physiological responses to aortic cross clamping?

An understanding of the physiological response to cross clamping of the aorta is a potential SAQ or SOE question and a clear account will be necessary to pass. This is very likely to be asked in any question on aortic aneurysms, whether elective or emergency.

When the aorta is clamped there is a sudden increase in systemic vascular resistance and blood pressure. This increase in afterload raises the left ventricular end-diastolic pressure (LVEDP) leading to an increase in myocardial work and a decrease of the coronary perfusion pressure. This can precipitate left ventricular ischaemia and failure. Increasing the depth of anaesthesia or administration of nitrates may be used to attenuate this response. It is important to maintain the intra-vascular volume in preparation for removal of the clamp, and intra-vascular fluid loading is required. This can be aided by using nitrates or anaesthetic agents to increase vasodilatation.

What happens when the clamp is removed?

When the clamp is removed there is a sudden drop in afterload. Metabolites from ischaemic tissues enter the circulation causing vasodilatation and myocardial depression. This can result in a lactic acidosis, a fall in blood pressure and CVP and increase in heart rate. Myocardial ischaemia can result and if not treated promptly this can lead to circulatory collapse. Arterial pressure should be maintained using intravascular volume expansion and vasoconstrictors or inotropes.

What is the significance of supra- or infra-renal clamps?

The position of the cross clamp depends on the position of the aneurysm and its relationship to the renal arteries. This will dictate whether the clamp needs to be positioned above or below the renal arteries. The relevance is that if the clamp is placed supra-renally then the kidneys are more likely to suffer ischaemic injury as their main blood supply is clamped off.

The role of the anaesthetist is to attempt to avoid worsening renal ischaemia by maintaining normotension and normovolaemia. Diuretics such as furosemide or mannitol can be given prior to cross clamping but there is no evidence they improve outcome. Nephrotoxic drugs such as NSAIDs and contrast should be avoided.

What are the surgical complications once the graft is in place?

Bleeding from the vascular anastomosis may occur after release of the clamp, and if severe, the clamp may be reapplied to allow further repair. Transfusing blood and clotting factors and achieving normothermia will reduce the risks of bleeding.

Thromboembolism may occur and micro-emboli may contribute to post-operative renal failure. For elective aneurysm repair, heparin is commonly given prior to cross clamping to reduce this risk but this is not routine in emergency repairs.

Infection is a significant risk and may be an early or late complication. Management will most likely be conservative initially with anti-biotics but may require further surgery.

What are the aims of post-operative care?

Post-operative care should take place on ICU. Patients should be warmed to normothermia, abnormal clotting corrected, adequate analgesia administered and artificial ventilation maintained until any metabolic acidosis is corrected. Fluid management should include appropriate maintenance fluids with timely fluid boluses to correct hypotension or low urine output.

Regular monitoring of renal function, haemoglobin and coagulation will be required. Cardiovascular or renal support may be necessary post-op.

Prolonged ileus commonly occurs and total parenteral nutrition may be indicated. Patients are at high risk of developing abdominal compartment syndrome and intra-abdominal pressure should be monitored.

You mentioned abdominal compartment syndrome – what is it exactly?

This is just an example of how the examiners may pick you up on what you say.

Abdominal compartment syndrome occurs when intra-abdominal pressures are equal or above 20 mmHg. It may be preceeded by intra-abdominal hypertension, which is when pressures are equal or above 12 mmHg. It can lead to poor blood flow, particularly poor renal and bowel perfusion and multi-organ failure. Risk factors for abdominal compartment syndrome include:

- Acidosis
- Fluid over-load

- Anaemia
- Hypertension
- Cardiopumonary resuscitation (CPR).

The patient may require a surgical laparostomy with mesh closure, which should be considered as the primary method of closure in patients at risk of abdominal compartment syndrome.

How should patients be optimised prior to an elective AAA repair?

Patients should be advised to stop smoking. If they are diabetic their blood sugars should be well controlled. They should be prescribed statins and possibly β-blockers. If there is evidence of significant coronary artery disease they should have further cardiac investigation, which may include dobutamine stress test, echocardiography or coronary angiography. Patients with significant pulmonary disease should be reviewed and optimised by respiratory physicians.

What do you know about endovascular aneurysm repair (EVAR)?

Endovascular aneurysm repair or EVAR avoids the need for a laparotomy and is becoming increasingly popular. It is performed via a 23 French gauge femoral line. There is some evidence for elective aneurysm surgery suggesting that there is a lower mortality rate with EVAR compared with open repair. There are some centres performing EVAR as an emergency and this can be performed under local anaesthesia with or without sedation. A significant number of patients require conversion to general anaesthesia as they may develop severe back, abdominal or ischaemic leg pain when these aortic occlusive devices are used. Another problem is that patients may be unable to tolerate lying flat for the required time period, which may be several hours.

Further Reading

Endovascular Aneurysm Repair Trials. http://www.evartrials.org.

Leonard A, Thompson J. Anaesthesia for ruptured AAA. *Continuing Education in Anaesthesia, Critical Care & Pain*. 2008; **8**(1): 11–15.

Nataraj V, Mortimer A. Endovascular abdominal aortic aneurysm repair. *Continuing Education in Anaesthesia, Critical Care & Pain*. 2004; **4**(3): 91–94.

National Confidential Enquiry into Patient Outcome and Death. Abdominal aortic aneurysm: A service in need of surgery? NCEPOD 2005. http://www.ncepod.org.uk/2005report2/Downloads/AAA_report.pdf.

National Health Service. NHS Abdominal Aortic Aneurysm Screening Programme http://aaa.screening.nhs.uk/aboutus.

Sakalihasen N, Limet R, Defaive OD. Abdominal aortic aneurysm. *Lancet*. 2005; **365**: 1577–1589.

2.9.2. Anaesthesia for carotid endarterectomy – Emily K Johnson and Jessie R Welbourne

Questions about carotid endarterectomy feature in both the SAQs and structured oral examinations (SOEs). This is a reflection of the increase in the use of regional techniques instead of general anaesthesia for this procedure, and recent publications regarding the benefits and complications of the different anaesthetic options.

A 75-year-old man presents for a carotid endarterectomy. He had a myocardial infarc-tion 10 years ago and is a non-insulin dependent diabetic. He can walk up two flights of stairs with some breathlessness. His medication includes ramipril, aspirin and metformin.

What is a carotid endarterectomy?

Carotid endarterectomy is a vascular surgical procedure for treating asymptomatic or symp-tomatic carotid artery stenosis. It involves removing plaque from the lining of the internal carotid artery. Diseased intima and a portion of the media may be removed. It is aimed at reducing the incidence of an embolic stroke in high-risk patients.

What are the indications for surgery ?

Carotid endarterectomy is a prophylactic operation so careful evaluation of the risks and ben-efits is required. There are two large randomised controlled trials providing evidence guid-ing which patients should undergo surgery for carotid artery stenosis. They are the North American Symptomatic Carotid Endarterectomy Trial (NASCET) and the European Carotid Surgery Trial (ECST). The NASCET trial demonstrated that for every 6 patients treated, 1 major stroke was prevented at 2 years for symptomatic patients with 70–99% stenosis. Smaller benefit was demonstrated with patients with 50–69% occlusion, with a number needed to treat of 22 at 5 years.

NICE guidance published in July 2008 advises patients with non-disabling strokes or transient ischaemic attacks (TIAs) receive carotid imaging within a week of symptom onset. Stenosis is measured according to the criteria from either of the trials mentioned. Symp-tomatic stenosis of 50–99% according to NASCET criteria or 70–99% according to ECST criteria warrants referral and assessment for carotid endarterectomy, with the procedure ide-ally being undertaken within 2 weeks from onset of symptoms.

Discuss the risks associated with carotid endarterectomy.

The risks can be classified into those associated with the patient co-morbidities and those asso-ciated with the anaesthetic and the procedure itself.

Carotid endarterectomy is a high-risk procedure. The risks can be classified into those associated with the patients' co-morbidities and those related to the surgery.

Patients presenting with symptomatic stenosis commonly have widespread atheroscle-rotic disease. Therefore they are often elderly, hypertensive, smokers with diabetes, ischaemic heart disease and/or COPD.

Co-morbidity adversely affects the outcome, so patients with multiple medical problems have a higher post-operative mortality and morbidity and hence benefit less from the proce-dure.

The procedure itself carries considerable risk; peri-operative combined mortality and major stroke risk is 2–5%.

Other than stroke the procedure carries a risk of TIAs, myocardial infarction and ischaemia. Hypo- or hypertension may occur, haemorrhage can be potentially life threat-ening and haematomas can cause tracheal compression and laryngeal oedema. Damage to surrounding structures such as recurrent laryngeal nerve or hypoglossal nerve can occur dur-ing surgery. Another uncommon (0.3–1.2%) but potentially serious complication is cerebral hyperperfusion syndrome due to the sudden increase in perfusion of the vasculature distal to stenosis, which can cause post-operative headaches, seizures or intra-cranial haemorrhage.

Do you know any specific factors that increase the risk of peri-operative morbidity or mortality?

An increased risk is associated with:

- Females
- Age over 75
- Systolic hypertension
- Recent stroke or TIA.

Other less well-confirmed risks include:

- Cardiovascular disease
- Diabetes
- Smoking
- Hyperlipidaemia
- Contralateral stenosis.

Factors that decrease the risk of a cerebrovascular event include:

- Treatment with anti-platelet drugs
- Being asymptomatic
- Suffering purely ocular symptoms (amaurosis fugax).

What are the anaesthetic options available?

Carotid endarterectomy can be performed under local or general anaesthesia. Local anaesthetic techniques are deep and superficial cervical plexus block and local infiltration. Cervical epidural has also been described but is associated with significant risk.

What is the evidence for general anaesthesia or local anaesthesia for carotid endarterectomy?

The GALA trial, general anaesthesia versus local anaesthesia, was a multicentre randomised controlled trial comparing the primary endpoints of stroke, cardiac events and death following carotid endarterectomy between two groups randomised to have carotid endarterectomy under general or local anaesthesia. The risks of these events in the two groups were not shown to be statistically different and no differences were noted in quality of life or length of hospital stay. The conclusion was that the anaesthetist and surgeon should consult with the patient and decide upon suitable anaesthetic technique on an individual basis.

Can you tell me a little more about the nerves you would need to block to perform carotid endarterectomy under local anaesthetic?

It is necessary to block the dermatomes of C2, C3 and C4 for successful surgery. These are blocked using deep or superficial cervical plexus blocks.

The superficial cervical plexus consists of four main nerves:

1. Lesser occipital nerve
2. Greater auricular nerve
3. Transverse cervical nerve
4. Supra-clavicular nerve.

These nerves supply the skin over the lateral aspect of the neck, which cover the area of surgical incision. The deep cervical plexus supplies the deep muscles of the neck and diaphram.

Surgical retraction of submandibular tissues can cause pain in the region of the trigeminal nerve. The carotid sheath also has cranial nerve innervation. Local anaesthetic can be infiltrated into these two areas by the surgeon.

Describe the technique for performing a superficial cervical plexus block.

When asked to describe any nerve block do not forget to mention the preparations you would make. If the examiner is not interested in this they can stop you but it is important to demonstrate you are safe and thoughtful. If you can, quickly sketch a diagram to support your answer (Figure 2.9.2a).

Prior to performing any nerve block I would take a full history and examine the patient. Once establishing their suitability and ruling out any contraindications I would explain the procedure and risks and consent the patient. I would prepare my equipment and monitoring and have a trained assistant and emergency equipment to hand.

Firstly, I would gain intra-venous access, attach monitoring and administer oxygen, giving sedation if indicated. I would position the patient supine with some head up tilt and the head turned slightly away from the side of the block. The landmark is the mid-point of the posterior border of sternocleidomastoid muscle (SCM). Using a sterile technique I would insert a 21-gauge needle along the posterior border of SCM both cephalad and caudad, puncturing the first fascial layer, aspirating and injecting a total of 10 ml of 0.25% bupivacaine. I would expect a sausage shape to form along the posterior border of SCM.

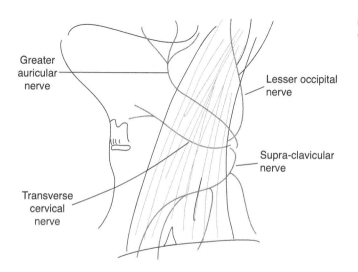

Figure 2.9.2a. Superficial cervical plexus.

Greater auricular nerve

Lesser occipital nerve

Supra-clavicular nerve

Transverse cervical nerve

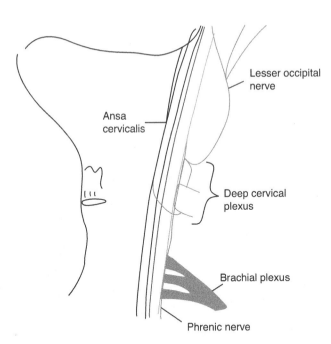

Figure 2.9.2b. Deep cervical plexus.

Lesser occipital nerve

Ansa cervicalis

Deep cervical plexus

Brachial plexus

Phrenic nerve

Describe the technique for performing a deep cervical plexus block.

I would prepare the patient as I mentioned and position the patient supine with some head up tilt and the head turned away from the side of the block. I would identify the landmarks, the posterior border of sternocleidomastoid muscle and feel for the inter-scalene groove behind the lateral border of SCM at the level of the thyroid cartilage, C4. Then, using aseptic technique I would use some local anaesthetic to the skin and insert a 5-mm needle towards the contralateral elbow, that is in a medial, caudal and dorsal direction until the patient feels paraesthesia or the bone of C4 transverse process is contacted. After careful aspiration I would inject 8–10 ml of 0.25% bupivacaine.

What are the risks associated with a deep cervical plexus block?

When asked the risks of any nerve block you can classify into the generic risks of local anaesthetic injection and those specific to the particular block.

The risks can classified into those due to local anaesthetic injection, such as local anaesthetic toxicity, anaphylaxis and nerve damage, and those specific to deep cervical plexus blocks.

These include:

- Intra-vascular injection (especially vertebral artery)
- Nerve palsies, specifically the phrenic nerve is often affected, and this block should never be performed bilaterally for this reason; recurrent laryngeal nerve can be damaged causing hoarseness from vocal cord paralysis; sympathetic block can occur giving a Horner's syndrome.
- Epidural spread of the local anaesthetic

- Intra-thecal injection or spinal cord damage
- Small risk of pneumothorax.

What are the risks and benefits of using a local anaesthetic technique?

As mentioned, the GALA trial has not shown any clear benefits in using local over general anaesthetic, so anaesthetic technique must be decided on an individual basis.

A regional technique has the advantages of avoidance of general anaesthesia in what is likely to be a high-risk patient group. The other main advantage to regional techniques is that cerebral function can be continuously assessed throughout surgery by maintaining verbal contact with the patient.

Disadvantages include potential poor compliance during a potentially long operation, discomfort of the patient and movement of the surgical field. Anxiety-related tachycardia and hypertension may make haemostasis more challenging as well as increasing the risk of myocardial ischaemia. Patient anxiety may also lead to an increased cerebral metabolic rate and therefore increased oxygen demand during a time when supply may be reduced. If the need arises to convert to a general anaesthetic due to an inadequate block for patient or surgical reasons this may present practical problems for the surgeon and anaesthetist. The complications of a deep cervical block are outlined above.

If you were to choose a regional technique, which would you choose?

Feel free to express your own opinions when asked a question about personal choice, however be prepared to justify your choices.

The technique I would choose is that with which I am familiar, a combination of a superficial cervical plexus block and infiltration at the incision site. There is a randomised controlled trial comparing deep and superficial block with superficial block alone. It demonstrated the techniques were comparable in the amount of supplemental local anaesthetic given by the surgeon. Anatomically, a superficial block alone would not be expected to block all the relevant nerves, however dye studies suggest that as long as the injection is below the investing fascia, local anaesthetic may spread from superficial to deep structures. A superficial block alone avoids the hazards of the deep cervical plexus block.

What are the principles of general anesthesia for carotid endarterectomy?

When using general anaesthetic for carotid endarterectomy it is important to establish invasive arterial monitoring prior to induction. A cautious intravenous induction should be undertaken with the use of an opioid prior to intubation. Many anaesthetists consider it essential to intubate the trachea as the airway will be inaccessible during surgery and a laryngeal mask may alter the anatomy and compromise surgical access. Throughout the procedure it is important to maintain cardiovascular stability and good oxygenation. The patient's cerebral circulation is dependent on a collateral circulation during carotid cross clamping, although a shunt may be used by the surgeon, the key principle of anaesthesia is the maintenance of an adequate perfusion pressure. A beneficial aspect of general anaesthesia is that it reduces the cerebral metabolic rate for oxygen ($CMRO_2$), which is important when cerebral blood flow may be compromised. TIVA techniques allow rapid control of changes in blood pressure, smooth emergence with less coughing (coughing is not desirable as it may precipitate surgical site bleeding) and allow rapid awakening for early neurological assessment.

How may cerebral perfusion be monitored during general anaesthesia?

Cerebral perfusion may be assessed using processed EEG monitoring, measuring jugular venous oxygen tension, transcranial Doppler (TCD) or carotid artery stump pressure.

The EEG gives a crude measure of the trend in brain electrical activity and is largely unspecific and dependent on correct application of surface electrodes. A low jugular venous oxygen tension indicates high oxygen uptake by the brain and so lower blood flow assuming the oxygen consumption by the brain remains stable.

Transcranial Doppler can be used to measure blood flow in the middle cerebral artery therefore can give an estimate of cerebral blood flow and also an indication of particulate emboli. Carotid artery stump pressure measurement is a crude method to estimate adequacy of perfusion. A mean pulsatile pressure of more than 50mmHg is accepted as sufficient to proceed without a shunt.

How would you manage cerebral ischaemia upon carotid cross clamping?

The initial management would be to administer supplemental oxygen and increase the mean arterial pressure, roughly 20% greater than the pre-operative level, in attempt at maintaining collateral perfusion. If cerebral ischaemia persists, insertion of a shunt is indicated, however an increased arterial pressure is required to maintain flow through a surgical shunt. Shunts are associated with many other problems including air and plaque embolisation, intimal tears, carotid dissection and late carotid restenosis. Even following shunt insertion, flow may be insufficient to meet cerebral oxygen requirements.

Where should these patients be looked after post-operatively?

Post-operative care should be provided on a high dependency unit (HDU) or a specialised area that can provide appropriate care. Post-operative problems that are significant to long-term outcome or which require rapid intervention are possible. For example, neurological deficit occurs in up to 7% and there may be headache, seizures or intra-cranial bleeding. Airway obstruction following bleeding into the surgical site may occur and this requires rapid intervention to manage the airway and stop the bleeding. Post-operative hypertension in response to pain or baroreceptor dysfunction is common.

Do you know of alternative treatments for carotid artery stenosis?

Carotid artery stenting is a developing procedure. The SAPPHIRE study compared carotid artery angioplasty and stenting using distal embolic protection with carotid endarterectomy in high-risk surgical patients. The incidence of the primary end-points of stroke, myocardial infarction and death at 3 years were not significantly different. However there are concerns that restenosis is more common following stenting and long-term efficiency in terms of preventing stroke is unknown.

Further Reading

GALA Trial Collaborative Group. General anaesthesia versus local anaesthesia for carotid surgery (GALA): a multicentre, randomised controlled trial. *Lancet* 2008; 372 (9656): 2132–2142.

Garrioch MA, Fitch W. Anaesthesia for carotid artery surgery. *British Journal of Anaesthesia*. 1993; 71: 569–579.

National Institute for Health and Clinical Excellence. Cartoid artery stent placement for symtomatic extracranial carotid stenosis. http://guidance.nice.org.uk/IPG191.

National Institute for Health and Clinical Excellence. Stroke: Diagnosis and initial management of acute stroke and transient ischaemic attack (TIA). http://guidance.nice.org.uk/CG68.

Paciaroni M, Eliasziw M, Kappelle LJ, et al. Medical complications associated with carotid endarterectomy. North American Symptomatic Carotid Endarterectomy Trial (NASCET). *Stroke*. 1999; **30**(9): 1759–1763.

Warlow CP. Symptomatic patients: the European Carotid Surgery Trial (ECST). *Journal des maladies vasculaires*. 1993; **18**(3): 198–201.

Spargo J, Thomas D. Local anaesthesia for carotid endarterectomy. *Continuing Education in Anaesthesia, Critical Care & Pain*. 2004; **4**(2): 62–65.

Stoneham MD, Knighton JD. Regional anaesthesia for carotid endarterectomy. *British Journal of Anaesthesia* 1999; **82**: 910–919.

Chapter

3.1

Emergency medicine

3.1.1. Acute poisoning – Ami Jones

You are called to the Emergency Department (ED) to review a 29-year-old woman with impaired consciousness who is suspected to have taken an overdose of tricyclic anti-depressants, benzodiazepines and paracetamol.

Describe your initial management of this patient

Having first established some brief details of her past and present medical history, I would first assess this patient in a systematic manner concentrating on the adequacy of her airway, breathing and circulation before making an assessment of her level of consciousness using the Glasgow Coma Scale (GCS).

The patient is maintaining her airway, has a respiratory rate of 20 breaths/min and an oxygen saturation of 99% on 15 L of oxygen via a non-rebreathing mask. Her pulse rate is 46 beats/min and her blood pressure is 90/60.

She is opening her eyes to painful stimulation, localises to pain and is confused and disorientated. What is her GCS score?

Her GCS score is 11 (2 for best eye response, 5 for best motor response and 4 for best verbal response.

What would your next steps be in this patient's management?

Now that I have ensured her basic vital functions are maintained and she is conscious enough to protect her own airway I would try to ascertain a more precise history of which drugs were taken, if possible, the exact doses and the timing of ingestion. I would also ask if she had been drinking alcohol.

Her mother has brought in several empty bottles of medication found at the scene. It is estimated that she has taken approximately 12 g of paracetamol, 100 mg of temazepam, 1.5 g of amitriptyline and half a litre of vodka about 5 hours prior to her arrival in the ED.

Dr. Podcast Scripts for the Final FRCA, ed. Rebecca A. Leslie, Emily K. Johnson,
Gary Thomas and Alexander P. L. Goodwin.   Published by Cambridge University Press.
© R. A. Leslie, E. K. Johnson, G. Thomas and A. P. L. Goodwin 2011.

What investigations would you like to order now?

I would order a full blood count, U&Es, glucose, liver function tests, coagulation screen, paracetamol and salicylate levels, an ECG and a chest X-ray. An arterial blood gas would be useful to assess her acid–base status.

Why have you have ordered an ECG and a chest X-ray?

The patient has taken a significant amount of a tricyclic anti-depressant (TCA). More than 1 g in a 70-kg adult can cause severe toxicity that often manifests with ECG abnormalities including an increased QRS duration, a long QT interval, an increased PR interval and AV block as well as ventricular arrhythmias. The chest X-ray may help to determine whether pulmonary aspiration has occurred.

Are there any other systems that can be affected by TCAs?

Many of the initial symptoms and signs are accociated with anti-cholinergic effects including a dry mouth, mydriasis and blurred vision. The central nervous system can also be involved with agitation, lethargy, myoclonus, hyperreflexia, seizures and eventually, coma. Central nervous system depression may cause hypoventilation. The patient may present with a sinus tachycardia, arrhythmias, hypertension or hypotension.

Is there any specific treatment for TCA overdose?

The management of tricyclic anti-depressant overdose depends upon the severity of the symptoms. Treatment is mainly supportive with the administration of oxygen, fluid maintenance and treatment of hypotension, arrhythmias and seizures. Magnesium sulphate may be useful in the treatment of arrhythmias.

The patient should be managed in a high-dependency area with continuous ECG monitoring.

TCAs become less protein bound if the patient has a metabolic acidosis. This increases the free fraction of the TCAs in the blood potentially enhancing their toxicity An infusion of sodium bicarbonate will increase the pH of the blood and raise the protein bound fraction of the drug.

Would activated charcoal be of use?

Activated charcoal should only be used if less than an hour has elapsed since the tablets were ingested.

This patient has also taken 12 g of paracetamol, is this of concern to you?

Yes. Metabolism is primarily in the liver. There are three main pathways: Conjugation with glucuronide and sulphate (70–80%) and hydroxylation. Cytochrome P450 enzyme system produces an alkylating agent NAPQI (*N*-acetyl-*p*-benzo quinone amine) that is normally irreversibly conjugated with the sulphydryl groups of hepatic glutathione. NAPQI is hepatotoxic when hepatic glutathione is depleted; this can occur when a large dose of paracetamol is ingested.

A toxic dose after a single ingestion is 150 mg/kg and so 12 g of paracetamol is a significant dose. This patient it at significant risk of developing severe liver damage if it is not effectively treated.

What are the symptoms and signs of an untreated paracetamol overdose?

In early stages (<24 hours), the patient may be asymptomatic. Non-specific symptoms of anorexia, nausea, vomiting and abdominal pain (right hypochondrium) may be a feature.

But if allowed to progress without specific treatment (12–48 hours: hypoglycaemia, coagulopathy, encephalopathy, metabolic acidosis and cerebral oedema may supervene.

Patients may progress to develop acute renal failure, arrhythmias and acute pancreatitis.

How should paracetamol overdose be treated?

Immediate treatment is essential in accordance with established guidelines.

If <1 hour since ingestion then activated charcoal should be given orally.

Plasma paracetamol levels should be measured at 4 hours or more after ingestion and treated with *N*-acetylcysteine (NAC) up to 24 hours after ingestion (maximal effect up to 8 hours post-ingestion).

The dose of NAC is then guided by using paracetamol concentration/time since ingestion nomograms. If evidence of hepatic failure, discuss with regional liver unit.

How does NAC work?

NAC acts as a precursor for glutathione, replenishing hepatic stores and therefore enhances the conjugation of paracetamol.

What is the dose of NAC?

The 150 mg/kg IV as a loading dose over 15 minutes, then 50 mg/kg over 4 hours, then 100 mg/kg over 16 hours. This is continued for 36 hours or longer until the INR is in normal limits.

Does NAC have any side effects?

Yes, it commonly causes nausea and vomiting as well as urticaria, fever and bronchospasm.

Where should this patient be looked after?

If she had only taken paracetamol then she could be managed on a medical ward, but since the amitriptyline overdose is associated with hypotension and a reduced GCS she should be cared for in a high dependency area.

You are called to the ED to assess a 54-year-old male who has been found unconscious in a fumed-filled car. He has been brought into hospital by the paramedics, who have also found a suicide note.

Describe your initial management of this patient

I would assess the patency of the airway, the adequacy of the breathing and the status of the circulation. I would also make a rapid assessment of the patient's Glasgow Coma Scale score.

The patient is making grunting respiratory efforts with seesawing of his chest and abdomen, what are your next actions?

The patient is showing signs of upper airway obstruction and therefore I would apply simple manoeuvres to establish a patent airway. I may also need to insert a guedel or nasopharyngeal airway. I would also give the patient 15 litres of oxygen via a non-rebreathing mask or give as close to 100% oxygen as possible.   .

This improves his respiratory pattern. His oxygen saturations are 100% on 15 litres of oxygen via a non-rebreathing mask. His blood pressure is 70/40 mmHg and his pulse rate is 50 beats/min. His GCS is 3.

How would you further manage this patient?

I would establish wide bore intra-venous access, commence fluid resuscitation and prepare to intubate and ventilate this patient. Given the history of entrapment in a fume-filled car, his reduced blood pressure, pulse rate and conscious level I suspect he may have severe carbon monoxide poisoning. I would send blood for routine biochemical and haematological investigations but would specifically request arterial blood gas analysis and measurement of carbon monoxide (CO) levels. I would also want to review an ECG, chest X-ray and a toxicology screen. I would perform a rapid sequence induction, intubate his trachea and ventilate him with 100% oxygen. He may also require vasoactive drugs if his hypotension remains refractory to fluid resuscitation.

What are the symptoms and signs of acute carbon monoxide poisoning?

Carboxyhaemoglobin concentrations in heavy smokers may range from 3 to 10%. Symptoms may be experienced in the 10–30% range and death can result from higher concentrations.

Mild poisoning often presents with non-specific symptoms of headache, nausea and visual disturbances. Moderate poisoning may present with confusion, hyperventilation, tachycardia and syncope. Higher concentrations lead to seizures, coma, hypotension, cardiac dysrhythmias, pulmonary oedema and eventually cardiorespiratory arrest.

What is the initial treatment for severe carbon monoxide poisoning?

The initial treatment is supplemental high flow oxygen at as high a concentration as is possible. Carbon monoxide's affinity for haemoglobin is 250 times greater than that of oxygen. The oxygen carrying capacity of the blood is reduced because oxygen is displaced. The resultant anaemic hypoxia, leftward displacement of oxygen-haemoglobin dissociation curve and inhibition of mitochondrial cytochrome A3 results in cellular hypoxia and acidosis. Administering 100% oxygen reduces the half-life of CO from 4–6 hours to 60–90 minutes.

Are there any other treatment options?

Hyperbaric oxygen has two theoretical advantages. It reduces the half-life of CO to 23 minutes and significantly increases the oxygen content of the blood by enhancing its solubility in plasma. Only a few limited case reports have suggested that hyperbaric oxygen therapy helps to prevent permanent neurological damage.

Hyperbaric oxygen therapy should be considered in patients who have moderate to severe CO toxicity associated with neurological impairment. There are relatively few hyperbaric oxygen chambers in the United Kingdom. This has anaesthetic implications for managing a critically ill patient on a long-distance transfer and then in an unfamiliar environment.

What other toxic gas is associated with smoke inhalation?

Cyanide also causes cytotoxic hypoxia. It is released when materials such as wool, silk and plastic undergo combustion. It is common in household and industrial fires.

What are the symptoms and signs of cyanide poisoning?

Mild toxicity can cause dizziness, headache, drowsiness and dyspnoea with progression to confusion, agitation and seizures. Eventually coma and cardiorespiratory arrest may follow.

How would you manage a patient who presented with cyanide toxicity?

The treatment options are initially supportive but specific antidotes can then be considered. I would administer 100% oxygen to the patient and if necessary intubate and control ventilation. Hypotension can be managed with fluid resuscitation and vasopressor agents. I would send a blood sample for cyanide levels, blood gases and lactate concentrations. There is likely to be a severe metabolic acidosis.

There are a number of specific antidotes available, which vary depending on which country you are working in. In some countries a cyanide antidote package exists which consists of sodium and amyl nitrates and sodium thiosulphate. The nitrites oxidise haemoglobin to methaemoglobin, which has a high affinity for cyanide and forms cyan-methaemoglobin which the liver then metabolises.

A more commonly used and less complicated antidote is hydroxycobalamin. Hydroxycobalamin displaces cyanide from cytochrome oxidase in the mitochondria and forms cyanocobalamin, which is then excreted.

Do you know of any treatments given in a hospital environment that can actually cause cyanide toxicity?

Rapid or prolonged administration of the vasodilator, sodium nitroprusside (SNP) can cause toxicity significant enough to cause a metabolic acidosis. The metabolites of SNP include cyanide ions. Prolonged or high-dose sodium nitroprusside therapy can therefore lead to iatrogenic cyanide poisoning.

Further Reading

Joint Formulary Committee. *British National Formulary.* 58th edition. London: British Medical Association and Royal Pharmaceutical Society of Great Britain, 2009.

Ward C, Sair M. Oral poisoning: an update. *Continuing Education in Anaesthesia, Critical Care & Pain.* 2010; **10**(1): 6–11.

3.1.2. Burns and drowning – Helen L Jewitt

These are potentially life-threatening situations, the initial management of which you will be expected to be confident of. Apply an airway, breathing, circulation approach and add the details specific to the particular scenario you are given.

A 25-year-old male is brought into the Emergency Department following a house fire.

Describe your initial assessment

I would make an initial assessment of the patient according to an airway, breathing and circulation approach aiming to identify potentially life threatening problems and make an estimation of the extent of the burn. I would simultaneously take a brief history including the timing and circumstances of the injury, consumption of alcohol or recreational drugs and relevant past medical history.

I would firstly assess the patency of the airway, listening for any added sounds such as stridor, which may indicate upper airway compromise. Cervical spine control must be maintained if there is any history of trauma. High flow humidified oxygen should be given via a non-rebreathing bag and facemask

I would make an assessment of the respiratory system by observation of the chest for respiratory movements, determination of respiratory rate, auscultation of the chest and measurement of oxygen saturations. The extent of any burns on the chest should also be noted.

Circulation would be assessed by feeling the warmth of the peripheries and measuring central capillary refill time, heart rate and blood pressure. I would obtain intra-venous access with two large bore cannulae and commence fluid resuscitation.

Assessment of the neurological system would consist of determination of Glasgow Coma Scale score or AVPU score and assessment of the pupils. I would cautiously administer intravenous morphine to the patient if pain was an issue, provided there were no contraindications.

The patient should then be exposed to allow the extent of the burn to be estimated.

How is the severity of a burn graded?

Burns can be graded both on the depth of the injury and the percentage surface area that is affected. The depth of a burn can be subdivided into superficial or deep. Superficial burns affect the epidermis only. They appear red, can blister and are painful. Deep burns cause damage to the dermis and have a white appearance. There is loss of pinprick sensation due to destruction of the nerve endings.

Percentage surface area can be estimated using the "rule of nines", whereby areas of the body are assigned a surface area based on multiples of nine. This rule is not applicable to children as they have small limbs in comparison to their head and trunk. Alternatively the area of the patient's own palm can be used to represent 1% of their total surface area.

What further investigations are appropriate for this patient?

Blood tests should be performed including full blood count and urea and electrolytes. Alcohol levels and drug toxicology may be indicated depending on the history. Arterial blood gases should be obtained. Co-oximetry allows accurate determination of carboxy-haemoglobin levels. A chest X-ray should also be performed at this stage.

What would alert you to the possibility that this patient may have suffered an inhalation injury?

Features from the history and clinical examination would raise the possibility of an inhalational injury. In the history evidence of prolonged exposure to smoke such as entrapment in a burning building or loss of consciousness at the scene are worrying features.

Evidence on examination of soot around the nostrils or inside the mouth, facial burns, respiratory distress, stridor, soot staining of the sputum or oropharyngeal oedema are markers of possible inhalational injury.

What is the appropriate course of action if inhalational injury is suspected?

The airway should be secured by endotracheal intubation immediately. The reason for this is that swelling of the airway can progress rapidly leading to complete obstruction. A range of endotracheal tube sizes should be immediately to hand as the oedema may be advanced by the time of presentation to hospital. A full-length endotracheal tube should be used to allow for the development of facial oedema. A nasogastric tube may be inserted at the same time to permit early enteral feeding.

How is the fluid requirement of this patient calculated?

There are several different formulae available for estimating the fluid requirement for resuscitation following a major burn. One of these is the Parkland formula. The information needed to make the calculation is the patient's weight, the percentage area of the burn and the approximate time of the injury.

The patient should receive 4 ml/kg of crystalloid solution per percentage area of the burn in the first 24 hours following the burn injury. Half of this total volume should be administered in the first 8 hours and the remainder in the following 16 hours. This formula only provides an initial guide for fluid resuscitation. Additional fluid may be necessary if the patient fails to respond.

What specific monitoring and investigations are indicated in the first 24 hours of admission?

The patient should be managed in a critical care environment. The airway is maintained by endotracheal intubation with adequate sedation. Invasive cardiovascular monitoring is indicated to assess the adequacy of ventilation and the response to fluid resuscitation. A urine output of 0.5–1 ml/kg/hr should be ensured. Haematocrit, urinary osmolality and serial plasma electrolytes can also be used to guide fluid replacement.

A full secondary survey is performed to detail the full extent of the burn and any other injuries. Circumferential burns can reduce chest wall compliance or distal limb perfusion and may therefore require urgent surgical escharotomy.

Strict attention should be paid to analgesia, gastric ulcer prophylaxis and nutrition.

What are the criteria for transfer of this patient to a regional burns unit?

Transfer should be arranged if this patient has a burn surface of more than 10% of total body surface area, has sustained burns to specific parts of the body including face, hands, feet, genitalia, perineum or major joints; or if there is an inhalational injury. Other criteria for transfer are greater than 5% surface area burns in children, electrical and chemical burns, circumferential burns to the limbs or chest and burns in patients with pre-existing medical conditions or at the extremes of age.

The patient has been transferred to a regional burns unit. He has a total burn surface area of approximately 20% affecting his right arm, flank and thigh. He does not have a significant inhalational injury.

Outline your peri-operative management of this patient for debridement and split skin grafting of his burn

Answer this in a structured way beginning with aspects of your pre-operative assessment, followed by intra-operative and post-operative issues. It is vitally important to mention an awareness of the possibility of massive blood loss, maintenance of the patient's temperature and provision of adequate analgesia.

In my pre-operative assessment of this patient, I would look at events since his admission to the burns unit to establish how stable he has been. In addition to this I would gather available information regarding past medical and anaesthetic history, medication and allergies. Appropriate preparation for this case include warming the theatre to 28–32°C and ensuring there are at least six units of crossmatched blood available.

I would plan to intubate the patient ensuring that suxamethonium was not used. This is because suxamethonium can precipitate an exaggerated increase in plasma potassium concentration due to a proliferation of extrajunctional acetylcholine receptors. This can precipitate life-threatening arrhythmias or cardiac arrest. It is considered to be unsafe to use suxamethonium for a 12-month period beginning 24 hours after a burn.

If not already in use, invasive arterial monitoring is appropriate for this case. An arterial line allows beat to beat monitoring of blood pressure and regular sampling of blood.

One of the potential problems I would anticipate in theatre is massive blood loss and cardiovascular instability. Debrided tissue bleeds significantly and it can be difficult to keep an accurate track of how much blood has been lost. Blood sampling at regular intervals will show a trend in haemoglobin. Packed cells should be transfused as indicated by the clinical findings and haemoglobin. Some units use monitoring techniques such as oesophageal Doppler utrasonography and arterial waveform analysis (LiDCO™) to help optimise fluid administration.

The patient should be actively warmed with a forced air device and fluid warmer. The temperature of the theatre should also be increased to above 25°C.

The post-operative care of the patient will take place in a specialised burns intensive care unit or general ITU. Strict attention should be paid to fluid balance, analgesia, prevention of infection and nutrition. The patient will need regular dressing changes for which they may require sedation and analgesia.

A 16-year-old male is brought into the Emergency Department having fallen into a river on an outdoor pursuits course. He is unconscious with no obvious external injuries and has a weakly palpable carotid pulse. His rectal temperature is 28°C.

This is an uncommon scenario but can be simplified by using advanced life support guidelines as the mainstay of your answer. Always remember and make clear in your answer that other injuries can co-exist in this type of patient. Appropriate precautions must be taken, for example cervical spine protection.

How do you define drowning and near-drowning?

Drowning is defined as death following asphyxia due to partial or complete submersion in water. Near-drowning is a term that has been used to describe evidence of recovery following submersion.

What is the initial management of this patient?

After a brief assessment of airway, breathing and circulation, the first step is to intubate the patient with cervical spine control. He should be ventilated with 100% oxygen. His cardiovascular system should be assessed for evidence of a spontaneous circulation. If this is absent cardiopulmonary resuscitation according to the ALS guidelines must be commenced. Intravenous access should be secured and administration of warmed intra-venous fluids commenced.

Further active rewarming measures should be taken. These include warmed inspired gases, forced air warming blankets and irrigation of the bladder or stomach with warm fluid. More invasive methods include peritoneal lavage with warm fluid and the use of extracorporeal warming.

What is the significance of hypothermia following this type of injury?

Hypothermia in this setting may provide a degree of protection from the harmful effects of hypoxia on the central nervous system. Resuscitation should not be discontinued until the patient's temperature is above 32°C.

What is the appearance of the ECG in hypothermia?

The ECG in hypothermia can show sinus bradycardia, various stages of heart block progressing to complete heart block. There may be J waves visible which appear as positive deflections after the QRS complex. There is a significant risk of arrhythmias particularly atrial fibrillation and ventricular fibrillation which may be refractory to defibrillation.

Can you list any predictors of patient outcome following a near-drowning?

There are a number of factors that indicate a poor prognosis. These include a prolonged immersion time of greater than 5–10 minutes, cardiac arrest at the scene, dilated unreactive pupils or pH less than 7 on arrival to hospital and lack of purposeful motor response after 24 hours.

What other issues may be important in the treatment of this patient?

The clinical picture may be complicated by intoxication with alcohol or recreational drugs or a co-existing acute medical condition such as epilepsy.

A distinction was commonly made between fresh water and salt water near-drowning. Absorption of fresh water from the lungs into the systemic circulation can provoke haemolysis and electrolyte disturbances. Both types of water produce a similar clinical picture of pulmonary oedema and hypoxaemic respiratory failure and the distinction is of limited clinical value.

In the longer term, near-drowning victims are at risk of developing an acute lung injury and/or sepsis. The latter is a particular issue if the injury took place in contaminated water.

Further Reading

Hilton P, Hepp M. The immediate care of the burned patient. *Continuing Education in* *Anaesthesia, Critical Care & Pain.* 2001; **1**(4): 113–116.

Intensive care

3.2.1. The high-risk surgical patient – Matt Thomas

This topic would be most likely to appear as part of either a long or short clinical case, as it allows ample opportunity to discuss common clinical problems.

Have you any idea of mortality rates after surgery in the UK?

Data from National Confidential Enquiry into Patient Outcome and Death (NCEPOD) puts 30-day mortality somewhere between 0.7 and 1.7% for all operative procedures. Using a sample of over 4 million operations between 1999 and 2004 from ICNARC (Intensive Care National Audit & Research Centre) and CHKS, overall 30-day mortality after elective surgery is approximately 0.5%, and 5.5% after emergency surgery. These data also indicated that a small group of patients accounted for the majority of deaths. About 1 in 8 patients were in this high-risk group that had a crude mortality rate after all surgery of 12.5%. Interestingly, in absolute terms, this group accounted for over 80% of the total number of deaths, but fewer than 15% of them were admitted to an ICU.

Which groups of patients have higher mortality rates?

There are patient and surgery related factors. NCEPOD have shown that mortality increased with age: patients with an age of more than 70 have 25% of all operations but suffer 75% of all deaths. Existing comorbidities, especially heart failure, and current physiological status are also important. With regard to surgical factors, mortality increases with emergency surgery and with major and major-plus procedures (i.e., laparotomy or thoracotomy). These operations are generally longer and result in more tissue damage. Anaesthetic related factors might influence post-operative outcome. There are data to suggest that fluid management, location of post-operative care and even analgesic technique influence mortality in high-risk patients.

How would you define high-risk?

Risk is difficult to define and means different things to different people, so this is somewhat subjective. Practically speaking, a common threshold is to consider a patient or procedure high-risk if mortality is estimated at over 5%, or twice the usual mortality associated with

Dr. Podcast Scripts for the Final FRCA, ed. Rebecca A. Leslie, Emily K. Johnson, Gary Thomas and Alexander P. L. Goodwin.   Published by Cambridge University Press.
© R. A. Leslie, E. K. Johnson, G. Thomas and A. P. L. Goodwin 2011.

that procedure. More NCEPOD data indicate that surgeons miss 1 in 3 high-risk patients if asked to identify them pre-operatively.

So how can these patients be identified beforehand?

It would be better to use more objective means of assessment than personal opinion. There are a number of assessment and prediction tools that can be applied in the pre-operative clinic or at the bedside to estimate risk. Both patient factors and surgical risk need to be evaluated, but the latter should be easier as there are more national data on complication rates including mortality available to use as a benchmark.

What assessment and prediction tools do you know?

There are checklists and scoring systems based on a clinical history, examination and simple laboratory tests, and then there are those that involve more sophisticated investigations. The Goldman and Detsky scores each use slightly different factors weighted in slightly different ways to produce estimates of the risk of cardiac death or cardiac complications postoperatively, whereas the POSSUM score estimates mortality and all, not just cardiac, morbidity. Several authors have devised criteria for identifying high-risk patients, but with less accurate estimates of risk.

Cardiac investigations have dominated the field of risk prediction in non-cardiac surgery, with the exception of thoracic surgery where lung function testing is well established. Echocardiography, stress echocardiography, nuclear investigations and even angiography are all used, but these are tests for the presence or absence of cardiac disease and are not preoperative screening tests.

Recently, interest has grown in functional tests of the cardiorespiratory system, such as quantification of activities of daily living (ADLs), using metabolic equivalents (METs), 6 minute or shuttle walks, or cardiopulmonary exercise (CPX) testing.

Why is this?

What is seen as more important is the functional ability of the heart, not merely the presence or the absence of coronary artery disease. Even the Goldman index reflects this, as the highest weighting for any score is for heart failure. Individual patient risk depends on individual physiological reserve and this cannot be assessed by history and clinical examination alone.

Why identify these patients pre-operatively?

Firstly, the patient can be given accurate information about the likely risks of the procedure and secondly, additional resources can be used to reduce these risks and increase the chances of survival. These resources, for example ICU beds, are expensive and scarce so must be used to greatest effect.

What do you understand by the terms "optimisation" and "goal directed therapy"?

Goal directed therapy is a term used widely in anaesthesia and critical care that usually refers to more-or-less protocolised care aimed at achieving a set of predominantly haemodynamic goals that have been associated with improved outcome in a clearly defined group of patients. Optimisation refers more specifically to this process in the context of peri-operative care.

What is the principle behind goal directed therapy?

It was first noticed over 40 years ago that patients who could not increase their cardiac output post-operatively had a higher mortality, and in the 1980s, was noted again by Shoemaker in trauma patients. It was thought that cardiac ischaemia and organ failure was caused by low cardiac output and reduced oxygen delivery, so it was hypothesised that increasing cardiac output and oxygen delivery to the levels attained by survivors would lead to reduced mortality. In a landmark trial he was able to show that achieving oxygen delivery goals with oxygen, fluids and inotropes, post-operative mortality was significantly reduced but there are some methodological concerns. His findings have not been consistently replicated.

So what is current thinking?

The modern concept of goal directed therapy also concentrates on oxygen supply–demand imbalance, but less on cardiac ischaemia. The stress response to surgery imposes the extra oxygen demand for adequate mitochondrial generation of ATP, required primarily for wound healing and the post-operative inflammatory response. This is met by increasing cardiac output and oxygen extraction. Patients with the inability to respond to this increase in demand are those who are at risk of developing complications because mitochondrial function is affected by prolonged reductions in oxygen delivery. The patients are therefore at risk of developing post-operative myocardial ischaemia and infarction. Mitochondrial dysfunction may lead to immunosuppression and is thought to underlie multi-organ failure. It also explains why heart failure is so significant, why lower central venous saturation identifies a high-risk group, and why functional tests like CPX testing are good at predicting post-operative complications.

For further details on CPX testing see Chapter 1.2.1. "Pre-operative assessment and management of patients with cardiac disease".

You are asked to anaesthetise an 81-year-old woman who has presented for an elective abdomino-perineal resection. She has chronic obstructive pulmonary disease and is known to have moderate left ventricular dysfunction. The results of a CPX test show an anaerobic threshold (AT) of 10.5 ml/kg/min without ischaemia.

What are the anaesthetic implications of this result?

The combination of a major operative procedure and an AT of <11 ml/kg/min indicate that the patient has a high risk of developing post-operative complications.

Prior to admission this patient's medical therapy should be reviewed by her consultant physician and optimised and an ICU bed should be arranged for post-operative care. I would plan to use goal directed therapy, so I would use full haemodynamic monitoring, including cardiac output monitoring, as relying on MAP and CVP alone does not allow calculation of oxygen delivery and both may be normal when cardiac output is insufficient. In an ideal world the ICU bed would be available pre-operatively, so that the monitoring and therapy could be started in advance, but this is rarely possible. In practice, most patients achieve the targets with fluid supplementation alone and a minority will need inotrope therapy. The highest risk time for problems is intra-operatively and within the first 8 hours post-operatively. Although the stress response continues for longer than this, effective therapy during this period prevents complications days after surgery.

What cardiac output monitoring would you use?

A recent NHS technology assessment concluded that oesophageal Doppler ultrasound monitoring to guide intra-operative fluid therapy is both clinically and cost effective in this situation. That said, there is no evidence to suggest that one cardiac output monitor is any better than another, and successful protocols using alternatives such as pulse contour analysis using lithium dilution (LiDCO^{TM}) are reported. Similarly, dobutamine, dopexamine and adrenaline have all been used successfully. I would probably use dobutamine as an inotrope as it is the drug with which I'm most familiar for that indication. What seems to be important is the achievement of appropriate targets before organ failure supervenes.

Are there any problems associated with goal directed therapy?

As with any medical intervention there are risks and benefits. There are risks associated with the insertion of intra-vascular catheters, with the fluids and drugs used, and with use of the cardiac output monitoring device itself. The main problem seen with the drugs is tachycardia, which increases myocardial oxygen demand, and this is a common reason for failure to achieve the goals. There are risks with the technique applied, particularly if a pulmonary, artery (PA) catheter is used. If the cardiac output monitors are incorrectly set up or not calibrated, the data produced may be unreliable or misinterpreted. Finally, if goal directed therapy is started too late, that is after organ failure is established, complications may be increased.

Tell me about the role of β-blockers in high-risk patients?

There is considerable interest in β-blockers in high-risk patients, mainly because of their effects on reducing myocardial oxygen demand and increasing plaque stability, and the 2009 guidelines from the American Heart Association (AHA) suggest that they should be used in high-risk patients or high-risk surgery after consideration of individual risks and benefits. It must be said that none of these recommendations are based on evidence from multiple randomised controlled trials (RCTs), and the recent POISE (peri-operative ischaemic evaluation) study casts more doubt on widespread use of β-blockers.

What was the POISE trial?

POISE was a randomised multi-centre trial with over 8000 patients having non-cardiac surgery. A β-blocker (metoprolol) or placebo was started 2 to 4 hours before surgery and continued for 30 days. Although fewer patients in the metoprolol group had a myocardial infarction, more patients had a stroke or died.

When do you think β-blockers should be used?

Patients who are already taking β-blockers should remain on them, and those with an independent indication should start, preferably well in advance of their operation. For those patients at high risk of cardiac complications, or undergoing high-risk surgery, the decision to start a β-blocker is less clear. At present there is not enough evidence to make firm recommendations, but there may well be groups of patients who will benefit from β-blockers as long as hypotension and bradycardia are avoided. They should not be started *de novo* in the day or two prior to high-risk surgery and in the emergency setting a cause for tachycardia should be sought and corrected before even cautious use of β-blockers is considered.

Could you combine β-blockers and goal directed therapy?

There is a practical problem, in that patients taking β-blockers will be less susceptible to the effects of inotrope therapy, although there may still be beneficial β2 effects. There is no other reason why they could not be combined, and arguably they should as high-risk patients may have multiple pathologies and benefit from multiple therapies. Withdrawal of β-blockers is also associated with significant morbidity and mortality. Patients on long-term β-blocker therapy have the cardiac adaptations of increased stroke volumes at lower heart rates that are ideal for the peri-operative period. Overall, the risks and benefits are likely to be related to the haemodynamic effects of β-blockers, especially if used acutely. More fluid may be required, and greater attention to detail, but that is no bad thing. There could be a role for new inotropes such as levosimendan.

Tell me about the effects of statins in the peri-operative period?

Statins have a number of advantageous effects that are independent of their lipid lowering properties. They are anti-inflammatory, reduce thrombosis, endothelial activation and platelet activation. They also reduce ischaemia-reperfusion injury, enhance fibrinolysis and vasodilatation in the microcirculation. Several cohort studies show increased cardiac morbidity and mortality risk if statins are stopped peri-operatively. A single small RCT showed a reduction in death or cardiac complications after vascular surgery in a group given atorvastatin. Although there is sufficient evidence to test the utility of statins in high-risk patients, however there is not enough evidence yet to recommend initiation in those not already taking them.

Why do you think goal directed therapy is not more widely practised?

There are three main reasons. First, there is confusion because of conflicting trial evidence and some scepticism about positive trials relating to their methodology and therefore validity. Second, there is the problem of a limited number of critical care beds, both ICU and HDU. Finally, there is reluctance to use PA catheters or other cardiac output monitoring devices, which may also be affected by availability of and familiarity with the appropriate equipment in theatres.

Further Reading

Agnew N. Preoperative cardiopulmonary exercise testing. *Continuing Education in Anaesthesia, Critical Care & Pain.* 2010; **10**: 33–37.

Kohl B, Deutschman C. The inflammatory response to surgery and trauma. *Current Opinion in Critical Care.* 2006; **12**: 325–332.

Lees N, Hamilton M, Rhodes A. Goal directed therapy in high risk surgical patients. *Critical Care.* 2009; **13**: 231.

National Health Service (NHS) Technology Adoption Centre. Doppler Guided Intraoperative Fluid Management. http://www.technologyadoptionhub. nhs.uk/doppler-guided-intraoperative-fluid-management/evidence-base. html.

POISE Study Group, Devereaux PJ, Yang H, Yusuf S, et al. Effects of extended-release metoprolol succinate in patients undergoing non-cardiac surgery (POISE trial): a randomised controlled trial. *Lancet*. 2008; **371**: 1839–1847.

Powell-Tuck J, Gosling P, Lobo DN, et al. British Consensus Guidelines on Intravenous Fluid Therapy for Adult Surgical Patients (GIFTASUP). 2008. http://www.asgbi.org.uk/en/search-result/index.cfm/str/GIFTASUP/category/doc.

Tote S, Grounds R. Performing perioperative optimization of the high-risk surgical patient. *British Journal of Anaesthesia*. 2006; **97**: 4–11.

Williams G, Rhodes A. Pre-operative care of the high-risk surgical patient. *Continuing Education in Anaesthesia, Critical Care & Pain*. 2002; **2**: 178–182.

3.2.2. Management of multi-organ failure – Matt Thomas

This is an extremely wide topic and could go almost anywhere. If asked about management, be reassured that there is unlikely to be one right way to do things and as long as you are safe, sensible and can justify your actions you will be unlucky to fail. You can help yourself by thinking of patients and clinical problems you have encountered and how they were managed.

What do you understand by the term multi-organ failure (MOF)?

The term is associated with critically ill patients in the ICU. In one sense, it just means failure of more than one organ, but is usually used in the context of acute severe illness and refers to new organ failures requiring advanced organ support techniques, for example ventilation and haemofiltration. There is no one accepted definition of multi-organ failure, and it can be difficult to decide if, say coagulopathy and thrombocytopenia should be considered as liver or blood failure for example.

Do you think this is a useful concept?

The term is very non-specific, and really says nothing detailed about the cause of the problem, the organs involved and the severity, or the overall prognosis. Organ failure itself can be difficult to define, as it is often a matter of degree, not an all-or-nothing phenomenon.

Are there any more specific descriptions of organ dysfunction?

There are two ways of looking at individual organ dysfunction. First, there are definitions that do reduce it to a simple question of failure or no failure, for example brain failure or delirium that is either present or absent. Then there are scores which recognise that organ failure is a matter of degree, for example the difference between acute lung injury and adult respiratory distress syndrome (ARDS) using the $PaO_2 : FiO_2$ ratio. ARDS is likely if the ratio is <200 and acute lung injury <300.

Further examples include the Child-Pugh score for liver dysfunction or the GCS for conscious level.

There are consensus definitions of organ failure, produced by European and American societies of intensive care medicine, as part of the updated sepsis definition in 2001, but these tend to focus on either the presence or absence of failure of organs. However there are elements of organ dysfunction included in prognostic scores such as acute physiology and chronic health evaluation (APACHE).

Table 3.2.2. The SOFA scoring system

	1	2	3	4
Respiratory: PaO_2/FiO_2 **(mmHg)**	<400	<300	<200 and mechanically ventilated	<100 and mechanically ventilated
CVS: MAP or vasopressor	MAP < 70 mmHg	dop <= 5 or dob (any dose)	dop > 5 OR epi <= 0.1 OR nor <= 0.1	dop > 15 OR epi > 0.1 OR nor > 0.1
CNS: GCS	13–14	10–12	6–9	<6
Coagulation: Platelets $(\times 10^3/mm^3)$	<150	<100	<50	<20
Hepatic: Bilirubin (mg/dl)	1.2–1.9	2.0–5.9	6.0–11.9	>12.0
Renal: Creatinine (mg/dl) (or UO)	1.2–1.9	2.0–3.4	3.5 – 4.9 (or <500 ml/day)	>5.0 (or <200 ml/day)

Have you heard of any composite scores of organ dysfunction relating more directly to multi-organ failure?

Sepsis-related organ failure assessment (SOFA) is a well-established and validated scoring system that was developed in Europe in the mid-nineties (Table 3.2.2). It uses daily assessments of function in six organ systems and assigns a value to each depending on the deviation from normal, where higher numbers mean worse function. The advantage of SOFA is that the progress of organ dysfunction can be followed from day to day, both overall and within each of the six organs monitored. It has been shown that mortality is related to the total score as well as the change in the score, where a particularly poor prognostic sign is an increase in the SOFA score after the first 24 hours. These scores are increasingly used as outcome measures in clinical trials in the ICU.

What are the drawbacks of the SOFA scoring system?

This scoring system works well, but there are a number of issues. First, there is the issue of case mix. For example, the SOFA score was developed by consensus to apply to septic patients and must not be assumed to apply to all critically ill patients, particularly in specialist areas, although in fact, validation of SOFA score has been performed in populations of trauma, cardiac surgery and bone marrow transplant patients among others, and appears robust in each. The problem of lead-time bias is less with daily scores than with the general prognostic scores that use only admission data.

It is not developed as an outcome measure tool and there is some scepticism regarding the relevance of a sudden fall in the SOFA score must be maintained. Also there does not seem to be a simple bedside way of quantifying cardiac dysfunction independent of therapy. SOFA currently uses dose of vasoactive drugs, but in future, the measurement of brain B-natriuretic peptide and troponins might aid prognostic scoring.

What causes multi-organ failure?

Multi-organ failure is seen with all the illnesses that present to intensive care – medical, traumatic and surgical. It is the endpoint of a severe systemic inflammatory response whatever the trigger. When it develops after some time in the ICU the most likely trigger is infection.

Is there a final common pathway at cellular level?

There are several theories of the origin of cell dysfunction in multi-organ dysfunction, which may just reflect the large number of triggering events rather than the cell processes responsible for organ failure which are more likely to be stereotypical (this is not clear). Examples of triggers include sepsis, trauma, or ischaemia especially with reperfusion injury. Each induces a pro-inflammatory response that includes local and systemic leucocyte and endothelial activation and activation of innate immune and coagulation systems.

So how does this actually lead to organ failure?

This process leads to microvascular occlusion within organs that in turn results in cellular hypoxia and dysfunction even if global haemodynamics and oxygen transport appear relatively normal. There is certainly evidence of microvascular dysfunction in systemic inflammatory response syndrome (SIRS) and multi-organ failure especially secondary to sepsis. One step further, others have noted the lack of evidence of infarction in affected organs and their potential for complete recovery, and have proposed that multi-organ failure is a form of adaptive cellular hibernation triggered by periods of cytopathic hypoxia (diminished ATP production despite normal oxygenation) maintained by the hormonal and metabolic changes induced by systemic inflammation. What has not been explained is why some develop multi-organ failure and others do not, and why a particular organ might be affected in one individual and not another.

What treatments are available for multi-organ failure?

Treatment of the cause, if it can be identified, is essential, but as yet there are no specific treatments for multi-organ failure, although Singer's hypothesis of hibernation may generate some interesting therapies. At the moment the focus is on prevention, support and avoiding secondary insults. Ensuring adequate early resuscitation and control of the trigger for SIRS are the basis of prevention. Maintaining oxygen delivery to mitochondria early in the critical illness in theory prevents the "switch off" that underpins cell and organ dysfunction. If MOF does occur then the patient must be supported until recovery of function occurs. In this period avoidance of secondary insults, notably infection, but also hypoxia, hypotension, hyperglycaemia, will reduce the period of organ failure.

Is this true in every case?

There is the odd situation, such as fulminant hepatic failure, where single-organ transplantation is a treatment for multi-organ failure, but the general principle of supporting organs and maintaining homeostasis does apply to all.

What specific organ support techniques are available?

Mechanical devices are available to support lungs, heart, kidneys and liver although some are more effective than others, or more suitable for long-term use. Drugs are also available for support of cardiovascular function, with there being no really effective pharmacological support of other organs.

The gut may be supported by enteral or parenteral feeding or drug therapy of motility disorders. Blood products, erythropoietin, vitamin K and haematinics are used to support haematology and coagulation, and dressings and grafting to protect the skin. Endocrine support currently consists of insulin and glucocorticoids in selected patients, although this may be an area that can be developed in the future. There is no substitute for the brain, although a range of drugs can be used to alter function, usually depressing it to reduce oxygen demand ($CMRO_2$) thus protecting against ischaemia.

Are these support techniques benign?

Drug therapies have side effects that may be unpredictable in the context of critical illness, or there are unintended consequences. For example, iron supplementation may help prevent anaemia and avoid transfusion, but the same iron may promote bacterial overgrowth. Catecholamines are widely used for haemodynamic support, but increase myocardial oxygen demand, have metabolic consequences and enhance bacterial growth. Blood products carry risks of immunosuppression, incompatibility and infection. Catheters are associated with complications of insertion, infection and if intra-vascular, thrombosis. Ventilation, the supportive therapy that distinguishes intensive care, has the potential to cause further lung injury when used inappropriately. It is also often forgotten that many interventions in ICU are painful if nothing else. Before starting any therapy the benefits, risks, alternatives and consequences of doing nothing must be considered.

Are there any other important adjuncts to supportive therapy?

DVT and stress ulcer prophylaxis are essential in the absence of contraindications. Good nursing care and physiotherapy are also important in general supportive care. Infection control and good hygiene are vital, as patients with MOF have increased susceptibility to infections.

What is the mortality associated with multi-organ failure?

It is very difficult to predict individual outcome, and models such as APACHE scores are intended for population and not personal use. A very rough guide is approximately 20% risk of mortality per organ failure, although this will vary with the cause, co-morbidity, organs failed and initial response to therapy.

Are there any particularly ominous signs?

Some organ failures have a particularly high associated mortality. Liver failure in the context of multi-organ failure (MOF) is a poor sign, so hypoglycaemia with high bilirubin and lactate is worrying. The presence of disseminated intra-vascular coagulation (DIC) is similarly ominous, and a simple DIC score using INR, platelets, fibrinogen and D-dimers has good predictive accuracy for mortality. The response to therapy is also important, and any failure to improve or deterioration after support has started is a poor sign. The response to treatment may be tracked sequentially using SOFA scores.

How long would you continue organ support?

Active treatment should continue for as long as the risks and burdens were outweighed by the benefits, i.e., the possibility of survival with a quality of life meaningful to the patient. Each decision is made on an individual basis considering the clinical context and the wishes of the patient if they are known or can be ascertained. The relatives can give useful information bearing on the patient's best interests and their wishes should also be taken into consideration. It remains a medical decision, although the recent Mental Capacity Act contains guidance on how to proceed when considering the best interests of incompetent patients.

What are the long-term effects on survivors?

Long-term effects can be considered in two groups: those that are present in hospital and those that persist after discharge home. Some sequelae of MOF are slow to resolve and lead to problems within hospital and indeed delay discharge home. In particular, critical illness polyneuropathy and polymyopathy are associated with MOF and perhaps could be considered part of neurological system failure. Muscle weakness is the most obvious manifestation and leads to prolonged dependency because of poor mobility and muscle strength. Even feeding oneself may be difficult or impossible and nutritional supplements or nasogastric/jejunal feeding may be needed for some time.

Is there anything else?

Many things that we take for granted, such as sleep or bowel and bladder function, may take time to return to normal after MOF. Delirium is another neurological failure that can be very subtle and slow to resolve, and may be mis-attributed to memory impairment or considered a normal response to the events surrounding critical illness. For some, particularly the elderly, any of these effects may prevent a return to home or independence.

Tell me about mortality and morbidity after discharge

Overall mortality is increased after discharge from hospital. This is affected by age and co-morbidity, but there is a clear effect of MOF that lasts for a year or more. Of those who survive, between 25 and 50% need assistance with activities of daily living at 1 year, although it is much less than this at 3 years; again this is affected by age and previous functional status. Few will require long-term respiratory support, and less than 10% develop the need for long-term renal support for example, but testing will reveal sub-clinical deficits. After ARDS a restrictive deficit with reduced diffusing capacity is present for months. Studies of cognitive function suggest that problems persist for months or years afterwards across several domains such as attention, memory, task planning and execution.

What are the social implications for these patients?
And how do they feel about it?

This can cause problems with return to work, relationships and general quality of life. Using validated questionnaires, most patients report a lower quality of life than matched controls, but most would undergo the ICU episode again.

Are there any other problems that arise from a long-term ICU stay?
How can patients with problems be identified and treated?

There are many other problems that can result, but there are insufficient data to make confident estimates of the size of the problem in the UK. Chronic pain, chronic fatigue and sleep problems occur, as does anxiety, depression and post-traumatic stress disorder. These may be difficult to diagnose or may not be attributed to time spent in ICU with multi-organ failure. As attention turns from simple mortality based statistics to patient related outcome measures such problems are likely to be better identified, and recent NICE guidance emphasises the importance of multidisciplinary rehabilitation after critical illness. An ICU follow-up clinic is one way in which patients can be identified earlier and appropriate support and treatment organised.

Further Reading

Department for Constitutional Affairs (DCA). Mental Capacity Act 2005 – Summary. http://webarchive.nationalarchives.gov.uk/+/www.dh.gov.uk/prod_consum_dh/groups/dh_digitalassets/@dh/@en/documents/digitalasset/dh_4108596.pdf.

Hofhuis J, van Stel H, Schrijvers A, et al. Health related quality of life in critically ill patients. *Current Opinion in Critical Care*. 2009; **15**: 425–430.

National Institute for Health and Clinical Excellence (NICE). Rehabilitation after critical illness. 2009. http://www.nice.org.uk/nicemedia/live/12137/43526/43526.pdf.

Singer M, De Santis V, Vitale D, Jeffcoate W. Multiorgan failure is an adaptive endocrine-mediated metabolic response to overwhelming systemic inflammation. *Lancet*. 2004; **364**: 545–548.

Strand K, Flaatten H. Severity scoring in the ICU: a review. *Acta Anaesthesiologica Scandinavica*. 2008; **52**: 467–478.

Vincent JL, Moreno R, Takala J. The SOFA (Sepsis-related Organ Failure Assessment) score to describe organ dysfunction/failure. On behalf of the Working Group on Sepsis-Related Problems of the European Society of Intensive Care Medicine. *Intensive Care Medicine*. 1996; **22**: 707–110.

3.2.3. ARDS and ventilation difficulties – Matt Thomas

The management of ARDS is a core topic in intensive care, and will also be relevant to all who will have to anaesthetise high-risk and critically ill patients. In the structured oral examinations (SOEs) it may be a clinical scenario or follow a discussion of respiratory physiology, for example, the different causes of hypoxia.

What are the causes of hypoxia and give me clinical examples of each?

Even if you are not asked to define a particular term it is worth stating briefly what you understand by it so that you (a) demonstrate knowledge to the examiners and (b) allow any possible misunderstanding of the question to be clarified before you have gone too far.

Hypoxia is an inadequate tissue oxygen supply or use and has four main causes:

- Hypoxic
- Anaemic
- Ischaemic/stagnant
- Cytopathic/histotoxic.

Hypoxic hypoxia is a reduction of oxygen uptake by the lung, for example after pneumonia. Anaemic hypoxia results from reduced arterial oxygen content secondary to loss of haemoglobin, or presence of abnormal haemoglobins; examples are major haemorrhage and carbon monoxide poisoning respectively. Ischaemic hypoxia results from a reduced oxygen delivery secondary to reduced cardiac output or local vascular occlusion, for example cardiogenic shock or arterial thromboembolism. Cytopathic hypoxia results from disrupted cellular metabolism, for example cyanide poisoning of mitochondrial respiratory chain enzymes. Different types may coexist.

What are the causes of hypoxic hypoxia?

There are several causes:

- Reduced inspired oxygen concentration (FiO_2)
- Hypoventilation.
- Ventilation/perfusion (V/Q) mismatch
- Shunt with venous admixture
- Reduced diffusing capacity.

Tell me a little more about V/Q mismatch and shunt?

The alveolus is the functional unit of gas exchange and if we assume that the cardiac output and inspired oxygen concentration (FiO_2) are in a steady state then the PaO_2 is determined by the balance between ventilation and perfusion across all alveoli. A disturbance of this normal balance is called V/Q mismatch.

A shunt refers to blood entering the arterial circulation and has not taken part in gas exchange. Examples of a true shunt include bronchial and thebesian venous drainage and congenital heart disease with right to left shunt. Unlike V/Q mismatch the administration of 100% will not increase the PaO_2.

What is the significance of diffusion impairment?

In most pathological conditions gas exchange is not diffusion limited since the alveolar–capillary barrier is so gas permeable. Equilibration between alveolar gas and pulmonary capillary blood is normally very fast, normally one-third of the contact time of 0.75 seconds in the capillary. However, if the alveolar membrane is thickened or capillary transit times are quick (high cardiac output states), then this may contribute towards hypoxia.

Can you explain how hypoxia may arise from V/Q mismatching?

Full saturation of mixed venous blood requires a sufficiently high alveolar PO_2. In poorly ventilated well-perfused alveoli there is insufficient oxygen delivered to the alveoli to saturate pulmonary venous blood fully. In cases of true shunt, where there is no ventilation and perfusion is maintained, no oxygen is taken up into the pulmonary venous blood. So, as the number of units with low V/Q ratio increases, the total oxygen content of pulmonary venous blood will fall. Incidentally, this is also how hypoventilation causes hypoxaemia since alveolar O_2 falls and CO_2 rises, and is also important if dead-space volume approaches tidal volume.

If the dead-space increases then a greater portion of the tidal volume does not participate in gas exchange. The effective alveolar minute ventilation is reduced, and this means that alveolar CO_2 rises and also, in poorly ventilated alveoli, V/Q ratio falls. Overall alveolar oxygen content falls and therefore so does pulmonary oxygen uptake.

Are you aware of any clinical conditions in which dead-space fraction is related to mortality?

The two clinical conditions where this has been demonstrated are pulmonary embolism and ARDS.

What is the generally accepted definition of ARDS?

The generally accepted definition is that of the American–European consensus conference in 1994. It has four components: an acute onset, bilateral infiltrates on chest X-ray, absence of left atrial hypertension and a $PaO_2 : FiO_2$ ratio of less than 200 mmHg, or 26.7 kPa.

Are there any difficulties with this definition?

First there is an element of subjectivity in assessing infiltrates on chest X-rays. Secondly it can be difficult to exclude left atrial hypertension clinically, and a pulmonary artery occlusion pressure of more than 18 may coexist with ARDS. Finally the $PaO_2 : FiO_2$ ratio may be significantly affected by parameters set up on a ventilator and some argue the definition should specify standard settings.

What are the causes?

There are many, conveniently considered in two categories: pulmonary and extra-pulmonary. Pulmonary causes result from direct insults to the lung and include:

- Pneumonia
- Aspiration
- Smoke inhalation
- Pulmonary contusion.

Extra-pulmonary or indirect causes include:

- Sepsis
- Severe trauma
- Transfusion reactions
- Burns
- Acute pancreatitis
- Drug reactions.

Does this classification help?

There is a lot of debate about whether or not pulmonary and extra-pulmonary ARDS are different diseases, and I don't think this has been resolved. For practical purposes most treat them in the same way.

Tell me about the pathophysiology of ARDS?

There are two stages that may be distinguished histologically: the exudative phase followed by the fibroproliferative phase. First there is an acute inflammatory reaction in the lung, and the alveoli fill with neutrophils, blood and a protein-rich pulmonary oedema. There is associated alveolar epithelial and capillary endothelial damage, with loss of alveolar cells and structural integrity and capillary thrombosis. Days or weeks later, chronic inflammation, fibrosis and neovascularisation occur.

How does ARDS cause hypoxia? Can you relate this to our earlier discussion?

There is widespread and profound V/Q mismatching as a result of the inflammatory reaction, which may be superimposed on a direct lung injury. Both shunt and dead-space increase, as alveoli and capillaries respectively are occluded. If severe, right ventricular failure and low cardiac output contribute further to venous admixture and hypoxia.

I would like you to consider this scenario

You are asked to review a previously fit 25-year-old man who is unwell in recovery following a femoral nailing under general anaesthesia. He has received a transfusion of 4 units of allogeneic blood. His respiratory rate is 30 breaths/min and has an oxygen saturation (SpO_2) of 91% on 15 L of O_2 via a reservoir mask. Apart from obvious respiratory distress and a sinus tachycardia, examination is unremarkable. What could be the problem?

Some opening statements might seem too obvious, but do serve to tell the examiner that you are able to recognise a critically ill patient promptly and appreciate situations calling for urgent action. If asked for a differential diagnosis in these scenarios, start with the most likely given the history.

This young man is clearly extremely unwell, given his very high respiratory rate and low SpO_2. It is possible that post-operative respiratory distress could arise from incomplete reversal of neuromuscular blockade and should be excluded using a peripheral nerve stimulator.

Other causes of acute respiratory distress should be considered and these include:

- Pulmonary aspiration
- Fat embolism syndrome
- Transfusion-related-acute-lung-injury (TRALI)
- Pneumothorax
- Lung contusions
- Bronchospasm.

The history, clinical examination and investigations suggest a diagnosis of ARDS. How will you proceed?

This patient should be referred to the critical care team for further management. In some centres, non-invasive ventilation might be attempted initially but this patient is most likely to require intubation and ventilation.

How are you going to set up the ventilator?

If you are going to quote any trials to support what you say then you must have a clear idea of what the trial showed and any major criticisms, though a full critical appraisal is not required.

Working on the assumption that this patient has an acute lung injury I would be guided by a lung-protective strategy used in the ARDSnet trial using low tidal volumes. I would use pressure-controlled ventilation to aim for a tidal volume of 6 ml/kg of ideal body weight, providing plateau pressures are less than 30 cm of water. I would set PEEP to 10–12 cm H_2O and titrate the FiO_2 aiming for a PaO_2 of 8 kPa. If the $PaCO_2$ became raised I would increase respiratory rate but would not aim for a normal CO_2.

What level of PEEP should be used?

The level of PEEP is guided by the ARDSnet table. There are more complicated ways based on transpulmonary pressures or compliance curves but as yet no firm evidence to show these are better than the ARDSnet strategy.

Did the ARDSnet trial use pressure-controlled ventilation?

Volume controlled ventilation was used. Many believe pressure-controlled ventilation allows better control of plateau pressures and has gas exchange benefits.

What are the principles of management of ARDS in the ICU?

There is specific and supportive care. Specific care includes treating the cause of ARDS and preventing further lung damage with a lung protective ventilatory strategy. Fluid balance is important as the ARDSnet fluids and catheters study suggests that keeping the lung dry is associated with better outcomes. Supportive care includes DVT and ulcer prophylaxis, enteral feeding, tight control of blood glucose and elevation of the head of the bed.

Are there specific treatments for ARDS itself?

As yet there is no proven therapy for established ARDS. There are two small studies where enteral feeding with omega-3 fatty acids (derived from fish oil), anti-oxidants and physiological amounts or arginine improve oxygenation and clinical outcomes, there is however, conflicting evidence. Other therapies under investigation include exogenous surfactant to replace the endogenous deficit, and fibrinolytics or activated protein C to reduce alveolar and capillary thrombosis. A recent randomised placebo controlled trial using intravenous β-agonists (salbutamol) to help reduce extravascular lung water was stopped because of arrhythmias.

Is there a role for steroid therapy?

There is conflicting evidence and considerable controversy regarding steroids in ARDS. If given at moderate doses within the first week or ten days and tapered slowly there appear to be benefits in gas exchange and reduced time on the ventilator. Given later, any benefit is outweighed by the risks of neuromuscular problems, immunosuppression and increased mortality.

What does a lung-protective ventilation strategy aim to avoid?

It is a ventilation strategy that is based on the premise that ventilation causes injury to the sick lung in a number of ways. The major causes of injury are volutrauma, barotrauma, atelectrauma and biotrauma.

What do these terms mean?

In ARDS not all the lung is equally involved in the pathological process. Essentially excessive tidal volume and inflation pressure over-distend healthy alveoli, hence volu- and barotrauma, and the lungs are subjected to cyclical opening and closing, hence atelectrauma. The damage to the alveolar–capillary barrier leading to increased permeability, release of inflammatory mediators and translocation of pathogens, hence biotrauma.

Despite optimal management of this patient, his gas exchange continues to deteriorate. What are your options?

The initial diagnosis might need to be reconsidered, but complications such as pneumothorax, pneumonia or heart failure should be excluded. Boluses of neuromuscular blocking agents are useful to decrease chest wall compliance and may have additional benefits in reducing inflammation (cisatracurium), although the precise mechanism is unclear. Following neuromuscular blockade, alveolar recruitment manoeuvres can then be applied. I would also accept a lower target PaO_2 and review the ventilator settings with a senior colleague, thinking about reviewing the PEEP.

The patient's oxygenation continues to deteriorate?

The first line rescue strategy is prone ventilation. Although there is little evidence of an effect on mortality, a significant number of patients' oxygenation will improve due to alterations of V/Q relationships within the lungs. This is best considered at an early stage and maintained for long periods, up to 18 to 20 hours at a time.

What problems are associated with prone ventilation?

The main problems relate to the process of turning and the prone position itself. Turning a patient in a controlled fashion will require numerous staff.

The most common manoeuvre-related complications are:

- Airway obstruction or accidental extubation
- Transient hypoxia
- Hypotension and arrhythmias
- Vomiting
- Accidental loss of drains or central venous lines.

Nursing in the prone position can be difficult (suction/mouth care etc.) and practical procedures such as urinary catheterisation, insertion of central, peripheral and arterial lines can be impossible. Patients often develop facial oedema. Care must be taken to prevent ocular, joint and peripheral nerve injuries.

What other methods can be considered to improve oxygenation?

As with the prone position, other rescue therapies are largely unsupported by evidence with respect to overall mortality or suitability for specific patients or situations. They include steroids as mentioned earlier, inhaled nitric oxide or prostacyclin, high frequency oscillation, the interventional lung assist device or full extra-corporeal membrane oxygenation (ECMO). Whichever rescue strategy is chosen it should ideally be started within 96 hours to reduce the risk of ventilator induced lung injury (VILI). There is also recent evidence to suggest centres seeing high numbers of ventilated patients have a better outcome, although regional referral centres for ARDS do not exist in the UK.

However, The Glenfield Hospital in Leicester has the national ECMO centre, but is not a referral centre for ARDS *per se*. Their CESAR trial and the Australian experience with ECMO for pandemic flu, have raised the profile of this rescue treatment, though the trial methodology and results have been questioned. It is probably fair to say that used early, in appropriately selected patients, in centres with experience, ECMO is a useful strategy for severe ARDS.

What is the mortality associated with ARDS?

In recent randomised controlled trials the mortality has been around 25–30%, but community surveys show mortality of about 35–40%. This may reflect the difficulty of translating research findings into clinical practice.

What are the predictors of outcome?

The age of the patient and the number of non-pulmonary organ failures are the best predictors. Elderly patients with shock do badly, as do those with hepatic failure. Surprisingly the initial $PaO_2 : FiO_2$ ratio is not predictive, unless it is under 50 or fails to improve during the first week.

What is the mode of death in ARDS?

Death is usually due to other organ failures and sepsis. It is rarely intractable severe hypoxia itself.

What is function like in survivors of ARDS?

There are persistent problems in many survivors. Lung function deficits are present in most, although this is rarely a problem in day-to-day life and return to nearly normal within the first year. Cognitive and neuromuscular complications can be frequent and severe and more likely to prevent return to work or precipitate loss of independence. Survivors do have a reduced health related quality of life.

Further Reading

Gattinoni L, Vagginelli F, Chiumello D, Taccone P, Carlesso E. Physiologic rationale for ventilator setting in acute lung injury / acute respiratory distress syndrome patients. *Critical Care Medicine*. 2003; **31**(Suppl): S300–304.

Peek GJ, Mugford M, Tiruvoipati R, et al. CESAR Trial Collaboration. Efficacy and economic assessment of conventional ventilatory support versus extracorporeal membrane oxygenation for severe adult respiratory failure (CESAR): a multicentre randomised controlled trial. *Lancet*. 2009; **374**(9698): 1351–1363.

Rodrigues-Roisin R, Roca J. Mechanisms of hypoxaemia. *Intensive Care Medicine*. 2005; **31**: 1017–1019.

The Acute Respiratory Distress Syndrome Network. Ventilation with lower tidal volumes as compared with traditional tidal volumes for acute lung injury and the acute respiratory distress syndrome. *New England Journal of Medicine* 2000; **342**: 1301–1308.

Wheeler A, Bernard G. Acute lung injury and the acute respiratory distress syndrome: a clinical review. *Lancet*. 2007; **369**: 1553–1565.

3.2.4. The management of severe sepsis – Gareth J Gibbon

You are most likely to have to confront this topic as part of a case-based discussion.

You are asked to urgently review a 47-year-old man who is in respiratory distress and hypotensive.

How would you approach this patient?

The examiner is looking for a safe, systematic approach to managing a sick patient. It is sensible to have a generic answer to start every similar question – this gives you time to think and makes sure you don't miss out on any easy marks.

I would approach this patient as I would every potential medical emergency. I would assess the airway, breathing and circulation, apply high flow oxygen through a non-rebreathing mask and, if concerned, would call for help sooner rather than later. I would ensure large bore intra-venous access is secured and, providing there is no obvious con-traindication, I would start intra-venous fluids. I'd set up basic monitoring: a pulse oximeter, frequent non-invasive blood pressure measurements and, if available, ECG telemetry.

When safe to do so I would attempt to make a diagnosis through a history, examination and by requesting relevant investigations. These would include a 12-lead ECG, a chest X-ray and blood investigations: a full blood count, urea and electrolytes, clotting, two sets of blood cultures and an arterial blood gas including a lactate level.

What would you like to know about him?

It is always sensible to start from the beginning. It gives you time to formulate your thoughts. It also may help to imagine yourself in that situation.

My first concern is his airway. Is he able to talk to me?

Yes. He is however struggling to complete sentences

What is the respiratory rate and his oxygen saturation? He is already receiving high flow oxygen via a non-rebreathing mask. I would continue to think about his breathing and listen to his chest.

You can hear coarse crepitations over the right side of his chest but his left chest sounds clear. His oxygen saturation is 93% on the mask you've put on and his respiration rate is 40 breaths per minute.

I would like to proceed to assess his circulation. What is his blood pressure? Is there a 12-lead ECG? Has he had an arterial blood gas sampled? Are there any blood results? Is he able to tell me a history? Does he feel hot to touch? Is he pyrexial?

His blood pressure is 74/45 mmHg, his ECG shows a sinus tachycardia, his blood gases show a metabolic acidosis and his chest X-ray shows right lower lobe shadowing. He has a temperature of 39°C and feels very flushed. He's able to tell you that he has been unwell for the past 48 hours with a worsening cough, fevers and breathlessness. He has no other significant medical history.

What are your thoughts?

Remember – you might also be given a copy of the investigations and asked to describe them. Ensure you have a systematic way of doing so. Usually, you will see the relevant investigations before the SOE.

This is a sick, young man with right lower lobe air space shadowing on his chest X-ray and my initial feeling is that this all ties in with severe sepsis from a right lower lobar pneumonia. There is a broader differential, but the history and chest X-ray changes don't really tie in with a pulmonary embolism, and the lack of any ischaemic ECG changes infers that a primary cardiac problem is unlikely. I see his haematocrit on the blood gas is 0.4 and there is no history of acute blood loss.

Are you able to classify how you diagnose severe sepsis and septic shock?

A good examiner will always steer you to where points might be scored. Diagnosing sepsis has recently been changed from the SIRS criteria documented in the 2004 surviving sepsis campaign. SIRS was not specific enough, and so an even more sensitive definition of sepsis has been adopted. The guidelines are now more directed at severe sepsis and septic shock.

Sepsis
Sepsis is defined as infection with the systemic manifestations of infection. These can be general variables including temperature, heart rate, mental state, or inflammatory variables beyond normal ranges such as white cell counts and CRPs.

Severe sepsis
In severe sepsis there is organ dysfunction including hypoxaemia, oliguria, a significant increase in creatinine, a coagulopathy, thrombocytopenia, ileus or hyperbilirubinaemia or hyperlactataemia.

Septic shock
In septic shock, hypotension persists despite adequate fluid resuscitation.

How would you manage this patient?
Having commenced fluid resuscitation and administered oxygen I would ensure two sets of blood cultures were taken and broad-spectrum anti-biotics were administered as soon as possible. This is most likely to be a community acquired pneumonia and so you would need to cover pneumococcus, haemophilus and atypical organisms. In my hospital we would administer intra-venous augmentin and clarithromycin. This man is sick and probably in septic shock. His lactate is 4.4 mmol/L – this is a marker of significant tissue hypoperfusion and puts him in a high-risk group. He will require "level II" care at the very least. I would arrange for safe transfer from his current location to a critical care unit with resuscitation ongoing.

What else would you do for him?
With a working diagnosis of severe sepsis then he will need a central line. This will help guide fluid resuscitation and allow us to administer vasopressors should his blood pressure not respond to fluids – this would be if his mean arterial pressure (MAP) was less than 65 mmHg despite his CVP being above 8 mmHg. It would also allow us to measure his central venous oxygen saturation (SvO_2) levels. These should be above 70%. I would also site an arterial line to enable constant arterial blood pressure monitoring and sampling to gauge how he's responding to treatment.

What would you do if his mean arterial pressure remained lower than, as you said, 65 mmHg despite what you thought was adequate fluid resuscitation?

If I was confident in my diagnosis of vasodilatory shock then I would start a noradrenaline infusion centrally titrated to response, running up to 0.5 μg/kg/min. In the event of low central venous saturations (that is less than 70%) then dobutamine should be run concurrently to optimise cardiac output and tissue oxygenation. This, again, should be titrated to response. The maximum therapeutic dose of dobutamine is 20 μg/kg/min.

Other things to consider would be to ensure that the haematocrit was over 30%. If the hypotension proved refractory to higher doses of vasopressors then low-dose steroids should be considered. In the centre where I work at the moment then vasopressin is used in septic shock refractory to noradrenaline. Other therapeutic options to consider would be using activated protein C, initiating insulin therapy to keep blood glucose levels less than 10 mmol/L, prophylactic low molecular weight heparin and stress ulcer prophylaxis.

You've mentioned a lot of therapeutic interventions for managing sepsis. Do you know of any recent publications or guidelines?

The Surviving Sepsis Campaign was formed in Barcelona in 2002 and is an international campaign developed to improve the diagnosis, treatment and outcome from sepsis. They have recently published revised guidelines in 2008 outlining an international expert committee review of the current literature recommending optimal management for sepsis. There are two "bundles" a resuscitation bundle at 6 hours and a management bundle at 24 hours where changes can be targeted for improvement.

The resuscitation bundle describes seven tasks that should begin immediately:

- The measurement of lactate
- The taking of blood cultures prior to anti-biotics
- The timely administration of anti-biotics
- The administration of 20–40 ml/kg of fluid
- The administration of vasopressors
- Achieving an adequate central venous pressure
- Adequate central venous oxygen saturations.

The management bundle describes four interventions that should be applied in the first 24 hours:

- Low-dose steroids administered by a standard unit policy
- Activated protein C administered by a standard unit policy
- Adequate glycaemic control
- Preventing excessive inspiratory plateau pressures in mechanically ventilated patients.

What do you know about early goal directed therapy?

Rivers in 2001 published a study showing that one life was saved for every seven patients with severe sepsis or septic shock presenting to an emergency department treated with early goal directed therapy. All patients were resuscitated to achieve a CVP of 8–12 mmHg, a MAP of 65 mmHg and a urine output greater than 0.5 ml/kg/hr. In the control group this was under critical care consultation and patients admitted as soon as possible. The treatment groups were managed in the Emergency Department for 6 hours, a central line was sited and SvO_2 measured with the haematocrit. If after achieving targets the SvO_2 remained <70% then the haematocrit was raised to 30% with a transfusion, and should it still be <70% then dobutamine titrated to a maximum dose of 20 μg/kg/min. The dobutamine was decreased or stopped if the MAP fell below 65 or the heart rate was greater than 120 bpm. Patients whose oxygen delivery couldn't be achieved were sedated, intubated and ventilated. This led to the recommendations in the resuscitation bundle of placing a central line, measuring and treating reductions in SvO_2 and measuring the lactate in patients with sepsis. A lactate of greater than 4 mmol/L was an inclusion criteria into the study.

Steroids in sepsis are controversial aren't they? What do you know about that?

I think that the two most important trials to date are the Annane study from 2002 and the more recent CORTICUS study published in 2008. Annane demonstrated that for every seven patients in septic shock and a low or absent response to a short Synacthen test treated with low-dose hydrocortisone and fludrocortisone that one more person left hospital. Of note these patients also had a systolic blood pressure of less than 90 mmHg for one hour despite fluid replacement and inotropes. The international multi-centre CORTICUS trial, however, has more recently shown no benefit of starting regular hydrocortisone. There was quicker resolution of the need for vasopressor support, but this was offset with an increased incidence of significant infection. The short Synacthen test result bore no influence on 28-day mortality. It could be that the patients in Annane's original study were sicker. The surviving sepsis campaign states that low-dose steroids could be considered in cases of septic shock refractory to vasopressors.

What is your view on using recombinant activated protein C?

I know about the controversial PROWESS study published in 2001 where for every 16 patients with severe sepsis treated with activated protein C (APC) within 24 hours there is one less death at 28 days. This was a large multicentre international trial stopped after second interim analysis because of significant difference between groups. It was the first new treatment to show any improved outcome in severe sepsis and led to its inclusion in the 2004 Surviving Sepsis Campaign guidelines. The results were particularly significant for patients who were sicker with higher APACHE 2 scores for whom it has been licensed.

But criticisms have been made about the influence and sponsorship from Lilly, the makers of APC, of these original guidelines and also about the validity of the study. The blinding has been criticised because the control solution was changed part way through the study, several centres were dropped and several more recruited part way through the study, the most significant improvement was in patients aged 80–90 with significant cardiovascular comorbidity, there was an unexplained reduction in do not resuscitate (DNR) orders in the treatment group and there was no significant difference in the number of patients who survived to hospital discharge home. Coupled with no proven benefit in the ADDRESS trial in patients at low risk of death, an increased harm in bleeding in the ENHANCE study of paediatric patients and no clearly improved survival in retrospective data following the introduction of APC its use has reduced in popularity.

Of interest, studies show that patients with low protein C levels have a worse outcome in septic shock. APC might improve outcome in those patients with low serum protein C levels with severe sepsis and I believe that there is an ongoing clinical trial recruiting at the moment. It is thought that protein C has anti-inflammatory effects and that, in the context of severe sepsis, the anti-coagulant properties are an unfortunate side effect. At the moment the Surviving Sepsis Campaign state that patients with APACHE scores higher than 16 probably warrant treatment.

Further Reading

Abraham E, Laterre PF, Garg R, et al. Administration of Drotrecogin Alfa (Activated) in Early Stage Severe Sepsis (ADDRESS) Study Group. Drotrecogin alfa (activated) for adults with severe sepsis and a low risk of death. *New England Journal of Medicine.* 2005; **353**: 1332–1341.

Annane D, Sebille V, Charpentier C, et al. Effect of treatment with low doses of hydrocortisone and fludrocortisone on mortality in patients with septic shock. *Journal of the American Medical Association.* 2002; **288**: 862–871.

Bernard GR, Vincent JL, Laterre PF, et al. Recombinant Human Protein C Worldwide Evaluation in Severe Sepsis (PROWESS) Study Group. Efficacy and safety of recombinant human activated protein C for severe sepsis. *New England Journal of Medicine.* 2001; **344**: 699–709.

Rivers E, Nguyen B, Havstad S, et al. Early Goal-Directed Therapy Collaborative Group. Early goal-directed therapy in the treatment of severe sepsis and septic shock. *New England Journal of Medicine.* 2001; **345**: 1368–1377.

Society of Critical Care Medicine. Surviving Sepsis Campaign. www.survivingsepsis.org.

Sprung CL, Annane D, Keh D, et al. CORTICUS Study Group. Hydrocortisone therapy for patients with septic shock. *New England Journal of Medicine.* 2008; **358**(2): 111–124.

Vincent JL, Bernard GR, Beale R, et al. Drotrecogin alfa (activated) treatment in severe sepsis from the global open-label trial ENHANCE: further evidence for survival and safety and implications for early treatment. *Critical Care Medicine.* 2005; **33**: 2266–2277.

3.2.5. Oxygen toxicity – Emily K Johnson and Jessie R Welbourne

As anaesthetists, our most used drug is probably oxygen. However its use is not without problems. Therefore you may have an SAQ or structured oral examination (SOE) asking about the adverse effects of oxygen therapy or more specifically about oxygen toxicity.

What are the potential problems associated with oxygen therapy?

Take your time and gather your thoughts. With a broad question like this it is vital you classify your answer. Don't rush into an answer about free radicals you may later regret! If the examiner wants to know about the mechanisms of oxygen toxicity they will lead you down this path of questioning in due course. It is important to show a logical approach and mention the common problems first.

The problems with oxygen therapy can be divided into general problems and the specifics of oxygen toxicity.

General problems:

- Hypoventilation
- Absorption atelectasis.

Specific problems:
- Central nervous system toxicity
- Pulmonary oxygen toxicity
- Ocular conditions such as paediatric retrolental fibroplasia.

Tell me a little more about the problems of hypoventilation and absorption atelectasis.

Oxygen may cause hypoventilation in a sub-group of patients with a chronically raised $PaCO_2$ and an established hypoxic drive to ventilation. These patients should be given no more than 28% O_2 unless being mechanically ventilated with a mandatory mode, or if their hypoxia is imminently life threatening.

Absorption atelectasis occurs as a result of high solubility of oxygen in the blood compared with nitrogen. Therefore, when administered in high concentrations, it leaves the alveoli "unsplinted" and vulnerable to collapse. When breathing air, the insolubility of nitrogen in blood results in nitrogen "splinting" the alveoli open. Removal of nitrogen, by administration of high concentrations of oxygen, causes oxygen to be absorbed faster than it can be replaced by ventilation, with consequent loss of alveolar volume.

Can you tell me more about the specific problem of oxygen toxicity?

Classify to add structure to your answer. You can classify by system affected, that is central nervous system, respiratory system and ocular, or into acute and chronic toxicity. The latter form of classification will allow you to demonstrate your understanding in the context of a clinical situation.

Oxygen toxicity can be divided into acute and chronic toxicity.

Acute toxicity can occur in patients exposed to very high concentrations of oxygen for a short duration, for example in hyperbaric oxygen therapy. This acute form of toxicity has mainly the central nervous system effects.

Chronic toxicity occurs in patients who are exposed to lower concentrations of the gas for a longer duration and they usually suffer the pulmonary effects.

Describe the pulmonary effects of oxygen toxicity.

Pulmonary toxicity can occur due to prolonged exposure or high concentrations of oxygen causing damage to the pulmonary epithelium and inactivating surfactant. This leads to intra-alveolar oedema and interstitial thickening, which progresses to fibrosis.

Three phases have been described:
1. Tracheobronchitis
2. ARDS
3. Pulmonary interstitial fibrosis.

Bronchopulmonary dysplasia can occur in infants.

The development of toxicity is time and dose related although there is a lot of individual variation.

The threshold is 12 to 24 hours of exposure to oxygen above 50 kPa. At sea level 100% oxygen can be tolerated for 24 to 48 hours, after which definite tissue injury occurs. Higher partial pressures lead to more rapid development of toxicity.

The symptoms and signs include:

- Tracheal irritation
- Dry cough
- Chest pain
- Reduced vital capacity
- Pulmonary oedema.

You mentioned bronchopulmonary dysplasia, can you tell me more about it?

Bronchopulmonary dysplasia occurs in mechanically ventilated children, usually premature neonates. It occurs in 10–20% of those with respiratory distress syndrome and is defined as an increased oxygen demand for more than 30 days in the presence of typical radiological changes. These are a diffuse fine reticular ground glass appearance of the lung. The incidence is related to the severity of the respiratory distress syndrome, the degree of prematurity and the high and prolonged oxygen concentrations. The condition improves with age and alveolar growth improves respiratory function and reserves.

Describe the effects of oxygen toxicity on the central nervous system.

Central nervous system toxicity is a concern to those encountering oxygen at greater than atmospheric pressures, such as divers. It is due mainly to oxidation and polymerisation of enzymes leading to their inactivation and resulting in cellular damage.

Symptoms occur above a threshold of 150 kPa of oxygen and include:

- Visual changes – particularly tunnel vision
- Tinnitus
- Nausea
- Twitching
- Irritability
- Dizziness
- Tonic–clonic seizures
- Unconsciousness.

There are several factors which predispose to CNS toxicity and they are:

- Exercise
- Cold
- Stress
- Fatigue
- Elevated $PaCO_2$
- Dietary deficiency of trace elements
- Nitrogen narcosis.

At rest in a dry environment patients can tolerate up to 280 kPa of oxygen given intermittently.

What are the ocular effects of oxygen toxicity and when do they occur most commonly?

Ocular or retinopathic conditions include:

- Reversible constriction of the peripheral field of vision
- Progressive reversible myopia
- Delayed cataract formation
- Retrolental fibroplasia in neonates.

Ocular effects are more common when the entire eye is exposed to high ambient oxygen concentrations and pressures, for example in an oxygen tent or hyperbaric chamber, rather than when there is hyperoxia of the arterial circulation.

What is retrolental fibroplasia?

Retrolental fibroplasia was previously known as retinopathy of prematurity or ROP. It is the formation of an opaque membrane behind the lens. Usually retinal vascularisation continues after birth but if vasoconstriction occurs, blood vessel lumens become obliterated due to anoxic endothelial damage. The temporal portion of the retina is worst affected as this is usually the last to be vascularised. Once revascularisation occurs, new vessel growth extends beyond the retina into the vitreous humour. High oxygen levels promote this new vessel growth. These vessels are prone to dilatation and rupture that subsequently leads to vitreous and retinal haemorrhages, fibrosis and adhesions, causing retinal detachment and blindness. Retrolental fibroplasia is one of the leading causes of blindness in childhood.

The main risk factor for development of retrolental fibroplasia is prematurity. Premature infants of less than 30 weeks or 1.5-kg birth weights are at greatest risk. Many other factors can influence the disease progression including general health and the stage of disease at diagnosis. Supplemental oxygen exposure is a risk factor, but restricting oxygen will not necessarily reduce the rate of progression and may have systemic implications. Concentrations of above 40% for 1–2 days after birth may be implicated and for neonates who develop retrolental fibroplasias a PaO_2 of greater than 10.4 kPa for more than 6 hours may cause progressive damage, so an oxygen saturation of 90% is aimed for.

Are there any other toxic effects of oxygen you know about?

The main effects have been covered, this is small print and you are doing well if you are asked this!

Oxygen toxicity can also affect red blood cell morphology. A reduction in red cell mass can occur and haemolysis has been seen following hyperbaric oxygen therapy.

Serous otitis media and dysbaric osteonecrosis have been observed in astronauts and are thought to be partially attributable to high oxygen concentrations whilst in space flights.

What levels of oxygen carry risk?

At atmospheric pressure, oxygen toxicity is related to the dose and time. However, there is a lot of individual variation in the development of toxicity. As a rough guide, 12 hours is the maximum length for a patient to be on 100%, 24 hours on 80%, 36 hours on 60% and indefinitely on 50%. The safest policy is to wean patients off high oxygen concentrations as early as possible without compromising oxygen delivery.

What are the mechanisms of oxygen toxicity?

The proposed mechanisms of toxicity are complex and not fully understood. However oxygen-derived free radicals are the likely aetiological factors in toxicity development.

Free radicals are produced as a result of several processes:

- Mitochondrial oxireductive processes
- By xanthine oxidase at extra-mitochondrial sites
- By auto-oxidative reactions
- By phagocytes during bacterial killing.

The free radicals have a number of harmful effects:

- Lipid peroxidation in cell membranes
- Inactivation of cellular enzymes
- Nucleic acid inhibition
- Protein synthesis inhibition.

Under normal conditions, anti-oxidant enzymes such as glutathione peroxidise and catalase and superoxide dismutase protect the body from these free radicals, but hyperoxic situations allow increased free radical production that exceeds anti-oxidant capacity.

Oxygen toxicity can also occur due to cellular metabolic alteration or enzyme inhibition that is not mediated by free radicals.

What are the indications for hyperbaric oxygen therapy?

Hyperbaric oxygen is oxygen administered at higher than atmospheric pressure.

It is used in a number of clinical scenarios:

- Carbon monoxide poisoning
- Decompression sickness
- Respiratory distress of newborn
- Anaerobic infections such as gas gangrene caused by *Clostridium welchii*
- Refractory chronic osteomyelitis with draining lesions
- Infected superficial burns
- To sensitise tumours to radiotherapy.

The toxic effects are predominantly central nervous system effects.

Under hyperbaric conditions, oxygen toxicity is again dose dependeant and is the main limitation to treatment. It affects the CNS, lung, myocardium, liver, kidneys and visual system.

After 8 hours of receiving 100% oxygen at a pressure of 2 atmospheres, subjects may experience a decreased vital capacity, facial twitching, abnormal taste and smell and tonic-clonic siezures. It may cause cardiovascular problems including vasoconstriction and myocardial depression.

Further Reading

Brubakk A, Neuman T. *Bennett and Elliott's physiology and medicine of diving*. Fifth Revised Edition. Edinburgh, New York: Saunders, 2003.

Patel DN, Goel A, Agarwal SB, Garg P, Lakhani KK. Oxygen toxicity. *Journal, Indian Academy of Clinical Medicine*. 2003; 4(3): 234–237.

Pitkin A, Davis N. Hyperbaric oxygen therapy. *British Journal of Anaesthesia. CEPD Reviews* 2001; **1**(5): 150–156.

Taneja R, Vaughn R. Oxygen. *British Journal of Anaesthesia. CEPD Reviews* 2001; **1**(4): 104–107.

3.2.6. Renal replacement therapies – Emily K Johnson

You are called to ITU to review a 46-year-old man. He is a known intra-venous drug abuser and alcoholic who had been brought into the Emergency Department 24 hours previously. He had been found by a neighbour, unconscious and lying on the floor of his hallway. On admission his Glasgow Coma Scale (GCS) score was 8 and his temperature 34°C. He was resuscitated. His blood results are as follows:

Sodium	141 mmol/L
Potassium	6.4 mmol/L
Urea	35.6 mmol/L
Creatinine	760 µg/L
Haemoglobin	8.5 g/dl
White cell count	18.0×10^9/L
Platelets	150×10^9/L
Creatinine kinase (CK)	15 600 IU

He has an ECG demonstrating a rate of 64 beats per minute, an increased PR interval and tall tented T waves.

This is a good example of a long clinical case you may be faced with. There are many potential routes of questioning and often numerous abnormal results with potential for discussion. You will have 10 minutes to study the case and make notes, use this time wisely, the information will be available at the exam table too so you do not need to copy it out. The examiners will lead you along their structured line of questioning but they will start by asking you for a summary. It is crucial you come across well at this stage and a SUCCINCT summary is advisable. It is worth taking a few minutes to prepare your summary.

Can you summarise the case?

This is a 46-year-old male who is a known substance abuser and has been found collapsed on a floor for an unknown length of time. He has acute renal failure and life-threatening hyperkalaemia, which are most likely to be secondary to acute rhabdomyolysis.

It is better to give a short summary and let the examiner lead the questioning than go into the finer details of the case. It is likely a discussion about the investigations, particularly the causes of any abnormalities will follow.

What could be the causes of his acute kidney injury?

Acute kidney injury, previously known as acute renal failure, can be classified into pre-renal, intrinsic and post-renal causes. The most likely cause in this scenario is acute rhabdomyolysis. The patient has a history suggesting muscle damage may have occurred. This is associated with a significantly raised creatinine kinase, a biochemical marker of muscle damage.

However, the differential diagnosis would include:

Pre-renal causes:

- Severe dehydration or haemorrhage causing hypovolaemia
- Hepato-renal syndrome
- Thromboembolic disease
- Sepsis.

Intrinsic renal causes:

- Toxins
- Deterioration of pre-existing renal disease.

Post-renal causes:

- Obstruction of the urinary tract.

Do you know of any classifications for acute kidney injury?

If you don't know then just say so. Don't try to make up an answer to a question like this – it is unlikely that such a question alone is a pass or fail question.

As far as I am aware there are no universally accepted classifications for acute kidney injury. I am aware of two recently proposed classifications.

1. The RIFLE criteria, which helps diagnose and define the severity of acute kidney injury. RIFLE is an acronym for Risk, Injury, Failure, Loss and End-stage renal disease.

   · Risk is if the creatinine is raised 1.5 times or the urine output is less than 0.5 ml/kg for 6 hours.
   · Injury is if the creatinine is raised 2.0 times or urine output is less than 0.5 ml/kg for 12 h.
   · Failure is if the creatinine is raised 3 times or urine output is less than 0.3 ml/kg for 24 hours.
   · Loss is persistent acute renal failure or complete loss of kidney function for more than 4 weeks.
   · End-stage renal disease is complete loss of kidney function for more than 3 months.

2. The Acute Kidney Injury Network (AKIN) staging of acute kidney injury. This divides the severity into stage 1, 2 and 3 based on the rise in serum creatinine and the urine output.

When this patient was first admitted, what are the treatment priorities?

My priorities in the treatment of this patient are initially administration of oxygen and stabilisation of any upper airway, respiratory and circulatory abnormalities. Cervical spine immobilisation will be required as he may have sustained trauma and he would need a full secondary survey. Treatment of his hyperkalaemia should be undertaken immediately as his potassium is dangerously high and he has ECG changes. He should also be actively warmed as he is hypothermic.

The underlying cause of his unconciousness should be sought and appropriately treated and while a secondary survey may help identify this, his history indicates blood toxicology may also be helpful.

How would you manage his hyperkalaemia?

I would initially manage his hyperkalaemia with 10 ml of 10% calcium gluconate to help stabilise the myocardium by raising the threshold potential to excitation. I would commence an infusion of insulin (10 units in 50 ml of 50% dextrose) over 30 minutes to help drive K^+ back into cells. Salbutamol 5 mg via a nebuliser would also have this effect. I would then recheck his serum potassium and if it is not responding to conservative treatment I would consider haemofiltration.

What are the indications for starting haemofiltration?

The main indications for starting haemofiltration are:

- Hyperkalaemia
- Fluid over-load
- Metabolic acidosis
- Symptomatic uraemia, the symptoms include peri-carditis, blood dyscrasias or encephalopathy
- Drug toxicity if the drug in question is cleared by dialysis
- Hyperthermia.

There are no universally agreed levels at which haemofiltration is commenced and there is variation between units. Generally speaking hyperkalaemia with potassium above 6.5 or an acidosis with pH less than 7.1 would guide a clinical decision to commence haemofiltration, although I believe there is some evidence available showing lower morbidity with early and aggressive continuous renal replacement in critically ill patients.

As mentioned above, less common indications for haemofiltration include cooling a hyperthermic patient, inducing deliberate hypothermia or rewarming a hypothermic patient. It can also be used in the management of systemic inflammatory response syndrome (SIRS) or endotoxic shock to reduce the plasma levels of inflammatory mediators. Finally, haemofiltration can be employed for the treatment of dysnatraemias and for plasmapheresis.

Can you give examples of drugs cleared by dialysis?

Drugs that have a low volume of distribution, low molecular weight and low plasma protein binding are more likely to be removed from plasma by dialysis.

Examples include:

- Ethylene glycol
- Methanol
- Aspirin
- Vancomycin
- Theophylline
- Lithium.

Can you classify the types of renal replacement therapies?

Renal replacement therapies can be classified into intermittent and continuous techniques. Intermittent dialysis can be either intermittent haemodialysis or peritoneal dialysis. Continuous renal replacement therapies are more commonly used in the critical care setting. They consist of continuous veno-venous haemofiltration (CVVH), continuous veno-venous haemodialysis (CVVHD), continuous veno-venous haemodiafiltration (CVVHDF) and slow continuous ultrafiltration (SCUF).

Can you tell me a bit more about the intermittent techniques of renal replacement therapy?

This is unlikely to be asked but it is helpful for your understanding of the subject.

Intermittent renal replacement therapies are most commonly used in chronic renal failure where the patients are haemodynamically stable.

Intermittent haemodialysis requires insertion of specialist dialysis catheters or the formation of an arterio-venous fistula. Dialysis takes place at regular intervals, depending on the degree of renal impairment, commonly three times a week. It involves large volumes of blood leaving the circulation at any one time so rapidly removes a solute or volume load, but is unsuitable if a patient is already haemodynamically compromised. The primary method of solute and fluid removal in haemodialysis is diffusion.

Peritoneal dialysis uses the peritoneum as the dialysis membrane and fluid can be introduced at regular intervals throughout the day, which is continuous ambulatory peritoneal dialysis (CAPD) or overnight using automatic peritoneal dialysis (APD). This form of dialysis requires a permanent peritoneal catheter, which carries a considerable risk of infection. It is also inefficient at removing large volumes of fluid or solute and would be inappropriate in critically ill patients as the increase in intra-abdominal volume could cause splinting of the diaphragm and ventilation difficulties.

What are the differences between the types of continuous renal replacement therapies?

The continuous renal replacement therapies are based on the transfer of solute and fluids across a semipermeable membrane by either diffusion, in the case of haemodialysis, or convection, in the case of haemofiltration, or a combination of the two processes in haemodiafiltration.

What is the difference between diffusion, osmosis, and dialysis?

Diffusion is the spontaneous movement of a substance across a semipermeable membrane from a region where it is in a high concentration to a region where its concentration is lower. The rate of diffusion is proportional to the concentration gradient.

Osmosis is the diffusion of a liquid solvent (water) from a weak solution across a semipermeable membrane into a stronger solution so that when equilibrium is reached the osmotic pressures on each side are equal.

Dialysis is the separation of substances in solution by means of their unequal diffusion through semipermeable membranes.

What determines the rate of dialysis?

In haemodialysis the rate of diffusion is driven by the differing concentrations of solute between the blood and dialysate. The higher the concentration gradient, the greater the rate of diffusion.

The other factors influencing the rate of diffusion include solute factors such as size of the particles, ionic charge and degree of plasma protein binding. The rate of diffusion is also dependent on the size and number of pores, thickness and surface area of the membrane used. Dialysis becomes more efficient as the rate of delivery of dialysate increases.

What is convection?

Convection is also described as "solvent drag" and occurs when a moving stream sweeps a solute molecule along causing it to pass through a membrane. A positive pressure is produced in the blood compartment and the solute molecules are pushed into the dialysate compartment where the fast flows create a negative pressure effectively pulling the solute along. This trans-membrane force that is created is the driving force for ultrafiltration. Therefore convection, unlike diffusion, is independent of concentration gradients across the membrane.

What factors influence the rate of convection?

The amount of convective transport is determined by the direction and magnitude of the trans-membrane force. The porosity of the membrane also influences the rate at which solutes are removed. The faster the flow rate of blood along the membrane the greater the rate of ultrafiltration and solute clearance. Also, the greater the negative pressures in the ultrafiltrate compartment the greater the rate of ultrafiltration. This means that increased hydrostatic pressure in the blood will increase trans-membrane pressure and speed up ultrafiltration, similar effects would occur with a reduction in the plasma colloid osmotic pressure.

Could you draw a simple circuit for continuous veno-venous haemofiltration?

This could well be expected, and it is recommended you spend a bit of time practising a simple diagram of a haemofiltration circuit (Figure 3.2.6). You need to understand the differences between CVVH and CVVHDF circuits and be able to illustrate these on your diagram. CVVH relies on the process of convection and CVVHDF relies on both convection and diffusion.

A CVVH circuit starts with large bore intra-venous access to the patient. A single cannula has a dual lumen for removal and return of blood. The removal flow may range between zero and 300 ml/min. This will pass through a pressure sensor to detect changes in pressure that may indicate cannula blockage. Then a volumetric pump drives the flow of blood through the haemofilter where the ultrafiltrate is removed and delivered into a collection bag. The filtered blood continues in the circuit through another pressure sensor. The blood then passes into a drip chamber where replacement fluids can be added. Blood is then returned to the patient via a final pressure sensor.

The rate of ultrafiltration, and therefore of the solute convection, depends on the speed of the pump and the resultant trans-membrane pressure generated.

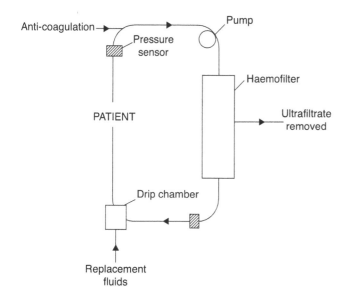

Figure 3.2.6. A continuous veno-venous haemofiltration circuit.

In summary the components of a CVVH circuit are:

- Double-lumen central venous catheter
- Afferent and efferent tubing
- Pressure sensors
- Volumetric pump
- Haemofilter and drip chamber
- Collection bag and tubing for ultrafiltrate
- Portal for anti-coagulants and replacement fluids.

Describe how this differs from continuous veno-venous haemodiafiltration

In CVVHDF there is dialysate entering the haemofilter. This is because dialysis is used in addition to filtration. Dialysate fluid is pumped through to maintain concentration gradients on either side of the semipermeable membrane and therefore allow solute transfer by diffusion. These two solutions must run in opposite directions to allow convection to occur as well. The pump blood flow is much higher, ranging from 200 to 400 ml/min making this a more efficient method of continuous renal replacement therapy.

Can you tell me what types of membranes are used in continuous renal replacement therapy?

There are two types of membrane used in renal replacement therapy, natural (cellulose) and synthetic (polyacrylonitrile). Modern haemofilters using synthetic membranes are preferred because they allow the clearance of larger molecules and they are more compatible with patients' blood.

What are the different types of replacement fluids commonly used?

The replacement fluids consist of balanced solutions containing phosphate and potassium with either lactate or bicarbonate as a buffer.

Lactate containing solutions are cheaper and have a longer shelf life but can cause hyper-lactataemia and a deterioration of metabolic acidosis. Patients with liver dysfunction are particularly at risk. Also, those with a pre-existing raised lactate or profound hypoperfusion should be considered for lactate-free replacement fluid. The bicarbonate solutions require pre-mixing as the bicarbonate is not stable in aqueous solution.

What are the options for anticoagulation when haemofiltering a patient on ICU?

Anti-coagulation is required for haemofiltration as the blood makes direct contact with the haemofilter circuit and membrane, having the potential to activate the clotting cascade. The aim of anti-coagulation is not only to extend the life of the haemofilter by preventing it clotting off but also to minimise the effects of systemic anti-coagulation. Heparin is the first line anti-coagulant used, initially to flush the filter and as a bolus to start the filter, then as an infusion whilst the filter is running. Unfractionated heparin can induce a thrombocytopaenia.

Another option is a prostacyclin (Flolan) infusion. This can be used in patients with pre-existing thrombocytopaenia and it acts by preventing platelet aggregation.

Alternatives to unfractionated heparin include:

- Low molecular weight heparin (less likely to cause a thrombocytopaenia)
- Fondaparinux
- Danaparoid sodium
- Citrate.

Citrate is thought to be advantageous as its effects are more confined to the haemofilter circuit, causing less systemic anticoagulation. It acts by chelating calcium ions causing inhibition of coagulation. The calcium is then replaced after filtering to reverse this effect and residual citrate is rapidly metabolised by the liver.

Patients with a pre-existing coagulopathy may not require anti-coagulation at all.

What are the potential complications of CVVH?

The complications of CVVH can be divided into those associated with the intra-venous catheter itself, those associated with anti-coagulation and those associated with the filtration process.

Catheter-related complications include:

Complications at insertion (these are site dependent and the same as those for a standard central line, bearing in mind the intra-venous catheters for haemofiltration are significantly larger bore than a standard central line).

These include:

- Bleeding
- Infection
- Damage to surrounding structures

- A-V fistulae
- Arrhythmias
- Pneumothorax
- Pain.

Anti-coagulation-related problems are:

- Bleeding
- Heparin-induced thrombocytopaenia.

General complications include:

- Cardiovascular instability and hypotension, particularly when starting filtration on a critically ill patient
- Hypovolaemia
- Hypothermia
- Electrolyte imbalance
- Metabolic abnormalities
- Air embolism
- Anaemia
- Reactions to the filter membrane and anaphylaxis.

Can you tell me more about the role of renal replacement therapies in sepsis?

There is a potential role for renal replacement therapies in sepsis. This is because most of the inflammatory mediators thought to be pathogenic in sepsis are medium-sized water-soluble compounds that can be removed by haemodiafiltration. It has been shown that the standard rates of haemofiltration of around 20 ml/kg/hr are not sufficient to reduce the concentration of inflammatory mediators in sepsis. However, high volume haemofiltration may result in significant reduction in the plasma concentrations of these mediators and there have been animal studies demonstrating improvements in outcomes.

Further Reading

Bellomo R, Kellum JA, Ronco C. Defining acute renal failure: physiological principles. *Intensive Care Medicine.* 2004; **30**: 33–37.

Hall N, Fox A. Renal replacement therapies in critical care. *Continuing Education in Anaesthesia, Critical Care & Pain.* 2006; **6**(5): 197–202.

Ricci Z, Cruz D, Ronco C. The RIFLE criteria and mortality in acute kidney injury: a systematic review. *Kidney International.* 2008; **73**: 538–546.

Anatomy

Chapter 4.1

4.1.1. Anatomy of central venous access – Poonam M Bopanna

What are the indications for central venous access?

Indications for short-term central venous access include:

- Administration of drugs which are irritant if given via a smaller peripheral vein
- Haemodialysis
- When peripheral access is difficult
- Transvenous cardiac pacing and cardiac catheterisation
- Measurement of central venous pressures.

Long-term access is predominantly for total parenteral nutrition and chemotherapy.

What are the common sites used for central venous access?

The most commonly used sites are the internal jugular, subclavian and femoral veins. Internal jugular is the preferred site due to low risk of complications; however the subclavian vein is the site which carries the least risk of infection. The femoral vein carries the highest risk of infection owing to its proximity to the perineum.

Can you describe the anatomy of the internal jugular vein?

Anatomy questions are best answered using a simple diagram (Figure 4.1.1a and b) and a systematic approach describing the bones, muscles, ligaments, nerves and vasculature.

The internal jugular vein is a continuation of the jugular bulb; it extends from the jugular foramen in the skull to a point behind the sternoclavicular joint where it joins the subclavian vein.

It lies within the carotid sheath alongside the carotid artery and vagus nerve. Its position in the sheath, relative to the artery changes throughout its course in the neck. Initially it lies behind the artery before moving laterally and then moving anterolaterally.

The following structures lie superficial to the carotid sheath:

- Sternocleidomastoid muscle (in the lower part of the neck)
- The platysma muscle

Dr. Podcast Scripts for the Final FRCA, ed. Rebecca A. Leslie, Emily K. Johnson, Gary Thomas and Alexander P. L. Goodwin.   Published by Cambridge University Press.
© R. A. Leslie, E. K. Johnson, G. Thomas and A. P. L. Goodwin 2011.

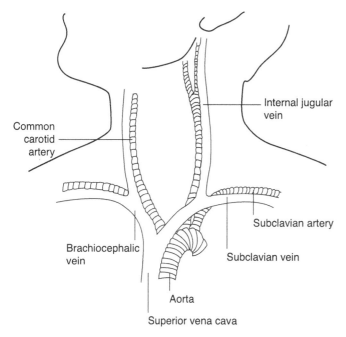

Figure 4.1.1a. Vessels of the head and neck. Reproduced with permission from Pinnock, C., Lin, T. and Smith, T. 1999. *Fundamentals of Anaesthesia.* Greenwich Medical Media Ltd. © Greenwich Medical Media Ltd 1999.

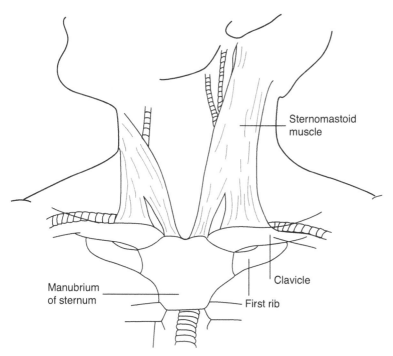

Figure 4.1.1b. Structures superficial to vessels of the head and neck. Reproduced with permission from Pinnock, C., Lin, T. and Smith, T. 1999. *Fundamentals of Anaesthesia.* Greenwich Medical Media Ltd. © Greenwich Medical Media Ltd 1999.

- Subcutaneous tissue
- Skin.

Posteriorly it is related to the prevertebral fascia, sympathetic chain, vertebral muscles and transverse processes of the cervical vertebrae. In the upper part of the neck it is related to the first cervical vertebrae. At the root of the neck the dome of the pleura lies close to the internal jugular vein. On the left side the thoracic duct lies posterior to the internal jugular vein.

The ninth (glossopharyngeal), tenth (vagus), eleventh (accessory) and twelfth (hypoglossal) cranial nerves, the common and internal carotid arteries, the trachea and oesophagus lie medial to the internal jugular vein through its caudal course.

What are the complications of central venous access?

They can be divided into immediate and delayed complications.
Immediate complications include:

- Bleeding from the site
- Carotid arterial puncture causing haematoma
- Pneumothorax
- Haemothorax
- Chylothorax (on the left side only)
- Air embolism
- Foreign body embolism (e.g., guide-wire or catheter fragment)
- Arrhythmias
- Complications associated with unrecognised catheter misplacement (intra-pleural infusion)
- Cardiac tamponade has been reported.

Long-term complications include:

- Local infection
- Line-related sepsis
- Thrombus formation.

How can these complications be minimised?

Position the patient head down to reduce the risk of air embolism.

The risk of pneumothorax and haemothorax are minimised by using a high approach.

An ultrasound-guided technique will reduce the risk of arterial puncture and catheter misplacement.

Performing a chest X-ray post-insertion to ensure appropriate catheter tip position may reduce the risk of thrombosis and cardiac tamponade.

One should avoid threading the guide wire into the right atrium. Continuous ECG monitoring should be in place to detect arrhythmias, withdrawing the guide wire should they occur.

How can the risk of infection be minimised?

Subclavian vein cannulation is associated with the lowest risk of infection. A full aseptic technique with sterile gown, gloves, hat, mask and drapes should be used. The chosen site should be prepared with a 2% aqueous chlorhexidine gluconate. It has been shown to have lower bloodstream infection rates compared with site preparation with 10% povidone-iodine or 70% alcohol.

Teflon or polyurethane catheters have been associated with fewer infectious complications than catheters made of polyvinylchloride or polyethylene.

A central venous catheter with the minimum number of ports or lumens required for the management of the patient should be used.

Use an anti-microbial- or anti-septic-impregnated central venous catheter in adults whose catheter is expected to remain in place >5 days.

A transparent dressing should be used to allow early identification of signs of infection. The need for central access should be reviewed daily.

All ports on the central line should be capped off at all times when not in use. Giving sets should be changed no more frequently than 72-hour intervals, unless catheter-related infection is suspected. Tubing used to administer blood, blood products, or lipid emulsions should be changed within 24 hours of initiating the infusion.

There should be local protocols and care pathways implementing the above procedures, together with regular staff education and monitoring of infection rates.

Further Reading

National Institute for Health and Clinical Excellence (NICE). Guideline TA49: Central Venous Catheters Ultrasound Locating Devices. The clinical effectiveness of ultrasonic locating devised for the placement of central venous lines. http://guidance.nice.org.uk/TA49.

4.1.2. Anatomy of the extradural space and spinal cord blood supply – Amy K Swinson

Describe the arterial blood supply to the spinal cord

The arterial supply to the spinal cord consists of the anterior and posterior spinal arteries. The single anterior spinal artery lies in the anterior median fissure of the cord. It is formed from branches of each vertebral artery at the level of the foramen magnum. It runs the whole length of the spinal cord. The anterior spinal artery supplies the anterior two-thirds of the spinal cord.

The posterior spinal arteries arise from the posterior inferior cerebellar artery at the level of the foramen magnum; they lie both anterior and posterior to the dorsal nerve roots.

There are important contributions to the spinal arteries from radicular branches at each spinal level. The anatomy of this is variable. Commonly there is a dominant radicular branch to the anterior spinal artery called the great anterior radicular artery of Adamkiewicz (adamker-vits). Typically it arises from a low intercostal or a high lumbar artery, but sometimes the major contribution can arise from the iliac artery. This variation can lead to the development of anterior spinal artery syndrome for example following cross clamping of the aorta during aortic surgery.

Anterior spinal artery syndrome is flaccid paralysis at the level of ischaemia or infarction and a spastic paralysis with decreased pain and temperature appreciation below the level of the lesion. There is relative sparing of the senses of proprioception and vibration, as the posterior columns are usually preserved.

What is the epidural or extradural space and what are its contents?

The epidural space is a continuous space within the vertebral column. It is the part of the spinal canal that is not occupied by the dural sac and its contents (i.e., the spinal cord!). It extends from the foramen magnum to the sacrococcygeal membrane at the lower end of the caudal canal.

The epidural space contains:

- Fat
- Lymphatics
- Loose connective tissue
- Nerve roots
- Arteries
- Venous plexus.

The pressure in the epidural space is usually found to be negative particularly in the thoracic region, although this may be related to stretching of the dural sac during extreme flexion of the back whilst performing an epidural.

What are the boundaries of the epidural space?

The posterior boundary is the ligamentum flavum and the periostium of the laminae. The ligamenta flava connect adjacent laminae of each vertebra, they become progressively thicker in lower interspaces. The ligamenta flava may be paired at each level or be one pair of continuous longitudinal ligaments – opinion varies. Posterior to the ligamentum flavum is the interspinous then the supra-spinous ligaments.

The anterior boundary is the bodies of each vertebrae and the intervertebral discs, which are covered by the posterior longitudinal ligament.

The lateral boundaries are the pedicles of the vertebral arches and the intervertebral foramina, which contain the nerve roots.

The superior boundary is the foramen magnum where the dura attaches to the cranium.

The inferior boundary is the sacral hiatus, which is covered by the sacrococcygeal membrane.

The spinal canal is triangular, with the base anteriorly. The space is deepest in the midline posteriorly. The epidural space is up to 3–4 times larger at the caudal as compared to the cephalad margin, so in cross section a saw tooth pattern will be seen. The epidural space is very thin anteriorly, but up to about 6mm deep posteriorly in the lumbar region.

There has been debate surrounding the presence of a midline dorsal band of connective tissue called the plica mediana dorsalis, which was thought to draw the dura closer to the ligamentum flava in the midline, narrowing the space in the midline. The most recent conclusion is that this does not exist. However there can be fibrous bands in the epidural space.

What are the important features of the venous system within the epidural space?

The veins of the epidural space run vertically but communicate freely. They are valveless and called the venous plexus of Batson. The plexus allows communication from the pelvic veins inferiorly to the cerebral venous system as well as to the azygos system. Air or drugs injected intra-venously in the epidural space can therefore reach the brain and heart directly. Pelvic infection or malignancy spread can occur via Batson's plexus to the brain or vertebrae.

If thoracic or abdominal pressure is increased, the veins become relatively distended, thus the likelihood of intra-vascular placement of epidural catheter is increased, for example during a uterine contraction.

There is connection with abdominal and thoracic veins via the intervertebral foramina, which can transmit changes in venous pressure. Chronic increased intra-abdominal pressure or venous obstruction, such as inferior vena cava compression occurring due to the gravid uterus, can increase the calibre of veins, thus increasing the likelihood of venous placement of epidural needle or catheter. The increased vascular surface area may also increase absorption of local anaesthetics and therefore increase the likelihood of toxicity.

What can you tell me about the relevance of epidural fat?

The fat of the epidural space is different to most in the body. Firstly, obesity is unrelated to amount of epidural fat. Secondly, the quantity of epidural fat declines with age, therefore elderly patients have a potentially larger epidural space. Finally, the fat is semi-liquid and contained within a capsule.

What are the features suggestive of a post-dural puncture headache?

The features of the headache are as follows:

- Severe
- Frontal and occipital
- Radiating to the neck and shoulders
- Worsened by an upright posture and neck movement
- Relieved by lying down
- Associated with neck stiffness, photophobia, tinnitus or visual disturbances
- Seen more commonly after dural puncture (recognised or otherwise) with needles of larger calibre and with cutting tips
- Increased frequency in parturients
- Decreased frequency in the obese
- Symptoms usually occur within 48 hours and last about 2 weeks.

Post-dural puncture headache can lead to cranial nerve palsies, convulsions, or even intra-cranial haemorrhage and death.

There should be a full assessment of the headache and a neurological assessment performed. Other causes of headache should be considered. MRI or CT can demonstrate CSF leaks, but in practice are not often used.

How should a post-dural puncture headache be managed?

Patients with significant symptoms can initially be managed conservatively with bed rest, analgesia, anti-emetic drugs and hydration.

There are a number of pharmacological agents that have been recommended to treat post-dural puncture headache, caffeine 500 mg orally or intra-venously once or twice a day has found to be an effective treatment. It is thought that it may act by vasoconstricting dilated cerebral vessels. Sumatriptan and ACTH have also been used in the past but there is no evidence to support their use.

Epidural blood patch is regarded as the definitive treatment and has a success rate of between 70 and 98% if carried out more than 24 hours after dural puncture. If the symptoms persist after the epidural blood patch, the procedure may be repeated.

4.1.3. Anatomy of the trachea and bronchi – Mari H Roberts

This is most likely to come up in the science structured oral exam. Diagrams will help you remember the anatomy, which can be quite cumbersome to learn. The examiner is likely to start with describing the anatomy before moving on to some applied clinical aspects.

How long is an average adult's trachea?

It is 10 to 15 cm long and extends from the cricoid cartilage at the level of C6 to the carina at T4–5. It may extend to T6 at full inspiration.

What is the trachea made of?

It is made of fibro-elastic connective tissue reinforced by 15 to 20 cartilaginous rings that are incomplete posteriorly. It is lined by ciliated columnar epithelium and mucus glands. There is also a smooth muscle layer posteriorly which runs both longitudinally and transversely. This is called the trachealis muscle.

What is its diameter?

The diameter is 1.5 to 2 cm, and it is flattened posteriorly.

What are its anterior relations?

You may want to draw a diagram or two to help you explain this. It is useful to learn the cross-sectional anatomy at two levels; in the neck, usually at the level of C6 and in the thorax usually at the level of T4. The examiner may want the anatomy at both levels, or only at one.

Take a minute to draw the diagrams before going through them (Figure 4.1.3a, b).

In the neck its anterior relations are, from outside in; skin and superficial and deep fascia, the anterior jugular vein, sternohyoid and sternothyroid muscles in the lower neck and pretracheal fascia. The isthmus of the thyroid gland lies anterior at the level of the second to fourth tracheal rings.

In the thorax the manubrium sterni lies anteriorly as does the thymic remnants and the inferior thyroid veins. Lower down in the thorax, the brachiocephalic artery and the left brachiocephalic vein crosses the trachea anteriorly as well as the aortic arch. The pulmonary bifurcation lies behind the carina.

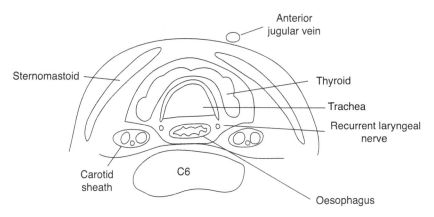

Figure 4.1.3a. Cross-section at C6.

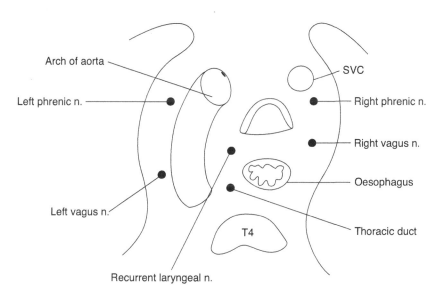

Figure 4.1.3b. Cross-section at T4.

What are its posterior relations?

Again you can refer to your diagrams.

In the neck its immediate posterior relation is the oesophagus with the recurrent laryngeal nerves lying in the grooves between trachea and oesophagus.

In the thorax, it is only the left recurrent laryngeal nerve and oesophagus which lies posteriorly. The right laryngeal nerve leaves the vagus as it crosses the subclavian artery which is at a higher level than where the left recurrent laryngeal nerve originates. It then ascends in the tracheo-oesophageal groove. The left leaves the vagus at a lower level, as it crosses the aortic arch and then ascends.

What are its lateral relations?

In the neck, the lobes of the thyroid and the carotid sheaths lie laterally. The carotid sheath contains the internal jugular vein, the common carotid artery and the vagus nerve.

In the thorax it is related on both sides by the pleura and the lung and the right and left vagus nerves respectively. On the right-hand side it is also related to the azygos vein and the superior vena cava. On the left lie the left common carotid artery and the aortic arch.

What is the nerve supply to the trachea?

The nerve supply is from the recurrent laryngeal nerve and sympathetic branches from the middle cervical ganglion.

Lets move down to the bronchi and bronchial tree.

What are the subdivisions of the bronchial tree from trachea to alveolus?

The subdivisions are bronchus, bronchioles, respiratory bronchioles, alveolar ducts, alveolar sacs and then alveolus.

Can you describe to me the anatomy of the right main bronchus? How long is it?

It is about 3 cm long which is shorter than the left. It is also wider.

At what angle does it leave the trachea?

It leaves the trachea at an angle of 25–30 degrees which is more vertical than the left.

What are its relations?

It passes under the azygos vein and lies initially above and then behind the right pulmonary artery.

What about the left main bronchus? Can you describe its anatomy?

The left main bronchus is about 5 cm long. It leaves the trachea at an angle of 45 to 50 degrees.

What are its relations?

The left main bronchus passes under the aortic arch, in front of the oesophagus and descending aorta. It then passes to lie initially below and then behind the left pulmonary artery.

Let's concentrate on the right-hand side first. How many lobes are there on the right?

The examiner is probably going to talk you through explaining the anatomy of the bronchi and bronchial tree. Again a diagram will help you remember and explain this (Figure 4.1.3c).

The right lung has three lobes, which are supplied by three lobar bronchi, the upper, middle and lower lobes.

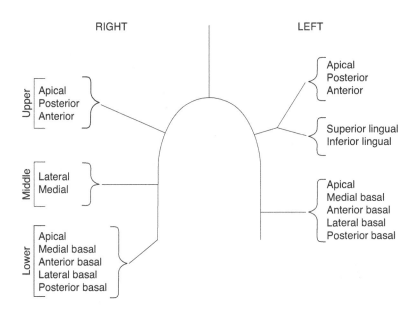

RIGHT   LEFT

Upper
- Apical
- Posterior
- Anterior

Middle
- Lateral
- Medial

Lower
- Apical
- Medial basal
- Anterior basal
- Lateral basal
- Posterior basal

Apical
Posterior
Anterior

Superior lingual
Inferior lingual

Apical
Medial basal
Anterior basal
Lateral basal
Posterior basal

Figure 4.1.3c. The bronchial tree.

Can you explain the anatomy of the bronchi and bronchial tree on this side?

The right upper lobe bronchus comes off the right main bronchus first, usually about 2.5 cm from the carina, but this may vary. It is therefore the right upper lobe that is most at risk of occlusion from a tracheal tube or a right-sided double-lumen tube. The right upper lobe bronchus then divides within 1 cm of its origin into apical, anterior and posterior segments.

The middle lobe bronchus is the next to come off the right main bronchus. This is directed downwards and forwards and splits into lateral and medial segmental bronchi.

The right lower lobe bronchus has an apical branch that comes off just below the origin of the middle lobe bronchus. The main stem of the lower lobe bronchus continues downwards before splitting into medial basal, anterior basal, lateral basal and posterior basal segments.

So how many bronchopulmonary segments are there on the right?

There are 10 bronchopulmonary segments on the right.

It is often difficult to remember the names of the bronchopulmonary segments. On the right they can be remembered by learning the acronym "A PALM A MALP".

Apical, posterior and anterior form the upper lobe; lateral and medial form the middle lobe and apical, medial, anterior, lateral and posterior form the lower lobe.

What about the left? How many lobes are there?

There are two main lobes, the upper and lower lobes and also a lingual which is thought of as part of the upper lobe.

Can you describe the anatomy of the bronchial tree on this side?

There are a lot of similarities between the anatomy on the right and on the left. It is a good idea to learn one side and then what is different on the other. Again refer to your diagram.

The acronym to remember the bronchopulmonary segments on the left side is "A PASI A MALP".

The left main bronchus is longer than the right and terminates in two lobar bronchi, the upper and lower, after about 5 cm. The left upper lobe bronchus divides into a superior division and a lingular division. The superior division splits into apical, posterior and anterior segmental bronchi. This is similar to the upper lobe on the right-hand side.

The lingular division splits into superior and inferior segmental bronchi.

The anatomy of the left lower lobe is similar to that of the right lower lobe. The left lower lobe bronchus gives off apical, medial basal, anterior basal, lateral basal and posterior basal segmental bronchi. However, the anterior and medial basal bronchopulmonary segments are often together.

So how many bronchopulmonary segments are there on the left?

There are 10 segments.

Remember A PASI A MALP.

Apical, posterior and anterior form the upper lobe; superior and inferior form the lingular and apical, medial, anterior, lateral and posterior basal form the lower lobe.

However since the anterior and medial bronchopulmonary segments are often together some would say that technically there are only nine.

The structured oral exam is now likely to turn to some applied clinical aspects.

From your knowledge of the bronchial tree, can you predict which part of the lung is most likely to be contaminated during aspiration if the patient is lying supine and explain to me why?

In the supine position, the apical segments of the lower lobes are most likely to be contaminated since the apical bronchi project posteriorly from the lower lobe bronchi.

What about if the patient was in the lateral position?

In the lateral position gastric content is more likely to enter the upper lobe bronchus of the side the patient is lying on since these bronchi project laterally.

What about if the patient was sitting up?

In this position, the most likely areas to be contaminated are the posterior basal and the lateral basal bronchopulmonary segments since the bronchi to these segments project downwards.

What if the patient was lying prone?

In the prone position gastric content is more likely to enter the middle lobe on the right and the lingular on the left. This is because the bronchi that supply the middle lobe and the lingular run downward and forward.

If you are doing well the examiner may move on to another clinical area. You may be asked about performing a tracheostomy, which is covered in another podcast, or about double-lumen endobronchial tubes.

What are the indications for a double-lumen tube?

A double-lumen tube may be used to facilitate one-lung ventilation. The indications can be classified as absolute and relative.

Absolute indications are firstly, airway soiling. This may be from bronchiectasis, bleeding, a lung abscess or an empyema with a bronchopleural fistula. The second absolute indication is a gas leak. A gas leak may occur from a giant lung cyst, a bronchopleural fistula, a tracheobronchial rupture or following bronchial surgery.

The relative indications are all to improve surgical access. The types of surgery where this may be of benefit are pulmonary, oesophageal, anterior spinal and great vessel surgery.

What sizes of double-lumen tubes do you know?

Double-lumen tubes are measured in French gauge. Left-sided tubes are normally 28 or 32 french gauge. Right sided tubes available include 35, 37, 39 and 41 french gauge.

Would you prefer to use a left- or a right-sided tube?

A left-sided tube.

Why is this?

The right upper lobe bronchus comes off the right main bronchus within about 2.5 cm from its origin therefore there is a significant risk of it being occluded by a right-sided tube. Left-sided tubes can be used for most procedures.

How would you insert a double-lumen tube?

After inducing anaesthesia and allowing adequate time to ensure muscle relaxation a double-lumen tube is initially inserted as a tracheal tube with the bronchial curve facing anteriorly. Once the tip of the tube is through the larynx the tube should be rotated 90 degrees so that the bronchial part is directed to the correct side. The tube is then connected to the breathing circuit via a double catheter mount. The tracheal cuff is then inflated until the air leak stops and both sides of the chest are auscultated to check for ventilation. The catheter mount to the tracheal lumen is then clamped and the tracheal lumen opened to air. The lung is now being inflated via the bronchial lumen only and the bronchial cuff should be inflated until no air leak is heard via the tracheal lumen. Only the selected lung should now be ventilating. The tracheal lumen should then be reconnected and ventilation should be checked on both sides.

How would you confirm the placement of a double-lumen tube?

Its placement should be confirmed clinically and by using bronchoscopy.

There are a number of clinical checks that should be done. Firstly, as with an endotracheal tube we should monitor for carbon dioxide (CO_2). Secondly we should inspect the rise and fall of the chest and auscultate both lung fields with both cuffs inflated. Thirdly the length of the tube should be carefully inspected. For a patient whose height is 170 cm the average depth of insertion to the incisors is 29 cm. For every 10-cm difference in the height of the patient the average depth of insertion of the tube changes by 1 cm. For example if the patient is 160 cm, on average the depth will be 28 cm. Fourthly, both lungs should be auscultated alternatively by clamping and releasing each side in turn.

Clinical assessment can be unreliable and therefore bronchoscopy should always be used to confirm placement.

What are you looking for when using bronchoscopy to confirm its placement?

We are looking to see the upper surface of the bronchial cuff lying immediately distal to the carina.

4.1.4. The anatomy of the autonomic nervous system – Gareth J Gibbon

This topic comes up a lot – take your time because it is very easy to tie yourself up in knots.

Tell me what you know about the autonomic nervous system

Start generally. Define and classify and try to be systematic in your answer.

The autonomic nervous system maintains homeostasis in the body and is not under conscious control. There's a sympathetic and a parasympathetic component. These differ anatomically, pharmacologically and physiologically.

Firstly, the anatomy – Generally, efferent outflow comes from autonomic centres in the hypothalamus, medulla and brainstem. The autonomic nerves, unlike the somatic nervous system, leave the central nervous system and synapse before reaching the effector organ. Myelinated first order nerves synapse onto unmyelinated second order nerves, which in turn supply the effector organ. Sympathetic nerves generally synapse distant to their effector site, whereas parasympathetic nerves synapse close to the target organ.

Pharmacologically the predominant effector neurotransmitter for the sympathetic nervous system is noradrenaline, whereas for the parasympathetic system it is acetylcholine. Acetylcholine is the neurotransmitter at all the synapses between first order and second order neurons. Of note the principle exception to this is the sympathetic supply to the sweat glands, which is cholinergic.

Physiologically the sympathetic nervous system is responsible for the fight or flight response.

Can you draw a diagram of the sympathetic nervous system?

The examiner will stop you if you are heading away from where the points are scored. If asked to draw a diagram; keep it as simple as possible, utilise the whole sheet of paper, don't be overly concerned keeping things to scale and talk whilst you are constructing it (Figure 4.1.4). It's all about demonstrating your knowledge of the principles and not about winning the Turner prize.

This is a cross section of the spinal cord at the thoracic level. The sympathetic outflow is from T1 to L2 or 3 of the cord. The first order neurones have their cell bodies in the lateral horn. They then run with the anterior nerve root but leave shortly after the root exits the intervertebral foramen to run anteriorly to the sympathetic chain. These myelinated nerves connect from the cord to the sympathetic chain via white rami communicantes. Usually they synapse here onto second order grey rami communicantes. These are unmyelinated fibres which can then run back towards the spinal nerve and follow its course.

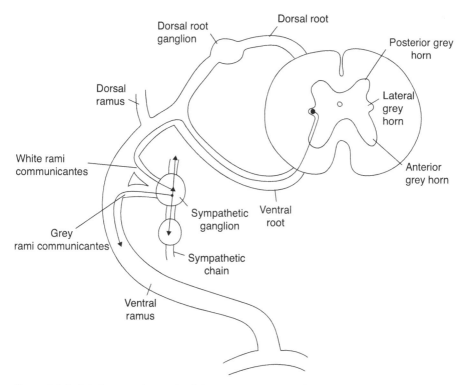

Figure 4.1.4. Spinal nerve at thoracic level showing sympathetic outflow.

Is there anything else that can happen to these neurones once they leave the spinal cord?

There are three possible fates of the first order neurones:

1. They can synapse in the chain before running back to follow the path of their originating spinal nerve.
2. They can run up or down the sympathetic chain to synapse in a more distant ganglion within the chain.
3. They can pass without synapse through the chain towards a peripheral ganglion.

This latter course occurs with the sympathetic supply to the abdominal and pelvic organs. These preganglionic sympathetic fibres run in the splanchnic nerves. The greater splanchnic nerve arises from the T5 to T9 segments of the sympathetic chain. The lesser splanchnic nerve runs from the T10 and T11 segments. Sometimes there is a third least splanchnic nerve from T12. All supply the coeliac plexus, which is where they synapse onto unmyelinated nerves.

After they have synapsed, all the sympathetic second order unmyelinated nerves tend to follow the arterial supply to their effector organs.

How is the adrenal gland innervated?

The adrenal innervation is different. White myelinated fibres pass through the coeliac ganglion towards the adrenal gland and innervate the adrenal medulla. Here they release acetylcholine to stimulate the secretion of adrenaline and noradrenaline from the medulla. Embryologically the adrenal medulla and the sympathetic nerves share a common origin.

You've mentioned the coeliac plexus; do you know of any other plexuses?

Yes. All the thoracic and abdominal organs are innervated via plexuses. These plexuses are simply clusters of postganglionic nerves. There is a cardiac plexus supplied from T1 to T4. The cardiac plexus supplies the heart. It also supplies the lungs via a pulmonary plexus. In the abdomen there is an aortic plexus formed from the postganglionic fibres of the coeliac plexus. This supplies further plexuses, named after the organs which they supply, again following the blood supply. The hypogastric plexus forms from the aortic plexus and the lumbar sympathetic trunks. This feeds right and left pelvic plexuses and the pelvic organs.

Tell me more about the coeliac plexus?

This is the largest of the sympathetic plexuses and is at the level L1, originating where the coeliac artery branches off the aorta. It acts as a conduit for the sympathetic supply to most of the abdominal organs. It can be blocked to stop pain pathways from the pancreas and upper GI tract.

Have you ever seen a coeliac plexus block?

No, but I know the principles. You will need an image intensifier or CT scan. The patient is positioned prone. At L2, 8–10 cm from the midline below the twelfth rib a needle is directed towards the body of L1. You should target the anterolateral border of the vertebra. On the left side you should feel the aorta pulsating when you are in the correct place. On the right side you can advance the needle slightly further anterior to the anterolateral border of the vertebra. You need to confirm you are not in a vessel and in a reasonable tissue plane before you inject. Contrast medium may be injected first.

What is the stellate ganglion?

The efferent supply to the sympathetic chain comes exclusively through the thoracic and upper lumbar nerve roots. The chain however, runs cranially to supply the head and neck via cervical ganglia. It also runs caudally towards the sacrum through, usually, four ganglia as the lumbar sympathetic chain. There are three cervical ganglia: superior, middle and inferior. The inferior cervical ganglion is usually fused with the first thoracic ganglion forming the stellate ganglion.

Where would you find the stellate ganglion?

The stellate ganglion sits anterior to the disc space between C7 and L1. The surface landmark for performing a stellate ganglion block is Chassaignac's tubercle – the transverse process of C6. This is found at the level of the cricoid cartilage with the neck extended, the mouth partially open and the carotid artery and sternocleidomastoid muscle retracted laterally. A needle is passed to touch the transverse process. Then it is withdrawn by 2 to 3 mm, aspirated and the block administered slowly following a test dose. The block is confirmed by the development of a Horner's syndrome.

Why and how would you perform a lumbar sympathectomy?

It would be fair for the examiner to ask about any of the blocks you have spoken about in more detail. Always have a systematic approach to discussing any procedure – it ensures you don't miss out on any easy marks.

The aim of a lumbar sympathectomy is to block the distal lumbar sympathetic outflow as well as impair any conduction through afferent pain fibres that can relay through the sympathetic chain. Local anaesthetic can be used for short-lasting effect, and phenol or alcohol can be used if a longer duration of symptomatic treatment is felt appropriate. There are indications, contraindications and complications. Indications include circulatory insufficiency, complex regional pain syndromes, phantom pain and frostbite to the lower limb. Contraindications, as with most procedures, would be infection over the site of instrumentation, lack of patient consent, allergy to any of the agents to be used and coagulopathy. Complications would include those caused by the procedure, and those resulting from the procedure. There might be damage to and bleeding from intercostal vessels, the aorta or inferior vena cava. Local haematoma and infection might also complicate the procedure. As a result of the injection, the ipsilateral leg will become subjectively and objectively warmer and more erythematous. Post-sympathectomy neuralgia occurs commonly manifesting as pain in the thigh or groin. There is also the potential for sexual dysfunction problems, especially if the block is bilateral. There is always the risk that the block fails.

As with every procedure I would see the patient on the ward, ensure that the potential benefit of the procedure outweighed the risk, establish the absence of contraindications and ensure that full consent has been ascertained. Personally, I would perform a lumbar sympathetectomy under skilled supervision as I have never attempted this procedure before. I would ensure trained anaesthetic staff were present, that my emergency drugs were drawn up and full monitoring had been applied. I would maintain strict asepsis. As with the coeliac plexus block, this procedure is usually performed under X-ray or CT guidance with the patient in the prone position. The L2 vertebra is identified and a needle inserted 10–12 cm from the midline. This time, however, the body of the L2 vertebra is targeted and the needle is aimed towards the anterolateral border of the body of L2. Radio-opaque contrast can be injected to confirm that the injection will be made in the correct tissue plane. I understand that neurolytic blocks are made more effective by repeating the procedure at the L3 and L4 vertebrae.

What about the parasympathetic nervous system – how does that differ from the sympathetic nervous system?

The parasympathetic nervous system differs anatomically, pharmacologically and physiologically.

Anatomically the parasympathetic efferents leave the CNS to synapse onto second order neurones close to the target organ. There is a cranial component and a sacral component.

The cranial component is conveyed in cranial nerves III, VII, IX and X from specific nuclei in the brainstem. These follow the course of the respective cranial nerves to synapse at four ganglia. The sacral component efferents are termed the nervi erigentes and arise from S2, 3 and 4. These join the pelvic plexuses and are distributed to the pelvic organs. Small ganglia in the visceral walls relay the postganglionic fibres.

Pharmacologically, the neurotransmitter is acetylcholine which acts on muscarinic receptors at both the ganglion and effector organs.

Physiologically the parasympathetic system antagonises the effects of the fight or flight sympathetic system. It causes constriction of the pupils, bradycardia, bronchoconstriction, mucus production, peristalsis and stimulates the production of pancreatic and gastric secretions. The nervi erigentes are nerves of emptying and controlling bladder and bowel function.

Do you know where the ganglia are for the cranial nerve outflow?

The third nerve transmits fibres from the Edinger-Westphal nucleus towards the ciliary ganglion in the orbit. Stimulation leads to pupillary constriction.

The seventh nerve transmits fibres from the superior salivatory nucleus to two ganglia. One is via the greater petrosal nerve to the pterygopalatine ganglion in the pterygopalatine fossa which then runs on to supply the lacrimal glands. The other is via the chorda tympani to the secretomotor supply to the salivary glands through the submandibular ganglion. The submandibular ganglion is closely related to the lingual nerve in the floor of the mouth.

The ninth nerve transmits fibres from the inferior salivatory nucleus to the otic ganglion via the lesser petrosal nerve. The otic ganglion lies below the foramen ovale. It supplies secretomotor fibres to the parotid gland.

And the vagus?

The vagus conveys the most widely distributed parasympathetic supply. The parasympathetic neurons arise from the dorsal nucleus in the medulla oblongata. They are carried with the vagus nerve and distributed through the cardiac, pulmonary and other organ plexuses. Again, the first order myelinated nerves pass through these plexuses to small ganglia in the walls of the target viscera. It is responsible for parasympathetic autonomic tone in all abdominal and thoracic viscera from the neck to the transverse colon. The majority of the neurones running in the vagus are afferent, conveying sensory information from the viscera. Significantly for anaesthetists it controls the motor and sensory supply to the larynx and vocal cords.

Can you describe its path in more detail?

See 4.1.5. "Cranial nerve anatomy" for a description of the course of the vagus.

4.1.5. Cranial nerve anatomy – Poonam M Bopanna

The anatomy of the cranial nerves is rather dry and cumbersome to remember. The following podcasts aim to give a concise description of the main cranial nerves relevant to anaesthetists.

Describe the anatomy of the optic nerve

The optic nerve is the second cranial nerve (CN II) and is the sensory nerve to the retina. Its fibres originate from the innermost layer of the retina called the stratum opticum. These fibres are axons of the cells in the retina and pierce the sclera to form the optic nerve. It is surrounded by the cranial meninges, containing an extension of the subarachnoid space. The optic nerve runs through the optic canal and enters the cranial cavity where it joins with the nerve from the other side, forming the optic chiasma. In the optic chiasma the fibres from the nasal half of the retina cross the median plane and enter the optic tract of the opposite side. However the temporal fibres remain and enter the optic tract on the same side. The decussation of the nerve fibres in the chiasma means that the right optic tract conveys impulses from the left visual field whilst the left optic tract conveys impulses from the right visual field. The optic tracts then continue backwards to terminate in the lateral geniculate body of the thalamus. From these nuclei, axons are relayed to the visual cortices of the occipital lobe of the brain.

Tell me about the motor supply to the eye

The third cranial nerve (CN III) is the oculomotor nerve and is the motor supply to all the extraocular muscles except the superior oblique and the lateral rectus. In addition, it also carries parasympathetic supply to the sphincter pupillae and the ciliary muscles. The nerve arises in upper midbrain, where the nuclei lie in the periaqueductal grey matter. Fibres then pass between the cerebral peduncles, pierce the dura mater and run in the lateral wall of the cavernous sinus. CN III exits the skull via the superior orbital fissure to enter the orbit. Within the superior orbital fissure it divides into the superior branch that supplies the superior rectus and levator palpebrae superioris and the inferior division that supplies the medial rectus, inferior rectus and the inferior oblique.

The trochlear nerve (CN IV) supplies the superior oblique muscle. It arises from a nucleus in the periaqueductal grey matter of the lower midbrain. Fibres pass through the posterior cranial fossa following the edge of the tentorium just lateral to CN III. Next, the fibres pass through the middle cranial fossa in the lateral wall of the cavernous sinus before entering the orbit through the superior orbital fisssure.

The abducent nerve (CN VI) supplies the lateral rectus muscle. The nucleus of the abducent nerve lies in the inferior pons. Fibres then pass through the posterior and middle cranial fossa, through the cavernous sinus and into the orbit through the superior orbital fissure. CN VI has a very long intra-cranial course and is susceptible to damage by stretching in patients with raised intra-cranial pressure.

What are the clinical signs of a third nerve palsy?

The clinical signs of a complete nerve palsy include:

- Ptosis
- Loss of pupillary light reflexes
- Dilatation of the pupil
- Downward and outward gaze due to unopposed action of the superior oblique and lateral rectus muscles
- Loss of accommodation.

If a patient has a fourth nerve palsy what will the patient complain of?

With a fourth nerve palsy the patient will experience diplopia on looking downwards because the eye is pulled down only by the inferior rectus and therefore moves slightly differently to the other side.

Describe the anatomy of the trigeminal nerve

The trigeminal nerve is the fifth cranial nerve and provides sensory supply to the face, nasopharynx, nasal and oral cavities, paranasal air sinuses and the anterior part of the scalp. Its motor branch supplies the muscles of mastication.

It has three sensory and one motor nucleus. The three sensory nuclei are:

- The **principle sensory nucleus** which lies in the upper pons and receives fibres transmitting touch sensation.
- The **mesencephalic nucleus** which lies in the midbrain and receives proprioceptive fibres
- The **nucleus of the spinal tract** of the trigeminal nerve which lies deep to a tract of descending fibres running from the pons to the substantia gelatinosa of the spinal cord. This nucleus receives pain and temperature fibres.

The motor nucleus is situated in the upper part of the pons and lies just medial to the principle sensory nucleus.

The nerves that originate from the above nuclei pass forward to the trigeminal ganglion (also called the semilunar ganglion due to its shape), which lies near to the apex of the petrous temporal bone. The sensory fibres pass through the ganglion whereas the motor fibres pass below the ganglion. The three main sensory divisions of the nerve emerge from the anterior border of the trigeminal ganglion and are the ophthalmic division (V1), the maxillary division (V2) and the mandibular division (V3).

The ophthalmic division (V1) of the trigeminal nerve divides into the lacrimal, nasociliary and frontal branches just before the superior orbital fissure. The frontal nerve further divides into the supra-orbital and supra-trochlear nerves. V1 also transmits some sympathetic and parasympathetic fibres. The ophthalmic division supplies the skin of the nose, the forehead, eyelids, scalp, conjunctiva, lacrimal apparatus and the globe.

The maxillary division (V2) runs below the ophthalmic division and leaves the base of the skull via the foramen rotundum. After traversing the pterygopalatine fossa it becomes known as the infra-orbital nerve, which passes through the infra-orbital foramen to supply skin to the surrounding areas of face.

The mandibular division (V3) also carries the motor fibres of the trigeminal nerve. It leaves the skull via the foramen ovale and subsequently divides into sensory and motor branches. The motor root supplies the muscles of mastication. The sensory branches are the meningeal, buccal, auriculotemporal, inferior alveolar and lingual. These branches supply the lower third of the face and floor of the mouth.

Tell me about the facial nerve

The facial nerve is the seventh cranial nerve (CN VII) and carries:

- Visceral motor fibres: to the facial muscles of expression
- Visceral sensory fibres: taste sensation from the anterior two thirds of the tongue
- Visceral parasympathetic fibres: secretomotor to salivary glands and lacrimal gland.

The facial nerve leaves the pons and passes through the internal auditory meatus to the facial ganglion. At the facial ganglion the parasympathetic fibres leave the rest of the facial nerve and travel in the greater petrosal nerve to the pterygopalatine ganglion. The remaining facial nerve turns posteriorly and descends through the bony canal in the posterior wall of the middle ear then emerges through the stylomastoid foramen. Just above the stylomastoid foramen the chorda tympani nerve arises, which joins with the lingular nerve to convey taste from the anterior tongue, parasympathetic innervation for the submandibular gland and some motor fibres. The remaining facial nerve has only motor actions and as it passes through the parotid gland it divides into the temporal, zygomatic, buccal, mandibular and cervical branches. These branches supply the muscles of facial expression, buccinators and platysma.

What does the vagus nerve innervate?

The vagus nerve has many different components:

- Parasympathetic fibres to the heart, lungs and alimentary canal
- Sensory fibres from the heart, lungs and alimentary canal
- Motor fibres to the larynx, pharynx and palate
- Sensory fibres from the larynx, pharynx and palate
- Somatic sensory fibres from the external acoustic meatus and tympanic membrane.

Describe the course of the vagus nerve

The vagus nerve (CN X) has the most extensive course compared to any other cranial nerve. It emerges from the medulla and exits the skull via the jugular foramen, alongside the glossopharygeal nerve, accessory nerve and internal jugular vein. The vagus nerve descends through the neck invested in the carotid sheath and lying between the internal jugular vein and internal and common carotid arteries. In the root of the neck the right vagus nerve descends in front of the subclavian artery to enter the thorax, whilst the left vagus nerve descends between the common carotid and left subclavian arteries. The two vagus nerves then pass posteriorly to each main bronchus to form the pulmonary plexus. Next they converge onto the oesophagus to create the oesophageal plexus. The anterior and posterior vagus nerves emerge from the oesphageal plexus and travel asymmetrically through the thorax and abdomen to supply the alimentary tract.

Tell me what the ninth, eleven and twelve cranial nerve innervate

The ninth cranial nerve (CN IX) is the glossopharyngeal nerve and has both general and visceral sensory, motor and parasympathetic fibres. The general sensory fibres supply the middle ear, pharynx, posterior two thirds of the tongue and the carotid sinus and carotid body. The visceral sensory fibres carry taste sensation from the posterior third of the tongue. The parasympathetic fibres supply the parotid gland. The motor fibres supply the stylopharyngeus. To test the integrity of CN IX a gag reflex can be tested. It will be absent on the side of the lesion.

The accessory nerve (CN XI) supplies the sternocleidomastoid and trapezius muscles resulting in a weakened shrugging of the shoulders and rotation of the neck.

The hypoglossal nerve (CN XII) supplies all the intrinsic and extrinsic muscles of the tongue except palatoglossus. It can be injured during tonsillectomy and results in ipsilateral paralysis of the tongue. Thus when the tongue is protruded it will deviate to the side of the lesion.

Further Reading

Craven J. The cranial nerves. *Anaesthesia and Intensive Care Medicine.* 2007; **8**(12): 499–503.

Moore KL, Agur AMR. *Essential clinical aanatomy.* Second edition. Philadelphia: Lippincott Williams & Williams, 2002.

Regional anaesthesia

Chapter

4.2

4.2.1. Brachial plexus, inter-scalene and axillary blocks – Pascal J Boddy

What clinical approaches do you know to block the brachial plexus?

For a complete answer to this question a demonstration of an understanding of the anatomy of the brachial plexus is important. This could be aided by a diagram (see Figure 4.2.1.) The examiners may interrupt, in which case there are four well-recognised approaches you should mention:

1. Inter-scalene
2. Supra-clavicular
3. Infra-clavicular
4. Axillary.

The brachial plexus is formed from the anterior primary rami of C5 to T1 and provides all motor and sensory innervation to the upper limb. The nerves that make up the plexus lie in a sheath that extends from the tubercles of the transverse processes of the cervical vertebrae to the axilla; it is within this sheath that we would inject our local anaesthetic. As these five roots pass between scalenus anterior and medius, C5 and 6 join to form the upper trunk, the root of C7 continues as the middle trunk and C8 and T1 unite to form the lower trunk. The inter-scalene approach aims to anaesthetise the trunks of the plexus.

The three trunks continue downwards and laterally in the posterior triangle of the neck to cross over the first rib, the supra-clavicular approach allows injection of local anaesthetic at this point.

At the lateral border of the rib the trunks each divide into anterior and posterior divisions (six divisions in total) and continue beneath the clavicle into the apex of the axilla to form the cords of the brachial plexus. As the divisions travel beneath the clavicle they can be blocked via the infra-clavicular approach.

Within the axilla, the anterior divisions of the upper and middle trunks form the lateral cord, which eventually forms the lateral head of the median nerve and the musculocutaneous nerve. The anterior division of the lower trunk forms the medial cord from which the ulnar nerve and medial head of the median nerve are formed. The posterior cord is made up of the

Dr. Podcast Scripts for the Final FRCA, ed. Rebecca A. Leslie, Emily K. Johnson, Gary Thomas and Alexander P. L. Goodwin.   Published by Cambridge University Press.

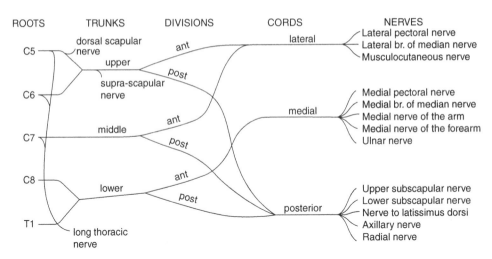

Figure 4.2.1. The brachial plexus.

posterior divisions of all three trunks and its main branch is the radial nerve. The names of the cords correspond to their relationship to the axillary artery. The axillary approach provides the ability to block the plexus at its most distal point.

For what type of surgery would an inter-scalene brachial plexus block be appropriate?

An inter-scalene block provides good analgesia for shoulder and upper arm surgery and provides good relief from tourniquet pain. Frequently the lower trunks are missed by the local anaesthetic, which makes this approach less suitable for hand surgery.

You have a patient listed for shoulder surgery, how would you perform an inter-scalene block?

I would firstly obtain informed consent from the patient and make sure the surgical site is marked and corresponds to the shoulder being operated on. I would ensure that full monitoring is established, I have a trained assistant and that resuscitation equipment is easily available. I would then site an intra-venous cannula in the contralateral arm.

The patient should be positioned supine, tilting their head slightly away from the side to be blocked. I would ensure asepsis by wearing a gown and sterile gloves and cleaning the skin with an appropriate cleaning solution. I would then palpate for the inter-scalene groove at the level of the cricoid cartilage. If it was difficult to identify I could ask the patient to sniff which would make the scalene muscles appear more prominent. I could also scan the area using ultrasound, which would allow me to identify the inter-scalene groove with the plexus trunks lying one on top of another between scalenus anterior and medius. After anaesthetising the skin, I would pass a short bevelled region block needle attached to a nerve stimulator perpendicular to all planes. I may feel a "pop" as the needle passes through the sheath at a depth of between 1 and 3 cm and should elicit muscle contractions in the biceps brachialis. At this point I would inject between 20 and 30 ml of local anaesthetic, ensuring that the injection was not intra-neural by noting that there should be minimal resistance to injection and there should be minimal discomfort to the patient.

You should try and make it sound that you are used to performing practical procedures and have a routine of following basic safety and infection control procedures. Mentioning consent and monitoring etc. also gives you some "thinking time" before embarking on the description of the procedure. The same pre-amble can be used for almost any practical clinical task.

What are the complications of an inter-scalene block?

Due to the level of the injection and the proximity of major cervical structures, complications can be very serious and life threatening. They include:

- Cervical epidural or intra-thecal injection
- Intra-vascular injection, particularly vertebral artery, carotid artery, external and internal jugular veins.

Less serious complications arise from the close proximity of other nerves and occur so frequently that they could be considered as effects of an inter-scalene block, and include:

- Phrenic nerve palsy
- Cervical sympathetic block (Horner's syndrome).

How would you reduce the risk of these complications?

- Angling the needle slightly towards the patient's feet, so that it would hit the superior border of a transverse process, minimises the risk of cervical neuraxial blockade or injury.
- Being aware of the depth of the plexus at this level, it is rarely deeper than 3 cm and is sometimes palpable in thin individuals.
- Only injecting once muscle contractions have been elicited and not introducing the needle any further once a "pop" has been felt.
- Recent NICE recommendations suggest the use of ultrasound to aid needle placement in regional anaesthesia.

Could you employ another approach to anaesthetise the shoulder?

The supra-clavicular approach can be used for shoulder surgery but as the supra-scapular nerve (sensory to the shoulder joint) arises from the upper trunk, it may be missed if the injection is too lateral or if the nerve branches off earlier than normal. However analgesia can be supplemented by a separate supra-scapular nerve block.

How is a supra-clavicular block performed?

With the patient supine and head turned away from the site of injection, the inter-scalene groove is palpated until the subclavian artery pulsation is felt. The injection is made just lateral and posterior to the subclavian artery, just superior to the border of trapezius. The angle of the needle is directed towards the ipsilateral foot with care not to advance the needle medially as this increases the likelihood of puncturing the pleura or artery. A pop should be felt as the needle pierces the sheath and nerve stimulation will lead to contraction of muscles in the forearm and hand. The volume of local anaesthetic required is usually between 20 and 30 ml. The first rib lies beneath the plexus at this point and serves a useful purpose in preventing the needle going too deep. In experienced hands the needle can be manipulated gently within the sheath to elicit ulnar, radial and median nerve stimulation in the forearm and hand. Again, ultrasound is useful to identify the plexus and direct the needle away from pleura and the subclavian artery, which lies just anterior and inferior to the plexus.

What problems can arise from a supra-clavicular block?

- Pneumothorax due to the proximity of the dome of the pleura the incidence can be as high as 1–2%, although by using ultrasound this is reduced dramatically.
- Peri-vascular injection is also a common complication, again reduced by the use of ultrasound.
- Diaphragmatic paralysis can still occur due to the proximity of the phrenic nerve although the incidence is less than for inter-scalene blocks.
- Partial ulnar nerve block. The lower trunk can be difficult to approach using this technique.
- Supra-scapular nerve can be missed and may need to be anaesthetised separately for shoulder surgery.

In what circumstances would you use a supra-clavicular block?

Any upper limb surgery, as this technique provides good analgesia of the forearm and hand as well as providing relief from tourniquet pain.

How is an axillary block performed?

The patient is positioned supine with their arm abducted to 90° and the elbow flexed. The patient's hand is either held aloft or rests behind their head. The axillary artery is palpated and the needle is inserted just superior to the artery at the lateral border of pectoralis major. The response elicited with a nerve stimulator should be finger flexion (median nerve). Gentle distal pressure is applied to encourage medial spread of local anaesthetic and 30–40 ml are usually required. It is possible to identify and block the ulnar and occasionally the radial nerve in the axilla, but it can be time consuming, risks arterial injury and does not give a better result than a single large volume injection. It is, however, important to block the musculocutaneous nerve separately by injecting local anaesthetic into the coracobrachialis just superior to the axillary artery, or by infiltrating anaesthetic subcutaneously around the upper arm.

In what circumstances is an axillary block useful?

An axillary block is relatively easy to perform and is useful for providing analgesia in patients with forearm and hand injuries. The main limitation to its use is that the lateral aspect of the forearm is often not anaesthetised due to inadequate block of the musculocutaneous nerve. The perivascular approach used in this block can lead to vascular injury within the axilla. It is however superior to the other approaches to the brachial plexus in that there is no danger of causing a pneumothorax.

What do you know about the infra-clavicular approach to the brachial plexus?

If the structured oral exam is going well you could be asked about topics that you are less familiar with and may never have seen. Having even a basic knowledge of an unfamiliar and less common procedure is likely to impress the examiners.

The infra-clavicular approach is less commonly performed in the UK, but is a popular approach on the continent and in America. The advantages are that it is less likely to cause a pneumothorax if performed correctly whilst providing blockade of the musculocutaneous nerve and radial nerve, which are often not anaesthetised when performing a single-shot axillary block. The point of injection is 3 cm inferior and at right angles to the mid-point of a line drawn from the medial end of the clavicle and the coracoid process. With the patient lying supine, the arm is abducted and elbow flexed and the needle, attached to a nerve stimulator, is passed in a vertical direction until muscle contraction in the forearm and hand are elicited. The depth of the needle should never be more than 4–5 cm. This block provides excellent analgesia for elbow, forearm and hand surgery, but is unsuitable for shoulder and upper arm analgesia.

What current would you accept on your nerve stimulator when identifying the brachial plexus?

A response with a current of 0.3–0.4 mA suggests that the tip of the stimulator needle is in close proximity to the target. A higher current would indicate that the target is still some distance from the needle tip and may not be anaesthetised after local anaesthetic injection. A higher current can also produce required responses with the needle still being outside the plexus sheath. If a response is elicited at a current less than 0.2 mA there is a danger that the needle tip is within the nerve, injection at this point could lead to permanent nerve damage. It is important to realise that nerve stimulators cause muscles to contract if directly stimulated which can lead to misinterpretation of the response observed.

After performing a brachial plexus block, what can be done if the block is inadequate?

You should assess whether the block has failed completely or if there is an incomplete block. Complete failure should lead the operator to try an alternative type of anaesthesia, it is inadvisable to attempt the same block again as the anatomy may have been transiently disrupted making further attempts less likely to succeed. The dose of local anaesthetic already injected should be considered, as a repeat injection may lead to an excessive dose of local anaesthetic being given. Forearm and wrist blocks of the nerves not anaesthetised can supplement an incomplete block.

What are the contraindications to brachial plexus blocks?

Absolute contraindications include:

- Patient refusal
- Allergy to local anaesthetic
- Infection at the site of injection
- Severe coagulation disorders.

Relative contraindications include:

- Severe respiratory compromise. The high incidence of phrenic nerve palsy with root blocks such as inter-scalene and supra-clavicular blocks could result in decompensation and lead to respiratory failure.
- Mild to moderate coagulation disorders. The choice of approach may be governed by its proximity to major blood vessels, and how easy it would be to apply pressure to a bleeding point.
- Presence of anticipated technical difficulties such as anatomical variation.
- Lack of equipment.
- Inexperienced operators.

Further Reading

Al Haddad MF, Coventry DM. Brachial plexus blockade. *British Journal of Anaesthesia. CEPD Reviews* 2002; **2**(2): 33–36.

Carty S, Nicholls B. Ultrasound-guided regional anaesthesia. *Continuing Education in Anaesthesia, Critical Care & Pain.* 2007; **7**(1): 20–24.

Macfarlane A, Anderson K. Infra-clavicular brachial plexus blocks. *Continuing Education in Anaesthesia, Critical Care & Pain.* 2009; **9**(5): 139–143.

4.2.2. Stellate ganglion and coeliac plexus blocks – Jonathan J Gatward

Can you describe the anatomy of the stellate ganglion?

Before the SOE, learn to draw a simple line diagram to describe the anatomy. This will help you to remember the position and relations of the ganglion, and can be quickly reproduced in the exam, rather than trying to recall the information verbally (see Figure 4.2.2a).

The stellate ganglion consists of a fusion of the inferior cervical and first thoracic ganglia of the sympathetic chain. It lies adjacent to the vertebral column, between the carotid sheath and the fascia overlying the prevertebral muscles at the level of the seventh cervical and first thoracic vertebrae. It is closely related to the neck of the first rib, and importantly, the dome of the pleura and the vertebral artery which both lie anterior to it.

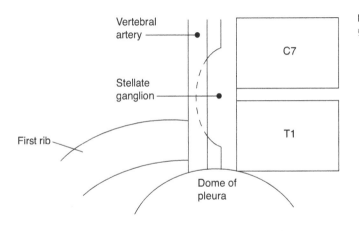

Figure 4.2.2a. The stellate ganglion.

Can you describe a technique for performing a stellate ganglion block?

You may not have performed a stellate ganglion block. You will find it easier to remember the surface anatomy if you have at least attempted to palpate Chassaignac's tubercle. Try it out!

The aim is to place local anaesthetic solution at C6 with caudal spread blocking the ganglion, because a direct approach risks entering the dome of the lung or the vertebral artery. I will describe the anterior approach to the ganglion. The patient is placed in the supine position, with the neck extended and rotated away from the side of the block. The carotid pulsation is palpated at the level of the cricoid cartilage. The sternocleidomastoid muscle and the carotid artery are displaced laterally so that the transverse process of C6 can be palpated. This is known as Chassaignac's tubercle.

After injecting local anaesthetic into the skin, a 25-gauge needle is inserted at 90 degrees to the skin and advanced towards the tubercle until bone is contacted. It is then withdrawn by 2 mm. Position should be confirmed fluoroscopically. It is very important to aspirate for blood before injecting 0.5 ml of solution as a test dose. An adrenaline containing test dose may be used to rule out intra-venous placement. If there are no adverse effects, 15 to 20 ml of low concentration local anaesthetic solution, such as 0.5% lidocaine or 0.125% bupivicaine is injected in 5-ml increments. It is best to sit the patient up to aid spread down towards the stellate ganglion.

Signs of a good block are the same as the signs of Horner's syndrome: ipsilateral ptosis, miosis, anhydrosis, conjunctival injection and enophthalmos. Patients may also get a blocked nose on the same side due to vasodilatation of the nasal mucosa (known as Guttman's sign). Warm, dry skin on the arm and hand suggests a good sympathetic block to the upper limb.

Can you name some indications for a stellate ganglion block?

Remember to categorise your answer.

Firstly, the stellate ganglion can be blocked in order to treat neuropathic pain, for example:

- Complex regional pain syndromes (CRPS) of the upper limb
- Acute herpes zoster and post-herpetic neuralgia
- Central pain following stroke
- Phantom limb pain.

The stellate ganglion block can also be used to treat ischaemic conditions in the upper limb such as:

- Vascular insufficiency
- Raynaud's disease
- After vascular or re-implantation surgery
- Inadvertent intra-arterial injection of thiopentone.

The ganglion can also be blocked for the treatment of visceral pain from the heart in refractory angina.

Why are sympathetic blocks thought to work in the treatment of neuropathic pain?

The sympathetic nervous system seems to have a role in the generation of pain. In certain pain states, there is an abnormal response of the primary nociceptive afferents to sympathetic stimulation. Peripheral and central sensitisation occurs, with reduced excitatory thresholds and the production of ectopic impulses. The afferent fibres also have increased adrenoceptor sensitivity, so that noradrenaline released from sympathetic nerve terminals causes further sensitisation. This sympathetically mediated pain is sometimes seen in CRPS. Sympathetic blocks are often used in CRPS for that reason, though only about a third of patients with the condition have sympathetically mediated pain.

Can you describe the specific side effects and complications of the stellate ganglion block?

The side effects of a stellate ganglion block include blocking other nearby nerves, such as the recurrent laryngeal nerve causing hoarseness, branches of the cervical or brachial plexus causing motor and sensory deficits, and phrenic nerve palsy, which is why bilateral blocks should not be performed at the same time.

Inadvertent injection can also occur, for example into the vertebral or carotid arteries causing seizures, and intra-thecal injection causing a spinal block.

Other complications include damage to blood vessels causing haematoma, damage to the vagus nerve or brachial plexus, the dome of the pleura causing pneumothorax, oesophageal puncture and chylothorax. Infection can also be introduced, causing abscess, osteitis or meningitis.

Let's move on to a different part of the body now. Can you describe the anatomy of the coeliac plexus?

Again, you may never have performed a coeliac plexus block but you need to know the anatomical relations of the plexus. Practise drawing a simple cross-sectional diagram of the abdomen at the level of the first lumbar vertebra (see Figure 4.2.2b).

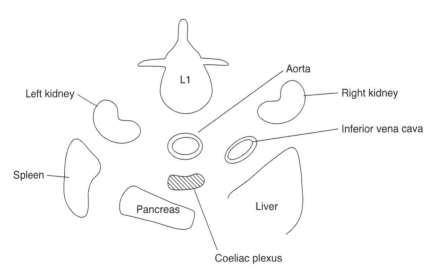

Figure 4.2.2b. The coeliac plexus.

The coeliac plexus is the main junction for autonomic nerves supplying the upper abdominal organs and consists of the bilateral coeliac ganglia with a network of interconnecting fibres. Some sympathetic preganglionic fibres do not synapse within the sympathetic chain, but exit the chain as a splanchnic nerve and synapse in prevertebral coeliac ganglia. The coeliac plexus is made up of fibres from T5 to 10, which form the greater splanchnic nerve, fibres from T9 to 11 which form the lesser splanchnic nerve, and fibres from T12 which form the least splanchnic nerve. The plexus also receives fibres from the vagus nerve. The coeliac ganglia lie anterior to the aorta on either side of the body of L1, and posterior to the pancreas.

Why might we want to perform a coeliac plexus block?

The sympathetic plexuses receive nociceptive impulses from all viscera via unmyelinated afferent fibres. These impulses can be blocked with local anaesthetic or neurolytic techniques. The coeliac plexus receives afferents from the pancreas, so the block is usually performed for pain associated with pancreatic cancer or pancreatitis. There is a risk of paraplegia of about 2 per 1000 blocks, so the risks and benefits must be balanced carefully. Also, the block may only last for a few months, and so may need to be repeated.

Do you know what a diagnostic block is?

A diagnostic block is performed with local anaesthetic only and is used to try to locate the source of pain or investigate how amenable it will be to treatment. If it is successful, there is the possibility of progressing to therapeutic or neurolytic treatment in the future.

What agents can we use in a therapeutic block?

We can use local anaesthetic agents with or without corticosteroids.

Why do therapeutic blocks with local anaesthetic alone last longer than the expected duration of action of local anaesthetic agent?

This may be due to the prevention of reflex muscle or sympathetic nervous effects, breaking the cycle of sympathetically mediated pain. Also, they may cause reduced sprouting of neurones in spinal ganglia, reduced ephaptic transmission (electrical transmission across the synapse which is not neurotransmitter mediated), and reduced hyperexcitability of pain fibres.

How can we achieve a neurolytic block?

We can use chemical, thermal or cryogenic techniques to destroy nerve tissue. The commonly used chemical agents are phenol 5 or 6% or ethanol 50 to 100%. These chemicals must be used with care, as they are obviously toxic to all tissue, not just the nerves we are targeting.

How would you prepare a patient for a coeliac plexus block?

Firstly, I would take a medical and anaesthetic history and perform a clinical examination. I would gain informed consent and discuss the risks and benefits of the treatment, including the potential side effects and complications. I would ensure that there are no contraindications, such as local infection or coagulopathy. I would secure intravenous access, fluid load the patient to reduce the risk of hypotension and make sure that full airway and resuscitation equipment was immediately available. I would attach the patient to standard monitoring and ensure that I had a skilled assistant. The block should be done under strict aseptic conditions, using anti-septic solution, sterile gloves, mask and gown, and sterile, disposable needles. The block also requires the use of an image intensifier with contrast to confirm correct needle placement.

Your patient is prepared and you are scrubbed, with a radiographer and image intensifier in position. Can you describe the technique for performing a coeliac plexus block?

The patient is in the prone position. The insertion point is just below the tip of the twelfth rib, approximately 8 cm lateral from the midline. The block is bilateral. After local anaesthetic infiltration of the superficial layers, a 100 to 150mm needle is inserted and directed medially towards the body of L1. The needle is inserted until it comes into contact with bone (the side of the body of L1) and then it is withdrawn and redirected anteriorly. It is then advanced a further 2 to 3 cm. Position is confirmed with radio-opaque dye spreading caudad and cephalad in the paracolic gutter, with no lateral spread. It is really important to aspirate before injecting. After a small test dose, 10 ml of local anaesthetic solution, with or without a neurolytic agent is then injected, under image intensifier guidance on each side.

What are the specific complications associated with the coeliac plexus block?

Remember to categorise your answers.

The complications can be divided into those associated with a misplaced needle and those caused by the drugs used. The needle can enter the inferior vena cava, the aorta or the coeliac artery, causing retroperitoneal haemorrhage. The kidneys or adrenal glands can be damaged, as can any upper abdominal organ, with abscess or cyst formation.

Complications caused by the drugs used include hypotension due to sympathetic blockade, even after unilateral block. Paraplegia can occur from injecting phenol into the arteries that supply the spinal cord. Sexual dysfunction is an important complication, which can occur if injected solution spreads to the sympathetic chain bilaterally. Finally, lumbar nerve root irritation can occur if injected solution tracks back towards the lumbar plexus.

4.2.3. Ulnar, median and radial nerve blocks – Poonam M Bopanna

The nerves of the arm can be blocked at a number of distal sites. You should have good knowledge of the anatomy and approaches for all the common peripheral nerve blocks. There are some considerations relevant to all blocks, so it is useful to learn a list and mention the points if you are asked about any block.

Points to consider when performing nerve blocks:

- Relevant medical and anaesthetic history including any drug allergies, airway assessment and aspiration risk
- Patient (and surgical) consent to the block
- Contraindications
  - History of infection at the site of injection
  - Anti-coagulation (may be relative or absolute contraindication)
  - Patient refusal
  - Allergy

- IV access required in the contralateral limb
- Full airway and resuscitation equipment must be available
- AAGBI recommended standard monitoring
- Trained assistant present.

How would you perform a mid-humeral block?

The mid-humeral block can be used for elbow, forearm or hand surgery.

The patient is positioned supine or semi-recumbent with the arm to be blocked flexed at the elbow and the shoulder abducted to 90 degrees. (Ask the patient to touch their head and then relax their arm back onto their pillow.)

The anatomical landmarks for this block are the brachial artery and the bicipital groove at the level of the deltoid muscle insertion. It is helpful to mark the brachial artery in the bicipital groove and to draw a line crossing the artery at the level of the insertion of the deltoid muscle.

The median nerve lies above and parallel to the artery. A 50-mm needle is inserted on the line drawn directly above the artery. Median nerve stimulation causes flexion of the middle and index fingers.

The musculocutaneous nerve lies above and lateral to the artery. It is blocked by advancing the needle deep to the median nerve, over the superior border of the humerus until elbow flexion is elicited with the nerve stimulator.

The ulnar nerve can be stimulated by withdrawing the needle and redirecting inferior to the artery. Thumb adduction and wrist flexion indicate ulnar nerve stimulation.

The radial nerve lies deep to the ulnar nerve and is found by advancing the needle around the inferior border of the humerus and eliciting finger and thumb extension.

All four nerves can be blocked with only one skin puncture. The 6–10 ml of local anaesthetic should be used to block each nerve. Post-operative analgesia can be provided by using a more concentrated local anaesthetic solution to block the nerve supplying the majority of the operation site.

The most common complication of mid-humeral block is brachial artery puncture.

Describe how to perform an elbow block?

Follow the safety and general precautions as above. It is a good idea to picture the anatomy of the antecubital fossa when describing this block as it is possible you may be asked to draw it (see Figures 4.2.3a, b).

Position the patient supine or semi-recumbent with their arm by their side, slightly abducted and supinated (palm uppermost). The elbow block is most commonly used for forearm and hand surgery and to supplement a patchy brachial plexus block.

The landmarks are the flexion crease of the elbow, the brachial artery, biceps tendon and the medial and lateral epicondyles.

To find the median nerve palpate the brachial artery and insert a 22-gauge 50-mm needle connected to a nerve stimulator just medial to the artery. You may feel a click as the needle passes through deep fascia. Finger flexion and thumb opposition indicate that the median nerve has been located. Inject 5 ml of local anaesthetic.

Infiltrating subcutaneously along the medial border of the biceps tendon after median nerve blockade, blocks the **medial cutaneous nerve of the forearm** that supplies the skin on the medial aspect of the forearm. A range of 5–8 ml of local anaesthetic should be used.

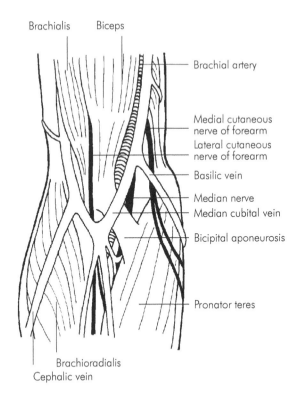

Brachialis — Biceps

Brachial artery

Medial cutaneous nerve of forearm

Lateral cutaneous nerve of forearm

Basilic vein

Median nerve

Median cubital vein

Bicipital aponeurosis

Pronator teres

Brachioradialis
Cephalic vein

Figure 4.2.3a. Superficial structures in the antecubital fossa. Reproduced with permission from Smith, T., Pinnock, C. and Lin, T. 2009. *Fundamentals of Anaesthesia.* Cambridge: Cambridge University Press. © Cambridge University Press 2009.

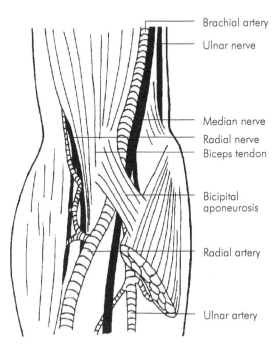

Brachial artery

Ulnar nerve

Median nerve

Radial nerve

Biceps tendon

Bicipital aponeurosis

Radial artery

Ulnar artery

Figure 4.2.3b. Deep structures in the antecubital fossa. Reproduced with permission from Smith, T., Pinnock, C. and Lin, T. 2009. *Fundamentals of Anaesthesia.* Cambridge: Cambridge University Press. © Cambridge University Press 2009.

To block the **radial nerve**, palpate the groove between biceps and brachioradialis tendons and insert the needle 2 cm above the flexion crease within this groove. The needle is directed towards the lateral epicondyle and thumb extension elicited. Inject 5 ml of local anaesthetic.

The **lateral cutaneous nerve of the forearm** can be blocked by infiltration along the lateral border of the biceps tendon, when withdrawing the needle from the radial nerve block. The 5–8 ml of local anaesthetic can be infiltrated.

Finally, to block the **ulnar nerve**, the arm should be flexed at the elbow and positioned across the patient's body. The ulnar groove is palpated and the needle inserted 1–2 cm proximal to the medial epicondyle inline with the ulnar groove. A motor response (flexion of the ring finger or adduction of the thumb) or paraesthesia are adequate identification of the nerve. The 5 ml of local anaesthetic is then injected.

The **posterior cutaneous nerve of the forearm** can subsequently be blocked by subcutaneous infiltration between the olecranon and lateral epicondyle. A range of 5–8 ml of local anaesthetic can be used.

How do you perform a wrist block?

Wrist blocks can be used, with wrist tourniquets, to perform hand surgery. They are more commonly used to supplement axillary blocks, as a supplement to general anaesthesia and to provide post-operative analgesia.

The patient is positioned supine or semi-recumbent with their arm by their side, slightly abducted and the hand supinated. The same safety considerations apply as for mid-humeral and elbow blocks.

A nerve stimulator is not normally used. A 25-gauge 25-mm needle is used rather than a regional block needle.

To block the **median nerve** insert a 25-gauge 25-mm needle in between the tendons of palmaris longus and flexor carpi radialis at the level of the palmar crease. (If palmaris longus is not present, insert the needle 5 mm medial to flexor carpi radialis.) As you pass through the flexor retinaculum, you feel a loss of resistance. At this point 3–5 ml of local anaesthetic is injected. Injecting a further 2–3 ml of local as the needle is withdrawn can block the **palmar cutaneous branch of the median nerve**.

The **ulnar nerve** is blocked by inserting the same needle on the medial aspect of the wrist underneath the tendon of flexor carpi unaris in a lateral direction. The 3 ml of local anaesthetic should be injected at a depth of approximately 1 cm. Further subcutaneous infiltration around the ulnar aspect of the wrist will block the **dorsal cutaneous branch of the ulnar nerve**.

The radial nerve has no motor function at the level of the wrist. A field block of the terminal branches can be achieved by infiltrating 5–8 ml of local anaesthetic over the radial aspect of the wrist. To make this block possible the arm should be abducted and the hand slightly pronated.

Further Reading

Nicholls B, Conn D, Roberts A. The Abbott pocket guide to practical peripheral nerve blockade. Abbott Laboratories, 2003.

The New York School of Regional Anesthesia. www.nysora.com.

4.2.4. Caudal block – Corinna J Hughes

Tell me about caudal analgesia?

Caudal analgesia is produced by injection of local anaesthetic into the caudal canal to block lumbar and sacral nerve roots. It is mainly used in paediatric anaesthesia.

Tell me about the anatomy?

Draw a sagittal section diagram (Figure 4.2.4).

The caudal space is the lowest part of the epidural space contained by the sacrum.
The sacrum consists of five fused sacral vertebrae.
It articulates with:

- Fifth lumbar vertebra superiorly
- The coccyx inferiorly
- The ilia laterally.

The dorsal roof has a median crest in the midline from fusion of the sacral spinous processes. Failure of fusion of S5 (and occasionally S4) leaves a defect called the sacral hiatus. The sacro-coccygeal membrane covers this. On either side of the sacral hiatus are sacral cornua. The sacral canal is accessed via the sacral hiatus.

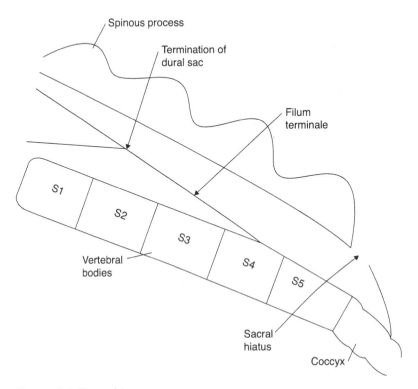

Figure 4.2.4. The caudal space.

What does the sacral canal contain?

The contents of the sacral canal are:

- The terminal part of the dural sac, which finishes at approximately S1–2 in adults and S3–4 in infants
- The cauda equina, which consists of five sacral and coccygeal nerves
- The filum terminale
- The venous plexus
- Epidural fat.

What operations can caudal analgesia be used for?

In adults, caudals are mainly used for operations on the perineum. In children they are used more extensively for operations below the umbilicus. These include inguinal hernia repair, hypospadias repair, orchidopexy and lower limb surgery.

Why are they used more extensively in children than in adults?

The fat within the sacral canal is loose in children allowing the spread of local anaesthetic making the block much more predictable. In adults the connective tissue forms a fibrous, closed mesh that leads to an unpredictable spread of local anaesthetic. The volume of the sacral canal also varies greatly in adults. The sacral cornua are more easily identifiable in children.

Can you describe your technique?

The examiners will probably move you on but don't forget to start by mentioning preparations such as pre-operative assessment, consent and all safety precautions. Make sure you have done some caudal blocks so you can speak convincingly about you own technique.

I would pre-operatively assess the patient, gain consent, obtain IV access and full monitoring, ensure I had a trained assistant and emergency drugs and equipment. I follow strict aseptic procedure. In children I perform the block after induction of anaesthesia.

The steps I follow to carry out the block are:

- Position the patient left laterally with knees flexed.
- Identify the landmarks by finding the posterior superior iliac spines and putting the left thumb and index finger on them. The sacral hiatus forms the third point of an equilateral triangle. It may not lie in the natal cleft. The sacral cornua can then be palpated by the left index finger.
- Use a 20- or 22-gauge cannula and insert the cannula at 45 degrees cranially, whilst feeling the sacral cornua.
- Proceed until a click is felt as the cannula goes through the sacrococcygeal membrane.
- Advance the cannula over the needle.
- Remove the needle.
- Exclude the presence of blood or cerebrospinal fluid by gently aspirating (not too hard as this may yield a negative aspiration due to collapse of the vein if the cannula is intra-venous).
- Slowly inject the local anaesthetic, ensuring there is no resistance, no subcutaneous swelling and intermittently aspirating.

What dose of local anaesthetic do you use?

In adults, 20–30 ml of bupivacaine 0.25–0.5% depending on the size of the patient. The volume of the sacral canal is normally 30–35 ml.

For children the volume depends on the level of block required.

For a sacral block	0.5 ml/kg 0.25% bupivacaine
For lumbar block	1 ml/kg 0.25% bupicacaine
For thoracolumbar block	1.25 ml/kg 0.19% bupivacaine

How do you get 0.19% bupivacaine?

Don't give information about things that YOU do without being able to back it up.

1 part normal saline to 3 parts 0.25% bupivacaine.

How long do caudal blocks generally last?

There is a lot of individual variety, if you don't know then guess! Giving information about additives looks like you've thought about how to prolong your block.

They normally last 4–8 hours. They can be extended by using a catheter technique or by using additives. These include:

- Clonidine (1 μg/kg)
- Opioids such as diamorphine at 30 μg/kg
- Preservative free ketamine at 0.5 mg/kg.

Any problems with these additives?

We must ensure that they are preservative free, as preservatives may be neurotoxic. Clonidine and opioids can cause sedation. Opioids may cause respiratory depression and urinary retention. I don't use additives for day-case procedures.

What complications are there?

Give figures if you can.

Severe complications are rare using a single-shot technique.

- Failure
- Urinary retention (4–8%)
- Leg weakness (4–8%)
- Proprioception loss (4–8%)
- Inadvertent intravenous injection (1:10 000)
- Inadvertant intradural injection
- Epidural abscess or haematoma.

4.2.5. Ankle and knee blocks – Matthew P Morgan

This topic would be well suited to the clinical sciences SOE.

What nerves supply the structures below the knee?

The nerve supply to structures below the knee is predominantly derived from the sciatic nerve, although the saphenous nerve supplies a variable portion of the medical calf. The sciatic nerve, derived from L4 to S3, divides approximately 6 cm above the popliteal skin crease into the tibial and common peroneal nerves. The tibial nerve subsequently divides into the medial and lateral plantar nerves beyond the medial malleolus and supplies the plantar surface of the foot. After passing around the neck of the fibula, the common peroneal nerve divides into the deep and superficial peroneal nerves. The superficial peroneal nerve supplies the majority of sensation on the dorsum of the foot, whilst the deep branch supplies a small area of skin webbing between the first and second toes.

Motor innervation of the ankle is derived from the common peroneal nerve, which causes dorsiflexion and eversion, whilst the tibial nerve results in plantar flexion and inversion. Finally, the sural nerve is formed from fibres of both the common peroneal and tibial nerves and supplies sensation of the lateral foot and calf.

What methods of nerve identification can be used in knee and ankle blocks?

Identification of the relevant nerves in an ankle block relies primarily on knowledge of anatomy applied to a landmark technique. Although paraesthesia has been used in the past to suggest correct placement, these blocks are now mostly performed under general anaesthesia. In addition, as few of the ankle nerves have a motor element, the use of a nerve stimulator would not be helpful. Increasingly, the availability of high-quality ultrasound devices can aid identification of these nerves even at the ankle. At the knee, a nerve stimulator can be combined with ultrasound to aid identification, although some anaesthetists will use ultrasound alone.

How do nerve stimulators used for the identification of peripheral nerves differ from those used for assessing neuromuscular blockade and why?

Due to the wide variation of tissue and hence impedance encountered as a nerve is approached by a stimulating needle, devices used for identification of peripheral nerves must be constant current generators. In addition, the delivered output should be clearly indicated on a digital display. The current duration, termed chronaxies, should be shortened to around 100 msec in order to preferentially stimulate A α-motor fibres and not A delta pain fibres. These devices use an insulated needle to maximise and pinpoint delivered current whilst minimising peripheral current loss. Incorrectly attaching the positive electrode to the needle will result in a cone of hyperpolarisation around the nerve and hence reduce effectiveness.

How would you perform a popliteal nerve block and what are the causes of sub-optimal intra-operative analgesia?

There are two main approaches to blocking the nerves of the popliteal fossa, a posterior and a lateral approach. Both approaches target the tibial and common peroneal nerves after they have divided from the sciatic nerve above the popliteal fossa. I am most familiar with the lateral approach and feel that it has advantages over the posterior approach as the patient is able to remain supine during placement. After inducing anaesthesia, checking all relevant equipment and using sterile precautions, I would insert a 5-cm insulated nerve stimulating needle approximately 7 cm above the lateral femoral epicondyle between the groove formed by biceps femoris and vastus lateralis. After contacting the femur, I would redirect the needle posteriorly until a motor response of the ankle is elicited at a current above 0.5 mA. After negative aspiration I would inject 30 ml of 0.5% bupivacaine in 5-ml increments.

Sub-optimal analgesia can result from a poorly working block or a poorly selected block. A nerve block may fail for a number of reasons:

- Local anaesthetic may have been deposited in the wrong location.
- Intravascular injection would result in a poor block.
- The nerve block selected may not cover an adequate area for the surgery. For example, surgery on the medical surface of the foot may additionally require a saphenous nerve block to ensure adequate analgesia.
- Using an above knee tourniquet would require additional analgesia or a more proximal nerve block.

You perform a popliteal block using a nerve stimulator on a patient with long-term diabetes. One week later you are told that she has paraesthesia over the outer aspect of her upper thigh.

What are the potential causes?

The causes of paraesthesia can be divided into those related to anaesthesia, those related to surgery and other causes. Lets start by considering those related to anaesthesia. The popliteal block will often be blamed for such problems, however the pattern of injury makes this very unlikely. The distribution of paraesthesia suggests involvement of the lateral cutaneous nerve of thigh at a point above where the previous block was performed. Damage to the lateral cutaneous nerve of thigh can often be traced to poor intra-operative positioning, especially in people with conditions increasing chances of neuropraxias such as diabetes. Poor positioning results in neuropraxias due to a combination of direct nerve compression, ischaemia and nerve stretching.

Surgical causes would include direct nerve trauma although in this case tourniquet damage would be more likely. Finally, the paraesthesia may be unrelated to recent events and represent a mononeuropathy from diabetes alone.

What are the advantages of a peripheral nerve block over those placed more centrally?

There are advantages to the technique itself and advantages to the patient. In general, the more peripheral a nerve is blocked the more superficial it can be found and therefore landmarks become simpler. Additionally, superficial nerves are often more amenable to ultrasound imaging and possibly easier to identify with a nerve stimulator.

Turning to advantages for the patient, central nerve blocks tend to be placed closer to vascular and neurological structures, and thus they carry greater risks. In addition, blocking nerves more peripherally will enable one to avoid some of the central effects of nerve blockade including urinary retention and dense whole limb weakness.

Should a popliteal nerve block be performed in a patient with a distal tibia fracture?

There are advantages and disadvantages to using peripheral nerve blocks. A traumatic tibial fracture is known to carry a risk of compartment syndrome, which persists even after surgical fixation. Some may argue that performing a long-lasting peripheral nerve block would make identifying a compartment syndrome difficult. However, even when a nerve block has been successful, the use of a tourniquet will often induce intra-operative physiological changes consistent with pain. There have been studies showing that this ischaemia type pain, common in compartment syndrome, will break through even a perfectly working peripheral nerve block. It has also been shown that good post-operative analgesia and hence early mobilisation can reduce the incidence of compartment syndrome. It could be argued that if surgeons are sufficiently concerned about the risks of compartment syndrome to advise avoiding a peripheral nerve block, then a different surgical technique or post-operative compartment pressure monitoring should be used. Overall, the decision to use a peripheral nerve block in these circumstances should be made jointly between the surgeon and the anaesthetist, and would be influenced by the safety of administering systemic analgesia to the patient in question.

When would you consider performing an ankle block?

I would consider an ankle block to provide surgical anaesthesia and post-operative pain relief for forefoot and digit surgery.

Which nerves are blocked in an ankle block?

There are five nerves that are blocked when performing an ankle block. Four of these nerves are terminal branches of the sciatic nerve:

- Tibial nerve
- Superficial peroneal nerve
- Deep peroneal nerve
- Sural nerve.

The remaining nerve, the saphenous nerve, is a branch of the femoral nerve.

Please tell me how you would block the superficial and deep peroneal nerves

I would position the foot so that it was at right angles with the tibia. I would then identify the tendon of the extensor hallucis longus by moving the big toe. The dorsalis pedis pulse is found lateral to the tendon. I would insert a 23- to 25-gauge needle 2–3 cm from the inter-malleolar line first medial and then lateral to the artery. I would advance the needle until contact is made with bone, I would then withdraw slightly and inject 2 ml on either side of the artery.

To perform a superficial peroneal nerve block I would withdraw the needle from the position it was in to perform a deep peroneal nerve block into the subcutaneous tissue. I would then infiltrate up to 10 ml of local anaesthetic laterally and medially across the dorsum of the foot to produce a weal of local anaesthetic to block the medial and lateral divisions of the superficial peroneal nerve.

How would you block the tibial nerve?

I would start by drawing a line between the medial malleolus and the posterior inferior border of the calcaneum. I would then palpate the posterior tibial pulse and mark a point on the line just posterior to the pulse. I would insert a 23-gauge, 50-mm needle at 90 degrees to the skin until either plantar-flexion of the toes is elicited by a nerve stimulator, or paraesthesia of the sole of the foot felt. A range of 6–10 ml of local anaesthesia is then injected.

How would you block the sural nerve?

The sural nerve is blocked by infiltrating 5 ml of local anaesthetic subcutaneously from the lateral malleolus to the lateral border of the Achilles tendon. A 23-gauge, 50mm needle should be used.

Finally, how would you block the saphenous nerve?

I would identify the saphenous vein anterior and proximal to the medial malleolus at the ankle. Using a 23-gauge needle, I would infiltrate 2 ml of local anaesthetic on either side of the saphenous vein. The total volume of local anaesthetic used should not exceed 4 ml and caution should be taken to avoid intravascular injection or trauma to the vein.

Further Reading

Grant CRK. Lower limb nerve blocks. *Anaesthesia & Intensive Care Medicine.* 2010; 11(3): 105–108.

Nicholls B. Lower limb nerve blocks. *Anaesthesia & Intensive Care Medicine.* 2007; 8(5): 132–136.

Nicholls B, Conn D, Roberts A. The Abbott pocket guide to practical peripheral nerve blockade. Abbott Laboratories, 2003.

The New York School of Regional Anesthesia. www.nysora.com.

4.2.6. Lumbar plexus, femoral and sciatic blocks – Jonathan J Gatward

Could you describe the anatomy of the lumbar plexus?

The easiest way to answer anatomy questions like this is to be able to draw a diagram. A simple line drawing of the lumbar plexus can be easily learnt and reproduced (see Figure 4.2.6a). A picture paints a thousand words!

The lumbar plexus arises from the anterior primary rami of L1 to 4. There is sometimes a contribution from T12.

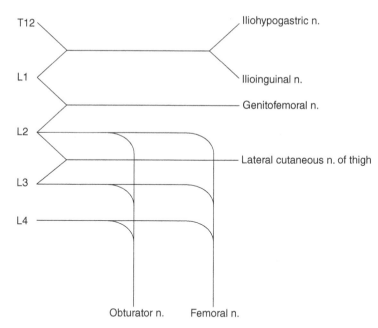

Figure 4.2.6a. The lumbar plexus.

L1 divides into the iliohypogastric and ilioinguinal nerves, and gives a contribution to the genitofemoral nerve.

L2 contributes the remainder of the genitofemoral nerve, and forms the lateral cutaneous nerve of the thigh with L3.

The obturator and femoral nerves are both formed from branches from L2 to 4.

When might we want to perform a lumbar plexus block?

We can use the lumbar plexus block for anaesthesia and post-op analgesia for surgery involving the hip, thigh, or upper leg, or after traumatic injury. We can use it in conjunction with a sciatic nerve or sacral plexus block for anaesthesia and analgesia of the leg. In a chronic pain setting, it can be used to treat cancer pain from the hip or upper femur. The sympathetic block achieved can also be useful in the treatment of ischaemic pain and complex regional pain syndrome.

How can the lumbar plexus be blocked? Do you know of any approaches?

The lumbar plexus can be blocked with a posterior approach (the "psoas compartment block"), and two inferior approaches; the "3 in 1" block and the "fascia iliacus" block.

Can you describe one of these approaches?

You are unlikely to be asked to describe all three, so just learn the one that you are most familiar with, and, ideally that you have actually performed. They are all included for the sake of completeness.

For the **psoas compartment block**, the patient is in the lateral position, with the side to be blocked uppermost. The insertion point is the intersection of two perpendicular lines, one running parallel to the spinous processes at the level of the posterior superior iliac spine and one joining the iliac crests. I use a nerve stimulator and a 100-mm insulated needle inserted at 90 degrees to the skin, aiming slightly caudally. The endpoint is quadriceps contraction, which should occur at a depth of about 8 to 10 cm. An alternative is the loss of resistance technique using a long Touhy needle. You can walk the needle off the inferior surface of the L4 transverse process, and then you get loss of resistance after a further 0.5 to 1 cm.

The **"3 in 1" block** aims to block the *femoral nerve*, the *obturator nerve* and the *lateral cutaneous nerve of the thigh* using a low anterior approach. The patient is in the supine position. The insertion point is 1 cm lateral to the femoral pulse and 2 cm below the inguinal ligament. I use a nerve stimulator and a 50-mm insulated needle, inserted at 45 degrees to the skin aiming proximally and parallel to the femoral artery. The endpoint is quadriceps contraction, which should occur at a depth of 30 to 50 mm. When the local anaesthetic is injected, you can apply distal pressure to help encourage cephalad spread. I usually block the lateral cutaneous nerve of the thigh separately by injecting 10 ml of local anaesthetic beneath the fascia lata at a point 2 cm medial and 2 cm inferior to the anterior superior iliac spine.

The **fascia iliacus block** is convenient because it does not require a nerve stimulator and can be done in the paralysed, anaesthetised patient. It may also be more effective at covering the lateral cutaneous nerve of the thigh than the "3 in 1" block. The patient is in the supine position. The insertion point is 1 cm inferior to the junction of the lateral and middle thirds of a line joining the pubic tubercle and the anterior superior iliac spine. I use either a 16-gauge or 18-gauge Tuohy needle or a blunt nerve stimulator needle. I insert the needle perpendicular to the skin and after penetrating the skin, advance until I feel two more "pops" as I puncture fascia lata and fascia iliaca. I then inject 30 to 40 ml of local anaesthetic. If using an epidural set, a catheter can be passed, leaving about 3–5 cm in the fascial compartment for continuous infusion of local anaesthetic.

How does the lumbar sympathetic block differ from the lumbar plexus block?

You've probably never performed a lumbar sympathetic block before. Just be familiar with a method, its complications and the safety measures that are employed when performing the block.

The lumbar sympathetic chains lie on the anterolateral aspect of the lumbar vertebrae, whereas the somatic nerves lie posterior and lateral to the psoas muscle and fascia. The anterior relations of the sympathetic chains are the aorta on the left and the inferior vena cava on the right. The aim is to place local anaesthetic solution around the lumbar sympathetic chain from the second to fourth lumbar vertebrae. This can either be achieved by a single injection at L3, or three separate injections at L2, L3 and L4. This block is used in the treatment of a variety of conditions, including lower limb ischaemia, complex regional pain syndrome of the lower limb, phantom limb pain and renal or urogenital pain.

How is the block performed?

The patient is positioned laterally with the side to be blocked uppermost. A point is marked 8 cm lateral to the midpoint of the spinous process of the desired lumbar vertebra. The block is done under image intensifier guidance. After local infiltration, a 12-cm, 22-gauge needle is inserted at 45 degrees to the skin, aiming medially towards the body of the vertebra.

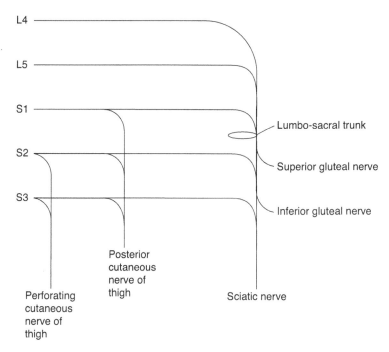

Figure 4.2.6b. The sacral plexus.

The body lies at a depth of about 8 cm. If bone is encountered at 4–5 cm, it is likely to be a transverse process, in which case the needle is redirected cranially or caudally to get past it. When the needle has come into contact with the body of the vertebra, it is redirected to pass just anterolaterally. You might feel a loss of resistance as the psoas fascia is penetrated. It is really important to aspirate for blood or cerebrospinal fluid, then a test dose of local anaesthetic mixed with radiographic contrast is injected. This should show a band of contrast along the vertebral column, covering the relevant lumbar vertebral levels. If contrast dissipates quickly, the needle may be in a vessel. Otherwise you may see contrast spreading into the retroperitoneal compartment or into the psoas muscle. Lateral and anteroposterior images should be obtained to make sure the needle is in the right place.

What specific complications of this block do you know?

Local anaesthetic toxicity can be caused by inadvertent intra-vascular injection into the aorta or inferior vena cava. Intra-thecal injection can occur, which would cause a profound motor block or permanent paralysis if neurolytic agents were used. The block can also cause profound hypotension, so intra-venous access, full monitoring and access to resuscitation equipment is mandatory. Other complications are ureteric damage and ejaculatory failure. Also, post-sympathectomy neuropathic pain can occur with neurolytic techniques.

Can you describe the anatomical course of the sciatic nerve?

While revising, practise drawing simple line diagrams of the sacral plexus, the sciatic nerve and its divisions, adding in some of its relations and landmarks to help you remember its course (see Figures 4.2.6b, c).

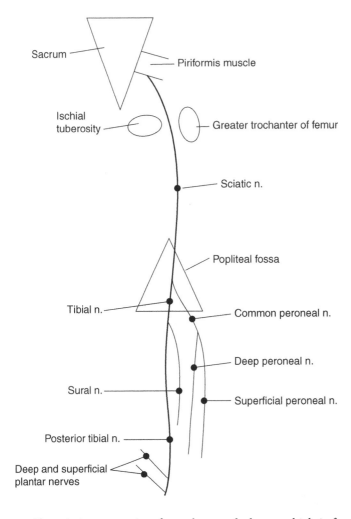

Figure 4.2.6c. The sciatic nerve.

The sciatic nerve arises from the sacral plexus, which is formed by the nerve roots of L4, L5 and S1–3. It passes anterior to the piriformis muscle and exits the pelvis through the greater sciatic notch. It passes into the posterior thigh between the ischial tuberosity and the greater trochanter of the femur. It then passes posterior to the femur, before dividing into the tibial and common peroneal nerves in the popliteal fossa. The tibial nerve passes medially and divides into the sural and posterior tibial nerves. The common peroneal nerve passes laterally and divides into the deep and superficial plantar nerves.

Can you describe the motor and sensory functions of the sciatic nerve?

The sciatic nerve is motor to:

- Hamstrings
- Soleus
- Gastrocnemius
- Peroneal muscles

- Tibialis anterior
- Muscles of the foot.

It is sensory to:

- Hip and knee joints
- Most of the leg except the medial side of the knee and calf, which are supplied by the saphenous nerve which is a branch of the femoral nerve.

When might we want to perform a sciatic nerve block?

The sciatic nerve block can be used alone to provide post-operative analgesia for ankle and foot surgery, or analgesia for fractures of the lower leg. In combination with a femoral nerve block, it can be used for analgesia for knee and lower leg surgery and amputations. In the chronic pain setting, it can be used for ischaemic pain and in CRPS.

What are the different approaches to the sciatic nerve block?

You are unlikely to be asked to describe more than one or two approaches. Again, they are all given for the sake of completeness. Draw a diagram if it helps you remember the anatomy!

There are three posterior, one anterior and one lateral approach to the sciatic nerve.

Labat's posterior approach is performed with the patient in the lateral position with the upper leg flexed at 90 degrees at the hip and knee. I draw two lines; one from the posterior superior iliac spine to the greater trochanter and the other from the greater trochanter to the sacral hiatus. I then drop a third line at 90 degrees from the upper line. The insertion point is where this perpendicular line hits my lower line. I use a 100-mm needle, inserted at 90 degrees. The endpoint I am looking for is plantar flexion, which I would expect at about 6 cm.

Another **posterior approach** occurs with the patient in the supine position, with the leg flexed at 90 degrees at the hip and knee. I draw a line from the greater trochanter to the ischial tuberosity. The midpoint of this line is the insertion point. I use a 100-mm needle, inserted at 90 degrees. The endpoint I am looking for is plantar flexion, which I would expect at about 6 cm.

The third posterior approach is the **popliteal fossa block**. This can be performed with the patient either prone with the leg straight, or supine with the hip and knee flexed at 90 degrees. The insertion point is 7 to 8 cm proximal, and 1 cm lateral to the midpoint of the skin crease of the knee. I use a 50-mm needle, inserted at 45 degrees proximally. The endpoint I am looking for is plantar flexion. However, the nerve may have already divided at this point, so I may get dorsiflexion caused by stimulation of the common peroneal nerve. If this occurs, I deposit half the local at this point and then redirect medially to locate the tibial nerve, looking for plantar flexion. I would deposit the rest of the local there.

The **anterior approach** to the sciatic nerve is performed with the patient in the supine position. I draw a line connecting the anterior superior iliac spine and the pubic tubercle. I then divide this into thirds, and drop a perpendicular from the junction of the middle and medial thirds of this line. The insertion point is where this line meets a parallel line at the level of the greater trochanter. I use a 100-mm needle, inserted at 90 degrees. The endpoint I am looking for is plantar flexion, which I would expect at about 8 to 10 cm. If I hit bone, I redirect medially.

The **lateral approach** is performed with the patient in the supine position. A line is drawn down the thigh from the posterior border of the greater trochanter. The insertion point is halfway between the knee and the greater trochanter. I use a 100-mm needle, inserted at 90 degrees. The endpoint I am looking for is plantar flexion, which I would expect at about 8 to 10 cm. If I hit bone, I redirect posteriorly.

What general safety measures do you employ when performing a regional block?

I take a full medical and anaesthetic history and ask about drug allergies. I secure intravenous access, and ensure that full airway and cardiovascular resuscitation equipment is immediately available. Patients should be fully monitored. I use a strict aseptic technique, with anti-septic solution, sterile gloves and sterile, disposable needles.

In general, what methods are available to identify nerves when performing blocks?
You can identify nerves in several ways:

- The most basic way is to use anatomical landmarks to find the insertion point. You can then insert the needle to a given depth, such as in the paravertebral block, or there may be an endpoint, such as a "pop" through fascia.
- Some anaesthetists elicit paraesthesiae in the distribution of the nerve concerned, though there is a risk of nerve damage.
- Loss of resistance techniques can be used, for example in epidural insertion, psoas compartment and paravertebral blocks. This can be the loss of resistance to the injection of air or saline.
- Another method is to transfix an artery lying within a nerve sheath such as the axillary artery, in axillary nerve blockade.
- Most anaesthetists now use nerve stimulation techniques, either with a non-invasive probe to help identify nerves, or with special insulated needles.
- Ultrasound-guided techniques are gaining popularity and may be combined with other techniques to try to improve accuracy. This allows visualisation of the nerve, surrounding structures and the block needle in real time. The spread of local anaesthetic around the nerve can also be seen and predicts a successful block.

What are the basic principles behind nerve stimulators? How do they work?

Electrical impulses are delivered via a needle to elicit either paraesthesiae or the muscle movement associated with the nerve concerned. They can help to reduce the incidence of nerve damage because the aim of the technique is to get the tip of the needle very close to the nerve without touching it. They still require a thorough knowledge of the relevant anatomy.

Talk us through how you would use a peripheral nerve stimulator

We'll assume you have IV access, monitoring, skilled assistance, and there are no contraindications.

I would connect the positive lead to an ECG electrode at least 20 cm from the needle insertion site and the negative lead to an insulated nerve stimulator needle of the required length. I remember which lead is which as I can remember that the patient is positive and the needle is negative. I set the duration of impulse at 100 msec or less and the frequency of impulse at 1–2 Hz. To start with, I set the delivered current at 1–2 mA.

I then prepare the area, inject some local anaesthetic into the skin with an orange needle, wait for it to work and then insert the stimulator needle. I look for synchronous muscle movement in the desired distribution and when I get it, I reduce the current. Movement should still be present at 0.5 mA, but should disappear at 0.2 mA, or the needle might be within the nerve. It is really important to aspirate at this point to check for intravascular placement. I then inject 1 ml of local anaesthetic, at which point the motor response should disappear as the nerve is displaced away from the needle tip.

Injection should be painless and without resistance. If not, I would consider re-positioning. I usually get an assistant to inject the local and get them to aspirate after each 5-ml increment. This is to check that the needle tip has not migrated into a blood vessel.

Could you compare and contrast lidocaine and bupivacaine when used for nerve blockade?

Both are amide local anaesthetic solutions commonly used in nerve blocks.

Lidocaine has a rapid onset and short duration of action. It causes vasodilatation at the site of injection, and so the addition of adrenaline 1:200 000 slows its systemic absorption and prolongs the duration of block. The maximum dose is 3 mg·kg^{-1} or 7 mg·kg^{-1} if adrenaline is added.

Bupivacaine has a slower onset of action and longer duration of action. It lasts two to three times longer than lidocaine. It does not cause vasodilatation, so the addition of adrenaline has no effect on its systemic absorption or its duration of action. The maximum dose is 2 mg·kg^{-1}. Levobupivacaine, the S-enantiomer of bupivacaine, is less cardiotoxic. Its maximum dose is also 2 mg·kg^{-1}.

What do you know about ropivacaine?

It has an onset of action similar to bupivacaine, but causes some vasoconstriction that may prolong its duration of action. Like bupivacaine, its maximum dose is 2 mg·kg^{-1}. It is marketed as causing less motor block and cardiotoxicity than bupivacaine, but this may just be due to lower potency.

4.2.7. Local anaesthetic toxicity – Andrew P Georgiou

What is a local anaesthetic agent?

You need to know an off-pat definition here in order to get the examiner on you side from the start.

A local anaesthetic agent is one that reversibly blocks neural transmission beyond its point of application, when applied locally.

All local anaesthetic agents are weak bases and can be subdivided into esters and amides, according to the chemical linkage between the hydrophobic aromatic ring structure and the hydrophilic chain.

Can you give me some examples of esters and amides?

Examples of amides include:

- Lidocaine
- Bupivacaine
- Prilocaine.

Examples of esters include:

- Cocaine
- Tetracaine
- Amethocaine.

Amides are more commonly used in clinical practice due to their increased stability, ease of heat sterilisation and longer shelf life.

How do local anaesthetic agents work?

Local anaesthetic agents work by blocking the voltage gated sodium channel from the cytosolic aspect of the receptor, that is from the inside of the cell. Inactivation of the sodium channel prevents the upstroke of the action potential and so inhibits depolarisation and therefore transmission of nerve impulses.

The drug accesses the receptor by crossing the neural membrane in its unionised form. It then becomes ionised in the relative acidic environment of the cytoplasm and it is the ionised form that is responsible for receptor blockade.

A secondary mechanism of action relies on disruption of impulse transduction due to the presence of unionised agent in the nerve cell membrane.

What factors determine the potency, the speed of onset and the duration of action of a local anaesthetic?

Potency is dependent on how **lipid soluble** the drug is, the more lipid soluble it is, the more potent it becomes.

The **onset of action** is related to the drug's **pKa**. A drug with a lower pKa will have a greater percentage present in the unionised form, which allows more rapid passage through the nerve cell membrane and a faster onset of action. So for example, lidocaine has a pKa of 7.9 and has a more rapid onset of action than bupivacaine which has a pKa of 8.1.

The **duration of action** is dependent on how **protein bound** the drug is. If a drug is highly protein bound, like bupivacaine, it will have a long duration of action.

What factors place a patient at risk of local anaesthetic toxicity?

Local anaesthetic toxicity results from the acquisition of a high or rapidly rising plasma local anaesthetic concentration. The factors which place a patient at risk of this situation developing are:

Firstly, the dose administered and the speed of injection, as large, rapidly administered doses raise the risk of high plasma concentrations developing.

Secondly, inadvertent vascular injection, for example through an epidural catheter, inadvertently placed into a vein in Batson's plexus, resulting in direct administration of local anaesthetic into the circulation.

Similarly inadvertent intrathecal injection will also produce toxic effects as an inappropriate intrathecal dose is likely to be administered.

Thirdly, the site of administration, as this affects the rate of absorption of local anaesthetic into the bloodstream. So for example, local anaesthetic is more readily absorbed into the bloodstream when it is administered via the intercostal or caudal site, compared to the subcutaneous or brachial plexus site. The performance of a pudendal nerve block (in obstetrics) is also highly likely to cause systemic toxicity due to the adjacent rich blood supply.

Related to this is the presence of vasoconstrictor in the injected solution. For example adrenaline may be co-administered with local anaesthetic agents producing localised vasoconstriction and limiting the absorption of local anaesthetic agent into the bloodstream. Adrenaline added to lidocaine increases the safe dose which may be given from 3 mg/kg to 6 mg/kg for this reason.

Fourthly, the type of local anaesthetic used as some types of local anaesthetic are inherently more toxic than others. For example, racemic bupivacaine is inherently more toxic than its pure S-enantiomer levobupivacaine. This is due to a reduction in the avidity of binding of the S-enantiomer to the sodium channels of the myocardium, and therefore less risk of the myocardial depressant effects of a toxic dose.

Fifthly patient heterogeneity and co-morbidity has an important bearing on the risks of toxicity. Patients with cardiac or hepatic disease and those who are critically unwell or pregnant as well as neonates and young infants are particularly at risk due to alterations in absorption, distribution, metabolism and excretion. These patients also have changes in their protein binding capacity, particularly to α-1 acid glycoprotein (where the levels are reduced), and therefore may well have increased free drug concentration, raising the risk of toxicity. In these situations the dose administered should be reduced.

Finally the acid–base status of the patient has a bearing on their risk of toxicity. Avoiding acidosis (so for example, ensuring patients are adequately ventilated) will reduce the risk of toxicity occurring.

Some patients are particularly at risk of a specific form of toxicity related to one of the amide local anaesthetic agents. Can you think of what that may be?

Prilocaine is metabolised to O-toluidine. Infants and those with methaemoglobin-aemia reductase deficiency are poorly able to metabolise O-toluidine and may develop methaemoglobinaemia, which results from the oxidation of the iron atom in haem from its ferrous to its ferric state. This produces a blue discolouration of the skin, which can produce errors in pulse oximeter analysis. Pulse oximeters may falsely read 85% leading the anaesthetist to believe the patient is hypoxic, where this may not be the case.

The oxygen carrying capacity of haemoglobin is reduced by the transformation in haem and in extreme cases this may result in tissue hypoxia.

How is this condition treated?

It can be treated with methylene blue at a dose of 1 mg/kg over 5 minutes.

It is important to remember however that prilocaine is relatively less toxic compared with bupivacaine, especially on the heart. This is why it is used for intra-venous regional anaesthesia.

Lets get back now to local anaesthetic toxicity in general. What are the symptoms and signs of local anaesthetic toxicity?

Most people can rattle off a list in answer to this question, but if you can bring in some basic science to your answer it looks like you really understand the concepts, making you a stronger candidate.

Local anaesthetic toxicity presents initially with central nervous system disturbance followed by cardiovascular system disturbance.

Toxic levels of local anaesthetic initially depress the depressant effects of the central nervous system, such that excitatory effects are initially seen.

These include headache, peri-oral paraesthesiae, tinnitus, vertigo, disorientation, visual and auditory disturbances, and a sense of impending doom. Shivering and tremors may be seen.

As the toxic effect progresses, both the depressant and the excitatory effects of the central nervous system are depressed. This may then lead to slurred speech, loss of consciousness and seizure activity, often manifesting as a grand mal type fit.

Escalating toxicity then results in respiratory depression and arrest and cardiovascular disturbances. This is initially hypotension from direct cardiac depression and vasodilation, followed by cardiac arrest with any number of dysrhythmias intervening. Sinus bradycardia, sinus arrest and resistant VF would be common examples.

What do you understand by the term "toxicity ratio"?

The toxicity ratio is the ratio between the plasma level of local anaesthetic required to produce cardiovascular symptoms to that required to produce central nervous system symptoms. It is expressed as a ratio for each local anaesthetic agent and gives an idea of the window between the onset of central nervous system symptoms and the onset of cardiovascular symptoms.

For example the toxicity ratio for lidocaine is 7 and for bupivacaine is 3, but for levobupivacaine is 5. This means that after CNS symptoms occur you need 7 times that plasma level of local anaesthetic to get cardiovascular symptoms with lidocaine, but only 3 times that plasma level to get cardiovascular symptoms with bupivacaine. In practical terms this means that the onset of central nervous system symptoms in bupivacaine toxicity means that cardiovascular symptoms are soon to follow.

So why is bupivacaine more toxic than lidocaine?

Bupivacaine is 4–16 times more cardiotoxic than lidocaine due to its increased protein binding and the avidity with which it binds myocardial tissue. It dissociates from myocardial sodium channels 10 times less readily then lidocaine producing a prolonged, refractory blockade. Reversal of this binding can be particularly difficult, especially in the face of cardiopulmonary arrest when hypoxia and acidosis may complicate the picture.

How would you manage a 28-year-old primigravida who has collapsed after complaining of tinnitus and vertigo following an epidural top up of 20 ml of 0.5% levobupivacaine? She is scheduled for a category 2 caesarean section

This is an emergency; the factors which pose the greatest threat to the mother's life should be managed first and without delay.

I would call for help immediately whilst placing the woman in a left lateral tilt of at least 15 degrees.

I would start by ensuring a patent airway and administer high flow oxygen via reservoir mask. Should the airway be compromised I would secure it with a cuffed endotracheal tube.

Whilst assessing the airway I would palpate a central pulse to exclude cardiac arrest, before going on to assess the breathing.

There is no palpable pulse, how would you proceed?

I would dedicate a member of staff to put out a cardiac arrest call and ask them on their return to bring the resuscitation trolley and more members of staff to assist. I would then allocate another member of staff to bring the 20% intra-lipid.

In the mean-time I would start advanced life support according to the Advanced Life Support guidelines. This involves cardiopulmonary resuscitation in the ratio of 30 compressions to 2 ventilations, or asynchronous compressions once the trachea is intubated. I would assume the role of cardiac arrest team leader and delegate team members to appropriate roles.

Discovery of the underlying rhythm is then essential to allow stratification to the VF/pulseless VT algorithm or to the asystole/PEA algorithm.

You mentioned intra-lipid. How is this administered in this setting?

On arrival of the 20% intra-lipid, I would immediately deliver a 1.5 mg/kg bolus IV and start an infusion of 0.25 mg/kg/min. The bolus injection may be repeated twice at 5-minute intervals. At 5 minutes after the third bolus of intra-lipid the infusion rate should be increased to 0.5 mg/kg/min.

It is worth bearing in mind that cardiac arrest due to local anaesthetic toxicity may be prolonged and refractory to treatment so I would persist with the resuscitation for over an hour if needed.

Although standard ALS protocols should be followed throughout, consideration should be given to the use of cardiopulmonary bypass where available, as the situation is potentially salvageable with prolonged life support.

Is there anything else that you may consider in this situation?

If after 5 minutes of CPR there has been no return of spontaneous circulation then a peri-mortem caesarean section should be undertaken, in order to optimise the efficacy of CPR and the chance of maternal survival.

Ventricular fibrillation should be treated according to standard ALS protocols. Magnesium should be considered at an early stage. Should the VF prove refractory to standard treatment and intra-lipid, then bretylium may be considered. It is not part of the standard resuscitation guidelines but in this situation there is a small chance it may be of benefit.

You mentioned bretylium. How does this drug work and what dose would you use?

Bretylium acts by inhibiting release of noradrenaline at the sympathetic nervous system and is administered by rapid IV injection at a dose of 5 mg/kg. If VF persists the dose may be increased to 10 mg/kg and given at 1- to 2-hour intervals. Bretylium is not commonly used and so its acquisition is unlikely to be rapid, hence the importance of all other aspects of resuscitation in this case.

Where is intra-lipid kept in your hospital?

You should know the answer to this, and if you don't, make it look like you do!

Intra-lipid is kept in areas where potentially toxic doses of local anaesthetic are administered. It is kept on the resuscitation trolley in theatre, on the resuscitation trolley on delivery suite, in the bag that the ICU registrar brings to arrest calls and it is available in the pharmacy store cupboard in theatres and from pharmacy.

What is the actual mechanism of local anaesthetic toxicity?

Local anaesthetic toxicity results from several processes, most commonly binding of the anaesthetic agent to the cytosolic aspect of the voltage gated sodium channel resulting in sodium channel blockade. Bupivacaine, one of the most toxic local anaesthetic agents, also interferes with almost all of the metabotropic and ionotropic cell transduction mechanisms studied. It also interferes with oxidative phosphorylation, perhaps most importantly the metabolism of carnitine, which is thought to be essential for the transport of fatty acids into the mitochondria. The transport of fatty acids into mitochondria is essential for the generation of ATP and so bupivacaine, in disrupting this process, limits the ability of cells to produce the energy they need to function normally. This disruption in ATP generation is particularly apparent in energy demanding cells, such as cardiac myocytes.

How does intra-lipid alter this process?

If you get a question like this, don't panic, it means you are doing well!

Twenty per cent intra-lipid has an avidity for local anaesthetic agents which may prevent the agent reaching the cell if administered reasonably soon after the toxic dose. It may have a potential role in drawing the agent out of the cell and removing it from its inhibitory action on metabotropic and ionotropic signalling, and restoring the action of carnitine on fatty acid transport in mitochondria.

This effect results in an apparent shift in the dose–response curve resulting in a higher plasma concentration of local anaesthetic agent required to induce asystole. Weinberg and colleagues, amongst others, have explored this in the experimental setting of rats and dogs and users of intra-lipid are encouraged to report cases to intra-lipid.org where case series are being compiled.

Further Reading

The Association of Anaesthetists of Great Britain & Ireland. Guidelines for the Management of Severe Local Anaesthetic Toxicity. http://www.aagbi.org/publications/guidelines/docs/latoxicity07.pdf.

Weinberg G. LipidRescue: resuscitation for cardiac toxicity. http://lipidrescue.squarespace.com/.

Chapter

4.3

Pain

4.3.1. Pain pathways – Michael B Clarke

Can you define pain?

There is a standard definition in answer to this question that is worth knowing.

Pain is an unpleasant sensory and emotional experience associated with actual or potential tissue damage, or described in terms of such damage.

Can you describe the different types of pain receptor?

Nociceptors are the sensory receptor for pain and are widespread. They are responsive to different types of stimuli; mechanical, thermal or chemical. Stimulation of these nociceptors results in propagation of an impulse to the spinal cord.

The primary afferent fibres involved in this impulse propagation can be divided into two classes:

1. Aδ fibres

    · Myelinated
    · 2 to 5 μm in diameter
    · Conduct rapidly (6 to 30 m/sec)
    · Responsible for localised, sharp pain sensations
    · Provoke the withdrawal reflex

2. C-fibres:

    · Unmyelinated
    · Smaller diameter (<1.5 μm)
    · Conduct less rapidly (0.5 to 2 m/sec)
    · Responsible for poorly localised, dull, burning-type pain.

How does stimulation of these nociceptors cause us to sense pain?

This question is dealing with the route the pain impulse takes to the somatosensory cortex. The answer is complex but detailed knowledge will not be expected. Just give a simple answer including the basic points and the examiner should be satisfied.

Dr. Podcast Scripts for the Final FRCA, ed. Rebecca A. Leslie, Emily K. Johnson,
Gary Thomas and Alexander P. L. Goodwin.   Published by Cambridge University Press.
© R. A. Leslie, E. K. Johnson, G. Thomas and A. P. L. Goodwin 2011.

Primary afferents have their cell bodies located in the dorsal root ganglia and synapse with secondary afferents in the dorsal horn. C-fibres tend to enter the dorsal horn laterally, whilst Aδ fibres tend to enter the dorsal horn more medially.

The grey matter of the dorsal horn is divided into laminae that run the length of the spinal cord. Aδ fibres synapse with cells principally in laminae I and V. C-fibres synapse with cells in laminae II and III, the substantia gelatinosa (Figure 4.3.1a).

There are two main classes of secondary afferents within the dorsal horn associated with further processing of the noxious stimulus. The first class is "nociceptive specific" or "high threshold". These are located within the superficial laminae and respond to noxious stimuli only. The second class is termed "wide dynamic range" or "convergent". These are located in the deeper laminae and respond to both noxious and non-noxious stimuli. Wide dynamic range neurones will fire in proportion to the intensity of the stimulus. Normally they do not signal pain, however, if they become sensitised and their activity exceeds a certain threshold, a normally non-noxious stimulus will be perceived as being painful, this is called allodynia.

From the dorsal horn, the main nociceptive pathway is the spinothalamic tract. Secondary afferents cross the cord and then ascend as the lateral spinothalamic tract. Afferents from here will terminate in various structures throughout the brainstem and thalamus, and then on to the somatosensory cortex. Areas of the cortex involved in pain processing include the post-central gyrus, the Sylvian fissure and the cingulate gyrus.

How is it possible then that we can receive a tissue injury and yet not experience pain, for example soldiers in battle who are unaware they have been injured?

This question concerns the modulation of pain signals and the perception of pain. A simple example of this is gate control in the dorsal horn and a diagram showing primary and secondary afferents with inhibitory interneurones and descending projections acting on interneuones will help you quickly answer this (Figure 4.3.1b).

The modulation of the nociceptive signal can occur at all levels of the pain pathway. The output from the dorsal horn of the spinal cord depends on the input from the periphery, regulation by interneurones and descending projections from the brain.

Descending projections from the periaqueductal grey matter and the locus ceruleus of the mid-brain play an important role. The periaqueductal grey matter receives input from the frontal cortex, the limbic system, the thalamus and the hypothalamus. It is involved in the production of endogenous opioids and its projections stimulate inhibitory interneurones in the dorsal horn.

Aβ afferents carry touch sensation from the periphery and can also stimulate inhibitory interneurones within the dorsal horn. The presence of interneurones means that the nociceptive signal can be "gated" and the relative activity of the Aβ-fibres and the Aδ- and C-fibres, plus the contribution of descending projections from the brain will either open or close the gate. If nociceptive input is greater than Aβ input, the gate will open and the nociceptive impulse will continue; if the Aβ input exceeds the nociceptive input, the gate is closed and the nociceptive signal is stopped (Figure 4.3.1b). This is why rubbing the skin can make a painful area "feel better".

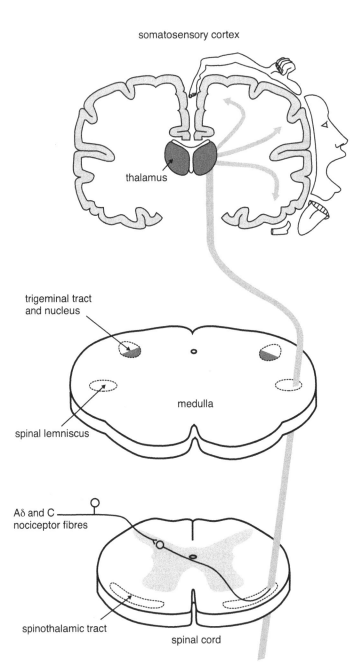

Figure 4.3.1a. Somatosensory pain pathway. Reproduced with permission from Smith, T., Pinnock, C. and Lin, T. 2009. *Fundamentals of Anaesthesia.* Cambridge: Cambridge University Press. © Cambridge University Press 2009.

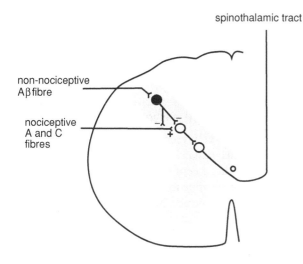

spinothalamic tract

non-nociceptive
Aβ fibre

nociceptive
A and C
fibres

Figure 4.3.1b. Gate mechanism. Reproduced with permission from Smith, T., Pinnock, C. and Lin, T. 2009. *Fundamentals of Anaesthesia.* Cambridge: Cambridge University Press. © Cambridge University Press 2009.

What is visceral pain and how does it differ from peripheral pain?

Visceral pain describes pain originating from the internal organs. It is poorly localised and associated with nausea and autonomic disturbance. It occurs with distension and ischaemia rather than thermal or mechanical trauma.

Nociceptors are present in the viscera but are less dense than in somatic structures, hence the poor localisation of pain. The cell bodies are located in the dorsal root ganglia and the afferent fibres reach the spinal cord via sympathetic and parasympathetic pathways. Secondary afferents travel in the spinothalamic tracts and project to the same areas of the somatosensory cortex as peripheral secondary afferents.

What is referred pain?

This is where pain originating from a viscus is felt in a somatic structure at a distance from the viscus, for example, diaphragmatic irritation causing shoulder-tip pain. It occurs because visceral and peripheral primary afferents converge upon the same secondary afferents and the brain cannot discern whether the pain is coming from the organ or the periphery.

If I cut my hand, why does the area around the injury also become red and painful?

A cut to the skin will not only activate nociceptors but will also release a number of inflammatory peptides, these include substance P and neurokinin A. Release of these chemicals causes local vasodilatation giving rise to the area of redness. They also stimulate the release of further inflammatory mediators from mast cells and platelets. These substances include histamine and serotonin. These then act to sensitise surrounding nociceptors, a process known as peripheral sensitisation. Now, pressure on the area immediately around the cut that would normally cause only slight pain or no pain at all will produce an exaggerated response and pain will be experienced. This is known as primary hyperalgesia.

Can sensitisation occur centrally?

Yes it can. Hyperalgesia in the uninjured skin further removed from the site of injury is called secondary hyperalgesia. Nociceptors in this area are not sensitised and so the mechanism for this is believed to be due to changes in the dorsal horn of the spinal cord, this is called central sensitisation.

What does this tell us about pain and the central nervous system?

The important point that this highlights is that in the presence of pain "plasticity" exists within the central nervous system. In other words, sustained nociceptive inputs have the ability to alter the functional properties of dorsal horn neurones. It has been shown that a painful stimulus will not only cause a dorsal horn neurone to fire but that the rate of firing will increase with the duration of the stimulus. This is termed "wind up" and it is an important part of central sensitisation.

There are other important features of central sensitisation. There is an expansion of the receptive field of neurones, meaning for any given noxious stimulus, more dorsal horn neurones will respond. There is an increase in the size and duration of the response to a noxious stimulus. Therefore the threshold for stimulation of dorsal horn neurones is decreased, so that normally non-noxious stimuli will activate dorsal horn cells.

Does this have implications for different types of pain?

Yes. It may be important in the development of chronic pain states.

Can you define chronic pain?

Chronic pain is defined as pain without apparent biological value that persists beyond normal tissue healing, usually taken to be 3 months.

Can you classify chronic pain?

Chronic pain can be described as inflammatory, neuropathic or dysfunctional.

Inflammatory pain is produced when tissues are damaged due to trauma or infection.

Neuropathic pain is due to a primary lesion or pathology of the peripheral or central nervous system. Examples include phantom limb pain, nerve entrapment pain, as in carpal tunnel syndrome, peripheral neuropathies secondary to diabetes and alcoholism, and central neuropathies due to spinal cord trauma and stroke.

Dysfunctional pain describes poorly localised pain that is not due to tissue inflammation or nerve damage and includes conditions such as fibromyalgia and irritable bowel syndrome.

Can you describe the pathways that produce chronic pain?

Since many of these pathways have not been elucidated the examiners should not expect too much detail.

It is not fully understood how pain signals can persist over long periods of time. A simple way of describing postulated mechanisms is to look at changes first in the periphery and then centrally.

Following an injury, nerves can become sensitised and discharge at lowered thresholds. C-fibres can develop new adrenergic receptors, which may help to explain the mechanism of sympathetically mediated pain. Damaged nerves also produce ectopic discharges, thought to be due to the formation of dysfunctional sodium channels.

Inflammatory mediators such as substance P and prostaglandins are released from damaged nerves. These can then spread to surrounding nociceptors activating them in turn.

Following a peripheral nerve injury, changes within the central nervous system can persist. This plasticity of the CNS is integral to the development of chronic pain states. Repetitive stimulation of C-fibres can result in the phenomenon of "wind-up", where the rate of firing of dorsal horn cells will increase with the duration of the stimulus. Repetitive episodes of wind-up may precipitate "long-term potentiation". Long-term potentiation is defined as a long-lasting increase in synaptic activity. The NMDA receptor is believed to play an important role in these sensitisation processes.

As well as changes at the spinal cord level, alterations in the descending pathways from the brainstem and higher centres will also play a role in the development of chronic pain states. This is highly complex but will involve the areas involved in the sensory-discriminative aspects of pain such as intensity and location, as well as centres involved in the affective-cognitive aspects of pain including anxiety, emotion and memory.

4.3.2. Neuropathic pain: complex regional pain syndrome, trigeminal neuralgia, post-herpetic neuralgia – Sarah J Love-Jones

These topics are well suited to the clinical sciences SOE, but equally they may come up as part of the clinical SOE.

What is neuropathic pain?

Neuropathic pain is pain that is initiated or caused by a primary lesion or dysfunction in the peripheral or central nervous system.

Neuropathic pain can also be called neurogenic pain. Neuropathic pain can be in a region of motor, sensory or autonomic nerve dysfunction. It is often described by patients as a burning, tingling or numb sensation, or as a sharp or shooting pain. Another common way that patients describe neuropathic pain is "like an electric shock" or "like a stabbing pain".

Can you give me any examples of neuropathic pain conditions?

There are seven types of neuropathic pain conditions, commonly seen in pain clinic. These are:

- Lumbar radicular pain
- Trigeminal neuralgia
- Post-herpetic neuralgia
- Complex regional pain syndrome (CRPS)
- Phantom limb pain
- Diabetic neuropathy
- Central pain syndromes.

Can you describe the clinical features of neuropathic pain?

Neuropathic pain can be associated with spontaneous pain, in the absence of any stimulus. This spontaneous pain may be continuous or paroxysmal. Neuropathic pain is also characterised by evoked pains such as allodynia, which is pain following an innocuous stimulus. Another evoked pain is hyperalgesia, which is pain of abnormal severity following a painful stimulus.

What are the treatments for neuropathic pain?

The treatment of neuropathic pain is difficult. No one treatment works for everyone and nothing works well. It is worth remembering that polypharmacy or the use of multiple therapies is rational in the treatment of neuropathic pain. The treatment of neuropathic pain can be divided into five categories:

- Drug treatment
- Injection treatments
- Neuromodulation therapies
- Physical therapies
- Cognitive behavioural therapy.

What drugs do you know can be used in the treatment of neuropathic pain?

Remember to classify the type of drug before launching into individual drug names, as there are many drugs used in the treatment of neuropathic pain.

Simple analgesics such as paracetamol, non-steroidal anti-inflammatory drugs and weak opioids such as codeine should always be tried first and this is usually done by the patient themselves or the GP.

The next class of drugs commonly used in pain clinics to treat neuropathic pain are the Tricyclic anti-depressants, such as amitriptyline and nortriptyline. Tricyclic anti-depressants act by blocking the reuptake of monoamines, and it is both the noradrenergic and serotonergic effects that are needed in the treatment of neuropathic pain. It is worth explaining to the patient when prescribing tricyclic anti-depressants that their analgesic effect is separate from their anti-depressant effect.

The membrane stabilising drugs such as the anti-convulsants carbamazepine, gabapentin and pregabalin and local anaesthetics such as lidocaine are also used to treat neuropathic pain. It is thought that the mechanism of action of gabapentin and pregabalin is that they bind to the $\alpha2\delta$ sub-unit of the voltage-dependent calcium channel and have calcium-channel blocking activity.

Topical treatments used in neuropathic pain include capsaicin cream, which is thought to deplete peptide neurotransmitters in the nerve endings. Lidocaine patches are also use for discreet painful areas and non-steroidal anti-inflammatory gels are sometimes helpful with neuropathic pain.

NMDA (N-methyl-D-aspartate) receptor antagonists such as ketamine and amantidine are sometimes used by infusion to treat neuropathic pain. Unfortunately their effect is short-lived and treatments need to be repeated. They also need to be given as an infusion in hospital with monitoring. Dextromethorphan is an orally administered NMDA antagonist but is not commonly used. Ketamine can also be used sublingually or intra-nasally.

Opioids can be helpful in the management of neuropathic pain, but their use must not be undertaken lightly. Patients should undergo an opioid trial, and sustained release, rather than immediate release, is preferable. There should be an agreed plan between the patient's GP and the pain clinic as to prescribing responsibility and the patient should be followed up regularly. The long-term side effects of opioids are not fully understood, but it thought there may be an effect on the immune system, and we know that tolerance and dependence develops.

What injection treatments are used in neuropathic pain?

Local infiltration with steroid and local anaesthetic can be performed either into joints or soft tissue. Facet joint injection with steroid and local anaesthetic under X-ray guidance is a common pain clinic procedure for back pain. Lumbar epidural or caudal with steroid and local anaesthetic is also commonly performed in the pain clinic for radicular leg pain. Nerve root injection can be performed at any level of the spine for nerve root pain in a single dermatome. This pain can occur due to nerve root compression or after surgery. Nerve root blocks can be both diagnostic and therapeutic. Soft tissue injections are performed for painful scar tissue, and into painful muscular trigger points.

Sympathetic blocks such as stellate ganglion block are used to moderate pain in the face and upper limb. Lumbar sympathetic block is used for sympathetically mediated pain in the lower limbs and is most useful for ischaemic leg pain, especially rest pain. Coeliac plexus block is most often indicated for the relief of pain from pancreatic carcinoma, but it can be used in managing pain from malignant disease of other viscera such as liver, stomach, spleen, kidney and colon.

What neuromodulation treatments do you know for chronic pain?

Transcutaneous electrical nerve stimulation or TENS is thought to work on the basis of the "gate theory" of pain. TENS aims to stimulate the large myelinated Aβ sensory fibres to block input from unmyelinated C-fibres. Pre-synaptic inhibition of C-fibres occurs with release of inhibitory neurotransmitters (such as GABA and glycine). Stimulation of the Aβ fibres may also activate descending inhibitory pathways within the CNS to effect pain relief.

Other neuromodulatory devices are spinal cord stimulators, which also work via stimulation of Aβ-fibres, but this time the large concentration of Aβ fibres in the dorsal columns are targeted, which is thought to cause inhibition of C-fibres and produce pain relief.

More recently deep brain stimulators have been used for chronic pain conditions and this involves neurosurgical implantation of electrodes via stereotactic positioning into areas of the thalamus.

How is physical therapy important in chronic pain conditions?

The traditional role of physiotherapy is important in chronic pain conditions in restoring the function and mobility of damaged muscles and joints and can be helpful in restoring mobility and relieving pain in stiff joints, back pain and limbs affected with complex regional pain syndrome. The physiotherapist is an important part of the multidisciplinary pain clinic staff, whose role is often to educate the patient in the active participation in managing their own pain.

How can the psychologist help in pain management?

Remembering that the definition of pain is a "sensory and emotional response" it is not uncommon for people with chronic pain to suffer so much that they are unable to function, with breakdown of relationships and loss of their job. The psychological effects of chronic pain are negative thinking, stress, disability, loss of control and impaired mental and physical performance. Psychologists are involved in pain management programmes which are effective in improving quality of life. The aim in the pain management programme is to bring about an understanding of pain and alteration of beliefs about pain, using cognitive behavioural therapy. The patient learns coping skills and the aim is to reduce stress and disability caused by chronic pain.

What is complex regional pain syndrome (CRPS)?

Don't be caught out if the examiners ask you what CRPS is and say "chronic" regional pain syndrome instead of "complex" regional pain syndrome.

CRPS is a chronic pain condition, where the key symptom is continuous, intense pain which is out of proportion to the severity of the injury. There are two types of CRPS. Type 1 was formerly known as reflex sympathetic dystrophy and occurs after a minor fracture or injury to a limb without direct injury to a nerve. CRPS type 2 was formerly known as causalgia and develops after injury to a major peripheral nerve.

What are the clinical characteristics of CRPS?

There are four categories of signs and symptoms associated with CRPS. The first category is abnormal sensory changes such as continuous burning pain of the affected extremity, and stimulus-evoked pains such as mechanical and thermal allodynia. The second category of CRPS characteristics is autonomic abnormalities such as changes in skin temperature, hyper or hypohidrosis and swelling of the distal extremity. The third category is trophic changes associated with CRPS such as abnormal nail and hair growth, fibrosis, osteoporosis and thin, glossy skin. The fourth category of characteristics associated with CRPS is motor abnormalities such as weakness, dystonia, tremor and neglect-like symptoms or symptoms of disturbed body perception of the affected extremity. In addition to these four categories there may be a component of sympathetically maintained pain, but this is not diagnostic.

What treatments do you know for CRPS?

Treatments for CRPS can be pharmacological, interventional, physical therapy or neurostimulatory. A multidisciplinary approach is important and treatment should start immediately after diagnosis. The pharmacological treatment of CRPS includes the tricyclic antidepressants, the anti-convulsants such as gabapentin and pregabalin and drugs used to treat sympathetically maintained pain such as guanethidine. Topical capsaicin has also been used in the pharmacological treatment of CRPS. Interventional treatments used for CRPS include the sympathetic blocks such as stellate ganglion block and lumbar sympathectomy and more recently guanethidine blocks. These blocks may help with the diagnosis of sympathetically mediated pain as well as being a treatment. Physical therapy is particularly important in the first few weeks of the diagnosis and patients must be encouraged to move the affected limb. Neurostimulatory treatments include TENS, spinal cord stimulation and deep brain stimulation.

What are the clinical features of trigeminal neuralgia?

Trigeminal neuralgia which is also known as tic douloureux is neuropathic pain in the distribution of the trigeminal nerve. Episodes of paroxysmal pain can occur in the eyes, lips, nose, scalp, jaw or forehead. The pain can be due to involvement of the gasserian ganglion or the peripheral branches of the trigeminal nerve. The pain is shooting or sharp in nature and the patient may describe it as "electric shock-like pain". Pain is typically provoked by innocuous stimuli such as light touch, eating, washing, talking or air currents on the face. It is commoner in patients with multiple sclerosis and in patients over 50 years, but can occur in young adults. The pain is usually unilateral, but can be bilateral in multiple sclerosis.

What is the cause of trigeminal neuralgia?

It is thought that vascular compression of the trigeminal nerve near the pons alters electrical activity in the trigeminal neurones. Many patients with trigeminal neuralgia have an aberrant micro vascular loop, pressing on the nerve which is seen on MRI scan. Other causes are micro vascular aneurysms, tumour, arachnoid cyst in the cerebellarpontine angle, or by traumatic events such as car accidents.

What treatments do you know for trigeminal neuralgia?

There are both drug treatments and surgical treatment for trigeminal neuralgia. The drug treatment of choice for trigeminal neuralgia is carbamazepine. If this fails gabapentin and pregabalin have had some success, and baclofen has also been used. The tricyclic anti-depressants have not proved so useful in trigeminal neuralgia as the anti-convulsants. Surgical treatments include micro-vascular decompression of the aberrant vessel, and about 75% of patients will have immediate pain relief following the procedure, although sometimes the pain does recur. Other surgical treatments include radio-frequency lesioning of the nerve, glycerol injection and balloon inflation into the foramen ovale. All the ablative treatments have the potential to cause anaesthesia dolorosa which is pain in an area of anaesthesia.

What are the clinical features of post-herpetic neuralgia?

Post-herpetic neuralgia is the persistence of pain in the affected dermatomes, after the resolution of an acute herpes zoster infection (also known as shingles). The diagnosis is usually given if the pain persists or arises at least 3 months after the skin lesions have healed. The commonest areas for shingles are the thoracic dermatomes and the ophthalmic division of the trigeminal nerve. The pain of post-herpetic neuralgia is described by patients as a constant, burning, tingling or numb sensation. Other symptoms included paraesthesia and sensory loss, and lancinating pain which is triggered by light touch or cold air. Often patients cannot bear their clothes touching the affected area. This is typical of neuropathic pain. The affected dermatomes in post-herpetic neuralgia often exhibit allodynia and hyperalgesia. Allodynia is the experience of pain following a normally non-painful or innocuous stimulus. Hyperalgesia is pain of abnormal severity following a painful stimulus. Post-herpetic neuralgia occurs in 9–34% of all patients with herpes zoster, the incidence being the same in men and women. The onset of post-herpetic neuralgia cannot be predicted by the severity of the acute herpes zoster infection, but we do know that post-herpetic neuralgia is more likely to occur with advancing age. In the over 70s about 50% of those suffering with post-herpetic neuralgia may have persistent pain even a year after the initial zoster infection.

What is the pathophysiology of post-herpetic neuralgia?

Following a varicella zoster or chicken pox infection, the virus settles in the dorsal horns of the sensory ganglia and remains dormant. That is until reactivation of the virus produces inflammation in the peripheral nerve and neural destruction. This then causes pain in the distribution of that nerve. Reactivation of the virus is thought to be caused by immunosupression, which is more likely with increasing age. Chronic pain is thought to arise due to the loss of nociceptive afferent neurones and A-β fibre demyelination.

What treatments do you know for post-herpetic neuralgia?

Treatments can be divided into 3 categories: oral drugs; topical treatments and Interventions or injections. Oral drugs used in the treatment of post-herpetic neuralgia include the amitriptyline and other anti-depressants; the anti-convulsants gabapentin and pregabalin; conventional analgesics and opioids. Occasionally intra-venous infusion of NMDA (n-methyl-D-aspartate) receptor antagonists such as ketamine is used. Topical treatments include the use of capsaicin cream, non-steroidal anti-inflammatory creams and more recently lidocaine patches. Interventional treatments for post-herpetic neuralgia include TENS (transcutaneous electrical nerve stimulation), sympathetic blocks such as stellate ganglion block and epidural steroid and local anaesthetic at the level of the affected dorsal root ganglion. The epidural steroid is thought to interrupt the mechanisms producing chronic pain.

Further Reading

Callin S, Bennett MI. Assessment of neuropathic pain. *Continuing Education in Anaesthesia, Critical Care & Pain*. 2008; **8**(6): 210–213.

4.3.3. Low back pain – Murli Krishna

How can we classify low back pain?

Low back pain can be classified on the basis of duration of symptoms into acute and chronic. It is defined as acute when symptoms have persisted for less than 6 weeks and chronic when symptoms last for longer than 3 months.

It can also be classified as "specific" and "non-specific". Specific low back pain is caused by specific pathophysiological mechanisms such as herniated disc, infection, tumour, osteoporosis, inflammation or fracture. Non-specific low back pain refers to those cases where no specific cause is found. Approximately 90% of such patients have non-specific low back pain.

What are the causes of low back pain?

Try to classify by thinking in terms of causes, i.e., structural or inflammatory.

How do you evaluate patients with low back pain?

Think in terms of aims of evaluation and targeted assessment/examination rather than head to toe examination (Table 4.3.3A).

TABLE 4.3.3.A.

Structural	Spondylosis or spondylolisthesis Prolapsed intervertebral disc Facet joint arthritis Spinal stenosis
Neurogenic	Prolapsed disc Spinal stenosis Failed back surgery syndrome (arachnoditis, epidural adhesions, recurrent herniations)
Inflammatory	Spondyloarthropathies Sacroilitis
Neoplasm	Primary or secondary (metastatic)
Infection	Osteomyelitis Discitis Abscess
Metabolic	Osteoporosis Paget's disease Vitamin D deficiency Hyperparathyroidism
Referred pain	From visceral structures (pancreas, bowel), aorta, hip, retroperitoneal structures (kidneys)
Other	Somatoform disorders Fibromyalgia

The aims of evaluation include:

- Identification of red flags (serious pathology)
- Identification of yellow flags (signs for chronicity)
- Identification of source of pain.

Assessment should include a focussed history including the nature of onset, duration, location of pain, radiation, neurological symptoms including bowel and bladder function, exacerbating factors and relieving factors. Ask specifically about rest pain and night pain as well as any history of trauma. Past medical history is very important especially a history of malignancy, steroids, immunosuppression and intra-venous drug abuse.

Examination should assess gait, posture, range of movements, tenderness on palpation and straight leg raise (SLR) test. Full neurological examination including tone, power, reflexes and sensory examination should be undertaken. Examination of other systems may be necessary in case of referred pain.

Investigations including blood tests, plain X-rays, MRI scans and bone scans as dictated by history, examination and findings.

Mnemonic worth remembering: OPQRST

Onset (spontaneous or triggered)
Pattern (location and timing)
Quality of pain
Relieving and exacerbating factors
Severity and systemic symptoms
Treatments

TABLE 4.3.3.B.

Red flag condition	Symptoms
Cauda equina syndrome	Motor weakness, numbness, progressive neurological deficit Sphincter disturbance (urinary retention, bowel or bladder incontinence) Saddle anaesthesia
Tumour or infection	Age > 50 years or < 17 years Severe pain at rest, night time pain Acute localised bone pain Unexplained weight loss Fever, night sweats Immunosuppression, HIV, IV drug use
Fracture	Significant trauma Osteoporosis
Acute abdominal aneurysm	Pulsatile abdominal mass

What are red flags and yellow flags?

Red flags suggest serious underlying pathology or nerve root pathology.

Think in terms of red flag conditions, rather than symptoms. It is easier to remember and looks more impressive. This is most likely to feature in SAQs and possibly MCQs.

Yellow flags are psychosocial barriers to recovery and indicate long-term chronicity and disability. They include:

- Belief that pain is damaging and activity is harmful
- Fear and avoidance behaviour
- Extremely high levels of pain
- Catastrophisation
- Low levels of activity
- Low mood, depression, social withdrawal
- Sickness behaviour (like extended rest)
- Tendency for seeking passive treatments
- Overprotective family or lack of support
- Problems at work, poor job satisfaction.

Are you aware of any other flags?

Blue flags refer to conditions in the workplace that may inhibit recovery. These include high work demands, poor relationship with colleagues, low degree of control, monotony and lack of job satisfaction.

Black flags refer to organisational obstacles to returning to work. These include social benefits, sickness policies and compensation claims.

Orange flags include serious mental health issues in conjunction with pain. Examples include very high levels of distress, major personality disorders, post-traumatic stress disorder, substance abuse and clinical depression.

What is the straight leg raise (SLR) test?

With the patient lying supine, the affected leg is raised with the knee fully extended. A positive test reproduces patient's leg pain (radicular pain) at between 30 to 70 degrees of elevation.

SLR tests the mobility of the dura mater and the dural sleeves of lower lumbar and sacral spinal nerves (L4 to S3). It has high sensitivity for radiculopathy but low specificity.

What are signs of nerve root irritation?

- Leg pain greater than back pain
- Radiation into foot or lower leg
- Numbness and paraesthesiae in dermatomal distribution
- Diminished leg reflexes
- Positive straight leg raising test (L4–S1 nerve roots)
- Positive femoral stretch test (L2–4 nerve roots)
- Leg pain exacerbated by coughing, sneezing, or Valsalva manoeuvre.

What is cauda euqina syndrome? How does it present and how should it be managed?

This is an important topic and could mostly likely feature in SAQs.

Cauda equina syndrome may result from any lesion that compresses the cauda equina nerve roots. This causes dysfunction of sacral and lumbar nerve roots in the vertebral canal. The syndrome is characterised by bladder (retention or incontinence), bowel or sexual dysfunction and perianal or saddle anaesthesia. Other clinical features include:

- Back pain
- Lower limb weakness
- Sensory changes in lower limbs
- Loss (or sluggish) of reflexes in lower limbs
- Unilateral or bilateral symptoms.

Patients can present either acutely as their first symptom of lumbar disc herniation, or after a long history of chronic back pain. It can also present insidiously with slow progression to numbness and urinary symptoms.

Features on examination include:

- Loss of perianal sensation
- Loss of anal tone
- Loss or diminution of lower limb reflexes
- Loss or diminution of bulbocavernosus reflex
- Motor weakness in lower limbs.

Describe your investigation and management of cauda equina syndrome

MRI is the investigation of choice for confirming cauda equina syndrome. Clinical diagnosis has high false-positive rates even in experienced hands. If MRI is unavailable, CT myelogram should be performed.

Surgical decompression is the treatment of choice for cauda equina syndrome. The timing of surgery remains controversial but retrospective analysis has shown that surgery within 24 hours is associated with a better outcome. The clinical outcome is poor in patients with urinary retention and the role of urgent surgery is less clear in these patients as shown by a recent meta-analysis.

What is the role of routine imaging in evaluation of low back pain?

There is no role for routine imaging in evaluation of low back pain. There is no evidence that routine plain radiography is associated with improvement in patient outcome in those with non-specific low back pain. In addition, there is no evidence of causal relationship between radiographic findings and non-specific low back pain. The amount of radiation from lumbar X-ray is also of concern (more than daily chest X-ray for a year). Similarly, up to 30% adults without low back pain have evidence of protruded disc on MRI scan.

Plain radiographs are recommended for initial evaluation of vertebral compression fracture in selected high-risk patients.

MRI scans or CT scans are recommended in patients with red flags (progressive neurological deficits, cauda equina syndrome, vertebral infection, cancer). Scans are also recommended if surgery or invasive treatment is planned.

What are the risk factors for chronicity in low back pain?

Always try to classify if possible.

Risk factors for chronicity can be divided in to three groups: individual factors, psychosocial factors and occupational factors.

Individual factors

- Obesity
- Low education level
- High levels of pain and disability

Psychosocial factors

- Distress
- Depressive mood
- Somatisation

Occupational factors

- Job dissatisfaction
- Heavy lifting
- Unavailability of light duties on return to work.

What treatment options are available for low back pain?

Try to answer this question by dividing treatments in to specific groups (non-pharmacological treatments, pharmacological treatments, interventional therapies and surgery).

1. Non-pharmacological treatments
   - Patient education: by providing evidence based information on low back pain, expected course, advise to remain active and effective self-care options (moderate quality evidence)
   - Intensive multidisciplinary rehabilitation: pain management programmes, back pack programmes (moderate evidence)
   - Exercise therapy
   - Acupuncture
   - Cognitive and behavioural therapy
   - TENS machine (no proven benefit)

2. Pharmacological treatments

   · Oral analgesics: paracetamol, NSAIDs, tramadol, strong opioids (controversial)
   · Muscle relaxants: indicated for short duration in acute back pain if significant muscle spasm present
   · Anti-depressants: tricyclic (amitriptyline, nortriptyline)- in low doses, more effective than placebo; SSRI- not effective; SNRI (duloxetine, venlafaxine)- have not been evaluated
   · Gabapentinoids: gabapentin and pregabalin for back pain associated with radiculopathy
   · Systemic corticosteroids: not recommended.

3. Interventional treatments (Cochrane review 2008 concludes that there is insufficient evidence to support injection therapy in chronic low back pain but specific sub-group of patients may respond to specific injections).

   · Epidural injection of steroids: short-term benefit in radicular pain, no long-term improvement in pain or function
   · Facet joint injections: evidence equivocal (ASA practice guidelines 2010)
   · Radiofrequency denervation of facet joints: better pain relief than sham interventions
   · Spinal cord stimulators: for neuropathic leg pain (NICE approved).

4. Surgery, in selected cases (less than 1% cases)

   · Discectomy/microdiscectomy
   · Spinal fusion
   · Spinal decompression.

Further Reading

Staal JB, de Bie R, de Vet HCW, Hildebrandt J, Nelemans P. Injection therapy for subacute and chronic low-back pain. *Cochrane Database of Systematic Reviews.* 2008 Issue 3. Art. No.: CD001824.

American Society of Anesthesiologists Task Force on Chronic Pain Management and the American Society of Regional Anesthesia and Pain Medicine. Practice Guidelines for Chronic Pain Management: an updated report by the American Society of Anesthesiologists Task Force on Chronic Pain Management and the American Society of Regional Anesthesia and Pain Medicine. *Anesthesiology.* 2010; **112**(4): 810–833.

4.3.4. Assessment of acute and chronic pain – Santhosh Gopalakrishnan and Sarah J Love-Jones

This topic can be asked as a part of the clinical sciences SOE. This is a tricky question, but a structured answer can get you through.

What can you tell me about pain assessment?

The IASP (International Association for the Study of Pain) definition of pain is "An unpleasant sensory and emotional experience associated with actual or potential tissue damage and expressed in terms of such damage". Pain is whatever the experiencing person says it is. Pain is commonly measured by pain measurement scales, which use aspects of patient reporting that can yield reproducible data. It should be easy to use and interpret over a wide variety of disease states and cultures.

What are the different methods of measuring pain that you know of?

A structured approach is vital to ensure that you do not forget any of the key points. It may be worth making a classification.

Pain is measured mainly using pain measurement scales.

They can be broadly classified into:

- Simple pain scales used to assess acute pain
- Multidimensional pain scales used to assess chronic pain.

What are simple pain scales and how do you interpret them?

Simple pain scales are widely used to measure acute pain intensity due to the ease of use. The commonly used scales are:

- Verbal rating scale
- Numerical rating scale and
- Visual analogue scale.

What is the verbal rating scale?

The verbal rating scale (VRS) has four points to describe pain. These are no pain, mild pain, moderate pain and severe pain. The verbal rating scale is commonly used in post-operative recovery rooms because it is simple to use. It is however insensitive to small changes in the patient's pain intensity.

What is the numerical rating scale (NRS)?

The numerical rating scale (NRS) takes two extremes of pain (no pain and worst imaginable pain) with numbers across the scale from zero to ten, making an eleven point scale. The patient is asked to translate their pain severity into a number where zero is no pain and ten is the worst pain they can imagine. The numerical rating scale is not very sensitive in measuring small changes in pain intensity, but is simple to use and can be translated into different languages.

What is the visual analogue scale (VAS)?

The visual analogue scale (VAS) is a simple pain scale, often used in research. The patient is shown a 10-cm line with the anchor words "no pain" written at one end and "worst pain imaginable" written at the other end. The patient is asked to put a cross on the line that best describes their pain. The distance from the "no pain" end is then measured in centimeters to give the pain score. This continuous aspect of the scale differentiates it from discrete scales. The visual analogue scale is sensitive to small changes in patient's pain.

What are multidimensional pain scales?

Simple pain scales do not separate the many factors associated with chronic pain. Chronic pain is of longer duration, is difficult to treat and often of unknown origin. Psychosocial factors play a large part in the development of chronic pain and the patient and their family will show distress and fear about the effects on life, work and money. The multidimensional pain scales analyse chronic pain by specific enquiry and can establish problems that do not just include pain intensity. The multidimensional pain scales include the McGill Pain Questionnaire, the Brief Pain Inventory, the Neuropathic Pain Scale and the Leeds Assessment of Neuropathic Symptoms and Signs.

Can you briefly describe the McGill Pain Questionnaire?

The McGill Pain Questionnaire consists of four major classes of word descriptors – sensory, affective, evaluative and miscellaneous – that are used by patients to specify subjective pain experience. It also contains an intensity scale to determine the properties of pain experience. The questionnaire was designed to provide quantitative measures of clinical pain. The three major measures are:

1. The pain rating index, based on two types of numerical values that can be assigned to each word descriptor
2. The number of words chosen
3. The present pain intensity based on a 1–5 intensity scale.

The McGill Pain Questionnaire provides quantitative information that can be treated statistically, and is sufficiently sensitive to detect differences amongst different methods to relieve pain. It also has a shorter version, with only 15 words, which is more commonly used nowadays.

Describe the short form McGill Pain Questionnaire (SF-MPQ)?

The main component of the SF-MPQ consists of 15 descriptors (11 sensory; 4 affective) which are rated on an intensity scale as 0 = none, 1 = mild, 2 = moderate or 3 = severe. Three pain scores are derived from the sum of the intensity rank values of the words chosen for sensory, affective and total descriptors. The SF-MPQ also includes the Present Pain Intensity (PPI) index of the standard MPQ and a visual analogue scale (VAS).

Describe the Brief Pain Inventory.

The Brief Pain Inventory assesses pain intensity at its best and worst and at the time of the test. It also assesses the percentage relief from medications and treatments for pain and the duration of relief. There are specific questions about patients' beliefs regarding their pain and questions about how their pain interferes with their daily activities such as work, relationships, rest and sleep.

Describe the Neuropathic Pain Scale.

The neuropathic pain scale specifically assesses neuropathic pain. It has eight descriptors of pain quality. These eight descriptors are sharp, hot, dull, cold, skin sensitivity, itching, surface and deep pain. It also measures the unpleasantness of pain on a scale of zero to ten.

What is the Leeds Assessment of Neuropathic Symptoms and Signs (LANSS)

The LANSS system identifies patients in whom neuropathic pain is the dominating part of their pain. It is based on five questions and a simple bedside examination of sensory dysfunction.

What are the adjunctive measurements of pain?

In chronic pain psychological distress and social function are important assessments. These adjunctive measurements can be divided into:

1. Assessment of mood
2. Quality of life.

Assessment of mood enables clinicians to tailor treatments for individual patients and evaluative questionnaires are often used. The commonly used ones are the Beck anxiety and depression inventories, hospital anxiety and depression score and Zung self rated depression score.

Quality of life assessments aim to evaluate the impact of the disease on the patient's life. The best known measure is the short form – 36 questionnaires.

How do you assess pain in children?

It is very difficult to assess pain in children. Scales for children must capture their imagination, be fun to use and must be reproducible.

Up to 3 years?

Neonates can feel pain contrary to old beliefs and theories. Effective pain scoring systems must rely on behavioural variables such as facial expression and crying or variables like cardiovascular parameters. The commonly used scales are the objective pain scale and the clinical scoring system.

3–7 years?

Most children above 3 years of age can report pain and its intensity effectively. Thus a verbal rating scale or a faces scale can be used. The faces scale is a series of cartoon faces that range from smiling to crying. A more detailed form of this is called the Oucher scale but it needs to be matched to cultural background. Visual analogue scales can also be used and better results can be obtained by using the colour graduation system and making the line vertical.

7 years +?

Conventional visual analogue scales can be used.

How can pain be assessed in the cognitively impaired?

It can be assessed using the behavioural pain assessment scale. Pain is scored from 0–10 and is based on the Face Score, Restlessness Score, Muscle Tone Score, Vocalisation Score and

Consolability Score. Zero = no evidence of pain. Mild pain = 1–3. Moderate pain = 4–5. Severe uncontrolled pain is ≥ 6.

Further Reading

Callin S, Bennett MI. Assessment of neuropathic pain. *Continuing Education in Anaesthesia,* *Critical Care & Pain.* 2008. **8**(6): 210–213.

4.3.5. Analgesic techniques – Michael B Clarke

Can you describe what is meant by the "analgesic ladder"?

The World Health Organisation (WHO) originally described a three-step approach to the administration of analgesics for cancer pain. If the patient's pain does not respond initially to weak peripherally acting non-opioid analgesics, the first rung of the ladder, then there are two further steps that allow the escalation of therapy. It has been adapted to encompass the management of acute pain by The World Federation of Societies of Anaesthesiologists (WFSA).

Pain is assessed and can be categorised as mild, moderate or severe. Treatment begins according to which level of pain the patient is experiencing; therefore, the treatment of a patient in severe pain need not start at the first step. If the pain becomes more severe or the analgesia is ineffective, then the patient moves up one step of the ladder to the next level of pain severity and is treated accordingly.

Can you describe the steps of the original ladder?

The three steps of the ladder ascend from non-opioids through weak opioids to strong opioids, according to the severity of the pain. For mild pain, non-opioid analgesics such as paracetamol and NSAIDs should be prescribed regularly. For moderate pain, weak opioids such as codeine are added, and for severe pain strong opioids such as morphine or fentanyl are substituted for the weak opioids.

In addition to analgesia, care must be taken to assess the patient for nausea and vomiting, sedation and respiratory depression.

What are the advantages and disadvantages of the analgesic ladder?

Advantages are:

- It is simple to use
- It is useful for a variety of clinical situations
- It employs commonly used drugs
- It emphasises a multi-modal approach to pain relief.

Disadvantages are:

- It is not easily applicable to different forms of chronic pain
- It may be inappropriate for some patients to take oral drugs
- The use of regional anaesthesia does not fit within the original ladder structure.

An ASA I, 45-year-old female has presented for an elective total abdominal hysterectomy.

How would you manage her post-operative pain?

This answer should not involve too much detail – the examiner will have further questions ready to tease out the finer points.

Abdominal hysterectomy usually involves a transverse incision below the umbilicus and is associated with moderate post-operative pain. My practice is to use a combination of oral and intra-venous analgesic drugs and peripheral nerve blocks that are performed following induction of anaesthesia.

Bilateral inguinal nerve blocks can be performed but I prefer to carry out a bilateral transversus abdominis plane (TAP) block. The latter can provide between 12 and 24 hours of pain relief.

The oral analgesics I prescribe regularly are paracetamol and diclofenac, providing there are no contraindications to their use.

I also prescribe intra-venous morphine via a PCA device, though it could be given as required using the intra-muscular route. A potential disadvantage of morphine in gynaecological surgery is a high rate of nausea and vomiting. An anti-emetic should also be prescribed to counteract this.

The epidural route is not commonly used but may be indicated in certain patients, for example, when trying to avoid morphine in patients with obstructive sleep apnoea.

You have mentioned a transversus abdominis plane block. Can you describe the anatomy relevant to this block and how you would perform it?

TAP blocks have become increasingly popular recently and so a good knowledge of the relevant anatomy would be expected.

The anterior rami of spinal nerves T7 to L1 innervate the anterolateral abdominal wall. Branches from the anterior rami include:

- The intercostal nerves (T7–11)
- The subcostal nerve (T12)
- The iliohypogastric and ilioinguinal nerves (L1).

At points in their course these nerves run in the plane between the transversus abdominis and internal oblique muscles before ending as cutaneous branches supplying the skin of the front of the abdomen.

A single injection will most likely block T10 to L1 and for an incision across the midline, as you would expect for an abdominal hysterectomy, bilateral blocks are required. The block can be performed using a landmark technique or using ultrasound. Classically, the point of entry is the "triangle of Petit" which is situated between the lower costal margin and iliac crest. When using the landmark technique, the end-point, a double pop, is felt as a blunt needle passes through the fascial layers of the external oblique and internal oblique. Use of ultrasound requires the probe to be placed in the transverse plane to the lateral abdominal wall in the mid-axillary line.

Success depends on a good spread of local anaesthetic and so 25–30 ml of local anaesthetic on each side should be used, adhering to the maximum safe dose.

What are the advantages and disadvantages of patient-controlled analgesia (PCA)?

Advantages of PCAs are:

- Provide an on-demand system minimising the delay between the experience of pain and receiving analgesia
- Provide a more consistent drug plasma concentration when compared to intra-muscular techniques and therefore better level of analgesia
- Reduction of nurses' workload
- Allows the patient to be in control which may contribute to a placebo effect and possibly better outcome
- Daily analgesic dose or number of demands can be used as an objective measure to monitor progress.

Disadvantages include:

- Need for expensive equipment
- Risk of patient harm from incorrect programming or equipment malfunction
- Cannot be operated by some patients, i.e., physical or cognitive impairment.

What other routes for the administration of analgesia do you know?

Analgesic drugs can also be given intra-nasally, sublingually and transdermally.

Tell me about transdermal delivery systems

The advantage of the transdermal route for drug delivery is that it avoids first pass metabolism and large variations in plasma drug concentration. Drugs suitable for transdermal adminis-tration must be able to penetrate the stratum corneum of the skin, i.e. they must be highly lipophilic. To this end, drugs must have a low molecular weight and high lipid solubility.

There are two types of transdermal patch available: the reservoir, or membrane-controlled system and the matrix system. In a reservoir patch, the drug is held in a gel or solution and a release membrane controls the rate of delivery of the drug to the skin. The matrix patch holds the drug as part of a polymer matrix. The matrix is applied directly to the skin.

Which analgesic drugs can be delivered via a transdermal patch and when are they indicated?

The most common analgesic dugs are buprenorphine and fentanyl. These opioid patches are not suitable for acute pain management because of the delay between patch application and the development of a desired minimum effective concentration. They are frequently pre-scribed to patients with chronic or cancer pain.

Tell me what you know about fentanyl patches

Fentanyl patches are more commonly of the matrix type. The patches deliver fentanyl at a constant rate and come in different strengths: 25 μg per hour up to 100 μg per hour. A steady state serum concentration is achieved after 24 hours and will continue as long as the patch is renewed. Each patch lasts for 72 hours.

Recently developed iontophoretic fentanyl drug delivery devices enable the patient to activate the delivery of a small dose of ionised analgesic transdermally using an electric current. In contrast to the reservoir and matrix patches, these are licensed for the treatment of acute post-operative pain.

What are the advantages and disadvantages of opioid transdermal patches?

Because the constant delivery of drug avoids the peaks and troughs of intermittent dosaging, the side effect profile of opioids, such as sedation, nausea and vomiting and respiratory depression is reduced. Patient compliance is also improved because of their convenience.

A problem common to all transdermal patches is skin irritation which can be solved by removing the patch. Respiratory depression and sedation can still occur and care must be taken when using other sedatives. Removing the patch will not immediately stop these problems and so patients and their carers have to be well educated as to the signs and symptoms of impending side effects.

Drug abusers have been known to extract the fentanyl from patches to inject intravenously.

What pharmacological adjuncts are used to treat pain?

Most adjuncts are used to treat chronic pain syndromes, in particular neuropathic pain. This should be emphasised at the start. The answer to this question then lends itself to a simple classification.

Acute inflammatory pain is usually well managed with a combination of paracetamol, non-steroidal anti-inflammatory drugs and morphine. These analgesics are often less effective when the patient is experiencing neuropathic pain. Drugs not developed to treat acute pain have been shown to be effective in the management of neuropathic pain. These include tricyclic anti-depressants, anti-convulsants, membrane stabilisers and other miscellaneous drugs.

Tricyclic anti-depressants (TCAs) such as amitriptyline have been used in low dosages to treat neuropathic pain. They work by inhibiting the reuptake of neurotransmitters noradrenaline and serotonin (5HT) and so potentiate the inhibitory pathways that occur in the dorsal horn of the spinal cord. The TCA mechanism of action may also involve sodium-channel blockade or N-methyl D-aspartate (NMDA) receptor antagonism.

Anti-convulsants are used to treat neuropathic pain; in particular, carbamazepine is the first line treatment for trigeminal neuralgia. Neuropathic pain is associated with ectopic discharge from sodium channels. Carbamazepine is also a sodium-channel blocker and this is thought to be why it can be effective. Gabapentin is also an anti-convulsant and is structurally related to γ-aminobutyric acid (GABA). Its site of action appears to be the α_2 δ-subunit of voltage-dependent calcium channels although its overall mechanism of action is not understood. It has been shown to be effective in the management of post-herpetic neuralgia and in particular diabetic neuropathic pain. Other anti-convulsants used in chronic pain syndromes include phenytoin, phosphenytoin and lamotrigine.

Membrane stabilisers such as lignocaine are used to treat chronic pain. Infusions of lignocaine are used to treat the pain associated with fibromyalgia syndrome and lignocaine patches are now licensed for use in the management of post-herpetic neuralgia. Its mechanism of action may again be through the suppression of ectopic discharges from sodium channels.

Miscellaneous drugs used in the treatment of chronic pain include:

- Baclofen: inhibition of the release of the excitatory neurotransmitters glutamate and aspartate
- Proglumide: inhibition of cholecystokinin (CCK)
- Ketamine: NMDA receptor antagonist
- Clonidine/dexmedetomidine: centrally acting α2-adrenoreceptor antagonists
- Capsaicin: reversible inhibition of substance P release from sensory nerve endings.

What non-pharmacological techniques can be used in the treatment of pain?

There are a number of non-pharmacological techniques that can be used to manage pain. They are rarely used as isolated interventions but are more often part of a multidisciplinary approach to pain management, particularly in the chronic pain setting.

Psychological intervention forms an important part of chronic pain management and can have a role in acute pain. Simple steps such as providing the patient with information about any forthcoming procedure has been shown to reduce pain scores and lengths of hospital stay. Relaxation training can be beneficial, as can hypnosis.

Cognitive-behavioural interventions focus on trying to alter targeted behaviours and utilise positive reinforcement of desired behaviours, pacing of behaviours and goal setting. It often occurs in a group setting and requires the patient to be an active participant in the process.

Transcutaneous electrical nerve stimulation, or TENS, is commonly used to help manage pain in the early stages of labour and is used to treat a variety of chronic musculoskeletal pains in chronic pain clinics. There are two theories proposed to explain its action. In the gate control mechanism, TENS stimulates large diameter Aβ fibres that inhibit the onward propagation of nociceptive signals via small diameter C-fibres within the dorsal horn of the spinal cord. The second theory is that TENS stimulates the release of endorphins that act on receptors within the central nervous system.

Acupuncture can be effective in the treatment of pain although its use and effectiveness remains controversial.

Index

Printed in the United States
By Bookmasters